Rehabilitation

FOR ❧ THE

POSTSURGICAL
ORTHOPEDIC PATIENT

Rehabilitation

FOR 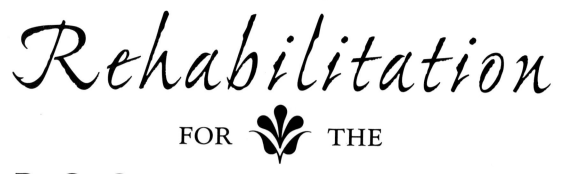 THE

POSTSURGICAL
ORTHOPEDIC PATIENT

Edited by

Lisa Maxey, PT
Staff Physical Therapist,
Sports Therapy,
Calabasas, California

Jim Magnusson, PT
Manager/Partner,
Pacific Therapy Services, Inc.,
Oxnard, California;
Co-Owner,
Performance Therapy Center Inc.,
Oxnard, Camarillo, and Thousand Oaks, California;
Team Physical Therapist,
Oxnard College,
Team Physical Therapist,
Pacific Suns Minor League Baseball Team,
Oxnard, California

with 40 contributors
with 225 illustrations

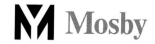 Mosby

A Harcourt Health Sciences Company

St. Louis   London   Philadelphia   Sydney   Toronto

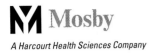

Editor: Kellie White
Developmental Editor: Christie M. Hart
Project Manager: Linda McKinley
Senior Production Editor: Jennifer Furey
Designer: Julia Ramirez
Cover Art: Angie Rovtar

Mosby, Inc.
A Harcourt Health Sciences Company
11830 Westline Industrial Drive
St. Louis, Missouri 63146

Printed in the United States of America

Library of Congress Cataloging in Publication Data

Rehabilitation for the postsurgical orthopedic patient / [edited by] Lisa Maxey, Jim Magnusson; with 40 contributors.
     p. ; cm.
   Includes bibliographical references and index.
   ISBN 0-323-00166-1
   1. Physical therapy.   2. Orthopedic surgery—Patients—Rehabilitation.
   3. Postoperative care.   I. Maxey, Lisa.   II. Magnusson, Jim.
     [DNLM: 1. Physical Therapy—methods.   2. Postoperative Care—rehabilitation.
   3. Orthopedic Procedures. WB 460 R3427 2001]
   RD736.P47 R44 2001
   615.8'2--dc21   00-051100

01   02   03   04   05   TG/MVY   9 8 7 6 5 4 3 2

Contributors

Kelly Akin, PT
Senior Hand Therapist,
Department of Physical Therapy,
Campbell Clinic,
Memphis, Tennessee

Mayra Saborio Amiran, PT
Physical Therapist,
HealthSouth,
Camarillo, California

James Andrews, MD
Clinical Professor of Surgery,
UAB School of Medicine, Division of Orthopaedic
  Surgery,
Birmingham, Alabama;
Clinical Professor of Orthopaedics & Sports Medicine,
University of Virginia Medical School,
Charlottesville, Virginia;
Clinical Professor,
Department of Orthopaedic Surgery,
University of Kentucky Medical Center,
Lexington, Kentucky;
Senior Orthopaedic Consultant,
Washington Redskins Professional Football Team,
Washington, DC;
Senior Orthopaedic Consultant,
Cincinnati Reds Professional Baseball Team,
Cincinnati, Ohio;
Medical Director,
American Sports Medicine Institute,
Orthopaedic Surgeon,
Alabama Sports Medicine & Orthopaedic Center,
Birmingham Alabama

Clive Brewster, MS, PT
Market Coordinator-Outpatient,
HealthSouth,
Los Angeles, California

Andrew A. Brooks, MD, FACS
Southern California Orthopedic Institute,
Los Angeles, California

Nora Cacanindin, PT
Director/Owner,
Pro-Active Therapy,
San Francisco, California

James Calandruccio, MD
Assistant Professor,
Orthopedic Department,
University of Tennessee-Campbell Clinic,
Chief Hand/Upper Extremity Service,
VA Hospital,
Memphis, Tennessee

Robert I. Cantu, MMSc, PT, MTC
Group Director,
Physiotherapy Associates,
Atlanta, Georgia;
Adjunct Instructor,
Institute of Physical Therapy,
University of St. Augustine for Health Science,
St. Augustine, Florida

Christina M. Clark, OTR, CHT
Hand Clinic,
Southern California Orthopedic Institute,
Van Nuys, California

James Coyle, MD
Spine Surgeon,
Midwest Spine Surgeons,
St. Louis, Missouri

Deborah Mandis Cozen, RPT
Physical Therapist,
Pasadena, California

Rick B. Delamarter, MD
Director,
The Spine Institute,
St. John's Medical Center,
Santa Monica, California

Robert Donatelli, PhD, PT, OCS
National Director of Sports Rehabilitation,
Physiotherapy Associates,
Memphis, Tennessee

Dan Farwell, PT, DPT
Adjunct Clinical Professor,
Department of Biokinesiology and Physical Therapy,
University of Southern California,
Los Angeles, California;
Owner/Director,
Body Rx Physical Therapy,
Glendale, California;
Instructor,
McConnell Institute,
Marina Del Rey, California

Richard Ferkel, MD
Clinical Instructor of Orthopedic Surgery,
UCLA,
Los Angeles, California;
Attending Surgeon and Director of Sports Medicine
    Fellowship,
Southern California Orthopedic Institute,
Van Nuys, California

Mark Ghilarducci, MD
Diplomate of the American Board of Orthopedic Surgery,
Fellow of the American Academy of Orthopedic
    Surgeons (AAOS),
Camarillo, California

Terry Gillette, PT, OCS, SCS
Administrator,
HealthSouth Rehabilitation Center of Woodland Hills,
Woodland Hills, California

David Girard, PT, CHT
Physical Therapist/Certified Hand Therapist,
Hands Plus Physical Therapy,
Northridge, California

Patricia A. Gray, MS, PT
Physical Therapist,
Visiting Nurse & Hospice,
California Pacific Medical Center,
San Francisco, California

Kristen L. Griffith, OTR/L
Occupational Therapist,
Department of Hand Therapy,
Campbell Clinic,
Germantown, Tennessee

Jane Gruber, PT, MS, OCS
Outpatient Supervisor,
Rehabilitation Services,
Newton Wellesley Hospital,
Newton, Massachusetts

Will Hall, PT, OCS
Clinic Director,
Physiotherapy Associates,
Cumming, Georgia

Wendy J. Hurd, PT
Director of Rehabilitation,
SouthWest Sports Medicine,
Phoenix, Arizona

Frank Jobe, MD
Associate,
Kerlan-Jobe Orthopaedic Clinic,
Clinical Professor,
Department of Orthopaedics,
University of Southern California School of Medicine,
Orthopaedic Consultant,
Los Angeles Dodgers,
Los Angeles, California;
Orthopaedic Consultant,
PGA Tour, Senior PGA Tour,
Palm Beach Gardens, Florida

Richard B. Johnston III, MD
Clinical Instructor,
Emory University;
Partner, Houghston Clinic, PC,
Atlanta, Georgia

Bert Mandelbaum, MD
Fellowship Director,
Santa Monica Orthopedic and Sports Medicine Group,
Santa Monica, California

Benjamin M. Maser, MD
Attending Plastic Surgeon,
Plastic Surgery,
Palo Alto Medical Foundation,
Palo Alto, California

David Pakozdi, PT, OCS
Director,
Kinetic Orthopaedic Physical Therapy,
Santa Monica, California

Mark Phillips, MD
Clinical Assistant Professor,
Department of Surgery-Orthopedic Surgery,
University of Illinois College of Medicine at Peoria,
Peoria, Illinois

Luga Podesta, MD
Physiatrist,
Ventura Orthopedic Hand and Sports Medical Group,
Oxnard and Thousand Oaks, California;
Physiatrist/Consultant,
Kerlan-Jobe Orthopedic Clinic,
Los Angeles, California;
Physician,
Major League Baseball Umpires,
New York, New York;
Team Physician,
Oxnard College,
Team Physician,
Pacific Suns Minor League Baseball Team,
Oxnard, California

Edward Pratt, MD
Facility Director,
Spine Memphis,
The Orthopaedic Clinic,
Memphis, Tennessee

Diane Schwab, BA, DipPT, MS, MPA
Owner,
Champion Rehabilitation,
San Diego, California

Jessie Scott, PT
Physical Therapist,
HealthSouth,
San Francisco, California

Paul Slosar, MD
Attending Surgeon,
SpineCare Medical Group;
Assistant Director of Surgical Research,
The San Francisco Spine Institute,
Daly City, California

Steve Tippett, MS, PT, SCS, ATC
Assistant Professor,
Department of Physical Therapy,
Bradley University,
Peoria, Illinois

†Geoffrey Vaupel, MD
Private Practice,
California Pacific Medical Center, Davies Campus,
Department of Orthopaedic Surgery,
San Francisco, California

Kevin E. Wilk, PT
National Director, Research and Clinical Education,
HealthSouth Rehabilitation,
Birmingham, Alabama

Julie Wong, PT
Co-Director,
Pro-Active Therapy,
San Francisco, California

James Zachazewski, MS, PT, ATC, SCS
Director of Rehabilitation Services,
Newton Wellesley Hospital,
Newton, Massachussets

Craig Zeman, MD
Board Certified Orthopedic Surgeon,
Ventura Orthopedic Sports Medical Group,
Oxnard, California

---

† Deceased.

This book is dedicated in memory of Dr. Geoffrey Vaupel.
Dr. Vaupel was a friend, educator, and advocate of physical therapy.
His patients benefited from his knowledge that physical therapy intervention was
an integral facet of a successful outcome. We will miss him dearly.

Nora Cacanindin and Julie Wong

To my parents for providing a loving home
and for being a wonderful example of goodness. I have no excuses.
To my friends for their encouragement and their help. To my children
for bringing more love into our lives. And to my husband
for his support, help, and commitment to our family.

Lisa Maxey

To my two children, Nicholas and Michelle.

Jim Magnusson

Preface ───────────────────────────────────

The practice of physical therapy has gone through many transformations over the past 50 years. It has evolved into a science that is continually being scrutinized by third-party payers challenging us to prove that what we do is effective and efficient. We are at a crucial point in our profession in which we need to justify how many treatments are necessary to treat a condition or ICD-9 code; at times this practice ignores the individual whom we are treating. This book is *not* a "cookbook" for success but rather a compass from which the clinician can find guidance. This text is our effort to provide a resource that the clinician can reference as a guideline in the rehabilitation of the postsurgical patient.

We feel this is a unique text in that we have brought together more than 30 authors from around the country. Many of the authors are well published and some are just plain good clinicians who are willing to share their experiential philosophy. We wanted the clinicians to be able to visualize the common surgical approaches to each case (through the physicians' portion) and then follow the therapist(s) guidelines to establish an efficient treatment plan. The prototype of this text has not been explored, to our knowledge, in this much depth (and with this many contributors), especially Appendix A, Transitioning the Throwing Athlete Back to the Field.

We expect that with progression and enhancement of surgical techniques, rehabilitation will evolve as well. Our hope is that this text will enhance our profession through the exchange of information and that subsequent editions can respond to the changing needs of the postoperative patient.

How to Use this Book

This book gives the physical therapist a clear understanding of the surgical procedures required for various injuries so that a rehabilitation program can be fashioned appropriately. Each chapter presents the indications and considerations for surgery; a detailed look at the surgical procedure, including the surgeon's perspective regarding rehabilitation concerns; and therapy guidelines to use in designing the rehabilitation program. Areas that might prove troublesome are noted, with appropriate ways to address problems.

The indications and considerations for surgery and the surgery itself are described by an outstanding surgeon specializing in each area. All of the information presented should be valuable in understanding the mechanics of the injury and the repair process.

The therapy guidelines section is divided into three parts:

Evaluation

Phases of rehabilitation

Suggested home maintenance

Every rehabilitation program begins with a thorough evaluation at the initial physical therapy visit. This provides pertinent information for formulating the treatment program. As the patient progresses through the program, assessment continues. Activities that are too stressful for healing tissues at one point are delayed, then reassessed when the tissue is ready for the stress. Treatment measures are outlined in tabular format for easy reference.

The phases each patient faces in rehabilitation are clearly indicated both as a way to break the program into manageable segments and to provide reassurance to the patient that rehabilitation will proceed in an orderly fashion. The time span covered by each phase and the goals of the rehabilitation process during that phase are noted. The exercises are carefully explained and photographs are provided for assistance.

Home maintenance for the postsurgical patient is an essential component of the rehabilitation program. Even when the therapist is able to follow the patient routinely in the clinic, the patient is still on his or her own for most of the day. The patient must understand the importance of compliance with the home program to maximize postoperative results. In the successful home maintenance program, the patient is the primary force in rehabilitation, with the therapist acting as an informed and effective communicator, an efficient coordinator, and a motivator. When the therapist successfully fulfills these obligations and the patient is motivated and compliant, the home maintenance program can be especially rewarding.

When the patient is not motivated or not compliant or possesses less than adequate pain tolerance, a nononsense and forthright dialogue with the surgeon, referring physician, rehabilitation nurse, or any other professionals involved is essential. Timely, accurate, and straightforward documentation also is significant in the case of the "problem" patient. Emphasizing active patient involvement in an exercise program at home is even more imperative in light of the prescriptive nature of current managed care dictums.

The keys to an effective home maintenance program are structure, individuality, prioritization, and conciseness. The term *structure* refers to exercises that are well defined in terms of sets, repetitions, frequency, resistance, and technique. The patient must know what to do and how to do it. Home programs with photographs or video demonstrations are helpful in assisting the patient to see what is intended. Some computer-generated home exercise programs also offer adequate visual descriptions of the desired exercises. Stick figures and drawings that the physical therapist makes are often unclear and confusing to the patient.

Individuality, in the clearest sense, involves prescribing exercises that address the specific needs of a patient at a specific point in time. It includes being flexible enough to allow the patient to work the home program into the daily schedule as opposed to following only an "ideal" treatment schedule. Other components inherent in the concept of individuality include assistance available to the patient at home, financial implications, geographical concerns that influence follow-up, and the patient's cognitive abilities.

Prioritization and *conciseness* involve maximizing the use of the patient's time to perform the exercises at home. If the patient is being seen in the clinic, home exercises should stress activities not routinely performed in the clinic. If the patient is constrained for time, the therapist can identify the most beneficial exercises and prescribe them. It is best not to prescribe too many exercises to be done at home. Ideally, the patient should have to concentrate on no more than five or six at a time. To help keep the number of exercises manageable, the therapist should discontinue less taxing exercises as new exercises are added to the program.

Lisa Maxey
Jim Magnusson
Steve Tippett

Acknowledgments

I would like to give my sincere appreciation to all the contributors for their commitment to their work and for sharing their time and knowledge with us for the benefit of patients. I also want to thank HealthSouth for providing some of the exercise photographs. Special thanks to Clive Brewster for his insights into book writing. Finally, thanks to my colleagues—I've been fortunate to have worked with good people.

"A smile must always be on our lips for any child to whom we offer help, for any to whom we give companionship or medicine. It would be very wrong to offer only our cures; we must offer to all our hearts."
—Mother Teresa of Calcutta

Lisa Maxey

In the course of a lifetime we meet people who have made impressions on us; good or bad it changes us and shapes our vision of who we want to become. I would be remiss by not including the obvious individuals (mother, father, and my two brothers). However, when I first embarked on a career in the medical field it was my grandfather, Dr. James Logie, who helped me understand the dedication of those who aspire to become the best in their profession. I studied some of his own hand drawings of the human anatomy when he was in school and have seen how through his dedication to serving his patients his life has been blessed. He has taught me the importance of patience and showed me the art of fly fishing.

In my experience (19 years) working in the field of physical therapy I also have worked with individuals who not only through clinical work but also through life experience have taught me the value of compassion, dedication, empathy, and respect. Although a number of physical therapists have individually helped, the ones I've singled out also have positively influenced countless other therapists: Dee LillyMasuda, Gary Souza, and Rick Katz.

The undertaking of a project such as this book (which requires countless hours) should be done by someone who has the utmost consent of their spouse. If an author is not married, I would highly suggest that he or she consider giving up any social life until deadline day. I thank God (and Dee) for helping me to find that special person in my wife, partner in life, and peer—Tracy Magnusson, PT.

Jim Magnusson

Contents ────────────────────────────────

PART ONE   Upper Extremity,   1

1   Soft Tissue Healing Considerations After Surgery,   2
Robert I. Cantu

2   Acromioplasty,   11
Mark Phillips, Steve Tippett

3   Anterior Capsular Reconstruction,   29
Frank Jobe, Diane Schwab, Clive Brewster

4   Rotator Cuff Repair and Rehabilitation,   46
Mark Ghilarducci, Lisa Maxey

5   Extensor Brevis Release and Lateral Epicondylectomy,   71
James Calandruccio, Kelly Akin, Kristen L. Griffith

6   Reconstruction of the Ulnar Collateral Ligament with Ulnar Nerve Transposition,   82
James Andrews, Wendy J. Hurd, Kevin E. Wilk

7   Carpal Tunnel Syndrome: Postoperative Management,   101
Benjamin M. Maser, Christina M. Clark, David Girard

PART TWO   Spine,   121

8   Lumbar Microdiscectomy and Rehabilitation,   122
Rick B. Delamarter, James Coyle, David Pakozdi

9   Lumbar Spine Fusion,   151
Paul Slosar, Jessie Scott

PART THREE   Lower Extremity,   171

10   Total Hip Replacement,   172
Edward Pratt, Patricia A. Gray

11   Open Reduction and Internal Fixation of the Hip,   188
Edward Pratt, Mayra Saborio Amiran, Patricia A. Gray

12   Anterior Cruciate Ligament Reconstruction,   206
Luga Podesta, Jim Magnusson, Terry Gillette

13   Arthroscopic Lateral Retinaculum Release,   227
Andrew A. Brooks, Dan Farwell

14   Meniscectomy and Meniscal Repair,   **243**
Andrew A. Brooks, Terry Gillette

15   Patella Open Reduction and Internal Fixation,   **257**
Craig Zeman, Dan Farwell

16   Total Knee Replacement,   **268**
Geoffrey Vaupel, Nora Cacanindin, Julie Wong

17   Lateral Ligament Repair,   **288**
Richard Ferkel, Robert Donatelli, Will Hall

18   Open Reduction and Internal Fixation of the Ankle,   **302**
Richard Ferkel, Robert Donatelli, Will Hall

19   Ankle Arthroscopy,   **314**
Richard Ferkel, Deborah Mandis Cozen

20   Achilles Tendon Repair and Rehabilitation,   **323**
Bert Mandelbaum, Jane Gruber, James Zachazewski

Appendix A   Transitioning the Throwing Athlete Back to the Field,   **350**
Luga Podesta

Rehabilitation

FOR ❧ THE

POSTSURGICAL
ORTHOPEDIC PATIENT

PART ONE

Upper Extremity

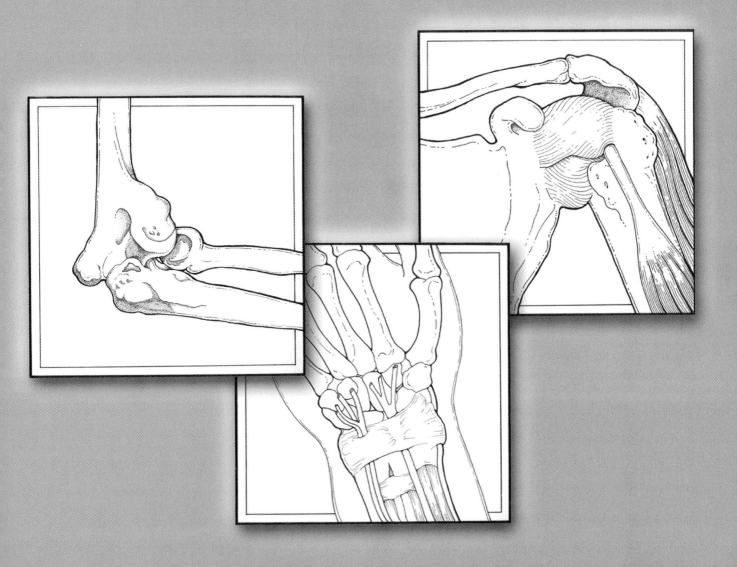

Soft Tissue Healing Considerations After Surgery

Robert I. Cantu

Physical therapists work daily on connective tissues that are dynamic and have the capacity for change. Changes in these tissues are driven by a number of factors, including trauma, surgery, immobilization, posture, and repeated stresses. The physical therapist must have a good working knowledge of the normal histology and biomechanics of connective tissue and understand the way connective tissue responds to immobilization, trauma, and remobilization. Both experienced and novice physical therapists can benefit from a good "mental picture" of connective tissues in operation.

Surgery Defined

Because this text primarily considers postsurgical rehabilitation, an operational definition of *surgery* is in order. For the purpose of considering injury and repair of soft tissues, surgery may be defined as *controlled trauma produced by a trained professional to correct uncontrolled trauma*. The reason for this unusual definition is that connective tissues respond in characteristic ways to immobilization and trauma. Because surgery is itself a form of trauma that is usually followed by some form of immobilization, the physical therapist must understand the way tissues respond to both immobilization and trauma.

This chapter begins by dealing with the basic histology and biomechanics of connective tissue. It then presents the histopathology and pathomechanics of connective tissues (i.e., the way connective tissues respond to immobilization, trauma, and remobilization). Finally it then addresses some basic principles of soft tissue mobilization based on the connective tissue response to immobilization, trauma, and remobilization.

Histology and Biomechanics of Connective Tissue

The connective tissue system in the human body is quite extensive. Connective tissue makes up 16% of the body's weight and holds 25% of the body's water.[9] The "soft" connective tissues form ligaments, tendons, periosteum, joint capsules, aponeuroses, nerve and muscle sheaths, blood vessel walls, and the bed and framework of the internal organs. If the bony structures were removed, a semblance of structure would remain from the connective tissues.

A majority of the tissues affected by mobilization are connective tissues. During joint mobilization, for example, the tissues being mobilized are the joint capsule and the surrounding ligaments and connective tissues. The facet joint space is merely a "space built for motion." Arthrokinematic rules are followed, but the tissue being mobilized is classified as connective tissue. Therefore a background knowledge of the histology and histopathology of connective tissues is essential for the practicing physical therapist.

Normal Histology and Biomechanics of Connective Tissue Cells

Connective tissue has two components: the cells and the extracellular matrix. The cell of primary importance is the fibroblast. The fibroblast synthesizes all the inert components of connective tissue, including collagen, elastin, reticulin, and ground substance.

The Extracellular Matrix

The extracellular matrix of connective tissue includes connective tissue fibers and ground substance. The connective tissue fibers include collagen (the most tensile), elastin, and reticulin (the most extensible). Collagen, elastin, and reticulin provide the tensile support that connective tissue offers. Extensibility or the lack of it is driven by the relative density and percentage of the connective tissue fibers. Tissues with less collagen density and a greater proportion of elastin fibers are more pliable than tissues with a greater density and proportion of collagen fibers.

The ground substance of connective tissue plays a very different role in the connective tissue response to immobility, trauma, and remobilization. The ground substance is the viscous, gel-like substance in which the cells and connective tissue fibers lie. It acts as a lu-

Table 1-1   **Classification of Connective Tissue**

Tissue Type	Specific Structures	Characteristics of the Tissue
Dense regular	Ligaments, tendons	Dense, parallel arrangement of collagen fibers; proportionally less ground substance
Dense irregular	Aponeurosis, periosteum, joint capsules, dermis of skin, areas of high mechanical stress	Dense, multidirectional arrangement of collagen fibers; able to resist multidirectional stress
Loose irregular	Superficial fascial sheaths, muscle and nerve sheaths, support sheaths of internal organs	Sparse, multidirectional arrangement of collagen fibers; greater amounts of elastin present

From Cantu R, Grodin A: *Myofascial manipulation: theory and clinical application,* Gaithersburg, MD, 1992, Aspen.

bricant for collagen fibers in conditions of normal mobility and maintains a crucial distance between collagen fibers. The ground substance also is a medium for the diffusion of nutrients and waste products and acts as a mechanical barrier for invading microorganisms. It has a much shorter half-life than collagen and, as will be discussed, is much more quickly affected by immobilization than collagen.[12]

Three Types of Connective Tissue

Connective tissue is classified according to fiber density and orientation. The three types of connective tissue found in the human body are dense regular, dense irregular, and loose irregular [6,13] (Table 1-1).

Dense regular connective tissue includes ligaments and tendons (Fig. 1-1). The fiber orientation is unidirectional for the purpose of attenuating unidirectional forces. The high density of collagen fibers accounts for the high degree of tensile strength and lack of extensibility in these tissues. Relatively low vascularity and water content account for the slow diffusion of nutrients and resulting slower healing times. Dense regular connective tissue is the most tensile and least extensible of the connective tissue types.

Dense irregular connective tissue includes joint capsules, periosteum, and aponeuroses. The primary difference between dense regular and dense irregular connective tissue is that dense irregular connective tissue has a multidimensional fiber orientation (Fig. 1-2). This multidimensional orientation allows the tissue to attenuate forces in numerous directions. The density of collagen fibers is high, producing a high degree of tensile strength and a low degree of extensibility. Dense irregular connective tissue also has low vascularity and water content, resulting in slow diffusion of nutrients and slower healing times.

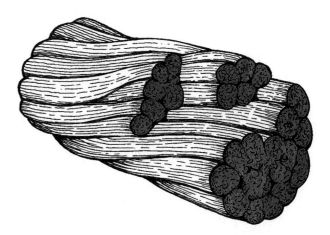

Fig. 1-1. Dense regular connective tissue. Note the parallel compact arrangement of the collagen fibers. (Modified from Williams P, Warwick R, editors: *Gray's anatomy,* ed 35, Philadelphia, 1973, WB Saunders.)

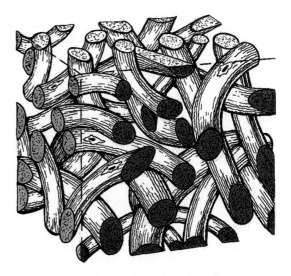

Fig. 1-2. Dense irregular connective tissue with multidimensional compact arrangement of collagen fibers. (Modified from Williams P, Warwick R, editors: *Gray's anatomy,* ed 35, Philadelphia, 1973, WB Saunders.)

Loose irregular connective tissue includes, but is not limited to, the superficial fascial sheath of the body directly under the skin, the muscle and nerve sheaths, and the bed and framework of the internal organs. Similarly to dense irregular connective tissue, loose irregular connective tissue has a multidimensional tissue orientation. However, the density of collagen fibers is much less than that of dense irregular connective tissue. The relative vascularity and water content of loose irregular connective tissue is much greater than dense regular and dense irregular connective tissue. Therefore it is much more pliable and extensible and exhibits faster healing times after trauma. Loose irregular connective tissue also is the easiest to mobilize.

Normal Biomechanics of Connective Tissue

Connective tissues have unique deformation characteristics that enable them to be effective shock attenuators. This is termed the *viscoelastic nature of connective tissue.*[15] This viscoelasticity is the very characteristic that makes connective tissue able to change based on the stresses applied to it. The ability of connective tissue to thicken or become more extensible based on outside stresses is the basic premise to be understood by the manual therapist seeking to increase mobility.

In the viscoelastic model two components combine to give connective tissues its dynamic deformation attributes. The first is the *elastic* component, which represents a temporary change in the length of connective tissue subjected to stress (Fig. 1-3). This is illustrated by a spring, which elongates when loaded and returns to its original position when unloaded. This elastic component is the "slack" in connective tissue.

The *viscous,* or plastic, component of the model represents the permanent change in connective tissue subjected to outside forces. This is illustrated by a hydraulic cylinder and piston (Fig. 1-4). When a force is placed on the piston, the piston slowly moves out of the cylinder. When the force is removed, the piston does not recoil but remains at the new length, indicating permanent change. These permanent changes result from the breaking of intermolecular and intramolecular bonds between collagen molecules, fibers, and cross-links.

The viscoelastic model combines the elastic and plastic components just described (Fig. 1-5). When subjected to a mild force in the midrange of the tissue, the tissue elongates in the elastic component, then returns to its original length. If, however, the stress pushes the tissue to the end range, the elastic component is depleted and plastic deformation occurs. When the stress is released, some permanent deformation has occurred. Note that not all the elongation is permanently retained, only a portion.

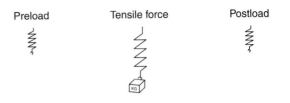

Fig. 1-3. The elastic component of connective tissue. (From Grodin A, Cantu R: *Myofascial manipulation: theory and clinical management,* Centerpoint, NY, 1989, Forum Medical Publishers.)

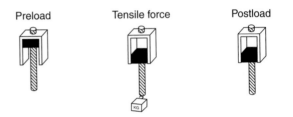

Fig. 1-4. The viscous, or plastic, component of connective tissue. (From Grodin A, Cantu R: *Myofascial manipulation: theory and clinical management,* Centerpoint, NY, 1989, Forum Medical Publishers.)

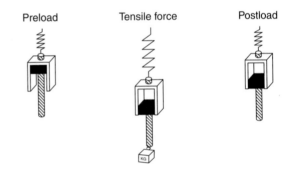

Fig. 1-5. The viscoelastic nature of connective tissue. (From Grodin A, Cantu R: *Myofascial manipulation: theory and clinical management,* Centerpoint, NY, 1989, Forum Medical Publishers.)

Clinically, this phenomenon occurs frequently. For example, a client with a frozen shoulder that has only 90 degrees of elevation is mobilized to reach a range of motion of 110 degrees by the end of the treatment session. When the client returns in a few days, the range of motion of that shoulder is less than 110 degrees but more than 90 degrees. Some degree of elongation is lost, and some is retained.

This viscoelastic phenomenon can be further illustrated by the use of stress/strain curves. By definition, stress is the force applied per unit area, and strain is the percent change in length. When connective tissue is initially stressed or loaded, very little force is required to elongate the tissue. However, as more stress is applied and the slack or spring is taken up, more force is required and less change occurs in the tissue (Fig. 1-6). When the tissue is subjected to repeated

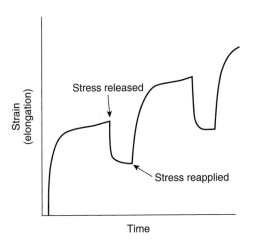

Fig. 1-6. Stress/strain curves indicating the progressive elongation of connective tissue with repeated stresses. (From Grodin A, Cantu R: *Myofascial manipulation: theory and clinical management*, Centerpoint, NY, 1989, Forum Medical Publishers.)

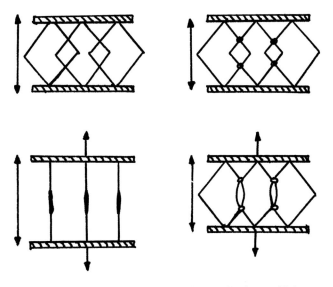

Fig. 1-7. The basket-weave configuration of connective tissue. With immobilization the distance between fibers is diminished, forming cross-link adhesions. (From Cantu R, Grodin A: *Myofascial manipulation: theory and clinical application*, Gaithersburg, MD, 1992, Aspen Publishers.)

stresses, the curve shows that after each stress the tissue elongates, then only partially returns to its original length. Some length is gained each time the tissue is taken into the plastic range. This phenomenon is seen clinically in repeated sessions of therapy. Range of motion is gained during a session, with some of the gain being lost between sessions.

Effects of Immobilization, Remobilization, and Trauma on Connective Tissue

Immobilization

Immobilization and trauma significantly change the histology and normal mechanics of connective tissue. A majority of the hallmark studies in the area of immobilization follow the same basic experimental mode.[1-5,15] Laboratory animals are fixated internally for varying periods. The fixation is removed and the animals are then sacrificed. Histochemical and biomechanical analyses are performed to determine changes in the tissues. In some studies the fixation is removed and the animals are allowed to move the fixated joint for a period before the analysis is performed. This is done to determine the reversibility of the effects of immobilization.[10]

Macroscopically, fibrofatty infiltrate is evident in the recesses of the immobilized tissues. With prolonged immobilization the infiltrates develop a more fibrotic appearance, creating adhesions in the recesses. These fibrotic changes occur in the absence of trauma. Histologic and histochemical analyses show significant changes primarily in the ground substance, with no significant loss of collagen. The changes in the ground substance

consist of substantial losses of glycosaminoglycans and water. Because a primary function of ground substance is binding water to assist in hydration, the loss of ground substance results in a related loss of water.

Another purpose of ground substance is to lubricate adjacent collagen fibers and maintain a crucial interfiber distance. If collagen fibers approximate too closely, the fibers will adhere to one another. These cross-links create a series of microscopic adhesions that limit the pliability and extensibility of the tissues (Fig. 1-7).

Furthermore, because movement affects the orientation of newly synthesized collagen, the collagen in the immobilized joints studied was laid down in a more haphazard, "haystack" arrangement. This orientation restricts tissue mobility further by adhering to existing collagen fibers (Fig. 1-8).

Biomechanical analysis reveals that as much as 10 times more torque is necessary to mobilize fixated joints than normal joints. After repeated mobilizations, these joints gradually return to normal. The authors of these studies implicate both fibrofatty microadhesions and increased microscopic cross-linking of collagen fibers in the decreased extensibility of connective tissues.

Remobilization

Available research seems to suggest that mobility and remobilization prevent the haystack development of collagen fibers and stimulate the production of ground substance. When connective tissue is stressed with movement, the tissue rehydrates, collagen cross-links are diminished, and new collagen is laid down in a more orderly fashion. The collagen tends to be laid down in the direction of the forces applied and in an appropriate length.

Additionally, macroadhesions formed during the immobilization period partially elongate and partially rupture during the remobilization process, increasing the overall mobility of the tissue. Both passive mobilization and active range of motion produce similar results.

Trauma

These studies have limited application because they involve the immobilization of normal, healthy joints.

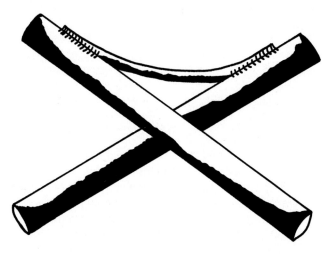

Fig. 1-8. The random haystack arrangement of immobilized scar tissue creating additional adhesions. (From Cantu R, Grodin A: *Myofascial manipulation: theory and clinical application,* Gaithersburg, MD, 1992, Aspen Publishers.)

To complete this discussion, we must superimpose the effects of trauma and scar tissue on immobilization.

Scar

Scar tissue mechanics differ somewhat from normal connective tissue mechanics. Normal connective tissue is mature and stable, with limited pliability. Immature scar tissue is much more dynamic and pliable. Scar tissue formation occurs in four distinct phases. Each of these phases shows characteristic differences during phases of immobilization and mobilization.[7,8]

The first phase of scar tissue formation is the inflammatory phase. This phase occurs immediately after trauma. Blood clotting begins almost instantly and is followed by migration of macrophages and histiocytes to start débriding the area. This phase usually lasts 24 to 48 hours, and immobilization is usually important because of the potential for further damage with movement. Some exceptions to routine immobilization exist. For example, in an anterior cruciate ligament (ACL) reconstruction in which the graft is safely fixated and damage from gentle movement is unlikely, there may be a great advantage in moving the tissue as early as the first day after surgery.

The second phase of scar tissue formation is the granulation phase. This phase is characterized by an uncharacteristic increase in the relative vascularity of the tissue. Increased vascularity is essential to ensure proper nutrition to meet the metabolic needs of the repairing tissue. The granulation phase varies greatly depending on the type of tissue and the extent of the damage. Generally speaking, the entire process of scar tissue formation is lengthened if the damaged tissue

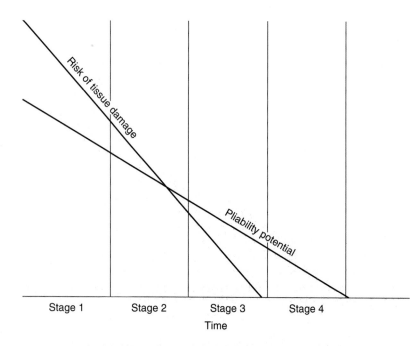

Fig. 1-9. Relationship of tissue pliability to relative risk of injury.

is less vascular in its nontraumatized state. For example, tendons and ligaments require more time for scar tissue formation than muscle or epithelial tissue. Movement is helpful in this phase, although the scar tissue can be easily damaged. The physician and therapist need to work closely to determine the extent of movement relative to the risk.

The third phase of scar tissue formation is the fibroplastic stage. In this stage the number of fibroblasts increases, as does the rate of production of collagen fibers and ground substance. Collagen is laid down at an accelerated rate and binds to itself with weak hydrostatic bonds, making tissue elongation much easier. This stage presents an excellent window of opportunity for the reshaping and molding of scar tissue without great risk of tissue re-injury. This stage lasts 3 to 8 weeks depending on the histologic makeup and relative vascularity of the damaged tissue. Scar tissue at this phase is less likely to be injured but is still easily remodeled with stresses applied (Fig. 1-9).

The final phase of scar tissue formation is the maturation phase. Collagen matures, solidifies, and shrinks during this phase. Maximal stress can be placed on the tissue without risk of tissue failure. Because collagen synthesis is still accelerated, significant remodeling can take place when appropriate mobilizations are performed. Conversely, if they are left unchecked, the collagen fibers can cross-link and the tissue can shrink significantly. At the end of the maturation phase, tissue remodeling becomes significantly more difficult because the tissue reverts to a more mature, inactive, and nonpliable status.

Surgical Perspective

Surgery has been defined in this chapter as *controlled trauma produced by a trained professional to correct uncontrolled trauma.* Postsurgical cases are subject to the effects of immobilization, trauma, and scar formation. However, they have the advantage of resulting from controlled trauma. The scar tissue formed by surgery is usually more manageable than scar tissue formed by uncontrolled trauma or overuse.

When dealing with scar tissue after surgery, the physical therapist should remember the following guidelines:
- Assess the approximate stage of development of the scar tissue. Although the timelines vary, vascular tissue matures faster than nonvascular tissue.
- Whenever possible, movement is helpful in controlling the direction and length of the scar tissue. Communicate with the referring physician regarding the amount of movement that is appropriate. In a study performed by Flowers and Pheasant,[11] casted joints regained mobility much faster than fixated joints. This is probably because a cast does not provide

the same immobilization as rigid fixation. The small amounts of movement allowed in casted joints may be enough to prevent some of the changes caused by rigid fixation.
- Recognize the window of opportunity to stress scar tissue, and keep in mind the associated risk of tissue injury or microtrauma (see Fig. 1-9). Although the potential to change scar tissue may be greater in earlier stages, the risk of damage is higher. The third stage appears to be the stage at which the reward of mobility work exceeds the risk. The therapist should proceed with caution in the second stage of scar tissue formation, recognizing that some risk may be necessary if optimal results are to be obtained.

Goals of Mobility Work

In 1945, John Mennell[12a] said "there are only two possible effects of any movement or massage: they are reflex and mechanical." The following summary emphasizes the goals of the mechanical changes of mobility work:
- Mobility work allows for the hydration and rehydration of connective tissues.
- Mobility work causes the breaking and subsequent prevention of cross-links in collagen fibers.
- Mobility work allows for the breaking and prevention of macroadhesions.
- Mobility work allows for the plastic deformation and permanent elongation of connective tissues.
- Mobility work allows for the laying down of collagen fibers and scar tissue in the appropriate length and direction of the stresses applied.
- Mobility work allows for the molding and remolding of collagen fibers during the fibroplastic and maturation stages of scar tissue formation.
- Mobility work prevents scar tissue shrinkage.
- Mobility work allows for the more generalized effects of increased blood flow, increased venous and lymphatic return, and increased cellular metabolism.

Principles for Mobilization of Connective Tissues

This section attempts to integrate the principles of basic scientific research and years of clinical experience into a series of techniques useful for the physical therapist in treating immobilized tissue.

The Three-Dimensionality of Connective Tissue

Connective tissue is three-dimensional. Especially after trauma and immobilization, the scar tissue can follow lines of development not consistent with the kinesiology or arthrokinematics of the area. Therefore the ability to feel the location and direction of the restriction becomes important in the mobilization of scar tissue.

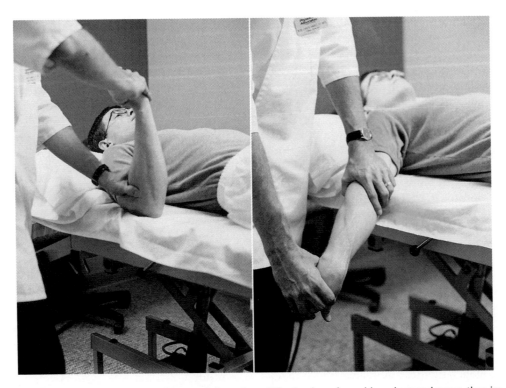

Fig. 1-10. The principle of short and long. Soft tissue immobilization is performed in a shortened range, then immediately elongated.

Creep

Creep is another term for the plastic deformation of connective tissue. Active scar tissue is more "creepy" than normal connective tissue (i.e., it is more easily elongated by external forces). Creep occurs when all the "slack" has been let out of the tissue. It is best accomplished with low-load, prolonged stretching but also can be accomplished with other manual techniques. Dynamic splinting is another technique used to elongate connective tissue. The tissue should be elongated along the lines of normal movement; however, at times the restrictive lesion may not follow the line of movement. The therapist must identify the direction of the restriction and mobilize directly into the restriction. This may be a transverse or horizontal plane. Mobilizing the scar in the direction of the restriction usually results in more movement along conventional planes.

The Principle of Short and Long

The principle of short and long is the idea that tissues mobilized in a shortened range often become more extensible when they are immediately elongated (Fig. 1-10). For example, in a lateral epicondylitis, cross-friction massage may be performed over the lateral epicondyle with the elbow passively flexed and the wrist passively extended. Immediately after the cross-friction in the shortened range, the tissue is stretched into the plastic range. In the shortened range, deeper tissues can be accessed. When tissue is taut, only the more superficial layers can be accessed. When the tissue has some slack, the deeper tissues can be accessed and prepared for stretching.

The principle of short and long has neuromuscular implications as well. If a muscle is guarded, shortening the muscle by mobilizing it has an inhibitory effect that makes immediate elongation easier.

Techniques for Mobilization of Connective Tissues

The following techniques and associated photographs illustrate some simple manual techniques effective in mobilizing soft tissues.

Muscle Splay

Muscle splay is a term that implies a widening or separation of longitudinal fibers of muscle or connective tissues that have adhered to one another (Fig. 1-11). These adhesions limit the ability of the tissue to be lengthened passively or shortened actively. When muscle bundles or connective tissue bundles stick together the muscle fibers become less efficient in their contractions. For example, muscle splay in the wrist flexors of-

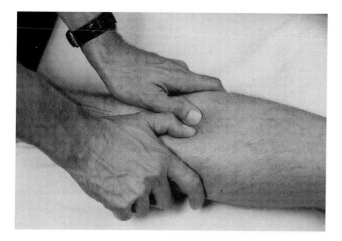

Fig. 1-11. The splaying, or longitudinal separation, of fascial planes.

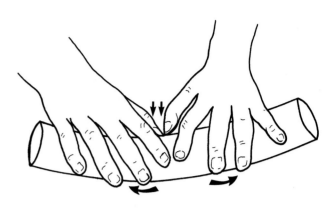

Fig. 1-13. Transverse movement of fascial planes.

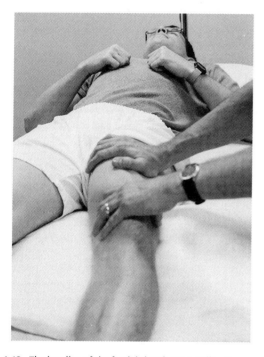

Fig. 1-12. The bending of the fascial sheath surrounding the muscles.

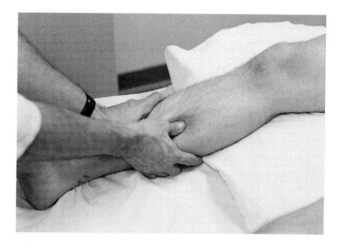

Fig. 1-14. Longitudinal stroke clearing fascia away from a bony surface.

ten produces a slightly greater grip strength immediately after soft tissue work. This is not greater strength, but greater muscle efficiency produced by increased soft tissue pliability. The muscle can contract more efficiently within its connective tissue compartments.

Transverse Muscle Bending

Transverse muscle bending takes the contractile unit and mobilizes it perpendicular to the fibers (Fig. 1-12). This perpendicular bending mobilizes connective tissues in a way similar to the bending of a garden hose (Fig. 1-13). The connective tissue sheath surrounding a muscle may be likened to the hose itself, with the muscle being analogous to the water inside it. If the connective tissue sheath is stiff and rigid, the muscle inside has difficulty contracting. The unforgiving sheath does not allow the muscle to expand transversely, creating a lack of efficiency and a low-grade "compartment syndrome." By mobilizing these muscle sheaths, overall mobility is enhanced along planes of normal movement.

Bony Clearing

Bony clearing is similar to muscle splay, except the mobilization is applied longitudinally along the soft tissues that border or attach to a bony surface (Fig. 1-14). A good example of this is longitudinal stroking of the anterior lateral border of the tibia in conditions such as shin splints. The connective tissues along the border of the tibia thicken and become adhered, and the therapist attempts to mobilize the tissues in this plane.

Cross-Friction

Cross-friction massage, which was developed and advocated by the late James Cyriax, is excellent for mobilizing scar tissue and nonvascular connective tissues. It is an aggressive form of soft tissue mobilization designed to break scar tissue adhesions and temporarily increase the blood flow to nonvascular areas. Ligaments and tendons struggling to heal completely are excellent candidates for cross-friction massage. This technique can be used on scar tissue as well and should be performed in many different angles to access fibers in all directions.

Summary

Basic principles and guidelines for soft tissue management after surgery have been outlined. The stages of scar tissue formation have been discussed. The time frames for these stages are variable based on the vascularity of the tissues and the surgical procedure performed. They are delineated in more detail in the following chapters.

The physical therapist must understand connective tissue responses to immobilization, trauma, remobilization, and scar remodeling to treat injured tissues effectively. Awareness of these principles along with good physician and client communication ensures consistently effective management of postsurgical rehabilitation.

REFERENCES

1. Akeson WH, Amiel D: The connective tissue response to immobility: a study of the chondroitin 4 and 6 sulfate and dermatan sulfate changes in periarticular connective tissue of control and immobilized knees of dogs, *Clin Orthop* 51:190, 1967.

2. Akeson WH, Amiel D: Immobility effects of synovial joints: the pathomechanics of joint contracture. *Biorheology* 17:95, 1980.

3. Akeson WH et al: Collagen cross-linking alterations in the joint contractures: changes in the reducible cross-links in periarticular connective tissue after 9 weeks of immobilization, *Connect Tissue Res* 5:15, 1977.

4. Akeson WH et al: The connective tissue response to immobility: an accelerated aging response, *Exp Gerontol* 3:289, 1968.

5. Akeson WH et al: The connective tissue response to immobilization: biochemical changes in periarticular connective tissue of the rabbit knee, *Clin Orthop* 93:356, 1973.

6. Copenhaver WM, Bunge RP, Bunge MB: *Bailey's textbook of histology,* Baltimore, MD, 1971, Williams & Wilkins.

7. Cummings GA: *Soft tissue contractures: clinical management continuing education seminar,* course notes, Atlanta, GA, March 1989, Georgia State University.

8. Cummings GS, Crutchfield CA, Barnes MR: *Orthopedic physical therapy series: soft tissue changes in contractures,* Atlanta, 1983, Stokesville Publishing.

9. Dicke E, Schliack H, Wolff A: *A manual of reflexive therapy of the connective tissue,* Scarsdale, NY, 1978, Sidney S. Simon.

10. Evans E et al: Experimental immobilization and mobilization of rat knee joints, *J Bone Joint Surg* 42A:737, 1960.

11. Flowers KR, Pheasant SD: The use of torque angle curves in the assessment of digital stiffness, *J Hand Therapy,* p. 69, Jan-March 1988.

12. Ham AW, Cormack DH: *Histology,* Philadelphia, 1979, JB Lippincott.

12a. Mennell JB: *Physical treatment by movement, manipulation and massage,* ed 5, London, 1945, Churchill.

13. Sapega AA et al: Biophysical factors in range-of-motion exercise, *Physician Sports Med* 9:57, 1981.

14. Warwick R, Williams PL: *Gray's anatomy,* ed 35, Philadelphia, 1973, WB Saunders.

15. Woo S et al: Connective tissue response to immobility, *Arthritis Rheum* 18:257, 1975.

Chapter 2

Acromioplasty

Mark Phillips
Steve Tippett

Before the broad topic of acromioplasty is addressed, the topic of subacromial impingement syndrome must be explored. In 1972 Neer described subacromial impingement as a distinct clinical entity in his landmark article.[41] He correlated the anatomy of the subacromial space with the bony and soft tissue relationships and described the impingement zone. Neer also described a continuum of three clinical and pathologic stages.[42] This study provides a basis for understanding the impingement syndrome, which ranges from reversible inflammation to full-thickness rotator cuff tearing. The relationships among the anterior third of the acromion, coracoacromial ligament, and acromioclavicular joint and the underlying subacromial soft tissues, including the rotator cuff, remain the basis for most of the subsequent surgery-related impingement studies. Many other researchers have contributed to current knowledge of the subacromial shoulder impingement syndrome. The works of Meyer,[40] Codman,[16] Armstrong,[4] Diamond,[17] and McLaughlin and Asherman[39] provide a historical perspective.

Surgical Indications and Considerations

Anatomic Etiologic Factors

Any abnormality that disrupts the intricate relationship within the subacromial space may lead to impingement. Both intrinsic (intratendinous) and extrinsic (extratendinous) factors have been implicated as etiologies of the impingement process. Nirschl[44] eloquently described the role of muscle weakness within the rotator cuff, leading to tension overload, humeral head elevation, and changes in the supraspinatus tendon, which is used most often in high-demand, repetitive overhead activities. Other authors[3,31,60] have described inflammation and thickening of the bursal contents and their relationship to the impingement syndrome. Jobe et al[30,31] studied the role of microtrauma and overuse in intrinsic tendonitis and glenohumeral instability and their implications for overhead-throwing athletes. Intrinsic degenerative tenopathy also has been discussed as an intrinsic cause of subacromial impingement symptoms.[48]

Extrinsic or extratendinous etiologic factors form the second broad category of causes of impingement syndrome. Rare secondary extrinsic factors (e.g., neurologic pathology secondary to cervical radiculopathy, supraspinatus nerve entrapment) are not discussed here, but the primary extrinsic factors and their anatomic relationships are of primary surgical concern. The unique anatomy of the shoulder joint sandwiches the soft tissue structures of the subacromial space (i.e., rotator cuff tendons, coracoacromial ligament, long head of biceps, bursa) between the overlying anterior acromion, acromioclavicular joint, and coracoid process and the underlying greater tuberosity of the humeral head and the superior glenoid rim. Bigliani's description of three primary acromial types and their correlation to impingement and full-thickness rotator cuff tears has been supported by Toivonen.[9,58] Acromioclavicular degenerative joint disease also can be an extrinsic primary etiology of impingement disease.[41,42] Many authors support Neer's original position on the contribution of acromioclavicular degenerative joint disease to the impingement process.[33,63] The os acromiale, the unfused distal acromial epiphysis, also has been discussed as a separate entity and a potential etiologic factor related to impingement.[8] Glenohumeral instability is a secondary extrinsic cause or contribution to impingement. Its relationship to the impingement syndrome is poorly understood, but it helps explain the failure of acromioplasty in the subset of young, competitive, overhead-throwing athletes with a clinical impingement syndrome.[21,23,31]

Diagnosis and Evaluation of the Impingement Syndrome

History and physical examinations are crucial in diagnosing subacromial impingement syndrome. Findings may be subtle and symptoms may overlap in the various differential diagnoses; therefore appreciating the impingement syndrome symptom complex may be difficult. The classic history has an insidious onset and a chronic component that develops over months, usually in a patient over 40 years old. The patient frequently describes repetitive activity during recreation, recreational sports, competitive athletics, and work. Pain is the most common symptom, especially pain with specific high-demand or repetitive away-from-the-chest and overhead shoulder activities. Night pain is seen later in impingement syndrome, after the inflammatory response has heightened. Weakness and stiffness may occur secondary to pain inhibition. If true weakness persists after the pain is eliminated, the differential diagnoses of rotator cuff tearing or neurologic cervical entrapment–type pathologies must be addressed. If stiffness persists, frozen shoulder–related conditions (e.g., adhesive capsulitis, inflammatory arthritis, degenerative joint disease) must be ruled out. Younger athletic and throwing patients need continual assessment for glenohumeral instability.

The physical examination of a patient with impingement syndrome focuses on the shoulder and neck regions. Physical examination of the neck helps rule out cervical radiculopathy, degenerative joint disease, and other disorders of the neck contributing to referred pain complexes in the shoulder area. The shoulder evaluation includes a general inspection for muscle asymmetry or atrophy, with emphasis on the supraspinatus region. Range of motion and muscle strength testing and generalized glenohumeral stability testing are emphasized during the evaluation. The Neer impingement sign[42] and Hawkins-Kennedy sign[26] are gold standard tests to help diagnose impingement. The impingement test, which includes subacromial injection of a Xylocaine-type compound and repeated impingement sign maneuvers, is most helpful in ascertaining the presence of an impingement syndrome. The acromioclavicular joint also is addressed during the shoulder evaluation. The clinician should note acromioclavicular joint pain with direct palpation and pain on horizontal adduction of the shoulder. Selective acromioclavicular joint injection also may be helpful. Long head biceps tendon pathology, including ruptures, are rare but may occur in this subset of patients. Physical examination will define the tendon's contribution to the symptom complex. Instability testing, especially in the younger athletic patient, also should be performed. The clinician should assess for classic apprehension signs and perform the Jobe relocation test, recording any positive findings.

Radiographic Evaluation

Standard radiographic evaluation is carried out with special attention to anteroposterior (AP), 30-degree caudal tilt AP, and outlet views of the shoulder.[24,49] These plain studies are helpful in demonstrating acromial anatomy types, hypertrophic coracoacromial ligament spurring, acromioclavicular joint osteoarthrosis, and calcific tendonitis. These views, in combination with an axillary view, can uncover os acromiale le-

sions. Magnetic resonance imaging (MRI) also is helpful in revealing relationships in impingement syndrome, especially if rotator cuff tear and other internal derangement pathologies (such as glenolabral or biceps tendon pathologies) are suspected.[7]

Surgical Procedure: Subacromial Decompression

Subacromial impingement syndrome that has not responded to rehabilitation techniques and nonoperative means may require surgery. If proven trials of rehabilitation, activity modification, use of nonsteroidal antiinflammatory agents (NSAIDs), and judicious use of subacromial cortisone injections are unsuccessful, acromioplasty and subacromial decompression (SAD) should be considered.

Historically, open acromioplasties produced excellent results and still have a significant role in surgical treatment.[8,41,54] Ellman[19] is credited with the first significant arthroscopic SAD techniques and studies, and many surgeons and investigators have developed techniques and arthroscopic SAD advancements for the surgical treatment of subacromial impingement syndrome.* Indications for surgery to correct subacromial impingement syndrome include persistent pain and dysfunction that have failed to respond to nonsurgical treatment, including physician- or therapist-directed physical therapy, trials of NSAIDs, subacromial cortisone or lidocaine injections, and activity modification.

The most controversial surgical indication topic concerns the amount of time that should elapse before nonoperative management is considered a failure.[8] Most surgeons and investigators recommend a trial period of approximately 6 months. However, this depends on the individual patient and pathologic condition and should be tailored to the circumstances. For example, a 42-year-old patient with a history of several months of progressive symptoms has an occupation or recreational activity that requires high-demand, repetitive overhead movement. In the absence of instability, with a hooked acromion (type III) and MRI-documented, partial-thickness tearing, this patient need not endure the 6-month trial period to meet surgical indications for the treatment of his condition. On the other hand, a noncompliant patient in a worker's compensation–related situation who has a flat acromion and equivocal, inconsistent clinical findings may never meet the surgical indications.

Procedure

Both open acromioplasty and the arthroscopic SAD procedure are discussed in the following sections. Open

---

*References 1, 20, 32, 35, 51, 55.

acromioplasty techniques have been well documented, their outcomes have been well researched, and their results have been rated as very good to excellent in numerous studies.[6,41,54] Because of these factors and the high technical demands of arthroscopic decompression, surgeons should never completely abandon this proven technique for the surgical management of persistent shoulder impingement. Surgeons also may resort to these open techniques in the event of arthroscopic procedure failure or intraoperative difficulties. Depending on surgical experience and expertise, an open procedure may be used in deference to an arthroscopic SAD procedure.

Arthroscopic SAD for the surgical treatment of impingement syndrome has a number of advantages. First, the arthroscopic technique allows evaluation of the glenohumeral joint for associated labral, rotator cuff, and biceps pathology, as well as assessment of the acromioclavicular joint and surgical treatment of any condition contributing to impingement. Second, this technique produces less postoperative morbidity and is relatively noninvasive, minimizing deltoid muscle fiber detachment. However, arthroscopic SAD is a technically demanding procedure whose "learning curve" can be higher than for other orthopedic procedures.

Many different arthroscopic techniques have been described, but the authors of this chapter recommend the modified technique initially described by Caspari and Thaw.[14] The patient is usually anesthetized with both a general and a scalene block regional anesthetic. In most community settings this combination has been highly successful in allowing patients to have this procedure done on an outpatient basis. A scalene regional block and home patient-controlled analgesia (PCA) provide acceptable pain control and ensure a comfortable postoperative course.

After the patient has reached the appropriate depth of anesthesia, the shoulder is evaluated in relationship to the contralateral side in both a supine and a semisitting beach chair position. Any concern regarding stability testing can be further assessed at this time, taking advantage of the complete anesthesia. Then, using the standard beach chair positioning, the surgeon begins the arthroscopic procedure. An inflow pressure pump (Davol) is used to maintain appropriate tissue space distention. Epinephrine is added to the irrigation solution to a concentration of 1 mg/L, thus enhancing hemostasis.

Specific portal placement is important to eliminate technical difficulties. Carefully addressing the palpable bony topography of the shoulder and marking the acromion, clavicle, acromioclavicular joint, and coracoid process greatly facilitate portal placement (Fig. 2-1). First, the sulcus is palpated directly posterior to the acromioclavicular joint. From this universal landmark, appropriate orientation can be obtained and con-

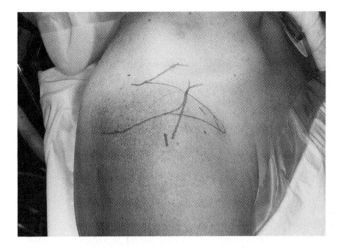

Fig. 2-1. The lateral portal is fashioned on the lateral aspect of the acromion just posterior and inferior to a line drawn by extending the topographic anatomy of the anterior acromioclavicular complex.

sistent reproducible posterior, anterior, and lateral portal placement achieved.

Using the standard posterior portal, the surgeon inserts the arthroscope into the glenohumeral joint. In a routine and sequential fashion, the glenohumeral joint is evaluated with attention directed to the biceps tendon and the labral and rotator cuff anatomy. Any incidental pathology can be addressed arthroscopically at this point. Subacromial space arthroscopy can now be performed.

For subacromial procedures a long diagnostic double cannula arthroscope is recommended. The cannula with blunt trocar is placed from the posterior portal superior to the cuff, exiting the anterior portal.

Using this cannula as a switch stick equivalent, the surgeon places a cannula with a plastic diaphragm over the arthroscopic instrument and returns it to the subacromial space. Gently retracting the arthroscopic cannula and inserting the arthroscope allows the inflow and arthroscopic cannulas to be close together. Adequate distention and maintenance of inflow and outflow are crucial for visualization and indirect hemostasis. This technique has been successful in achieving these goals. At this point the lateral portal is fashioned, generally on the lateral aspect of the acromion just posterior and inferior to a line drawn by extending the topographic anatomy of the anterior acromioclavicular complex (see Fig. 2-1). A spinal needle may assist in the accurate placement of this portal, which is crucial to instrument placement and subsequent visualization.

Starting from the posterior portal and using an aggressive synovial resector with the inflow in the anterior portal, the surgeon uses the lateral portal to perform a bursectomy and débride the soft tissues of the subacromial space. This is done in a sequential manner, working from the lateral bursal area to the anterior and medial acromioclavicular regions. Spinal needles can be placed in the anterolateral and acromioclavicular joint region to facilitate visualization and reveal spatial relationships. After the subacromial bursectomy and denudement of the undersurface of the acromion, the superior rotator cuff can be visualized along with the acromioclavicular joint and anterior acromial anatomy is more easily defined. The surgeon must take care not to violate the coracoacromial ligament during this initial bursectomy procedure.

At this point the surgeon inserts the arthroscope in the lateral portal for visualization. Using the posterior portal and following the posterior slope of the normal acromion, the surgeon performs sequential acromioplasty with an acromionizer instrument. In the technique described by Caspari,[14] the shank of the acromionizer is directed flat against the posterior acromial slope and acromioplasty is completed from the posterior to the anterior aspect. This accomplishes two goals. First, it provides a reliable and reproducible template to convert any abnormal hooked, sloped, or curved acromion to the therapeutic goal of a flat, type I configuration. Second, it allows for the removal of the coracoacromial ligament from its bony attachment with minimal chance for coracoacromial artery bleeding, thereby maximizing arthroscopic visualization and minimizing technical difficulties. At this point any further modification or "fine tuning" may be done through both the lateral and the anterior portals. Any residual coracoacromial ligament is removed from its acromial insertion while its bursal extension is excised.

The acromioclavicular joint also may be assessed at this stage, and minimal inferior osteophytes may be excised. Depending on the results of the preoperative evaluation, distal clavicle procedures can be performed at this point either through directed arthroscopic techniques or, as the authors of this chapter prefer, through a small incision located over the acromioclavicular joint region. If acromioclavicular joint symptoms are present with horizontal adduction and direct palpation, and/or if radiographs confirm the pathology, the surgeon should proceed with a distal clavicle excision. A T-type capsular incision is located over the acromioclavicular joint region, with the anterior and posterior capsular leaves elevated subperiosteally from the distal clavicle. Using small Homan retractors, the surgeon can excise the distal clavicle (usually 1.5 to 2 cm) at this point with an oscillating saw. The distal clavicle can then be easily palpated and rasped smooth. With a simple digital confirmation, the undersurface of the acromion also can be checked and any residual osteophytes rasped through this minimal incision technique.

The soft tissue is then closed in anatomic fashion with essentially no deltoid detachment. A routine subcuticular skin closure is used. The patient is placed in a postoperative pouch sling, and cryotherapy is frequently suggested. The patient is discharged to continue treatment as an outpatient or, if insurance or health demands require, overnight observation is used. Physical therapy may begin immediately on the first postoperative day and follows the standard program discussed in this chapter.

Outcomes

The surgical outcomes for arthroscopic SAD, partial acromioplasties, and distal clavicle excisions[8,35] have been most favorable. Many studies have compared open and closed techniques and obtained similar overall findings.[6,8,22] SAD procedures have three general goals:

1. To return the patient to a premorbid range of motion and strength perimeters
2. To eliminate pain
3. To eliminate the anatomic mechanical component of the impingement syndrome

Challenges and Precautions

The most common causes of surgical failures are associated with incomplete bone resection and not addressing acromioclavicular joint arthropathy. By carefully considering surgical techniques and including (if necessary) distal clavicle excision or combined open techniques, these common pitfalls can be eliminated. Another common reason for failure of arthroscopic SAD surgery is inappropriate diagnosis or patient selection. Again, with careful assessment, especially regarding instability, underlying lesions, and differential diagnoses, these failures can be dramatically lessened.

Rehabilitation Concerns: The Surgeon's Perspective

Therapists spend more time with postoperative patients than most surgeons do, and their input and direction are important in achieving a successful outcome. Their understanding of the procedure, postoperative pain, patient apprehension, and general medical concerns is vital. Physical therapy–directed early diagnosis of any wound problems (evidenced by erythema) or superficial infection can eliminate potential major complications. Postoperative inflammation also can be assessed with careful observation. Stiffness in frozen shoulder syndrome, although rare, can develop postoperatively and is addressed optimally with early diagnosis and progressive physical therapy.

Therapy Guidelines for Rehabilitation

The goal of the therapeutic exercise program after a SAD procedure is to augment the surgical decompression by increasing the subacromial space. Additional

---

Box 2-1   Components of the Physical Therapy Evaluation

Background Information
- Status of capsule
- Status of rotator cuff
- Status of articular cartilage
- Previous procedures
- Associated medical problems that can influence rehabilitation (e.g. cardiovascular concerns, diabetes mellitus)
- Work-related injury
- Insurance status
- Motivation
- Comprehension

Subjective Information
- Previous level of function
- Present level of function
- Patient's goals and expectations
- Intensity of pain
- Location of pain
- Frequency of pain
- Presence of night pain
- Assistance at home
- Access to rehabilitation facilities
- Medication (dose, effect, tolerance, compliance)

Objective Information
- Observation:
   Muscle wasting
   Resting posture
   Use of sling
   Wound status
   Swelling
   Color
- Range of motion (active/passive):
   Upper thoracic spine
   Scapulothoracic joint
   Sternoclavicular joint
   Acromioclavicular joint
   Scapulothoracic rhythm
- Strength:
   Rotator cuff
   Scapular upward rotators
   Scapular retractors
   Scapular protractors
   Deltoid
   Biceps

---

clearance for subacromial structures can be gained by strengthening the scapular upward rotators and humeral head depressors. Exercises to enhance the surgical decompression are straightforward. The challenge for the physical therapist is to implement the appropriate therapeutic exercise regimen without overloading healing tissue.

The postoperative rehabilitation program can be divided into three phases:

1. Phase one emphasizes *a return of range of motion.*
2. Phase two stresses *regaining muscle strength.*
3. Phase three stresses *endurance and functional progression.*

These three phases are not distinct entities and they do overlap. Together they serve as a template on which the physical therapist can build a management protocol for the post-SAD patient. An absence of pain is the primary guideline for progressing to more strenuous activities.[13] The phases are simply guidelines and should be adapted to each patient. Patients with significant rotator cuff involvement, articular cartilage defects, significant preoperative motion or strength loss, perioperative or intraoperative complications, and glenohumeral instability require special consideration and may not progress as rapidly as indicated in the standard rehabilitation program, which assumes that there is no glenohumeral instability and that the rotator cuff tendons are intact.

Signs that therapeutic activities are too aggressive include the following:
- Increased levels of referred pain to the area of insertion of the deltoid
- Night pain
- Pain that lasts more than 2 hours after exercising[46]
- Pain that alters the performance of an activity or exercise[46]

Evaluation

Every rehabilitation program begins with a thorough evaluation at the initial physical therapy visit. This evaluation provides pertinent information for formulating a treatment program. As the patient progresses through the program, assessment is ongoing. Activities that are too stressful for healing tissue at one point are reassessed when the tissue is ready for the stress. Measures to be included in the physical therapy evaluation are provided in Box 2-1.

Phase One

TIME: First 3 weeks after surgery.
GOALS: Emphasis on measures to control normal postoperative inflammation and pain, protect healing soft tissues, and minimize the effects of immobilization and activity restriction (Table 2-1).

Table 2-1 Acromioplasty

Rehabilitation Phase	Criteria to Progress to this Phase	Anticipated Impairments and Functional Limitations	Intervention	Goal	Rationale
Phase Ia Postoperative 1-2 days	Postoperative	• Pain • Edema • Dependent upper extremity (usually in a sling or airplane splint depending on degree of repair)	• Cryotherapy 20-30 minutes • Monitoring of incision site • Grip strength exercises (with arm elevated if swollen)	• Decrease pain • Prevent infection • Minimize wrist and hand weakness from disuse	• Self-manage pain and manage edema • Prevent complications during healing • Minimize disuse atrophy and promote circulation
Phase Ib Postoperative 3-10 days	No wound drainage or presence of infection	• As in phase Ia	Continue intervention as in Phase Ia with addition of the following: • PROM of shoulder as indicated • Isometrics—Submaximal to maximal internal and external rotation in sling or supported out of sling in neutral resting position • AROM—Scapular retraction/protraction (position as with isometrics) • Joint mobilization to the sternoclavicular (SC) and acromioclavicular (AC) joints as indicated	• Improve PROM avoiding aggravating surgical site • Produce fair to good muscular contraction of rotators • Restore/maintain scapula mobility • Reduce pain/joint stiffness	• Increase PROM preparing to advance AROM exercises • Minimize reflex inhibition of rotator cuff • Minimize disuse atrophy of scapula stabilizers • Use low-grade (resistance-free) mobilizations to decrease muscle guarding and progress grades as tolerated to restore arthrokinematics

| Phase Ic Postoperative 11-14 days | • Comfortable out of sling
• No signs of infection or night pain | • Intermittent pain
• Limited upper extremity use with reaching/lifting activities
• Limited ROM
• Limited strength | Continue as in Phases Ia & Ib:
• AROM—External rotation (at 60°-90° abduction)
Supine flexion
• AROM—Supine scapular protraction (elbow extended) "punches" side-lying (midrange) external rotation with support (towel) in axilla
Prone scapular retraction
• Pool therapy (with appropriate waterproof dressing if incision site not fully closed)
• Cardiovascular exercise (bike, walking program)
• Depending on job activities, return to limited work duties | • Flexion PROM to 150°
• External/internal rotation PROM to functional levels (or full ROM)
• Scapulothoracic PROM to full mobility
• Supine AROM flexion to 120°
• Symmetric AC/SC mobility
• Increase AROM tolerance in water to 100° flexion
• Minimize cardiovascular deconditioning
• Improve general muscular strength and endurance | • Increase capsular extensibility with flexion/elevation and rotation exercises
• Make rotator cuff ready for supine elevation
• Initiate strengthening of scapula stabilizers (proximal stability)
• Support axilla to allow for vascular supply to cuff during exercises
• Encourage AC/SC accessory motions required for full shoulder mobility
• Note that buoyant effects of water allow an environment where the water assists with flexion
• Prescribe lower extremity conditioning exercises to promote healing and improve cardiovascular fitness
• Provide ergonomic education early to prevent future complications |

Control of inflammation and pain. The surgeon may have prescribed NSAIDs to control normal postoperative inflammation and pain. These can be an adjunct to the other means the physical therapist employs to decrease inflammation (i.e., gentle therapeutic exercise, cryotherapy).

The therapist should determine whether a scalene block was performed in addition to the general anesthetic. If a block was performed, the onset of immediate postoperative pain may be delayed, and the patient should be monitored for signs of delayed motor return and prolonged or abnormal hypesthesia. If narcotics are used past the first few postoperative days, the therapist must undertake the therapeutic exercise program cautiously.

Cryotherapy can be used to help manage postoperative pain. Crushed ice conforms nicely to the shoulder, but commercially available cryotherapy and compression units (PolarCare, Cryocuff), although tedious to use, can be less messy. Sterile postoperative liners allow the source of the cold to be placed under the initial bulky dressing. The physical therapist should be aware of reimbursement practices for these units and use them accordingly.

Protection of healing soft tissues. Decreased use of the upper extremity is required to protect healing soft tissues after SAD. Depending on the surgeon's protocol and operative findings, a sling may be prescribed. The sling helps decrease the forces on the supraspinatus tendon by centralizing the head of the humerus in the glenoid fossa in a dependent position. Use of the sling is encouraged for the first 2 to 3 days after surgery in most cases, with the patient's level of discomfort dictating the degree of sling use.

Although the sling is used to minimize pain, it can add to the patient's discomfort. A "critical zone" of hypovascularity in the supraspinatus tendon initially described by Rathbun and McNab[53] may contribute to shoulder pain in a resting dependent position. The existence of this critical zone is debated by some, but recent work by Lohr and Ulthoff[37] corroborates Rathbun and McNab's initial findings. This critical zone corresponds to the anastomoses between osseous vessels and vessels within the supraspinatus tendon. Vessels in this critical zone fill poorly when the arm is at the side,[42] but this wringing out of the supraspinatus tendon is not observed when the arm is abducted.[15] If the patient experiences increased shoulder discomfort after prolonged periods with the arm at the side, he or she should place a small bolster (2 to 3 inches in diameter) in the axilla (resting the arm in a supported, slightly abducted position) to help decrease the pain.

Immobilization and restricted activities. While the sling protects the healing tissue around the glenohumeral joint, motion should be encouraged at proximal and distal joints. Scapular protraction, retraction, and ele-

vation can be performed in the sling. The patient should remove the arm from the sling at least three to four times daily to perform supported elbow, wrist, and hand range of motion (ROM) exercises.

The patient should always perform warm-up activities. This enhances the rate of muscular relaxation, increases the mechanical efficiency of muscle by decreasing viscous resistance, allows for greater hemoglobin and myoglobin dissociation in the time spent working, decreases resistance in the vascular bed, increases nerve conduction velocity, decreases the risk for electrocardiographic abnormalities, and increases metabolism.[64]

The physical therapist should educate the patient. Help him or her understand that discomfort experienced with passive stretching into external rotation comes from the capsule and occurs because the supraspinatus muscle is slack.

Patients with sedentary occupations who do not have lifting duties typically can return to work during phase one. Those returning to work should perform scapular, elbow, wrist, and hand exercises during working hours.

> **Q.** Carl arrives for therapy 5 weeks after a shoulder acromioplasty. He is having difficulty performing shoulder flexion and scaption exercises correctly. He occasionally demonstrates a mild shoulder hike with arm elevation exercises above 70 degrees of elevation. How can you sequence his exercises to maximize his ability to elevate his arm above shoulder height?

Phase Two

TIME: From 3 to at least 6 weeks after surgery.
GOALS: Emphasis on muscle strengthening, with continued work on rotator cuff musculature and scapula stabilizer strengthening (Table 2-2).

Many of the exercises used to strengthen the rotator cuff and scapular stabilizers have been assessed by electromyography (EMG).[12] EMG (both superficial and fine wire) has been used to document electrical activity in the rotator cuff and intrascapular musculature during the performance of various therapeutic exercises. McCann et al[38] evaluated the EMG output of rotator cuff musculature during the performance of more than 25 common exercises in normal subjects. Exercises were ranked from less to more strenuous based on the amount of electrical activity detected. A summary of these exercises is provided in Box 2-2.

Muscles of the rotator cuff (especially the supraspinatus) have relatively small cross-sectional areas and short lever arms. When working with them, the

Table 2-2   Acromioplasty

Rehabilitation Phase	Criteria to Progress to this Phase	Anticipated Impairments and Functional Limitations	Intervention	Goal	Rationale
Phase IIa Postoperative 3-6 weeks	• AROM to 120° flexion • AROM improving trend • Gait with normal arm swing • Strength of rotators to 4/5 (manual muscle test [MMT]—5/5 normal • Self-manage pain	• Limited reach and lifting abilities, especially above shoulder height • Limited strength and endurance of arm above shoulder height • Limited AROM	• Continue exercises from previous phases as indicated: • Progressive resistance exercises (PREs)—Elastic tubing exercises for internal rotation and scapular retraction At three weeks add external rotation and scapular protraction • Isotonics—Side-lying external rotation (with axilla support) with ½ to 1lb Standing scaption with shoulder externally rotated Standing shoulder flexion with ½ to 1lb Elbow and wrist PREs with appropriate weight • Assess lateral scapular slide	• PROM full in all ranges • Symmetric AROM flexion • Symmetric accessory motions of glenohumeral and SC/AC joints • AROM flexion in standing to shoulder height without substitution from scapulothoracic region • Symmetric strength scapula stabilizers and shoulder rotators	• Restore previous functional use and ROM of upper extremity • Begin strengthening; internal rotators (subscapularis) usually not affected by surgery • Initiate scapular retraction as long lever arm forces are minimal (versus protraction) • Progress exercise to include external rotators and scapula protraction as tolerance to exercises improves • Recognize that supraspinatus is secondary mover for straight plane external rotation • Strengthen upper quarter musculature • Accompany gravity-resisted shoulder flexion and abduction by substitution with scapular elevation

Continued

Table 2-2   Acromioplasty—cont'd

Rehabilitation Phase	Criteria to Progress to this Phase	Anticipated Impairments and Functional Limitations	Intervention	Goal	Rationale
Phase IIb Postoperative 6-8 weeks	Gravity-resisted flexion and abduction without scapulo-thoracic substitution Symmetric strength of external rotators	• Unable to work overhead for prolonged periods of time • Unable to participate in overhead-throwing athletics	• Continue with exercises from previous phases as indicated; maintain rotator cuff strength • AROM PREs—Standing scaption with shoulder internal rotation (empty can); perform below 70° scaption Prone or bent over horizontal abduction with shoulder at 100° abduction Begin exercises unresisted, then add weight, beginning with ½ lb Progress weight as indicated • Initiate throwing program as outlined in Appendix A • Begin gentle plyometrics	• Symmetric strength of supraspinatus and deltoid • Restoration of normal arm strength ratios (involved/uninvolved) • Return to previous levels of activities/sport as indicated by strength and tolerance • Prevention of poor mechanics with throwing • Preparation of upper extremity for advanced activities	• Continue to restore ROM and strength of upper quarter musculature • Strengthen supraspinatus as a prime mover • Advance strength demand on the scapula stabilizers • Progress resistance on a conservative basis • Progress activity on a sequential basis

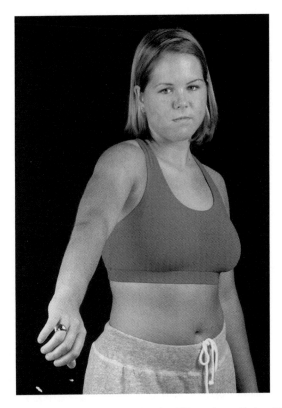

Box 2-2	**General Progression of Strengthening Exercises**

1. Supine:
   Active-assisted flexion
   Active-assisted external rotation
   Active flexion
2. Standing:
   Assisted extension
   Flexion with flexed elbow
   Flexion with elbow extended
   Abduction
   Resisted flexion
3. Isometrics
4. Elastic resistance:
   External rotation (elbow moving)
   External rotation (elbow fixed)
   Elevation

Fig. 2-2. Scaption with internal rotation should be performed below 90 degrees to prevent impinging subacromial structures.

therapist should apply minimal resistance, starting at 8 ounces, then increase to 1 pound, and then advance in $^1/_2$- or 1-pound increments as tolerated. Weights seldom have to exceed 3 to 5 lb for the supraspinatus. The infraspinatus and subscapularis can be stressed to a greater degree, and weights can be progressed from 5 to 8 lb. The therapist should emphasize scapular stabilizer efforts for proximal stability before addressing distal mobility.

Townsend[59] assessed the EMG output of three slips of deltoid, pectoralis major, latissimus dorsi, and the four rotator cuff muscles during 17 exercises. Findings from this study indicate that the majority of the muscles studied are most effectively recruited with the following:

- Scaption (with internal shoulder rotation)
- Flexion
- Horizontal abduction with external rotation
- Press-ups

Blackburn et al[10] first noted that 100 degrees of horizontal abduction is effective in recruiting the supraspinatus. Their findings were verified in both normal and abnormal subjects by Worrell et al.[67] Ballantyne et al[5] found greater EMG output in the infraspinatus than in the supraspinatus when the patient performed side-lying external rotation as opposed to prone external rotation and when the patient performed scaption with IR. In assessing exercises in both the sagittal and coronal planes, Pearl et al[52] noted similar EMG findings in straight plane movements and conical movements that encompassed all planes of motion. Howell et al,[29] using an isokinetic dynamometer, noted the supraspinatus and deltoid muscles were responsible for generating essentially all of the torque at the

shoulder for flexion and scaption. The variations of scaption, along with horizontal abduction, are demonstrated in Figs. 2-2 through 2-4.

Although isolation of specific muscles is vital to ensure a comprehensive strengthening program, work with muscles contracting in synchrony about a joint also is an important consideration. Wilk[65] notes that in overhead activities the subscapularis is counterbalanced by the infraspinatus and teres minor in the transverse plane, whereas the deltoid is opposed by the infraspinatus and teres minor in the coronal plane. As overhead movements are incorporated in the rehabilitation program, the physical therapist also should address the force couple of the upper and lower trapezius for scapular upward rotation.

When strengthening the shoulder internal rotators, do not work with the patient in a side-lying position. Lying on the involved shoulder often increases shoulder pain; therefore IR should be performed in the standing or prone position. When working on strengthening the supraspinatus and standing flexion and abduction in the same exercise session, perform the gravity-resisted elevation exercises before the strengthening ones. This sequence allows a non-fatigued supraspinatus to contribute effectively to achieve an adequate force couple.

Exercise combinations can be used effectively to strengthen the muscles of the shoulder girdle. Wolf[66]

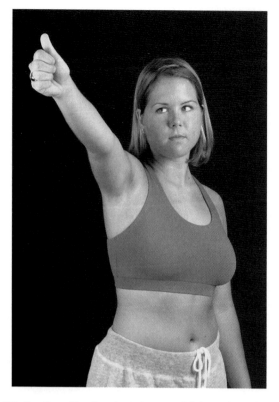

Fig. 2-3. Scaption with external rotation can safely be performed through full available ROM.

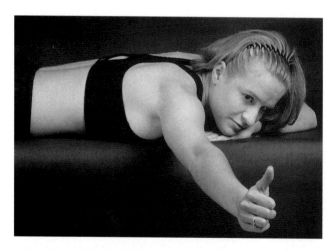

Fig. 2-4. Prone horizontal abduction with the humerus abducted to 100 degrees. The physical therapist should take care with patients with concomitant anterior glenohumeral instability.

Box 2-3	**Modified Kibler's Lateral Scapular Slide Test***

1. Patient stands with the arms resting against the sides.
2. Therapist palpates the spinous process immediately between the inferior angles of the scapula (usually T-7).
3. Therapist measures and records the distance from the spinous process to each scapular inferior angle.
4. Patient abducts the arms to 90 degrees.
5. Patient internally rotates the shoulders so that the thumbs point to the floor.
6. Therapist measures and records the distance from the spinous processes to each scapular inferior angle.

* Normal test is symmetry between right and left sides.

followed by rotator cuff stretching also can be used during phase two. The physical therapist should use care when performing flexibility exercises of the rotator cuff because horizontal adduction can reproduce or cause impingement symptoms.

Strong scapular stabilizers are required to provide a stable base for the glenohumeral joint, elevate the acromion, and provide for retraction and protraction around the thoracic wall.[34] The efficiency of the scapular stabilizers can be quantified with the lateral scapular slide test. This test, which was initially described by Kibler,[34] involves observing and measuring scapular motion during abduction of the shoulder. The steps of the modified lateral scapular slide test are described in Box 2-3. The lateral scapular slide is a valid tool to assess scapular motion.[56] Kibler[34] described side-to-side differences of 1 cm as an indicator of scapulohumeral dysfunction. Other authors assessing the reliability of the lateral scapular slide, however, note that a 1-cm difference cannot be used as an indicator of dysfunction[47] and that 1 cm can fall within intertester variability.[55]

Continue ROM efforts during phase two, especially if limited capsular extensibility detrimentally affects physiologic motion. In addition to aggressive stretching exercises and mobilization of the glenohumeral joint, self-mobilizations also may be of benefit.[27] Patients with glenohumeral laxity also require special consideration as ROM and strengthening exercises progress. For patients with anterior instability, exercises should not stress extremes of horizontal abduction and external rotation. Posterior glenohumeral instability requires care with horizontal adduction and IR. Strengthening programs for patients with glenohumeral instability are best performed in the plane of the scapula.

describes a "four square" combination of tubing-resisted flexion, extension, external rotation, and IR followed by stretching of the external rotators and abductors. A combination of "around the world" exercises of flexion, abduction, and horizontal abduction

Table 2-3   Acromioplasty

Rehabilitation Phase	Criteria to Progress to this Phase	Anticipated Impairments and Functional Limitations	Intervention	Goal	Rationale
Phase III Postoperative 9-12 weeks	Symmetric ROM and strength of upper quarter	• Decreased work- or sport-specific endurance	• Formal return to throwing and overhead activities	• Unrestricted overhead work and sporting activity	• Create a specific training principle to return the patient to the desired activity

A. If the patient is going to be strengthening the supraspinatus and performing shoulder elevation exercises (shoulder flexion, abduction, or scaption exercises), he should perform the gravity-resisted elevation exercises first. The supraspinatus works more efficiently, without fatigue, to achieve an adequate force couple, thereby helping Carl to execute the elevation exercises correctly.

Q. Drew is a 55-year-old plumber. He has a history of shoulder pain over the past 2 years and has a slouched posture. He had an acromioplasty performed 8 weeks ago. He still has minimal deficits with active ROM (AROM) for reaching overhead objects and cannot reach into his back pocket. On evaluation, Drew demonstrates near full passive ROM (PROM) for shoulder flexion. PROM for IR and a combined movement of IR with shoulder extension is limited. What are some essential points to address and treatment techniques to use during Drew's treatment?

Phase Three

TIME: Weeks 9-12
GOALS: Focus on enhancing kinesthesia and joint position sense, building endurance, strengthening the scapular stabilizer, and performing work-specific and sport-specific tasks (Table 2-3).

After the patient has progressed through the first two phases, the obvious deficits resulting from surgery (pain, limited motion, and decreased strength) have essentially been eliminated. Deficits in endurance and proprioception are not as readily apparent. Violation of the capsule, decreased use of the shoulder, and abnormal or restricted movement of the shoulder may decrease endurance and proprioception. One study[11] has demonstrated decreased proprioception in lax shoulders, with patients able to sense external rotation movements with greater ease than IR, especially at end range. Exercises to improve both passive detection of shoulder movement and active joint repositioning may help enhance kinesthesia and joint position sense, respectively. Voight et al[62] noted decreased glenohumeral joint proprioception with muscle fatigue of the rotator cuff.

Endurance training is addressed by decreasing the weight used with strengthening exercises and increasing the repetitions. Scapular stabilizer strengthening has been performed in sets of 30 repetitions to this point and repetitions can be increased as required. Work- and sport-specific tasks should be used as guidelines to the number of prescribed repetitions. The supraspinatus tendon is the one most frequently involved in the injury, so strengthen it last.

The physical therapist also can address proprioception by having the patient perform functional tasks and emphasizing the timing of muscle contraction and movement without substitution. When rehabilitating overhead-throwing athletes, Pappas et al[50] suggest timing muscle recruitment to correlate with the throwing sequence of active abduction, horizontal extension, and external rotation. Appropriate timing of muscle contraction also can be addressed using proprioceptive neuromuscular facilitation techniques.[36]

A functional progression program can be used to enhance the return of proprioception and endurance. Functional progression involves a series of sport- or work-specific basic movement patterns graduated according to the difficulty of the skill and the patient's tolerance. Providing a comprehensive functional progression program for every job or sport that a patient is involved in is impossible. Programs to return the patient to throwing, swimming, and tennis activities can be found in other sources.[2,57] Plyometric activities help restore endurance, proprioception, and muscle power.[25,61]

A. After correction of Drew's posture he was able to reach higher above his head. His slouched posture had previously restricted full active shoulder flexion. The shoulder capsule needs to be assessed immediately for restrictions. Emphasizing capsular mobilization of a restricted capsule allows for better joint arthrokinematics and increased ROM. The anterior, posterior, and inferior capsule were all restricted. General mobilizations were performed for all areas of the capsule, and specific mobilizations were performed for the anterior capsule. Drew then performed ROM and stretching to the shoulder, including stretches with the hand behind the back. A considerable increase in PROM and AROM for the hand behind the back was noted after this treatment.

Suggested Home Maintenance for the Postsurgical Patient

The home maintenance box on pages 25 to 26 outlines the shoulder rehabilitation the patient is to follow. The physical therapist can use it in customizing a patient-specific program.

Unlike more complex arthroscopic procedures or sophisticated open operative procedures, the need for structured clinic-based rehabilitation of the SAD patient should be the exception rather than the rule. Most of the rehabilitation for the patient after an uneventful SAD procedure can take place through a comprehensive home exercise program. Special cases may warrant a more formal and structured treatment program after the SAD procedure to detect problems. These special situations typically involve patients with the following conditions:

- Inadequate preoperative ROM
- Full-thickness rotator cuff pathology
- Biceps tendon or labral pathology
- Articular cartilage involvement
- Secondary "impingement"
- Tendency for excessive scarring
- History of regional complex pain syndrome or reflex sympathetic dystrophy (RSD).

Troubleshooting

1. *Scapulothoracic concerns.* If the patient cannot perform gravity-resisted flexion or abduction without substituting with scapular elevation, keep all efforts within the substitution-free ROM. Monitor scapular dynamic stability with the lateral scapular slide test. Because breakdown of the normal scapulothoracic muscle is more obvious with slow, controlled arm lowering, pay special attention to the eccentric component of gravity-resisted flexion and abduction.

2. *Appropriate exercise dosage.* Dye[18] has described the *envelope of function,* which is defined as the range of load that can be applied across a joint in a given period without overloading it. The challenge is to stress the healing tissue to maximize functional collagen cross-linking without exceeding the envelope of function. As functional levels are increased, alter the therapeutic exercise dosage. In cases of significant scapulothoracic dysfunction (long thoracic nerve neuropathy), scapulothoracic taping or figure-eight strapping may be used for additional stability.[28]

3. *Monitoring for complications.* Postoperative complications after SAD are rare, but you must guard against RSD. Pain disproportionate to the patient's condition should be construed as RSD until proven otherwise. Institute aggressive ROM and pain control efforts daily. Prolonged (more than 3 weeks after surgery) loss of accessory joint motions may predispose the patient to adhesive capsulitis. Give treatments three times a week for mobilization and aggressive ROM.

4. *Loading contractile tissue.* Progressively load contractile tissue. Stress healing tissue initially as a secondary mover (receiving assistance from other muscles) before using the tissue in its role as a prime mover.

5. *Prevention.* As the old adage goes, an ounce of prevention is worth a pound of cure. Preventing early primary impingement symptoms from becoming chronic may eliminate the need for surgery. Nirschl[45] notes the following factors as keys in preventing chronic impingement syndrome: relief of inflammation, strengthening (especially the external rotators, abductors, and scapular stabilizers), flexibility (especially shoulder internal rotators and adductors), general fitness, education, and proper equipment.

Summary

This chapter has discussed the surgical procedure of SAD along with principles that govern postoperative rehabilitation. A surgeon with sound diagnostic, management, and surgical skills, along with a physical therapist with the expertise to advance the patient through the postoperative phase, typically produces a favorable result. Of even greater importance is the rapport established between surgeon and therapist and the relationship between the health care providers and the patient.

Suggested Home Maintenance for the Postsurgical Patient

Week 1

GOAL FOR THE WEEK: Control pain and swelling and begin regaining range of motion for joints.

Days 0-2: Perform grip strength exercises. Elevate your arm if it is swollen.

Days 3-7: 1. Do pendulum exercises for 2 minutes, 3 to 4 times each day.
2. Go through the active range of motion for your elbow, wrist, and hand. Do 3 sets of 15 repetitions in all directions, 3 to 4 times each day.
3. Do IR and external rotation isometrics for 10 seconds each, with 10 repetitions 10 times each day.
4. Apply ice after you exercise.

Week 2

GOAL FOR THE WEEK: Prevent disuse atrophy.

Days 8-10: Continue your program from days 3-7 and add these exercises:
1. Active assisted supine flexion to tolerance. Do 3 sets of 15 repetitions, twice a day.
2. Supine scapular protraction at 90 degrees of flexion. Do 3 sets of 30 repetitions, twice a day.
3. Side-lying unresisted outward rotation to parallel with the floor. Do 3 sets of 15 repetitions twice a day.

Days 11-14: Discontinue the exercises you did on days 3-7 and only do the ones listed for days 8-10. Continue to apply ice after you exercise.

Week 3 (Only One Visit Required)

GOAL FOR THE WEEK: Prevent adhesive capsulitis and minimize disuse atrophy.

1. If passive range of motion is not within normal limits and symmetrical, institute organized outpatient treatment for mobilization. Schedule 3 times per week.
2. Begin tubing- or Theraband-resisted IR. Do 3 sets of 15 repetitions each twice a day.
3. Begin tubing- or Theraband-resisted scapular retraction exercises. Do 3 sets of 30 repetitions each twice a day.
4. Begin side-lying external rotation (support under arms) using 8-oz to 1-lb weights. Do 3 sets of 15 repetitions each twice a day.
5. Begin progressive resistance exercises (PREs) for elbow flexion and extension.
6. Assess lateral scapular slide.

Weeks 3-6 (Only One or Two Visits Required Over 3-Week Period)

GOAL FOR THE PERIOD: Supply added resistance for greater demand on scapular stabilizers.

1. Add tubing- or Theraband-resisted external rotation. Do 3 sets of 15 repetitions twice each day.
2. Do full range of motion unresisted exercises for standing forward flexion and abduction. Begin PREs using 8-oz or 1-lb weights.
3. Continue IR as previously, but decrease to daily, then every other day.
4. Add gravity-resisted scaption with the shoulder externally rotated and unresisted. Do 3 sets of 15 repetitions twice each day.
5. Add tubing- or Theraband-resisted scapular protraction exercises. Do 3 sets of 30 repetitions twice each day.
6. Continue scapular retraction exercises as previously described.

Continued

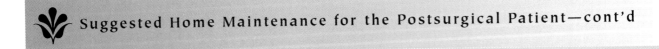

Suggested Home Maintenance for the Postsurgical Patient—cont'd

Weeks 3-6 (Only One or Two Visits Required Over 3-Week Period)—cont'd

7. Expand cardiovascular activities to include upper extremity use (e.g., using stair climbing machine, rowing machine, or upper extremity ergometer).

Weeks 7-8

GOALS FOR THE PERIOD: Return to normal work or sports (with restricted activities as needed) and normal dominant/nondominant muscle strength ratios.
1. Add scaption with shoulder internally rotated (use empty can) at no greater than 70 degrees of abduction. Begin with unresisted exercises, then add weight beginning with 8 oz and progressing in 8-oz to 1-lb increments. Do 3 sets of 15 repetitions twice each day.
2. Add prone and bent over horizontal abduction with the shoulder at 100 degrees of abduction. Begin unresisted exercises in the middle range. Do 3 sets of 15 repetitions twice each day.
3. Begin return to throwing program (Appendix A).
4. Begin gentle plyometrics.

Weeks 9-12 (Only One or Two Visits Required Over 4 Weeks)

GOALS FOR THE PERIOD: Obtain range of motion and muscle strength sufficient to reintroduce more aggressive occupational or sports demands.
1. Formal return to throwing and overhead activities.

REFERENCES

1. Altchek DW et al: Arthroscopic acromioplasty: technique and results, *J Bone Joint Surg Am* 72-A:1198, 1990.
2. Andrews JR, Whiteside JA, Wilk KE: Rehabilitation of throwing and racquet sport injuries. In Buschbachler RM, Braddom RL, editors, *Sports medicine and rehabilitation: a sport-specific approach*, Philadelphia, 1994, Hanley & Belfus.
3. Ark JW et al: Arthroscopic treatment of calcific tendinitis of the shoulder, *Arthroscopy* 8:183, 1992.
4. Armstrong JR: Excision of the acromion in treatment of the supraspinatus syndrome, report of ninety-five excisions, *J Bone Joint Surg Am* 31-B(3):436, 1949.
5. Ballantyne BT, O'Hare SJ, Paschall JL: Electromyographic activity of selected shoulder muscles in commonly used therapeutic exercises, *Phys Ther* 73(10):668, 1993.
6. Basamania CJ, Wirth MA, Rockwood CA, Jr: Treatment of rotator cuff tendonopathy by open techniques, *Sports Med Arthroscopy Rev* 3:68.
7. Beltran J: The use of magnetic resonance imaging about the shoulder, *J Shoulder Elbow Surg* 1:321, 1992.
8. Bigliani LU, Levine WN: Current concepts review. Subacromial impingement syndrome, *J Bone Joint Surg Am* 79-A(12): 8154, 1997.
9. Bigliani LU, Morrison DS, April EW: The morphology of the acromion and its relationship to rotator cuff tears, *Orthop Trans* 10:228, 1986.
10. Blackburn TA et al: EMG analysis of posterior rotator cuff exercises, *Athletic Training* 25(1):40, 1980.
11. Blasier RB, Carpenter JE, Huston LJ: Shoulder proprioception: effect of joint laxity, joint position, and direction of motion, *Orthop Rev* 23(1):45, 1994.
12. Bradley JP, Tibone JE: Electromyographic analysis of muscle action about the shoulder, *Clin Sports Med* 15(4):789, 1991.
13. Buuck DA, Davidson MR: Rehabilitation of the athlete after shoulder arthroscopy, *Clin Sports Med* 15(4):655, 1996.
14. Caspari R: A technique for arthroscopic S.A.D., *Arthroscopy* 8(1):23, 1992.
15. Chansky HA, Ianotti JP: The vascularity of the rotator cuff, *Clin Sports Med* 10(4):807, 1991.
16. Codman EA: Rupture of the supraspinatus tendon and other lesions in or about the subacromial bursa. In Codman EA, editor: *The shoulder*, Boston, 1934, Thomas Todd.
17. Diamond B: *The obstructing acromion: underlying diseases, clinical development and surgery*, Springfield, IL, 1964, Charles C. Thomas.
18. Dye SF: The knee as a biologic transmission with an envelope of function: a theory, *Clin Orthop* 323:10, 1996.

19. Ellman H: Arthroscopic subacromial decompression: analysis of one-to three-year results, *Arthroscopy* 3:173, 1987.

20. Esch JC et al: Arthroscopic subacromial decompression: results according to the degree of rotator cuff tear, *Arthroscopy* 4:241, 1988.

21. Fu FH, Harner CD, Klein AH: Shoulder impingement syndrome. A critical review, *Clin Orthop* 269:162, 1991.

22. Gartsman GM et al: Arthroscopic subacromial decompression. An anatomical study, *Am J Sports Med* 16:48, 1988.

23. Glousman RE: Instability versus impingement syndrome in the throwing athlete, *Orthop Clin North Am* 24:89, 1993.

24. Gold RH, Seeger LL, Yao L: Imaging shoulder impingement, *Skel Radiol* 22:555, 1993.

25. Goldstein TS: *Functional rehabilitation in orthopaedics,* Gaithersburg, MD, 1995, Aspen.

26. Hawkins RJ, Kennedy JC: Impingement syndrome in athletes, *Am J Sports Med* 8:151,1980.

27. Hertling D, Kessler RM: The shoulder and shoulder girdle. In Hertling D, Kessler RM, editors: *Management of common musculoskeletal disorders: physical therapy principles and methods,* ed 3, Philadelphia, 1996, Lippincott.

28. Host HH: Scapular taping in the treatment of anterior shoulder impingement, *Phys Ther* 75(9):803, 1995.

29. Howell SM, Imorsteg AM, Seger DH: Clarification of the role of the supraspinatus muscle in shoulder function, *J Bone Joint Surg Am* 68A(3):398, 1986.

30. Jobe FW: Impingement problems in the athlete. In Nicholas JA, Hershmann EB, editors: *The upper extremity in sports medicine,* St Louis, 1990, Mosby.

31. Jobe FW, Kvitne RS, Giangarra CE: Shoulder pain in the overhand or throwing athlete. The relationship of anterior instability and rotator cuff impingement. *Orthop Rev* 18:963, 1989.

32. Johnson LL: *Diagnostic and surgical arthroscopy of the shoulder,* St Louis, 1993, Mosby.

33. Kessel L, Watson M: The painful arc syndrome. Clinical classification as a guide to management, *J Bone Joint Surg Am* 59-B(2):166, 1977.

34. Kibler WB: The role of the scapula in the overhead throwing motion, *Contemp Orthop* 22(5):525, 1991.

35. Kuhn JE, Hawkins RJ: Arthroscopically assisted techniques in diagnosis and treatment of rotator cuff tendonopathy, *Sports Med Arthroscopy Rev* 3:60, 1995.

36. Lephart SM, Kocher MS: The role of exercise in the prevention of shoulder disorders. In Matsen FA, Fu FH, Hawkins RJ, editors: *The shoulder: a balance of mobility and stability,* Rosemont, IL, 1992, American Academy of Orthopaedic Surgeons.

37. Lohr JF, Ultoff HK: The microvascular pattern of the supraspinatus tendon, *Clin Orthop* 254:35, 1990.

38. McCann PD, Wooten ME, Kadaba MP: A kinematic and electromyographic study of shoulder rehabilitation exercises, *Clin Orthop* 288:179, 1993.

39. McLaughlin HL, Asherman EG: Lesions of the musculotendinous cuff of the shoulder. IV. Some observations based upon the results of surgical repair, *J Bone Joint Surg Am* 33-A:76, 1951.

40. Meyer AW: The minute anatomy of attrition lesions, *J Bone Joint Surg Am* 13:341, 1931.

41. Neer CS, II: Anterior acromioplasty for the chronic impingement syndrome in the shoulder. A preliminary report, *J Bone Joint Surg Am* 54-A:41, 1972.

42. Neer CS, II: Impingement lesions, *Clin Orthop* 173:70, 1983.

43. Nevaiser RJ, Nevaiser TJ: Observations on impingement, *Clin Orthop* 254:60, 1990.

44. Nirschl RP: Rotator cuff tendinitis: basic concepts of pathoetiology. In The American Academy of Orthopedic Surgeons, editors: *Instructional course lectures,* vol 38, Park Ridge, IL, 1989, The American Academy of Orthopedic Surgeons.

45. Nirschl RP: Rotator cuff tendinitis: basic concepts of pathoetiology. In Nicholas JA, Hershman EB, editors: *The upper extremity in sports medicine,* St Louis, 1990, Mosby.

46. O'Connor FG, Sobel JR, Nirschl RP: Five-step treatment for overuse injuries, *Phys Sport Med* 20(10)128, 1992.

47. Odom CJ, Hurd CE, Denegar CR: Intratester and intertester reliability of the lateral scapular slide test and its ability to predict shoulder pathology, *Athletic Training* 30(2):S-9, 1995.

48. Ogata S, Uhthoff HK: Acromial enthesopathy and rotator cuff tear. A radiologic and histologic postmortem investigation of the coracoacromial arch, *Clin Orthop* 254:39, 1990.

49. Ono K, Yamamuro T, Rockwood CA: Use of a thirty-degree caudal tilt radiograph in the shoulder impingement syndrome, *J Shoulder Elbow Surg* 1:246, 1992.

50. Pappas AM, Zawacki RM, McCarthy CF: Rehabilitation of the pitching shoulder, *Am J Sports Med* 13(4)223, 1985.

51. Paulos LE, Franklin JC: Arthroscopic S.A.D. Development and application: a 5 year experience, *Am J Sports Med* 18:235, 1990.

52. Pearl ML, Perry J, Torburn L: An electromyographic analysis of the shoulder during cones and planes of arm motion, *Clin Orthop* 284:116, 1992.

53. Rathbun JB, McNab I: The microvascular pattern of the rotator cuff, *J Bone Joint Surg Am* 52B:540, 1970.

54. Rockwood CA, Jr, Lyons FR: Shoulder impingement syndrome: diagnosis, radiographic evaluation, and treatment with a modified Neer acromioplasty, *J Bone Joint Surg Am* 75-A:409, 1993.

55. Snyder SJ: A complete system for arthroscopy and bursoscopy of the shoulder, *Surg Rounds Orthop* p. 57, July 1989.

56. Tippett SR, Kleiner DM: Objectivity and validity of the lateral scapular slide test, *Athletic Training* 31(2):S-40, 1996.

57. Tippett SR, Voight ML: *Functional progressions for sport rehabilitation,* Champaign, IL, 1995, Human Kinetics.

58. Toivonen DA, Tuite MJ, Orwin JF: Acromial structure and tears of the rotator cuff, *J Shoulder Elbow Surg* 4:376, 1995.

59. Townsend H, Jobe FW, Pink M: Electromyographic analysis of the glenohumeral muscles during a baseball rehabilitation program, *Am J Sports Med* 19(3):264, 1991.

60. Uhthoff HK et al: The role of the coracoacromial ligament in the impingement syndrome. A clinical, radiological and histological study, *Internat Orthop* 12:97, 1988.

61. Voight ML, Draovitch P, Tippett SR: Plyometrics. In Albert M, editor: *Eccentric muscle training in sports and orthopaedics,* ed 2, New York, 1995, Churchill Livingstone.

62. Voight ML, Hardin JA, Blackburn TA: The effects of muscle fatigue on and the relationship of arm dominance to shoulder proprioception, *J Orthop Sports Phys Ther* 23(6):348, 1996.

63. Watson M: The refractory painful arc syndrome, *J Bone Joint Surg* 60-B(4):544, 1978.

64. Wenger HA, McFayeden R: Physiological principles of conditioning. In Zachazewski JE, Magee DJ, Quillen WS, editors: *Athletic injuries and rehabilitation,* Philadelphia, 1996, WB Saunders.

65. Wilk KE: The shoulder. In Malone TR, McPoil T, Nitz AJ, editors: *Orthopaedic and sports physical therapy,* ed 3, St Louis, 1997, Mosby.

66. Wolf WB: Shoulder tendinoses, *Clin Sports Med* 11(4):871, 1992.

67. Worrell TW, Corey BJ, York SL: An analysis of supraspinatus EMG activity and shoulder isometric force development, *Med Sci Sports Exerc* 24(7):744, 1992.

Chapter 3

Anterior Capsular Reconstruction

Frank Jobe
Diane Schwab
Clive Brewster

Although it often goes undiagnosed, shoulder instability is the cause of shoulder pain in many patients.[1,2] The frequency of instability causing shoulder pain increases with the activity level of the patient and decreases somewhat with age. It is more likely in younger, more active patients—especially if they engage in overhead activities during vocational or recreational pursuits.[3] Understanding of the kinetics and root causes of shoulder pain is increasing; both factors must be addressed to redress the problem.

Surgical Indications and Considerations

Shoulder instability is not an isolated diagnosis, but rather one point on a continuum of pathology. It is often associated with impingement of either the "inside" or "outside" type and can be found in patients of all ages and activity levels. Group I patients are generally older; shoulder instability is seldom found in younger patients. A subset of this group also experiences impingement of the undersurface of the rotator cuff (Fig. 3-1).

Group II patients are usually younger than group I patients. They have instability and impingement, but their impingement is secondary to repetitive trauma. These patients are often engaged in overhead athletic sports. On clinical evaluation, both relocation and impingement signs are usually positive. Under anesthesia, the pass-through sign is seen and excessive anterior translation of the humeral head is often evident. Both the anterior inferior capsule and the posterior superior labrum show signs of repetitive trauma; a bare spot also may be seen on the posterior aspect of the humeral head. Other common findings are a tear on the undersurface of the supraspinatus or infraspinatus and laxity in the glenohumeral ligaments, especially in external rotation.

Young patients with generalized ligamentous laxity fall into group III. They too have a positive relocation test and internal impingement. Finally, group IV patients suffer from instability (usually subluxation, rarely dislocation) resulting from a traumatic episode. These patients show no evidence of impingement. They can have a positive relocation sign, but seldom a positive apprehension sign. Under arthroscopic examination a Bankart lesion and occasionally cartilaginous erosion of the posterior humeral head may be noted.

Younger, more active patients with shoulder pain and signs of impingement can fall into any of the four groups. Their activity demands test the limits of strength and endurance of their shoulders. If either is insufficient, brief episodes of anterior instability follow. Associated tightness of the posterior capsule can contribute another force vector driving the humeral head forward. The humeral head, now riding anterior and superior, causes posterior impingement and labral pathology. If left unchecked, the impingement can lead to a frank tear of the supraspinatus portion of the rotator cuff.

Some patients have signs of impingement or a diagnosis of rotator cuff tendinitis, bursitis, bicipital tendinitis, or arthritis and have been referred by an occupational medicine clinic or a gatekeeper in a managed care office. These patients have persistent pain and limitation of activity despite a course of care that may have included nonsteroidal antiinflammatory medication, other modalities (e.g., heat, ice, ultrasound, electrical stimulation), mobilization, exercise, and rest. They may have some temporary symptom relief but no lasting change in underlying difficulties. Some of these patients have subacromial decompression. Even after surgery they may report either no improvement or that the condition is worse than before the surgery.

All shoulder pain is not caused by anterior instability. Sometimes, the presence of a superior labral anteroposterior (SLAP) lesion complicates the clinical picture. Investigative arthroscopy may be necessary to determine the correct diagnosis if a conservative care program is not successful. Sometimes patients report relief of symptoms after rehabilitation. Because they have a normal shoulder under examination, they may return to their normal activities too early and consequently report recurring pain and difficulty. In these instances the therapist should determine whether faulty mechanics in their activities of choice is the culprit. It does not matter how well the patient's shoulder is rehabilitated if the offending stimulus is repeated.

However, when the diagnosis of anterior shoulder instability is the correct one and is made early during the pathologic course, as many as 95% of patients can

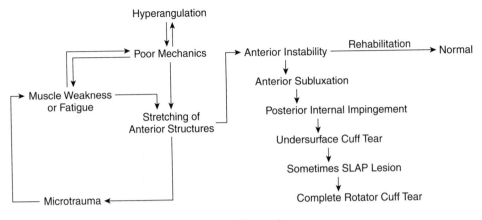

Fig. 3-1. Instability continuum.

return to their previous level of competition.[3] The later the diagnosis is made during the pathologic course, the lower the percentage of successful return with only conservative treatment. For any of these patients to return to their previous activities, the appropriate exercise program must be prescribed, supervised, and performed. While following this program the authors of this chapter have not needed to use mobilizations, massage, or modalities other than ice. The core group of exercises protects the anterior shoulder, strengthens the rotator cuff, and emphasizes the scapular muscles. Details of these exercises follow. Performing them only once or twice a week is futile. Performing them incorrectly is not beneficial and may even be harmful. Persistence and attention to detail are both essential to a successful outcome—the elimination of pain and a return to full activity without surgical intervention.

During this era of cost containment and rationed services, some may feel that this emphasis on supervision and performance detail is an unnecessary expenditure of medical dollars. However, by providing effective rehabilitation the physical therapist can relieve pain and restore function, saving medical dollars in the long run. If the therapist and patient are willing to accept lesser goals, less attention to rehabilitative detail will have to suffice.

When dysfunction persists despite the best efforts of orthopedist, therapist, and patient, an anterior capsulolabral reconstruction is the procedure most likely to eliminate pain while permitting the range of motion and strength needed for premorbid performance.[4,5] Traditionally, surgeons and therapists believed that any procedure that restabilized the shoulder (i.e., kept it from slipping out the front) would improve the patient's condition. Rehabilitation was prolonged and arduous after some of the more common procedures (Bankart repair, modified Bristow repair). Patients were managed with extended immobilization for weeks or months depending on the surgeon and the procedure. Full motion

was seldom regained after surgery. Stability was reestablished, but at the expense of flexibility; patients were never able to perform at the preoperative level again.

Surgical Procedure

In the anterior capsulolabral reconstruction (ACLR), an axillary incision is made 2 to 3 cm distal and lateral to the coracoid process and extending distally into the anterior axillary crease. The skin is undermined to provide access to the deltoid groove and allow visualization of the deltopectoral groove. This interval is then developed with blunt and sharp dissection. The clavipectoral fascia is incised along the lateral margin of the conjoined tendon from the inferior margin of the humeral head to the coracoid process. The surgeon dissects laterally to the fleshy portion of the coracobrachialis muscle, rather than medially at the lateral border of the tendinous short head of the biceps. The conjoined tendon is dissected bluntly and retracted medially.

External rotation of the arm brings the subscapularis into view. It is split longitudinally between the upper two thirds and lower third. After identifying the interval between the subscapularis and the capsule, the surgeon extends capsular exposure medially and laterally. The retractor should be placed under direct vision to avoid injury to neurovascular structures. The capsule is incised longitudinally and tag sutures are placed at the capsule margin just lateral to the labrum. The capsulotomy may be completed carefully down to the level of the glenoid labrum.

The glenoid labrum should be palpated carefully to assess for the presence of a Bankart lesion. The capsule must be palpated for integrity, volume, and ability to buttress the anterior inferior joint margin. The degree of capsular shift must be tailored to the degree of laxity. If a Bankart lesion is present, it is repaired by suture fixation to the prepared anterior scapular neck with Mitek bone anchors.

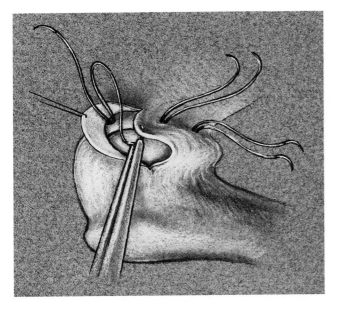

Fig. 3-2. The inferior lead is secured superiorly.

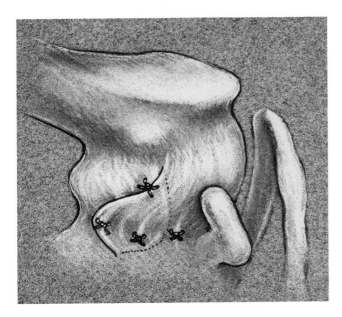

Fig. 3-3. The superior lead is secured inferiorly.

If the capsule is lax or incompetent, it is overlapped to obliterate the redundancy. The surgeon incises it down to the labrum and medial glenoid neck for subperiosteal elevation. The inferior leaf of the capsule contains most of the inferior glenohumeral ligament and is used to reconstruct it by advancing the tissue along the anterior glenoid rim and shifting it proximally. The superior portion of the capsule is brought over the inferior portion and labrum, resting along the anterior scapular neck. The reconstruction is fixed using #2 nonabsorbable sutures from the Mitek bone anchors. The inferior leaf is secured superiorly (Fig. 3-2) and the superior leaf is secured inferiorly (Fig. 3-3) using a vest-

over-pants technique with nonabsorbable sutures. If the labrum is intact, it does not require removal and repair. The surgeon can simply split the capsule and overlap it, thereby reducing the volume of the joint.

The anterior glenoid labrum may be absent or defective. In this case or in the presence of a Bankart lesion, the capsule must be affixed to the prepared anterior scapular neck. Usually, both a capsular shift and a reattachment must be performed.

After the capsule is closed, the surgeon takes the arm through a range of motion to note areas of tension on the repair. Immediately after surgery, the patient may begin active motion within this zone. The surgeon must communicate with the therapist for each patient to ensure that this safe zone is observed. Usually, avoiding abduction above 90 degrees in the scapular plane and external rotation beyond 45 degrees to 90 degrees is indicated. The palmaris longus may be used as a further capsular reinforcement in patients with hyperelasticity.

After determining safe postoperative motion, the surgeon reapproximates the subscapularis. All retractors are removed after a thorough irrigation of the operative field. Neither the deltoid nor the pectoralis muscles normally require surgical repair and the skin is closed subcuticularly, with the addition of adhesive strips (Steri-Strips). The arm is splinted in abduction and external rotation. The splint may be removed for bathing and postoperative range of motion assessment. If the patient has generalized ligamentous laxity, no splint is necessary—motion will be easy to reacquire.

Therapy Guidelines for Postoperative Rehabilitation

Because no muscles are cut in this reconstruction procedure, rehabilitation proceeds briskly with two familiar general goals:
1. Strengthen the dynamic glenohumeral and scapulothoracic stabilizers
2. Restore structural flexibility

The program primarily consists of active range of motion (AROM) exercises and resistive exercises. The therapist must monitor these exercises and enforce their correct execution for good progress to occur. This program includes concurrent exercises for all parts of the trinity of normalcy: range of motion, strength, and endurance. The key to success is to work on all three portions without waiting for completion of any one part. The therapist should not wait for full range of motion before strengthening or be overly aggressive in pushing for all movement early. Furthermore, the therapist should not wait for full strength before beginning endurance work, particularly in patients with hyperelasticity. The best plan is an integrated one. Programs to restore strength, motion, and endurance should overlap one another, rather than run in sequential phases.

Table 3-1   Anterior Capsular Reconstruction

Rehabilitation Phase	Criteria to Progress to this Phase	Anticipated Impairments and Functional Limitations	Intervention	Goal	Rationale
Phase I Postoperative 1 day–2 weeks	Postoperative	• Postoperative pain • Postoperative edema • Dependent upper extremity (UE) in a sling or airplane splint • Limited ROM • Limited strength • Limited reach, lift, and carry with UE	• Cryotherapy • Electrical Stimulation • Isometrics Shoulder—all movements in a neutral position • Assisted AROM—Shoulder—flexion, internal rotation, external rotation, and abduction, avoiding stress on the anterior capsule Wand exercises—Shoulder—Begin flexion after sling/splint is removed • AROM—Shoulder—Flexion, internal rotation, external rotation, and abduction, avoiding stress on the anterior capsule Elbow—Flexion, extension, pronation, supination Wrist—Flexion, extension	• Control pain • Manage edema • Produce good-quality contraction of shoulder muscles • Produce 135° of flexion in the scapular plane and 35° of external rotation • Allow activities of daily living below shoulder height with minimal difficulty, assisting with involved UE	• Educate patient to self-manage pain • Desensitize surgical site • Prevent atrophy of shoulder muscles • Allow early AROM as no muscles were torn or repaired • Provide assisted AROM initially to prepare muscles and joint for AROM • Take care to avoid stressing the anterior capsule with distraction stress and abduction or external rotation movements (speak with physician regarding limits of external rotation) • Regain functional movement of UE

Phase One

TIME: 1 day to 2 weeks after surgery (Table 3-1)

Shoulder

- The patient may be in an airplane-type abduction splint for a week or two. Patients with greater than normal tissue laxity may be in a sling instead. These patients will have no difficulty regaining their motion but need to tighten up before moving.
- AROM 1 day after surgery should consist of removing the arm from the sling or splint and flexing and abducting in the scapular plane. Use active assisted motion as needed.
- Strengthening begins when the splint is removed. Use active isometric contractions for internal rotation, external rotation, flexion, extension, and abduction (Fig. 3-4).
- After the splint or sling is removed, begin wand exercises for elevation. Make sure that the motion includes both flexion and abduction with external rotation. Do not stress the anterior capsule.

It is important to obtain necessary motion by 2 months after surgery. Avoid stressing the anterior joint capsule during the first postoperative month, then work gradually but insistently to get full range. After 2 months, it can be difficult to acquire additional motion. However, full range of motion is different for different patients. Improved function is the goal of the therapist. Function is different for a shipyard worker and for a baseball pitcher. The function of the opposite side may not be a reasonable yardstick either, depending on the patient's requirements.

Elbow, wrist, hand

- Active elbow flexion and extension may begin on postoperative day 1.
- Active forearm supination and pronation may begin on postoperative day 1.
- Active wrist flexion and extension may begin on postoperative day 1.
- Begin immediately squeezing a ball or plastic egg-shaped hand exerciser.
- Use cryotherapy for pain control.

Phase Two

TIME: 3 weeks to 3 months after surgery (Table 3-2)

Shoulder

- Resistive exercises may begin during week 3 after surgery. Emphasize the internal and external rotators of the rotator cuff. Use elastic band resistance and position the arm at the side. An axillary roll may be used to increase the emphasis on the teres minor. Eliminate the axillary roll to increase the emphasis on the infraspinatus muscle.

- Extension is best done prone on a table or standing and leaning forward from the waist. The elbow should be in full extension, and the extensor motion should end at the plane of the trunk (Fig. 3-5).
- Horizontal abduction begins in week 4, using the same starting position as for extension. Again, keep the elbow straight and make certain that motion does not continue beyond the plane of the trunk. Watch carefully to ensure that scapular adduction and trunk rotation are not substituted for true horizontal abduction.
- An axillary roll may be used to emphasize the teres minor muscle. By eliminating the axillary roll, emphasis is placed on the infraspinatus muscle.
- Horizontal adduction begins in week 4 or 5, supine, in the scapular plane. To get the arm in this position, use a towel or pillow under the humerus, ensuring that the start and finish positions are in front of the plane of the trunk (Fig. 3-6).
- Increase the difficulty of the rotation exercises; progress the external rotation to side-lying, using hand weights (Fig. 3-7). Put a bolster under the lateral chest wall for internal rotation.
- Supraspinatus exercises are done standing, within a pain-free range only. Start using only the weight of the arm as resistance and add hand weights only when both the form is perfect and the pain has disappeared.

Shoulder, elbow, wrist, hand

- Add upper body ergometer work for endurance training. Begin with low resistance for early sessions. Start with an easy 5-minute program such as the following:
  1 minute forward
  1 minute rest
  1 minute backward
  1 minute rest
  1 minute forward

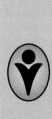

Q. John is a 35-year-old surfer. He had several episodes of shoulder dislocation while paddling his surfboard. He also complained of anterior shoulder pain. Conservative treatment failed, so he underwent an anterior capsular reconstruction 11 weeks ago. Passive range of motion (PROM) and AROM are good. John's main complaint is continuing anterior shoulder pain. The pain can be elicited by palpation over the biceps tendon and transverse humeral ligament. This symptom has delayed progress with strengthening. How should the patient be treated?

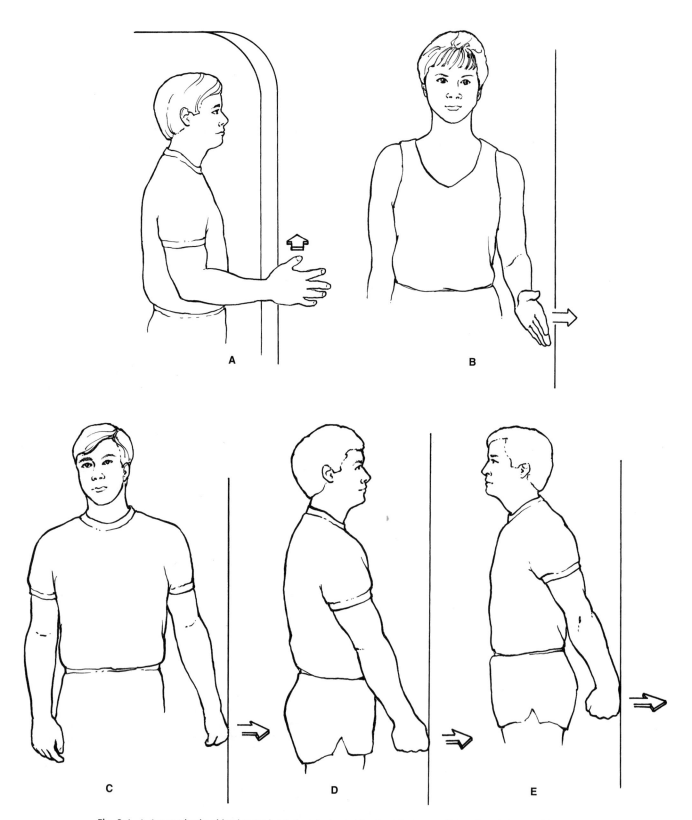

Fig. 3-4. **A,** Isometric shoulder internal rotation. **B,** Isometric shoulder external rotation. **C,** Isometric shoulder abduction. **D,** Isometric shoulder flexion. **E,** Isometric shoulder extension. (From Jobe FW: *Operative techniques in upper extremity sports injuries,* St Louis, 1996, Mosby.)

Table 3-2   Anterior Capsular Reconstruction

Rehabilitation Phase	Criteria to Progress to this Phase	Anticipated Impairments and Functional Limitations	Intervention	Goal	Rationale
Phase II Postoperative 3 weeks– 3 months	• No signs of infection • No increase in pain • Pain controlled with medication or modalities • No loss of ROM	• Out of sling or splint as appropriate • Limited ROM • Limited strength • Limited tolerance of UE for reach, lift, and carry activities	• Continue exercises as in Phase I • Resisted internal and external rotation using elastic bands • AROM—Shoulder— At 4 weeks add horizontal abduction At 5 weeks add supine horizontal adduction in scapular plane At 6 weeks add supraspinatus exercise using an empty can • Add exercises from Tables 2-1 and 2-2 inclusive of isotonics and elastic tubing	By 2 months the following should occur: • Shoulder AROM full • Strength 60%-70% • No pain during all activities of daily living • Lift 5 lb • Return to sedentary work By 3 months the following should occur: • Shoulder strength 80% • Carry 5 lb	• Progress rapidly after getting full ROM while avoiding stress on the anterior capsule • Strengthen scapula stabilizers and rotator cuff muscles • Increase tolerance of anterior shoulder muscles to movement • Avoid impingement while exercising rotator cuff • Strengthen entire UE and improve cardiovascular fitness in an effort to return patient to previous level of function

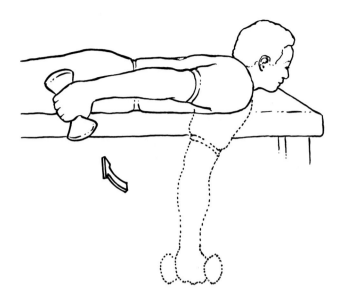

Fig. 3-5. Prone shoulder extension. (From Jobe FW: *Operative techniques in upper extremity sports injuries*, St Louis, 1996, Mosby.)

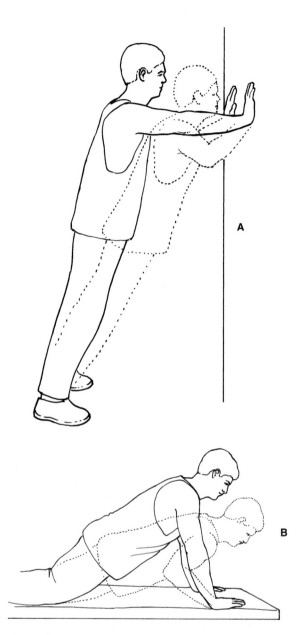

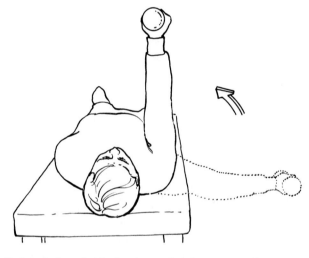

Fig. 3-6. Horizontal adduction. (From Jobe FW: *Operative techniques in upper extremity sports injuries*, St Louis, 1996, Mosby.)

Fig. 3-8. **A,** Wall push-ups. **B,** Modified hands-and-knees push-ups. (From Jobe FW: *Operative techniques in upper extremity sports injuries*, St Louis, 1996, Mosby.)

Phase Three

TIME: 3 to 4 months after surgery (Table 3-3)

Shoulder

- Add eccentric rotator cuff exercises
- Add serratus anterior work, beginning with wall push-ups and then move on to regular push-ups with a stop at a modified, hands-and-knees push-up (Fig. 3-8). The most important part of the push-up is at the end when the patient emphasizes scapular protraction.

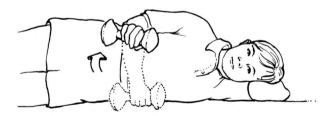

Fig. 3-7. Side-lying external rotation. (From Jobe FW: *Operative techniques in upper extremity sports injuries*, St Louis, 1996, Mosby.)

Table 3-3 Anterior Capsular Reconstruction

Rehabilitation Phase	Criteria to Progress to This Phase	Anticipated Impairments and Functional Limitations	Intervention	Goal	Rationale
Phase III Postoperative 3-4 months	Pain self-managed and primarily associated with increased activity No loss of ROM No loss of strength	• Limited strength and endurance of UE • Unable to perform sustained or repetitive reaching and overhead activities • Limited tolerance to carrying objects	Continue strengthening and ROM exercises as noted in phases I and II: • Progressive resistance exercises (PREs)—Eccentric rotator cuff exercises Wall push-up "plus" progressing to horizontal push-up "plus" (emphasizing scapular protraction at end of push-up) • Isokinetics for internal and external rotation at 200°/sec • Sport-specific drills when strength is 80% (see Appendix A)	• 80% overhead lifting strength compared with uninvolved extremity • 80% carrying strength below shoulder height	• Work on endurance of scapula and shoulder muscles before achieving full strength • Increase static and dynamic control of rotator cuff for return to previous activities • Strengthen and improve endurance of shoulder muscles using high-speed resistance training • Return to sport or activity safely and without injury

- Isokinetic training begins when the patient can lift at least 5 lb in side-lying external rotation and 10 to 15 lb in side-lying internal rotation without pain.
- Sport-specific drills do not begin until the involved side has 70% to 80% of the strength of the uninvolved side. The authors of this chapter use an isokinetic machine for strength testing at 120°/second for internal rotation and 240°/second for external rotation.
- If the patient has pain, reduce some or all of the following: number of throws, speed of the throw, distances thrown, or number of days spent throwing. Keep the speed below three quarters of maximum until 7 months after surgery. Full speed is reasonable after 1 year.
- Occasionally after beginning to throw, the patient will experience pain posteriorly. Check the teres minor for inflammation and the posterior capsule for tightness. Refer to the chapter on transitional throwing programs. Modified throwing programs for pitchers, throwing programs for position play-

ers, an exercise program for tennis players, and a rehabilitation program for golfers are detailed in Boxes 3-1 through 3-4. An additional throwing program is detailed in Appendix A.

Normal range of motion is relative. Again, function is the goal, and function is different for a shipyard worker than for a baseball pitcher.

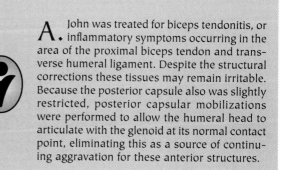

A. John was treated for biceps tendonitis, or inflammatory symptoms occurring in the area of the proximal biceps tendon and transverse humeral ligament. Despite the structural corrections these tissues may remain irritable. Because the posterior capsule also was slightly restricted, posterior capsular mobilizations were performed to allow the humeral head to articulate with the glenoid at its normal contact point, eliminating this as a source of continuing aggravation for these anterior structures.

Text continued on p. 44

Box 3-1   Rehabilitation Throwing Program for Pitchers*

Step 1: Toss the ball (no wind-up) against a wall on alternate days. Start with 25 to 30 throws, build up to 70 throws, and gradually increase the throwing distance.

Number of Throws	Distance (ft)
20	20 (warm-up phase)
25-40	30-40
10	20 (cool-down phase)

Step 2: Toss the ball (playing catch with easy wind-up) on alternate days.

Number of Throws	Distance (ft)
10	20 (warm-up)
10	30-40
30-40	50
10	20-30 (cool-down)

Step 3: Continue increasing the throwing distance while still tossing the ball with an easy wind-up.

Number of Throws	Distance (ft)
10	20 (warm-up)
10	30-40
30-40	50-60
10	30 (cool-down)

Step 4: Increase throwing distance to a maximum of 60 feet. Continue tossing the ball with an occasional throw at no more than half speed.

Number of Throws	Distance (ft)
10	30 (warm-up)
10	40-45
30-40	60-70
10	30 (cool-down)

Step 5: During this step, gradually increase the distance to 150 feet maximum.

Phase 5-1	Number of Throws	Distance (ft)
	10	40 (warm-up)
	10	50-60
	15-20	70-80
	10	50-60
	10	40 (cool-down)

Phase 5-2	Number of Throws	Distance (ft)
	10	40 (warm-up)
	10	50-60
	20-30	80-90
	20	50-60
	10	40 (cool-down)

*Patients start at the step that is appropriate for them. Postsurgical patients begin at step 1. Patients progress depending on the maintenance of their pain-free status and their strength and endurance.

Box 3-1 **Rehabilitation Throwing Program for Pitchers—cont'd**

Phase 5-3	Number of Throws	Distance (ft)
	10	40 (warm-up)
	10	60
	15-20	100-110
	20	60
	10	40 (cool-down)

Phase 5-4	Number of Throws	Distance (ft)
	10	40 (warm-up)
	10	60
	15-20	120-150
	20	60
	10	40 (cool-down)

Step 6: Progress to throwing off the mound at one-half to three-fourths speed. Try to use proper body mechanics, especially when throwing off the mound:
- Stay on top of the ball
- Keep the elbow up
- Throw over the top
- Follow through with the arm and trunk
- Use the legs to push

Phase 6-1	Number of Throws	Distance (ft)
	10	60 (warm-up)
	10	120-150 (lobbing)
	30	45 (off the mound)
	10	60 (off the mound)
	10	40 (cool-down)

Phase 6-2	Number of Throws	Distance (ft)
	10	50 (warm-up)
	10	120-150 (lobbing)
	20	45 (off the mound)
	20	60 (off the mound)
	10	40 (cool-down)

Phase 6-3	Number of Throws	Distance (ft)
	10	50 (warm-up)
	10	60
	10	120-150 (lobbing)
	10	45 (off the mound)
	30	60 (off the mound)
	10	40 (cool-down)

Phase 6-4	Number of Throws	Distance (ft)
	10	50 (warm-up)
	10	120-150 (lobbing)
	10	45 (off the mound)
	40-50	60 (off the mound)
	10	40 (cool-down)

At this time, if the pitcher has successfully completed phase 6-4 without pain or discomfort and is throwing approximately three-fourths speed, the pitching coach and trainer may allow the pitcher to proceed to step 7: up/down bullpens. Up/down bullpens is used to simulate a game. The pitcher rests between a series of pitches to reproduce the rest period between innings.

Step 7: Up/down bullpens: (one-half to three-fourths speed)

Day 1	Number of Throws	Distance (ft)
	10 warm-up throws	120-150 (lobbing)
	10 warm-up throws	60 (off the mound)
	40 pitches	60 (off the mound)
	Rest 10 minutes	
	20 pitches	60 (off the mound)
Day 2	Off	

Day 3	Number of Throws	Distance (ft)
	10 warm-up throws	120-150 (lobbing)
	10 warm-up throws	60 (off the mound)
	30 pitches	60 (off the mound)
	Rest 10 minutes	
	10 warm-up throws	60 (off the mound)
	20 pitches	60 (off the mound)
	Rest 10 minutes	
	10 warm-up throws	60 (off the mound)
	20 pitches	60 (off the mound)
Day 4	Off	

Day 5	Number of Throws	Distance (ft)
	10 warm-up throws	120-150 (lobbing)
	10 warm-up throws	60 (off the mound)
	30 pitches	60 (off the mound)
	Rest 8 minutes	
	20 pitches	60 (off the mound)
	Rest 8 minutes	
	20 pitches	60 (off the mound)
	Rest 8 minutes	
	20 pitches	60 (off the mound)

At this point the pitcher is ready to begin a normal routine, from throwing batting practice to pitching in the bullpen. This program can and should be adjusted as needed by the trainer or physical therapist. Each step may take more or less time than listed, and the program should be monitored by the trainer, physical therapist, and physician. The pitcher should remember that it is necessary to work hard but not overdo it.

From Jobe FW: *Operative techniques in upper extremity sports injuries*, St Louis, 1996, Mosby.

Box 3-2 Rehabilitation Program for Catchers, Infielders, and Outfielders

Note: Perform each step three times.
  All throws should have an arc or "hump."
  The maximum distance thrown by infielders and catchers is 120 feet.
  The maximum distance thrown by outfielders is 200 feet.

Step 1: Toss the ball with no wind-up. Stand with your feet shoulder-width apart and face the player to whom you are throwing. Concentrate on rotating and staying on top of the ball.

Number of Throws	Distance (ft)
5	20 (warm-up)
10	30
5	20 (cool-down)

Step 2: Stand sideways to the person to whom you are throwing. Feet are shoulder-width apart. Close up and pivot onto your back foot as you throw.

Number of Throws	Distance (ft)
5	30 (warm-up)
5	40
10	50
5	30 (cool-down)

Step 3: Repeat the position in step 2. Step toward the target with your front leg and follow through with your back leg.

Number of Throws	Distance (ft)
5	50 (warm-up)
5	60
10	70
5	50 (cool-down)

Step 4: Assume the pitcher's stance. Lift and stride with your lead leg. Follow through with your back leg.

Number of Throws	Distance (ft)
5	60 (warm-up)
5	70
10	80
5	60 (cool-down)

Step 5: *Outfielders:* Lead with your glove-side foot forward. Take one step, crow hop, and throw the ball.
  Infielders: Lead with your glove-side foot forward. Take a shuffle step and throw the ball. Throw the last five throws in a straight line.

Number of Throws	Distance (ft)
5	70 (warm-up)
5	90
10	100
5	80 (cool-down)

Step 6: Use the throwing technique used in step 5. Assume your playing position. Infielders and catchers do not throw farther than 120 feet. Outfielders to not throw farther than 150 feet (mid-outfield).

Number of Throws	Infielders' and Catchers' Distance (ft)	Outfielders' Distance (ft)
5	80 (warm-up)	80 (warm-up)
5	80-90	90-100
5	90-100	110-125
5	110-120	130-150
5	80 (cool-down)	80 (cool-down)

Step 7: Infielders, catchers, and outfielders all may assume their playing positions.

Number of Throws	Infielders' and Catchers' Distance (ft)	Outfielders' Distance (ft)
5	80 (warm-up)	80-90 (warm-up)
5	80-90	110-130
5	90-100	150-175
5	110-120	180-200
5	80 (cool-down)	90 (cool-down)

Step 8: Repeat step 7. Use a fungo bat to hit to the infielders and outfielders while in their normal playing positions.

From Jobe FW: *Operative techniques in upper extremity sports injuries,* St Louis, 1996, Mosby.

Box 3-3   Rehabilitation Program for Tennis Players

The following tennis protocol is designed to be performed every other day. Each session should begin with the warm-up exercises as outlined below. Continue with your strengthening, flexibility, and conditioning exercises on the days you are not following the tennis protocol.

Warm-Up
Lower extremity:
- Jog four laps around the tennis court.
- Stretches:
  Gastrocnemius
  Achilles tendon
  Hamstring
  Quadriceps

Upper extremity
- Shoulder stretches:
  Posterior cuff
  Inferior capsule
  Rhomboid
- Forearm/wrist stretches
  Wrist flexors
  Wrist extensors

Trunk
- Side bends
- Extension
- Rotation

Forehand ground strokes:
Hit toward the fence on the opposite side of the court.
Do not worry about getting the ball in the court.
During all of the strokes listed above, remember these key steps:
- Bend your knees.
- Turn your body.
- Step toward the ball.
- Hit the ball when it is out in front of you.

Avoid hitting with an open stance because this places undue stress on your shoulder. This is especially more stressful during the forehand stroke if you have had anterior instability or impingement problems. This is also true during the backhand if you have had problems of posterior instability.

On the very first day of these sport-specific drills, start with bouncing the ball and hitting it. Try to bounce the ball yourself and hit it at waist level. This will allow for consistency in the following:
- How the ball comes to you
- Approximating your timing between hits
- Hitting toward a target to ensure follow-through and full extension
- Employing the proper mechanics, thereby placing less stress on the anterior shoulder

Week 1
Day 1:   25 forehand strokes
         25 backhand strokes

Day 2:   If there are no problems after the first-day workout, increase the number of forehand and backhand strokes.
         50 forehand strokes
         50 backhand strokes

Day 3:   50 forehand strokes (waist level)
         50 backhand strokes (waist level)
         25 high forehand strokes
         25 high backhand strokes

Week 2
Progress to having the ball tossed to you in a timely manner, giving you enough time to recover from your deliberate follow-through (i.e., wait until the ball bounces on the other side of the court before tossing another ball). Always aim the ball at a target or at a spot on the court.

If you are working on basic ground strokes, have someone bounce the ball to you consistently at waist height.

If you are working on high forehands, have the ball bounced to you at shoulder height or higher.

Day 1:   25 high forehand strokes
         50 waist-height forehand strokes
         50 waist-height backhand strokes
         25 high backhand strokes

Day 2:   25 high forehand strokes
         50 waist-height forehand strokes
         50 waist-height backhand strokes
         25 high backhand strokes

Day 3:   Alternate hitting the ball cross court and down the line, using waist-high and high forehand and backhand strokes.
         25 high forehand strokes
         50 waist-height forehand strokes
         50 waist-height backhand strokes
         25 high backhand strokes

Week 3
Continue the three-times-per-week schedule. Add regular and high forehand and backhand volleys. At this point you may begin having someone hit tennis balls to you from a basket of balls. This will allow you to get the feel of the ball as it comes off another tennis racket. Your partner should wait until the ball that you hit has bounced on the other side of the court before hitting another ball to you. This will give you time to emphasize your follow-through and not hurry to return for the next shot. As always, emphasis is placed on proper body mechanics.

Day 1:   25 high forehand strokes
         50 waist-height forehand strokes
         50 waist-height backhand strokes
         25 high backhand strokes
         25 low backhand and forehand volleys
         25 high backhand and forehand volleys

From Jobe FW: *Operative techniques in upper extremity sports injuries,* St Louis, 1996, Mosby.

Continued

Box 3-3   Rehabilitation Program for Tennis Players—cont'd

Week 3—cont'd

Day 2: Same as day 1, week 3.

Day 3: Same as day 2, week 3, with emphasis on direction (i.e., down the line and cross-court). Remember, good body mechanics is still a must:
- Keep knees bent.
- Hit the ball on the rise.
- Hit the ball in front of you.
- Turn your body.
- Do not hit the ball with an open stance.
- Stay on the balls of your feet.

Week 4

Day 1: Continue having your partner hit tennis balls to you from out of a basket. Alternate hitting forehand and backhand strokes with lateral movement along the baseline. Again, emphasis is on good mechanics as described previously.

Alternate hitting the ball down the line and cross-court. This drill should be done with a full basket of tennis balls (100 to 150 tennis balls).

Follow this drill with high and low volleys using half a basket of tennis balls (50 to 75 balls). This drill also is performed with lateral movement and returning to the middle of the court after the ball is hit.

Your partner should continue allowing enough time for you to return to the middle of the court before hitting the next ball. This is to avoid your rushing the stroke and using faulty mechanics.

Day 2: Same drill as day 1, week 4.

Day 3: Same drills as day 2, week 4.

Week 5

Day 1: Find a partner able to hit consistent ground strokes (able to hit the ball to the same area consistently, e.g., to your forehand with the ball bouncing about waist height).

Begin hitting ground strokes with this partner alternating hitting the ball to your backhand and to your forehand. Rally for about 15 minutes, then add volleys with your partner hitting to you from the baseline. Alternate between backhand and forehand volleys and high and low volleys. Continue volleying another 15 minutes. You will have rallied for a total of 30 to 40 minutes.

At the end of the session, practice a few serves while standing along the baseline. First, warm up by shadowing for 1 to 3 minutes. Hold the tennis racquet loosely and swing across your body in a figure 8. Do not swing the racquet hard. When you are ready to practice your serves using a ball, be sure to keep your toss out in front of you, get your racquet up and behind you, bend your knees, and hit up on the ball. Forget about how much power you are generating, and forget about hitting the ball between the service lines. Try hitting the ball as if you are hitting it toward the back fence.

Hit approximately 10 serves from each side of the court. Remember, this is the first time you are serving, so do not try to hit at 100% of your effort.

Day 2: Same as day 1, week 5, but now increase the number of times you practice your serve. After working on your ground strokes and volleys, return to the baseline and work on your second serve: Hit up on the ball, bend your knees, follow through, and keep the toss in front of you. This time hit 20 balls from each side of the court (i.e., 20 into the deuce court and 20 into the ad court).

Day 3: Same as day 2, week 5, with ground strokes, volleys, and serves. Do not add to the serves. Concentrate on the following:
- Bending your knees
- Preparing the racket
- Using footwork
- Hitting the ball out in front of you
- Keeping your eyes on the ball
- Following through
- Getting in position for the next shot
- Keeping the toss in front of you during the serve

The workout should be the same as day 2, but if you emphasize the proper mechanics listed previously, you should feel as though you had a harder workout than in day 2.

Week 6

Day 1: After the usual warm-up program, start with specific ground-stroke drills, with you hitting the ball down the line and your partner on the other side hitting the ball cross-court. This will force you to move quickly on the court. Emphasize good mechanics as mentioned previously.

Perform this drill for 10 to 15 minutes before reversing the direction of your strokes. Now have your partner hit down the line while you hit cross-court.

Proceed to the next drill with your partner hitting the ball to you. Return balls using a forehand, then a backhand, then a put-away volley. Repeat this sequence for 10 to 15 minutes. End this session by serving 50 balls to the ad court and 50 balls to the deuce court.

From Jobe FW: *Operative techniques in upper extremity sports injuries,* St Louis, 1996, Mosby.

Box 3-3   Rehabilitation Program for Tennis Players—cont'd

Week 6—cont'd

Day 2:   Day 2 should be the same as day 1, week 6, plus returning serves from each side of the court (deuce and ad court). End with practicing serves, 50 to each court.

Day 3:   Perform the following sequence: warm-up; cross-court and down-the-line drills; backhand, forehand, and volley drills; return of serves; and practice serves.

Week 7

Day 1:   Perform the warm-up program. Perform drills as before and practice return of serves. Before practicing serving, work on hitting 10 to 15 overhead shots. Continue emphasizing good mechanics. Add the approach shot to your drills.

Day 2:   Same as day 1, week 7, except double the number of overhead shots (25 to 30 overheads).

Day 3:   Perform warm-up exercises and cross-court drills. Add the overhead shot to the backhand, forehand, and volley drill, making it the backhand, forehand, volley, and overhead drill.

If you are a serious tennis player, you will want to work on other strokes or other parts of your game. Feel free to gradually add them to your practice and workout sessions. Just as in other strokes, the proper mechanics should be applied to drop volley, slice, heavy topspin, drop shots, and lobs, offensive and defensive.

Week 8

Day 1:   Warm-up and play a simulated one-set match. Be sure to take rest periods after every third game. Remember, you will have to concentrate harder on using good mechanics.

Day 2:   Perform another simulated game but with a two-set match.

Day 3:   Perform another simulated game, this time a best-of-three match.

Day 3:   If all goes well, you may make plans to return to your regular workout and game schedule. You also may practice or play if your condition allows it.

Box 3-4   Rehabilitation Program for Golfers

This sport-specific protocol is designed to be performed every other day. Each session should begin with the warm-up exercises outlined here. Continue the strengthening, flexibility, and conditioning exercises on the days you are not playing or practicing golf. Advance one stage every 2 to 4 weeks, depending on the severity of the shoulder problem, as each stage becomes pain free in execution.

Warm-Up

Lower extremities: Jog or walk briskly around the practice green area three or four times; stretch the hamstrings, quadriceps, and Achilles tendon.

Upper extremities: Stretch the shoulder (posterior cuff, inferior cuff, rhomboid) and wrist flexors and extensors.

Trunk: Do sidebends, extension, and rotation stretching exercises.

Stage 1

Putt	50	3 times/week
Medium long	0	0 times/week
Long	0	0 times/week

Stage 2

Putt	50	3 times/week
Medium long	20	2 times/week
Long	0	0 times/week

Stage 3

Putt	50	3 times/week
Medium long	40	3 times/week
Long	0	0 times/week

Not more than $1/3$ best distance

Stage 4

Putt	50	3 times/week
Medium long	50	3 times/week
Long	10	2 times/week

Up to $1/2$ best distance

Stage 5

Putt	50	3 times/week
Medium long	50	3 times/week
Long	10	3 times/week

Stage 6

Putt	50	3 times/week
Medium long	50	3 times/week
Long	20	3 times/week

Play a round of golf in lieu of one practice session per week.

From Jobe FW: *Operative techniques in upper extremity sports injuries,* St Louis, 1996, Mosby.

Suggested Home Maintenance for the Postsurgical Patient

Because the correct execution of the exercises is vital the authors of this chapter do not give a home exercise program. Instead, we prefer to monitor the exercises in the clinic. When a patient graduates to a transitioning sports program, then home exercises may be given.

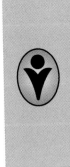

Q. Peter is a 20-year-old pitcher for a baseball team. He had right shoulder laxity and a painful shoulder secondary to impingement problems. He underwent capsular reconstruction on his right shoulder 9 weeks ago. His shoulder flexion and abduction with PROM is still limited by 15° for flexion and 20° for abduction. PROM for internal rotation also is limited by 20°. At this time, should decreased ROM be a concern? If yes, what techniques may be employed to improve ROM?

Troubleshooting Problems

Misapprehending Quality of Patient's Tissues

Patients with "normal" or tight connective tissue must work early and diligently to reacquire motion, while avoiding stress on the anterior joint capsule during the first postoperative month. The therapist should not push patients with hyperelasticity. They will reacquire motion quickly and should be allowed to heal before attempting extremes of motion.

Anterior Shoulder Pain

Despite surgery, some patients still have anterior shoulder pain on palpation of the proximal biceps tendon or transverse humeral ligament. This may be considered "leftover inflammation"; the structural problem may have been rectified surgically, but the residual inflammation does not disappear overnight. The therapist and patient should use modalities to reduce discomfort. Also, the physical therapist should ensure that the posterior cuff and capsule are stretched so that the humeral head can articulate with the glenoid at its normal contact point, eliminating this as a source of continuing irritation for these anterior structures.

Posterior Shoulder Pain

In addition to anterior shoulder pain, many patients also note pain in the posterior shoulder, especially with activity that requires elevation above 120° and motion that requires horizontal abduction posterior to the

frontal plane. Another potentially difficult motion is hyperextension posterior to the plane of the body. The therapist may note pain on palpation of the posterior cuff insertion, the posterior capsule, or the proximal third of the axillary border of the scapula and should ensure the patient has adequate excursion of the posterior capsule. Occasionally patients develop a tendinitis of the rotator cuff external rotators, specifically the teres minor. This tendinitis may be treated symptomatically with modalities, stretching (if necessary), and progressive strengthening.

Insufficient Range of Motion

If too much time elapses after surgery before the patient regains normal motion, adhesive capsulitis may develop. The best defense for this problem is a good offense: the physical therapist should know the patient's tissue type and encourage motion early. As noted earlier, normal range of motion differs for different patients. A baseball pitcher may require 130° of external rotation for function. Most other patients have more modest requirements.

Strength and Endurance

Often, rehabilitation programs concentrate on increasing strength. However, for most patients, including overhead throwers, endurance is probably much more important to overall function than strength. Endurance training is equally important for patients who are hurt on the job. With inadequate endurance, the patient substitutes muscles and alters mechanics for a given task or sport to continue functioning. Such substitutions and alterations are often the forerunners of tissue breakdown. The therapist should strengthen specific muscle groups and prescribe the appropriate exercises (e.g., separate programs for rotator cuff, scapular rotators, shoulder flexors and abductors) while paying special attention to the rotator cuff and the upward rotators of the scapula.

Stretching

Patients with anterior instability can have a tight posterior capsule. Despite surgical correction, the posterior tightness may remain and, if left untreated, lead to a recurrence of the original complaint. Sometimes, especially for older patients, the pectoralis minor is tight. The therapist should be suspicious if the patient has rounded shoulders and a protracted scapula. The goal should be to stretch the pectoralis minor and stretch the posterior capsule as shown in Fig. 3-9. The therapist must not stretch the anterior shoulder structures of any throwing athlete unless he or she is certain that tightness exists. By and large, all these patients can demonstrate anterior laxity in the dominant shoulder.

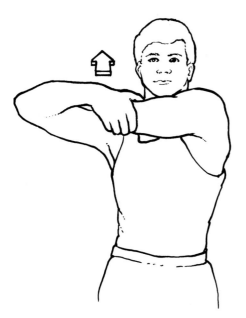

Fig. 3-9. Posterior cuff stretch. (From Jobe FW: *Operative techniques in upper extremity sports injuries,* St Louis, 1996, Mosby.)

Mechanics

Even though the patient may have good range of motion, strength, and endurance, important work remains to be done. Poor mechanics may be one of the reasons the patient was injured in the first place. Understanding the mechanics of the sport the patient is resuming is essential. For throwers, the physical therapist must ensure that the front foot is pointing toward the plate, the stride is not too long, the balance is correct, and the front foot does not hit the ground before the arm is ready to begin acceleration. An awareness of the mechanics of tennis, volleyball, swimming, and golf also is important.

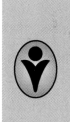

A. On further investigation a tight posterior capsule was noted. The therapist used posterior capsular mobilizations in the next treatment to increase shoulder flexion and internal rotation. The patient gained 10 to 15 degrees more for flexion and internal rotation and 5 to 10 degrees more for abduction. After mobilization and PROM were performed the patient executed AROM exercises for shoulder flexion, abduction, and internal rotation.

REFERENCES

1. Garth WP, Allman FL, Armstrong WS: Occult anterior subluxation of the shoulder in noncontact sports, *Am J Sports Med* 15:579, 1987.
2. Jobe FW, Moynes DR: Delineation of diagnostic criteria and a rehabilitation program for rotator cuff injuries, *Am J Sports Med* 10:336, 1982.
3. Jobe FW, Glousman RE: *Anterior instability in the throwing athlete,* instructional course lecture, Palm Desert, CA, June 1988, American Orthopaedic Society for Sports Medicine.
4. Jobe FW, Glousman RE: Anterior capsulolabral reconstruction. In Paulous LE, Tibone JE, editors: *Operative technique in shoulder surgery,* Gaithersburg, MD, 1992, Aspen.

Chapter 4

Rotator Cuff Repair and Rehabilitation

Mark Ghilarducci
Lisa Maxey

Rotator cuff disorders generally have a multifactorial etiology, including trauma, glenohumeral instability, scapulothoracic dysfunction, congenital abnormalities, and degenerative changes of the rotator cuff (Box 4-1). Intrinsic tendon degeneration and extrinsic mechanic factors have been described extensively and are primary contributors to rotator cuff pathology.

Surgical Indications and Considerations

Etiology

In 1931 Codman[19] suggested that degenerative changes in the rotator cuff lead to tears. Microvascular studies of the vascular pattern of the rotator cuff demonstrate a hypovascular zone in the supraspinatus adjacent to the insertion of the supraspinatus into the humerus.[47,54,56] Relative ischemia in this hypovascular zone leads to decreased tendon cellularity and the eventual disruption of the rotator cuff attachment to bone with aging.

Compression of the rotator cuff between the acromion and the humeral head may subject the cuff to wear as the supraspinatus passes under the coracoacromial arch. Neer[48,49] postulated that 95% of rotator cuff tears are caused by impingement of the rotator cuff under the acromion. Neer[48] classified three stages of rotator cuff injury on a continuum that leads to cuff tears:

  Stage I—Characterized by subacromial edema and hemorrhage of the rotator cuff; usually occurs in patients younger than 25 years

  Stage II—Includes fibrosis and tendinosis of the rotator cuff and occurs more commonly in patients 25 to 40 years old

  Stage III—A continued progression characterized by partial or complete tendon tears and bone changes; typically involves patients older than 40 years

Bigliani et al[9] described three types of acromion:

  Type I—Flat
  Type II—Curved
  Type III—Hooked

An increased incidence of rotator cuff tears are associated with a curved (Type II) or hooked (Type III) acromion.[10] Other sources of impingement include acromioclavicular (AC) osteophytes, the coracoid process, and the posterosuperior aspect of the glenoid.[28]

A rotator cuff tear may occur spontaneously after a sudden movement or traumatic event.[21] Ruptures of the rotator cuff have been estimated to occur in as many as 80% of persons older than 60 years who have glenohumeral dislocations.[52] Cuff tears usually occur late in the shoulder deterioration process (after secondary impingements) and in elderly persons.

Among athletes who participate in repetitive overhead activities (such as throwers, swimmers, and tennis players), small rotator cuff tears may appear late in the deterioration process as a result of secondary impingement. Instability of the glenohumeral joint or functional scapulothoracic instability causes this impingement.[14] The primary underlying glenohumeral instability may progress along a continuum from anterior subluxation to impingement to rotator cuff tearing. Treatment must be directed at the primary instability problem.[39]

The throwing athlete also can have secondary impingement caused by functional scapular instability. Fatigue of the scapular stabilizers from repetitive throwing leads to abnormal positioning of the scapula. As a result, humeral and scapular elevations lose synchronization and the acromion is not elevated enough to allow free rotator cuff movement.[14] The rotator cuff abuts the acromion, causing microtrauma and impingement. A tear may then occur either gradually or suddenly.

In summary, rotator cuff disease results from numerous causes, including vascular factors, impingement, degenerative processes, and developmental factors. Each of these contributes to the evolution and progression of rotator cuff disorders.

Clinical Evaluation

History. The majority of patients with rotator cuff dysfunction have pain. They also may complain of fatigue, functional catching, stiffness, weakness, and symptoms of instability. It is important to distinguish an acute or macrotraumatic condition from an overuse or microtrauma condition.

Pain is typically localized in the upper arm in the region of the deltoid tuberosity and anterolateral to the

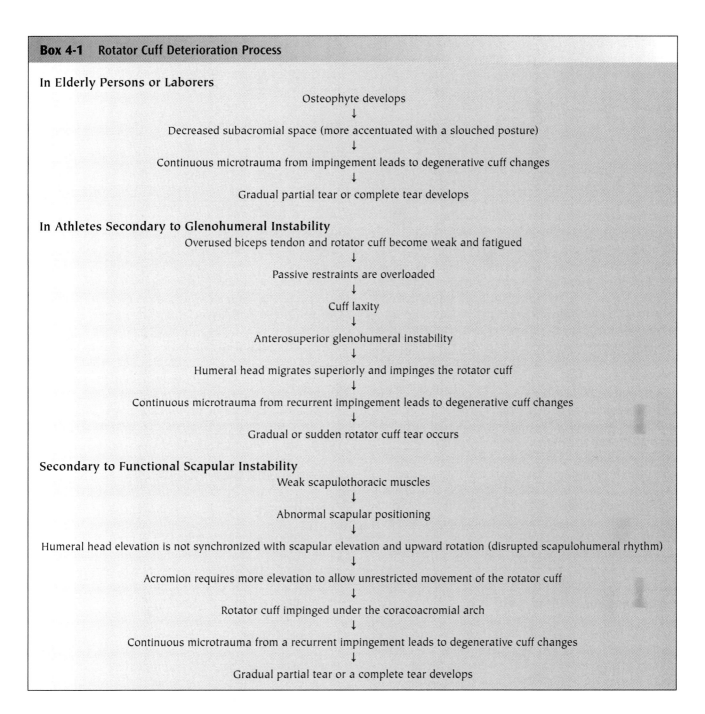

Box 4-1   Rotator Cuff Deterioration Process

In Elderly Persons or Laborers

Osteophyte develops
↓
Decreased subacromial space (more accentuated with a slouched posture)
↓
Continuous microtrauma from impingement leads to degenerative cuff changes
↓
Gradual partial tear or complete tear develops

In Athletes Secondary to Glenohumeral Instability

Overused biceps tendon and rotator cuff become weak and fatigued
↓
Passive restraints are overloaded
↓
Cuff laxity
↓
Anterosuperior glenohumeral instability
↓
Humeral head migrates superiorly and impinges the rotator cuff
↓
Continuous microtrauma from recurrent impingement leads to degenerative cuff changes
↓
Gradual or sudden rotator cuff tear occurs

Secondary to Functional Scapular Instability

Weak scapulothoracic muscles
↓
Abnormal scapular positioning
↓
Humeral head elevation is not synchronized with scapular elevation and upward rotation (disrupted scapulohumeral rhythm)
↓
Acromion requires more elevation to allow unrestricted movement of the rotator cuff
↓
Rotator cuff impinged under the coracoacromial arch
↓
Continuous microtrauma from a recurrent impingement leads to degenerative cuff changes
↓
Gradual partial tear or a complete tear develops

acromion. It is usually worse at night. Overhead activities often induce the patient's symptoms. Typical findings are loss of endurance during activities, catching, crepitus, and possibly weakness and stiffness.

Physical examination. A thorough examination of the shoulder should include evaluation of the cervical spine and an upper extremity neurologic assessment. The opposite shoulder must also be examined for comparison. Inspection, palpation for tenderness, and range of motion (ROM) testing should be completed. Palpa-tion should be used to evaluate the AC joint, sterno-clavicular joint, subacromial space, biceps tendon, and trapezius muscle. Impingement signs are induced to elicit pain. (Hawkins[31] described forward flexion to 90 degrees and internal rotation, and Neer and Welch[50] favored forward elevation and internal rotation.) If these tests produce pain they are considered positive signs of impingement and suggest rotator cuff dysfunction. The rotator cuff muscles are tested for strength. Examination for instability is performed. Apprehension, a positive relocation test, or the inferior sulcus sign indicates instability. Instability testing should be performed in different positions (seated and supine) to eliminate this as the cause of secondary impingement. Evidence of rotator cuff pathology includes painful impingement signs or weakness and a painful arc of motion.[48]

Diagnostic Testing

Diagnostic testing includes x-ray films, arthrograms or magnetic resonance imaging (MRI), and injections. An impingement test (injection into the subacromial space with 10 ml of 1% lidocaine) is invaluable. A physical examination should be completed several minutes after the injection and should include ROM testing and evaluation of impingement signs, strength, and instability. Resolution of symptoms without instability indicates primary rotator cuff pathology or impingement. Relief of pain with evidence of instability indicates possible primary instability with secondary rotator cuff changes resulting from altered shoulder mechanics.

Arthrography has been the gold standard for identifying rotator cuff tears. Although reliable for the diagnosis of complete rotator cuff tears, it is less reliable for the evaluation of partial-thickness rotator cuff tears. MRI provides an excellent noninvasive tool in the diagnosis of rotator cuff pathology and pathology of the shoulder labrum and is becoming the standard test for rotator cuff pathology. MRI provides information not available by other diagnostic testing, including amount of muscle atrophy, amount of rotator cuff retraction in full-thickness tears, extent of bursal swelling, and status of the AC joint and shoulder articular cartilage. MRI is less reliable for evaluation of partial-thickness or small, nonretracted full-thickness rotator cuff tears.[51]

Treatment Options

Initially, symptoms of rotator cuff dysfunction (e.g., tendinitis, partial or full-thickness tears) are usually treated in a nonoperative fashion. Nonsteroidal anti-inflammatory drugs (NSAIDs), heat, ice, rest, cortisone injections, and rehabilitation programs are used. The initial goal of treatment is restoration of a normal ROM. This is followed by a rotator cuff strengthening program. The use of stretch cords for resistance is initiated, followed by free weights as tolerated. To avoid aggravating the rotator cuff, initially all strength training should be done below shoulder level. Nonoperative treatment programs usually continue for 4 to 6 months, with success rates varying from 50% to 90%.[18,27,57,58,59] Approximately 50% of patients with symptomatic rotator cuff tears have satisfactory results with nonoperative measures, but these results may deteriorate with time.[34] This wide range of outcomes probably results from lack of uniformity in classification, indications, and treatment. Some individuals have rotator

cuff tears with no pain and normal function, whereas others may have debilitating pain. This demonstrates the need for a better understanding of the factors that lead to symptoms.

Indications for Surgery

Indications for rotator cuff surgery include failure of 4 to 6 months of conservative care or an acute full-thickness tear in an active patient younger than 50 years. Failure of treatment can be determined before an entire rehabilitation course is completed. Indications for earlier surgical treatment include return to full strength with persistent symptoms, failure to tolerate therapy because of pain, or plateau of initial improvement with persistent symptoms. Early surgical intervention also is indicated for patients who sustain acute trauma with full-thickness tears associated with significant rotator cuff weakness and posterior cuff involvement, particularly in young patients with higher functional demands. In addition, patients with acute tears or extension of chronic cuff tears may benefit from early surgery.[33] The duration of nonoperative treatment must be individualized based on the pathology involved, the patient's response to treatment, and individual functional demands and expectations.

Surgical Procedure

Surgical Goals

The primary goal of rotator cuff surgery is decreased pain, including resting pain, night pain, and pain with activities of daily living. Arrest of the progression of rotator cuff pathology and improved shoulder function are additional surgical goals.

Procedural Steps

Surgical management for impingement and partial-thickness rotator cuff tears generally involve open anterior acromioplasty as described by Neer[50] or arthroscopic subacromial decompression with release or partial release of the coracoacromial ligament.

Full-thickness tears. The mainstay of treatment for full-thickness tears is surgical repair. The type, pattern, and size of the tear, as well as the surgeon's preference, dictate whether the repair is a fully arthroscopic, partially open, or completely open procedure.

Small or moderately sized (3 cm or less) partial or full-thickness supraspinatus or infraspinatus tears may be repaired with the arthroscopic or partially open technique. Wide tears (3 to 5 cm) also may be repaired with the partially open technique if the cuff is mobile enough to allow anatomic repair. Large, immobile cuff

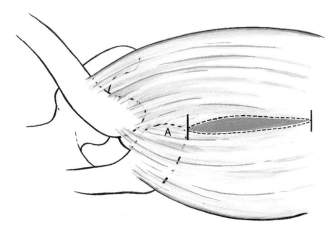

Fig. 4-1. Line of incision for partially open repair. The deltoid split begins at the lateral edge of the acromion *(A)* and should not extend more than 4 cm lateral to the acromion to avoid injury to the axillary nerve.

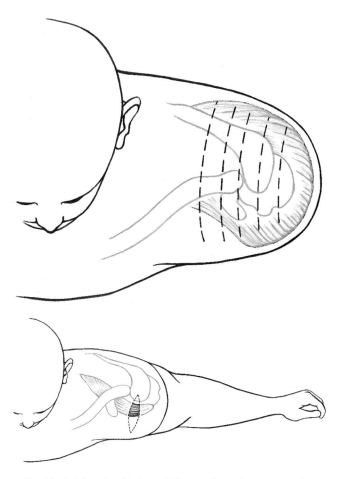

Fig. 4-2. Incision placed in Langer's lines produces the best cosmesis.

tears involving the subscapularis or teres minor, as well as tears of the musculotendinous junction, require an open approach. Massive, chronic, atrophic cuff tears should be considered for arthroscopic debridement to address pain control.

All the operative procedures discussed recently in the literature for primary repair of rotator cuff tears include an anteroinferior acromioplasty to decompress the subacromial space. Current preferences favor glenohumeral arthroscopy and subacromial bursoscopy on most patients undergoing surgery for cuff pathology. Shoulder arthroscopy and arthroscopic decompression are performed as previously described. After acromioplasty, the bursal surface of the rotator cuff is evaluated. With shoulder rotation the cuff can be completely visualized. Mobile tears are treated with the partially open technique. The lateral subacromial portal incision is extended either longitudinally or transversely to expose the deltoid fascia. The deltoid fascia is then split in line with its fibers directly over the tear. The anterior deltoid insertion on the anterior acromion is preserved. The deltoid fibers should not be split more than 4 cm lateral to the lateral acromion to avoid risking axillary nerve injury (Fig. 4-1). Rotation of the arm provides access to the tear. Digital palpation can be used to assess the adequacy of the acromioplasty. A bony trough is prepared in the greater tuberosity of the humerus. The rotator cuff may then be repaired through a bony bridge or with suture anchors with permanent sutures tied, pulling the rotator cuff down into its trough on the humerus.

Tears that are retracted but reparable are repaired with the open technique using principles developed by Neer.[48,49] An oblique incision is made in Langer's line from the anterior edge of the acromion to a point about 2 cm lateral to the coracoid process. The anterior deltoid is released from the anterior aspect of the acromion, preserving the coracoacromial ligament and splitting the deltoid no more than 4 cm lateral to the acromion (Fig. 4-2). The deltoid origin over the acromion is elevated subperiosteally. The coracoacromial ligament is released and the anterior acromion osteotomized. The acromion anterior to the anterior aspect of the clavicle is removed, and the undersurface of the acromion is flattened from anterior to posterior. The AC joint may be removed if it is arthritic and symptomatic. The distal clavicle is excised parallel to the AC joint so no contact occurs with adduction of the arm.

The cuff tear is visualized and mobilized. A bony trough is made that is 0.5 cm wide and parallel to the junction of the humeral articular cartilage and greater tuberosity of the humerus. The rotator cuff tear is repaired to bone with suture anchors or through a bony bridge in the greater tuberosity using permanent sutures (Fig. 4-3). The goal is to repair the cuff with minimal tension with the arm positioned at the side.

Watertight repairs are not necessary for good functional outcome. Excellent and good results have been shown in patients with residual cuff holes.[17,44] The an-

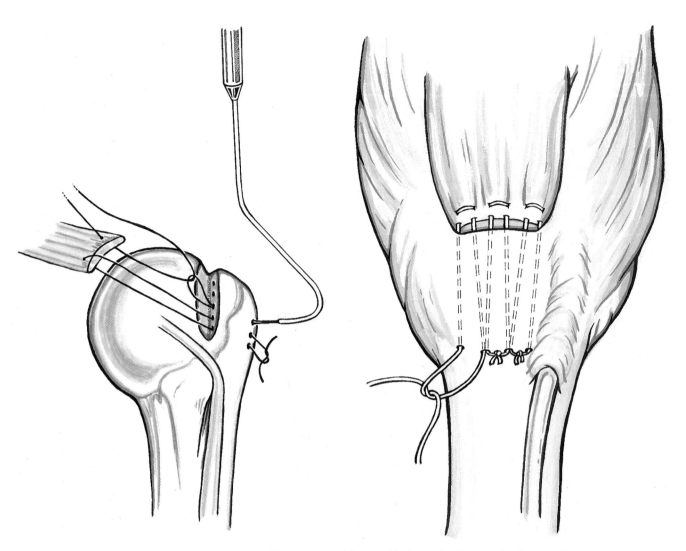

Fig. 4-3. Transosseous repair of rotator cuff tendon. A trough is created in the proximal humerus just lateral to the articular surface. Sutures are tied over the bone bridge in the greater tuberosity.

terior deltoid is repaired back to the acromion by preserved periosteum or through drill holes with permanent sutures. Routine skin closure is performed.

The postoperative management of cuff repairs must be individualized to address tear size, tissue quality, difficulty of repair, and patient goals. Passive motion is initiated immediately. Waist-level use of the hand can usually be started after surgery. Active range of motion (AROM) and isotonic strengthening start 6 to 8 weeks after surgery. Progression of strengthening is individualized, with full rehabilitation taking 6 to 12 months. Function can continue to improve for 1 year after surgery.

MANAGEMENT OF MASSIVE TENDON DEFECTS. The management of massive irreparable tendon defects remains controversial. Options include subacromial decompression and debridement of nonviable cuff tissue without attempt at repair, use of autogenous or allograft tendon grafts, and use of active tendon transfers.

Operations that require tendon transfer to nonanatomic sites to cover rotator cuff defects are likely to alter the mechanics of the shoulder unfavorably.[15] Debridement may be pursued using either an open or arthroscopic approach.

RESULTS OF TREATMENT OF FULL-THICKNESS ROTATOR CUFF TEARS. Satisfactory clinical results after rotator cuff repair for pain relief occur 85% to 95% of the time[30,31,48] and appear to correlate with the adequacy of the acromioplasty and subacromial decompression. Functional outcomes correlate with integrity of the cuff repair, preoperative size of the cuff tear, and quality of the tendon tissue. Poor outcomes are associated with deltoid detachment or denervation.[7]

The use of arthroscope-assisted partially open rotator cuff repair provides favorable clinical results and is increasing and advancing in popularity. In fact, results comparable with open cuff repair have been reported for small and moderate sized rotator cuff repair (less than 3 cm).[5,41,43] These studies have shown that the most important factor affecting outcome is cuff tear size. Small or moderate tears had better results. In a retrospective study Blevins et al[11] reported 83% good or excellent results regardless of cuff size. Most studies have shown a more rapid return to full activities with the arthroscope-assisted technique.

The preliminary reports on fully arthroscopic repair appear to show satisfactory results.[6,61,62] In the first prospective study comparing the partially open technique with full arthroscopic cuff repair for small rotator cuff tears, Weber[66] reported an increased incidence (14%) of the need for a second operation in the fully arthroscopic repair; partially open rotator cuff repairs had a rate of 2%.

A surgical technique that initially includes arthroscopy has the theoretical advantage of providing identification and treatment of intra-pathology (i.e., articular cartilage labrum, bicipital tendon). Additional theoretic advantages with the arthroscopic technique include decreased soft tissue dissection, improved cosmesis, and often preservation of the deltoid attachment. Unfortunately, rehabilitation cannot be accelerated for arthroscopic or partially open cuff repairs because the limiting factor—tendon-to-bone healing—is not influenced by the surgical technique.

No ideal surgical technique exists. Each surgeon must individualize treatment based on the type of lesion present as well as the physician's expertise. As the frequency of shoulder arthroscopy increases, it is expected that a transition from open to partially open to fully arthroscopic cuff repairs will proceed.

Therapy Guidelines for Rehabilitation

The general guidelines that follow are for the rehabilitation of a type 2 rotator cuff tear (a medium to large rotator cuff tear that is larger than 1 cm and smaller than 5 cm). The protocol is designed for active patients (i.e., recreational athletes). An older, more sedentary individual progresses through the stages more slowly and is not an appropriate candidate for the more aggressive exercises listed. These guidelines are designed to help guide therapists and provide treatment ideas. The therapist must choose the treatment ideas that are beneficial for each patient within the restrictions outlined by the operative surgeon.

Phase 1

TIME: 1 to 4 weeks after surgery
GOALS: Comfort, increasing ROM as tolerated, decreased pain and inflammation, minimal cervical spine stiffness, protection of the surgical site, and maintenance of full elbow and wrist ROM (Table 4-1)

To achieve pain control, use ice and electrical stimulation as needed. Gentle mobilizations using grades I and II help reduce pain, muscle guarding, and spasms. These mobilizations also help maintain nutrient exchange and therefore prevent the painful and degenerating effects immobilization produces: a swollen and painful joint with a limited ROM.[29] Passive ROM (PROM) and pendulum exercises are essential for increasing shoulder ROM. The passive exercises also provide nourishment to the articular cartilage and assist in collagen tissue synthesis and organization.[70] PROM exercises are done in guarded and protected planes, with the patient and therapist taking care not to overstretch healing tissues. Therefore horizontal adduction, extension, and internal rotation are not performed initially.

At 3 weeks after the operation, the patient can begin submaximal and subpainful isometric exercises to retard muscle atrophy. When performing isometric exercises, rotator cuff muscles generate the greatest electromyographic activity in neutral to mid-rotational positions.[35] Do not allow patients to perform isometrics at maximal effort until the repair site has had sufficient time for healing.

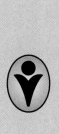

Q. Jim is a 38-year-old weekend athlete who sustained a large rotator cuff tear after falling onto an outstretched arm during a flag football game. At 3 weeks after rotator cuff repair surgery he complains of moderate shoulder pain that radiates through the upper trapezius area and into the superior medial scapular area. Jim also complains of neck stiffness that has worsened over the past few days. He remains guarded through most of his range when performing PROM. During today's session, what areas should be addressed by the therapist to improve the quality of movement and increase the ROM?

Phase 2

TIME: 5 to 8 weeks after surgery
GOALS: Protection of surgical site, improvement of ROM, increase in strength, decrease in pain and inflammation, maintenance of elbow and wrist ROM, and minimizing of cervical stiffness (Table 4-2)

During the second phase the patient should avoid stretching muscles into positions that could compromise the repaired tissues (e.g., horizontal adduction, internal rotation, shoulder extension). Strength should begin to improve, with the patient progressing from A/AROM to AROM movements against gravity. The therapist should incorporate active proprioceptive neuromuscular facilitation (PNF) patterns to mimic functional move-

Table 4-1   Rotator Cuff Repair

Rehabilitation Phase	Criteria to Progress to this Phase	Anticipated Impairments and Functional Limitations	Intervention	Goal	Rationale
Phase I Postoperative 1-4 weeks	Postoperative	• Limited ROM • Limited strength • Pain • Initially restricted to passive range of motion (PROM) of shoulder • Dependent upper extremity immobilized in sling or airplane splint	• Cryotherapy • Electrical stimulation • PROM—Pendulum exercises shoulder flexion, external rotation, internal rotation, and abduction in protected planes • Isometrics (at 3 weeks)—Submaximal (without increasing pain); shoulder flexion and internal rotation; elbow flexion and extension; at 4 weeks initiate shoulder abduction and external rotation • AROM—Elbow flexion, extension; cervical spine all ranges • Progressive resistance exercises (PREs)—Hand gripping, exercises with putty • Joint mobilization resistance free to the shoulder joint	• Decrease pain • Manage edema • Improve PROM and tolerance to movement • Increase quality of muscle recruitment • Maintain and improve ROM of joints proximal and distal to surgical site • Maintain and improve distal muscle strength • Control pain	• Pain control • Edema management • Prevention of joint stiffness • Promotion of healthy articular surface and collagen synthesis and organization • Prevention of further atrophy of upper extremity musculature • Prevention of associated weakness, stiffness, and dysfunction of neighboring joints • Gating of pain and preparation for stretches into resistance

Table 4-2 Rotator Cuff Repair

Rehabilitation Phase	Criteria to Progress to this Phase	Anticipated Impairments and Functional Limitations	Intervention	Goal	Rationale
Phase II Postoperative 5-8 weeks	Incision area well healed Decreased pain Improved PROM Improved sleep patterns	• Limited tolerance to ROM • Limited strength • Relatively dependent upper extremity	Continue phase I exercises and progress as indicated • A/AROM (supine) progressing to AROM • Shoulder proprioceptive neuromuscular facilitation (PNF) D1 and D2 patterns using elbow and wrist movements • Shoulder flexion, external rotation, abduction, and scaption (Fig. 4-4) • Soft tissue mobilization (after incision is healed) • Cardiovascular conditioning (bicycling, walking program)	• PROM Shoulder flexion/abduction 140°-165° external rotation 70° internal rotation 55° • A/AROM Reach above head height • Prevent increase of pain • Improve scar mobility; decrease pain • Improve fitness level	• Continuing phase I exercises to minimize stiffness of adjacent joints • Mimicing and strengthening of functional movements • Improvement of ROM and strength • Improvement of tolerance to movement and preparation for AROM • Performance of exercise to ease subacromial pressures • Normalization of skin mobility and desensitization of scar • Provision of a good healing environment and normalization of arm swing with gait

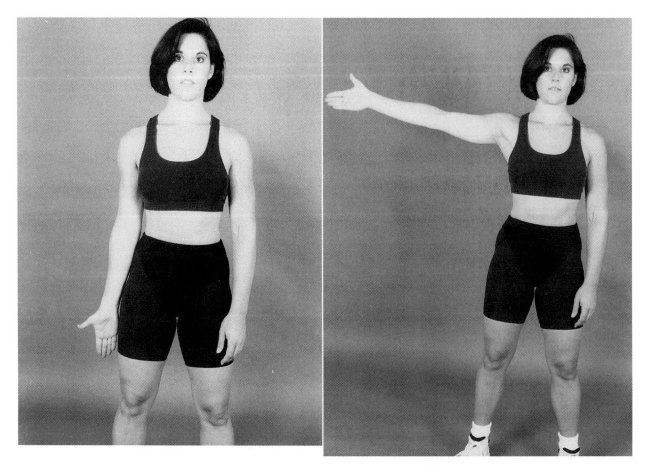

Fig. 4-4. Isotonic scaption exercises. These are elevation exercises done in the scapular plane. The patient holds the arm with the thumb up and the elbow straight and lifts the arm at a 45-degree angle to shoulder level. Patient progresses to full elevation and then gradually adds weight.

ments and strengthen the areas in functional planes.[53] Eventually active shoulder flexion, external rotation, and scaption exercises (Fig. 4-4) are performed. Active shoulder flexion and scaption are usually initiated between 0 and 70 degrees and progress according to the patient's ability to execute these exercises correctly.

Patients usually exhibit protective muscle guarding from the insult of the surgery and the preceding shoulder pathology. Muscle guarding is present in the cervical region and the shoulder musculature. Therefore patients perform cervical AROM exercises and stretches. Appropriate cervical spine mobilization techniques may be essential for decreasing cervical joint stiffness and muscle guarding, allowing more unrestricted movement of the shoulder complex.

After the incision is appropriately healed and closed, the therapist should apply soft tissue mobilization over the incision areas and instruct the patient in massaging the scarred area. Early movement minimizes tightness from scarring. Normal skin mobility allows normal movement to occur.[22]

Precautions at this stage include no heavy resisted exercises for 8 weeks. However, ROM exercises within pain tolerance can be performed. Marked increases in

swelling, pain, or wound drainage must be reported immediately and exercises should be discontinued.

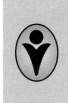

A. The cervical spine needs to be assessed to determine whether it may be contributing to some of the patient's complaints, particularly the neck stiffness and the superior medial scapular pain. If cervical spine joint stiffness or soft tissue tightness is noted, appropriate joint or soft tissue mobilizations may decrease these symptoms. As pain decreases, muscle guarding will lessen, allowing the shoulder to move more freely.

Q. Brent is a 27-year-old who had a rotator cuff repair for a large tear. He has progressed nicely with PROM. At 9 weeks after surgery, Brent can elevate his arm above his head with little effort. However, he demonstrates a mild shoulder hike with elevation above 70 degrees. How much weight should Brent begin lifting when performing elevation exercises to 90 degrees?

Phase 3

TIME: 9 to 12 weeks after surgery
GOALS: Expansion of ROM, avoidance of impingement problems, gaining of full ROM, increased strength, alleviation of pain, increased function, and decreased soft tissue restrictions and scarring (Table 4-3)

During the period from 9 to 12 weeks after surgery, the patient's ROM should progress toward full ROM. The repaired tissues are now strong enough to tolerate stretching within the patient's tolerance level. Passive stretching of the internal and external rotators is important. Tightness in these areas could promote abnormal shoulder mechanics, particularly in throwing. Tight external rotators lead to anterior translation and superior migration of the humeral head, which can produce impingement problems.[13]

AC joint pain is common in many patients who have undergone rotator cuff repair. The symptoms may result from a previous trauma, be caused by primary generalized osteoarthritis, or follow abnormalities in the glenohumeral joint such as degeneration and rupture of the rotator cuff.[20] When the AC joint is hypomobile and symptomatic, mobilization can help alleviate a portion of the symptoms and allow greater mobility (Fig. 4-5).

It is now safe to begin resisted exercises gradually. However, the patient should demonstrate correct active movements before resistance is added and be able to perform resisted exercises correctly. Isotonic exercises are important for strengthening and promoting dynamic shoulder stabilization. The supraspinatus, infraspinatus, teres minor, and subscapularis muscles pull the humeral head securely into the glenoid and control humeral rotation to allow the head of the humerus to maintain good alignment with the glenoid.[2] Resisted external and internal rotator exercises using exercise tubing can provide a constant loading to the musculotendinous unit.[2] The therapist should place an axillary roll under the shoulder to avoid a fully adducted position, which can cause avascular stress on the supraspinatus and biceps tendons. The supraspinatus and infraspinatus muscles (also referred to as decelerators) produce slow, controlled movements. These muscles are subjected to larger stresses and also are injured more frequently in overhead sporting activities.[3] Through the use of electromyographic (EMG) studies, Blackburn found that the best isolation for the infraspinatus and teres minor muscles occurs during prone exercises incorporating horizontal abduction and external rotation. An optimal exercise for glenohumeral congruity and stability is prone external resistance with the shoulder at 90 degrees abduction and the elbow flexed to 90 degrees. These exercises should be performed at a functional speed.[23] Resisted exercises also are performed in PNF patterns to strengthen the muscles in

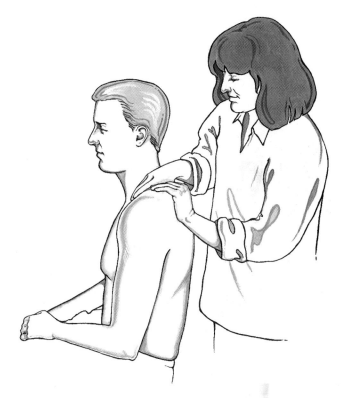

Fig. 4-5. AC mobilization through posteroanterior (PA) movement. The therapist stabilizes the mid-clavicle while applying a PA pressure through the spine of the scapula.

functional patterns. A frequently used pattern is the extension/adduction/internal rotation pattern (D_2) using both concentric and eccentric contractions. This is particularly effective in throwers. Scapular strengthening exercises also are initiated (Figs. 4-6 and 4-7). Rowing is excellent for all portions of the trapezius, levator scapula, and rhomboids. These muscles help maintain the scapula in good alignment during shoulder movements. Occasionally older patients with large tears have difficulty progressing to active shoulder flexion against gravity. Eccentric shoulder flexion exercises help provide these patients with a transition to active shoulder flexion.

Strengthening of the trunk and legs is important for athletes. Numerous studies indicate that the trunk and legs are responsible for more than 50% of the kinetic energy expended during throwing.

Endurance training also begins during this phase. Patients begin on the upper body ergometer (UBE) with short-duration and low-intensity bouts, then progress to longer durations and higher-intensity bouts. The therapist should continue soft tissue massage if needed. Modalities are seldom used during this stage. Pain is generally minimal but may increase with moderate to dramatic changes in activity levels. Therefore the therapist and patient should use modalities only as needed.

Table 4-3   Rotator Cuff Repair

Rehabilitation Phase	Criteria to Progress to this Phase	Anticipated Impairments and Functional Limitations	Intervention	Goal	Rationale

Phase III Postoperative 8-12 weeks	Steady improvement in ROM and strength (tolerance to movement) Pain controlled with therapy and medication	• Limited AROM
		• Limited tolerance to use of upper extremity
		• Limited reaching
		• Limited lifting
			Continue exercises from phases I and II as indicated.
			• AROM—Wand exercises (flexion, extension, abduction) progress to independent use of wand
			• PREs (elastic tubing)—Shoulder external rotation and internal rotation with axillary roll
			  Isotonics—
			  • Shoulder flexion and abduction
			  • Modified military press
			  Scapula exercises
			  • Reverse rows
			  • Horizontal abduction (see Fig. 4-6)
			  • Prone at 90°
			    Abduction external rotation
			  • Scaption
			    Perform with no weight initially, then progress
			  • Body Blade exercises
			  • Manual resistance added to PNF patterns
				• Increase exercises that patient can perform at home
				• Full PROM
				• Strength of shoulder to 65% to 70% (dependent on extent of repair)
				• Minimal pain associated with overhead activity
				• Able to perform self-care activities using involved upper extremity
					• Promotion of self-management
					• Transition to AROM program with emphasis as appropriate on PROM
					• Strengthening of shoulder and upper quarter musculature with a variety of resistance devices and positions
					• Scapula exercises to promote proximal stability for distal mobility
					• Progression from AROM to PREs as tolerance to activity improves
					• Performance of cuff stabilization exercises with pain-free ranges

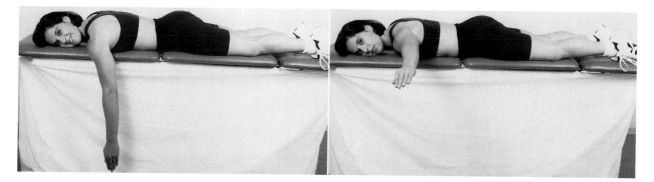

Fig. 4-6. Horizontal abduction in neutral, prone position with external rotation of the humeral head. Patient lies prone with elbow extended and arm hanging down. Therapist instructs patient to abduct the arm horizontally. Patient can start without weights, then gradually add resistance.

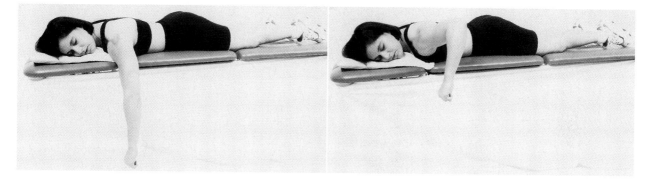

Fig. 4-7. Prone rowing. Patient hangs arm over edge of table, pulls hand upward while bending the elbow and tightening the scapular muscles, and slowly releases.

Precautions are necessary when initiating isotonic shoulder elevation exercises. Patients must be able to elevate the arm correctly without substitution patterns. All exercises should be performed with little or no shoulder joint pain. Complaints of muscle discomfort are acceptable and even desirable.[60] If the patient complains of pain through particular ranges, the therapist should modify exercises.

A. Brent should not lift any weights above 70 degrees during shoulder elevation until he can execute the exercise correctly. He should practice maintaining voluntary humeral head depression with active elevation in front of a mirror. He should only do resisted exercises through the range he can correctly perform. Brent also can continue to perform appropriate resisted strengthening exercises for the serratus anterior muscle and the rotator cuff muscles. When he can elevate the arm correctly above 70 degrees, he can begin adding weight for resisted elevation above 70 degrees.

Phase 4

TIME: 13 to 16 weeks after surgery
GOALS: Maintenance of full ROM, increased strength and endurance, improved function (Table 4-4)

The patient should have full ROM by 13 to 16 weeks. If this is not the case, the therapist should emphasize more aggressive mobilization using grades +3 and +4 on the glenohumeral capsule to normalize arthrokinematics at the glenohumeral joint. These mobilizations also can be performed near the physiologic end ROM. Adequate capsule laxity is necessary to allow normal roll-gliding between the bony surfaces of a joint.[69] Patients should continue the necessary stretches to gain and maintain ROM in restricted areas. (Figs. 4-8 through 4-10 illustrate some of the suggested stretches.) Strengthening exercises are progressed with PREs. Serratus anterior strengthening is incorporated to encourage humeral head depression with shoulder elevation (Figs. 4-11 and 4-13). Closed chain exercises are used to promote co-contractions and enhance dynamic joint stability (Fig. 4-12).[37] Isokinetic exercises may be initiated with ath-

Table 4-4　Rotator Cuff Repair

Rehabilitation Phase	Criteria to Progress to this Phase	Anticipated Impairments and Functional Limitations	Intervention	Goal	Rationale
Phase IV Postoperative 13–16 weeks	Close to if not full ROM Pain controlled and self-managed No loss of strength with addition of phase III exercises No increase in night pain	• Limited tolerance to overhead activities • Pain with activities involving prolonged use of upper extremity • Limited strength of rotator cuff	Exercises for phase III continued and progressed as appropriate • PROM Corner wall stretch (see Fig. 4-8a and 4-8b) Posterior capsule stretch if restricted (see Fig. 4-9) Hand-behind-back (see Fig. 4-10a and 4-10b). • PREs—Closed chain exercises Wall push-ups "plus" Seated push-ups "plus" (see Fig. 4-11a and 4-11b) • Shoulder girdle depressions using a Swiss ball (Fig. 4-13) • Plyometrics if appropriate • Isokinetics at 200°/sec[12] • UBE • Trunk and leg strengthening exercises for return to previous level of functioning • Joint mobilization to cervical and thoracic spine as appropriate	• Self-management of home exercises • Full AROM • Strength of 75% to 80% (dependent on extent of repair) • Self-management of pain associated with overhead activity • Reach in front and to side for light-weight objects • Carry light weight for short periods (grocery shopping)	• Preparation of patient for discharge and continued self-management • Improvement of capsular mobility • Strengthening of upper quarter, especially scapula stabilizers in a stable but challenging environment • Co-contraction exercises to enhance dynamic joint stability • Preparation of patient for activity-specific demands • Maintenance and improvement of cardiovascular fitness incorporating upper extremities • Restore end-range joint arthrokinematics

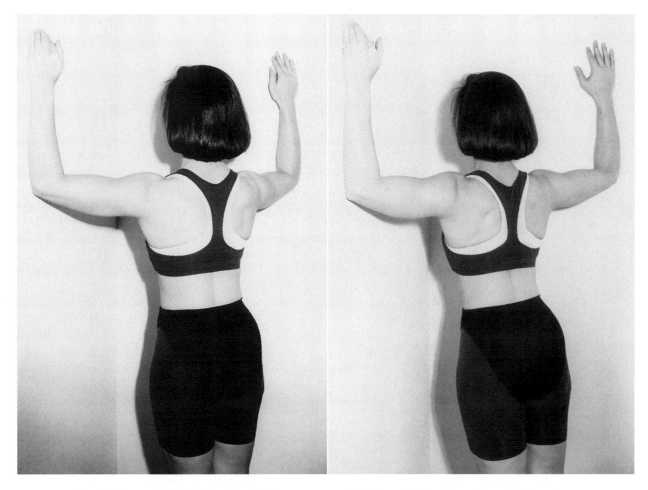

Fig. 4-8. Corner wall stretch. Patient stands facing a corner approximately one stride length away. The patient then places the forearms on the wall, keeping the elbows at shoulder height. The therapist instructs the patient to lean into the corner until he or she feels a stretch on the anterior portion of the shoulders.

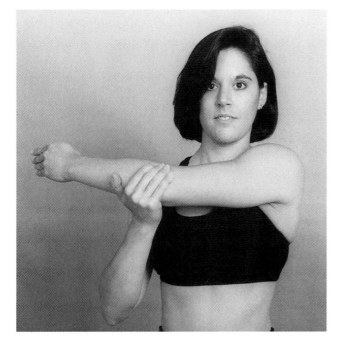

Fig. 4-9. Posterior capsular stretch. Patient horizontally adducts arm across body and then uses the other hand to pull the affected arm into further horizontal adduction.

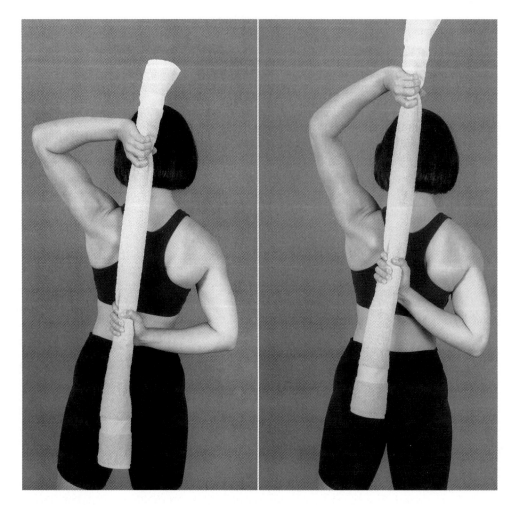

Fig. 4-10. Hand-behind-back stretch. Patient stands with towel in both hands and places the involved arm behind the buttock or low back. Patient places the uninvolved arm behind the head and slowly pulls with the superior hand up the back until he or she feels a stretch.

letes when they are able to lift 5 to 10 lb in external rotation and 15 to 20 lb in internal rotation without pain or significant edema. The patient should begin strength and endurance training at 200 degrees/sec.[12] Athletes and other appropriate patients can begin plyometric exercises, which involve a stretch-shortening cycle of the muscle. All sporting movements involve this explosive stretch-shortening cycle (jumping, throwing, running, swimming).[69] These exercises are excellent progressive steps between traditional strengthening exercises and training activities before initiating throwing drills.[68]

Phase 5

TIME: 17 to 21 weeks after surgery
GOALS: Maintenance of full ROM, increased strength and endurance, improvement of neuromuscular control, return to functional activities, initiation of sport-specific activities (Table 4-5)

The therapist should continue the stretching program and instruct the patient in self-mobilization techniques if indicated. The patient should maintain a shoulder strengthening program and continue PREs. Initiate sports-specific drills for athletes along with an interval sport program. (Refer to Appendix A.) Progressive plyometric exercises may be used with appropriate patients. Older, sedentary patients should work on specific activities of daily living (ADLs). As appropriate, patients may progress to more difficult tasks.

Phase 6

TIME: 22 and more weeks after surgery
GOAL: Return to normal activities, maintenance of full ROM, continued strengthening and endurance, gradual return to full activities. Athletes can return to their sports usually between 6 and 12 months.

Table 4-5   Rotator Cuff Repair

Rehabilitation Phase	Criteria to Progress to this Phase	Anticipated Impairments and Functional Limitations	Intervention	Goal	Rationale
Phase V Postoperative 17-26 weeks	Progression through phase IV without loss of strength or increase in pain Potential to return to high-level functional use of the upper extremity (i.e., competitive athletics)	• Limited strength and endurance of rotator cuff muscles • Continued manageable pain with overhead activities	Continuation of phase IV exercises as indicated • Joint mobilization as appropriate • PREs—Initiate strengthening in sport-specific activity Initiate throwing program when appropriate (see Appendix A)	• Pain-free with overhead activity • Able to perform activities of daily living without increased pain • Return to previous level of functioning	• Strengthening of rotator cuff in specific ranges (overhead and reaching to the side) • Provision of optimal ROM for the client to perform the associated activity • Provision of a vehicle for the client to return at or close to the previous level of functioning

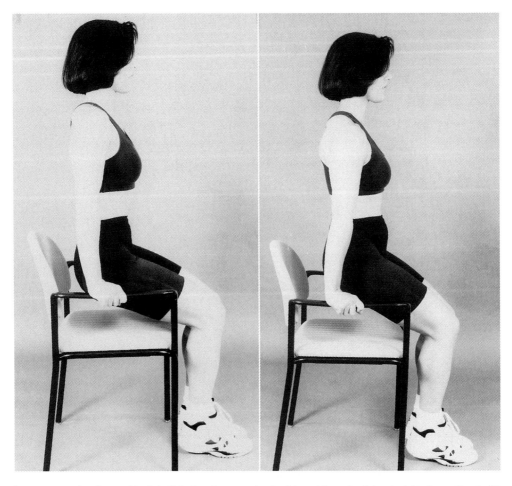

Fig. 4-11. Seated push-ups with a "plus". Patient depresses the shoulders while maintaining straight elbows, thereby lifting the torso. Patient then slowly lowers torso, attempting to avoid excessive superior translation of the humeral head.

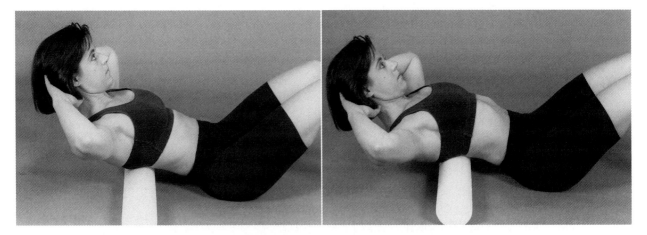

Fig. 4-12. Thoracic extension on foam roll or using tennis balls. Patient lies supine with both knees bent and places roll or balls at the middle thoracic spine levels. Patient then places hands under head and slowly leans back (taking care not to arch over the roll or balls) until a stretch is felt.

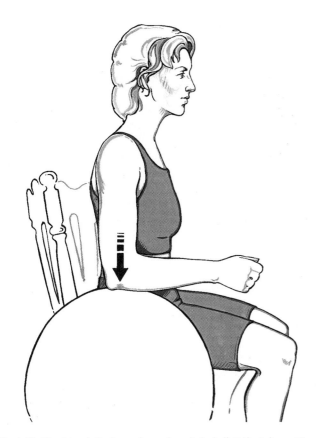

Fig. 4-13. Shoulder girdle depressions using a Swiss ball. Patient sits next to Swiss ball and places elbow on the ball. Patient maintains a 90-degree bend in the elbow while depressing the scapula to push the elbow down into the ball. This exercise is good for those who cannot or should not perform seated push-ups with a "plus" (e.g., elderly patients).

During weeks 22 to 26 patients maintain a stretching and strengthening program. Athletes continue on a sports interval program, and others gradually progress to recreational activities. Older individuals continue to progress with PREs and work on more advanced ADLs. After 26 weeks patients continue with their stretching and strengthening program as long as they anticipate using the shoulder aggressively in ADLs or sports.

Suggested Home Maintenance for the Postsurgical Patient

The home maintenance box on pages 67 to 68 outlines the rehabilitation the patient is to follow after rotator cuff repair. The physical therapist can use it in customizing a patient-specific program. Patients require a program that suits their needs and abilities. Some exercises may be appropriate for certain patients but not for others. Some patients progress slower than others. The therapist must take into account the patient's age, the condition of the repaired tissues, the size of the tear, the rate of healing, and the patient's abilities and previous level of function.

Troubleshooting

Considering influential factors outside the glenohumeral joint during treatment will aid the therapist in helping the patient progress more efficiently. General suggestions are given; however, it is beyond the scope of this book to instruct therapists in the use and application of techniques. The following areas are addressed:

- Cervical spine
- Thoracic spine
- Adverse neural tension
- AC joint
- Sternoclavicular joint
- Scapulothoracic joint

Cervical Spine

Evaluation of the cervical spine may prove vital in addressing cervical issues that may be inhibiting progress. Although the cervical spine is not the primary cause of shoulder dysfunction when dealing with rotator cuff repairs, it may be a contributory factor. Often cervical spine disorders occur in conjunction with a traumatic shoulder injury (e.g., falling onto the upper extremity may cause injury to the shoulder and the cervical spine). Furthermore, prolonged muscle guarding secondary to the shoulder injury or pathology affects the cervical area. Muscles in spasm originating or inserting along the cervical spine can lead to cervical symptoms. Thus a patient may present with a combination of cervical and shoulder signs and symptoms. Treatment to the appropriate cervical joint area can alleviate a portion of the symptoms and signs, thereby decreasing the complaints of pain and potentially allowing more glenohumeral movement and function. Clinicians may notice that after treating cervical spine dysfunctions, treatment of the shoulder is more effective.

Common patterns in cervical pathology are addressed to assist clinicians with differentiating shoulder and cervical symptoms because they frequently occur together. Spinal disorders may cause referred pain (Fig. 4-14). Joint movement disorders may cause joint pain and be associated with an altered range of cervical spine joint movement or shoulder movement. Therefore the cervical spine should be assessed for additional joint disorders that may be causing local pain or pain that is referred into the shoulder/arm region.[20]

Treating the cervical spine may diminish pain in the shoulder area and alleviate factors that are contributing to lack of progress with rehabilitation. Treating the dysfunctional or stiff cervical spine along with shoulder treatment decreases the complaints of shoulder pain and muscle guarding, leading to further gains in range of motion. (Suggested reading for treatment of the cer-

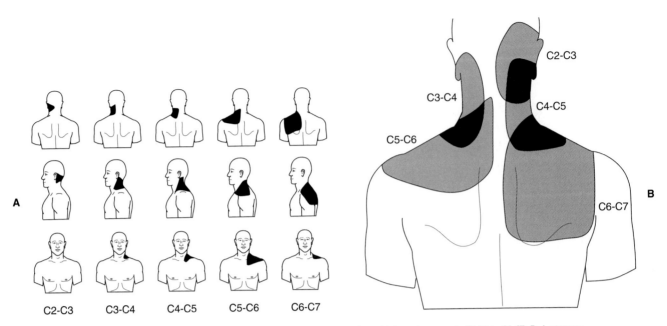

Fig. 4-14. **A**, Patterns of pain evoked by stimulating the zygapophyseal joints at segments C2-C3 to C6-C7. **B**, A composite map depicting the characteristic distribution of pain from zygapophyseal joints at segments C2-C3 to C6-C7. (From Dwyer A, Aprill C, Bogduk N: Cervical zygapophyseal joint pain patterns I: a study in normal voulunteers, *Spine* 15(6):453, 1990.)

vical spine are *Practical Orthopedic Medicine* by Corrigan and Maitland[20] and *Vertebral Manipulation* by Maitland.[46]

Thoracic Spine

Thoracic mobility affects shoulder mobility. During unilateral shoulder flexion, contralateral side flexion of the spine occurs; bilateral shoulder flexion produces spinal extension.[36] Therefore decreased thoracic extensibility or increased thoracic kyphosis can inhibit shoulder ROM.[4]

Postural education is important, especially with patients who can voluntarily correct and maintain good posture. Maintaining an erect posture while performing upper extremity activities allows greater ROM at the shoulders. Better posture decreases the amount of impingement, which a patient can see in the following maneuver:

1. Have the patient flex the shoulder through its available ROM while in a seated slouched position.
2. Ask the patient to flex the shoulder while seated with good posture.

The patient will be able to lift the arm higher when maintaining a more upright posture. A slouched position causes depressed forward-displaced shoulders and glenohumeral internal rotation. The potential for shoulder impingement increases with this type of posture.[4]

Evaluation and treatment of the thoracic spine may prove helpful for patients having difficulty progressing in ROM in the latter stages. Addressing issues of hypomobility and decreased ROM of the thoracic spine

and treating them appropriately allows for better progress. Mobilization of a hypomobile thoracic spine and ROM exercises to increase thoracic extension (e.g., supine on a Swiss ball) can be beneficial. A foam roll also may be used when appropriate to increase thoracic spinal extension and mobility (see Fig. 4-12). (*Vertebral Manipulation*[46] offers instruction on evaluation and treatment of the thoracic spine.) With regard to positioning, the therapist also must consider protection of the shoulder and the surgery site.

Adverse Neural Tension

The nervous system can be directly mobilized through tension tests and their derivatives.[16] Adhesions in neural tissue can limit shoulder movement and may influence the patient's progress after surgery. Evaluating and addressing positive adverse neural tension (ANT) issues can help relieve some of the patient's symptoms and potentially improve ROM. Treatment to the nervous system should only be performed by clinicians trained in neural tissue mobilization.

When performing ANT evaluations and administering techniques for mobilization, the therapist must remember to plan for protection of the shoulder and the surgery site. Therefore, standard upper limb tension tests (ULTTs) as described by Elvey[25] is inappropriate during the first 8 weeks after surgery.

Later, when the positioning required for a ULTT is safe, the clinician can evaluate for signs of ANT. Modifications can be made for patients who have restricted movements by placing the shoulder within the pain-free range before completing the other movements. These modifications will decrease the sensitivity of the test, but more susceptible ANT issues maybe provoked.

Precautions. It is often easy to forget the other structures that could be affected by tension testing and thereby cause injury or aggravation. In testing for spinal stenosis or spondylosis a neural response is more likely to occur earlier in the range.[16] The nervous system can be easily irritated and is particularly reactive because it is more mechanosensitive and chemosensitive than other structures. The therapist should exercise caution in the presence of neurologic signs, dizziness, or circulatory disturbances. Finally, he or she should respect pathologic conditions that affect the nervous system (e.g., diabetes, leprosy, acquired immunodeficiency syndrome [AIDS], multiple sclerosis) and protect the surgical area by maintaining all necessary restrictions.[16]

Contraindications. Among the contraindications to treatment are the following signs and symptoms:
- Recent onset or worsening of neurologic signs
- Injury to the spinal cord
- Cauda equina lesions

Acromioclavicular Joint

Osteoarthritis (OA) in the AC joint is not uncommon.[24] It may result from previous trauma or be part of a primary generalized OA, impingement, or capsulitis. OA in the AC joint also may follow other abnormalities in the glenohumeral joint (e.g., degeneration and rupture of the rotator cuff) that allow the head of the humerus to sublux upward.[20] In the experience of the authors of this chapter, many patients with repaired and unrepaired rotator cuff tears have some symptoms arising from a hypomobile AC joint.

Because the movement of the shoulder complex is affected by the movement of all the joints, it is essential to evaluate and treat the entire shoulder complex to improve upper extremity function.[42] Table 4-6 shows all the joint movements that occur within the shoulder complex. Restrictions in one area will affect other areas of the shoulder complex.

Complaints of AC joint pain are usually localized over the joint. An active movement that may best implicate this joint as a source of pain is horizontal adduction of the arm across the chest. The therapist may determine whether the AC joint is hypomobile or hypermobile by passive accessory movement tests of the joint.[64] If the AC joint is stiff and tender, its mobilization often relieves a portion of the symptoms and promotes better shoulder ROM.

Accessory movements can be applied to the clavicle or acromion. When applied to the clavicle they affect only the AC joint, but when applied to the acromion they affect both the AC and glenohumeral joints.[64] Accessory AC joint movements should be used within the limits of pain. To increase motion at the AC joint, the therapist should use an anterior glide to the acromion through the posterior spine of the scapula while stabilizing the mid-clavicle. This allows mobilization of the AC joint without direct manual pressure over the joint or inflamed tissues. As the available shoulder ROM progresses this same technique can be applied with the shoulder in some degree of available flexion or in horizontal adduction (see Fig 4-5).

Corrigan and Maitland[20] describe a similar technique for the AC joint. In this method an anteroposterior movement is produced by applying pressure over the anterior surface of the outer third of the clavicle with counterpressure along the spine of the scapula.

Sternoclavicular Joint

Degenerative changes are not found as commonly in the sternoclavicular joint as in the AC joint but may occur as the result of trauma or overuse of the shoulder.[38] Movements such as shoulder abduction or flexion may increase pain originating from this joint because of rotation of the inner end of the clavicle. Sternoclavicular joint pain is usually localized to the sternoclavicular area, but it may radiate to other areas. Signs that implicate the sternoclavicular joint as a contributing factor include reproduction of pain with horizontal flexion and passive accessory movements of the sternoclavicular joint. The capsule and surrounding ligaments are likely to be thickened and tender.[64]

Treatment of the sternoclavicular area includes rest, modalities, and mobilization, depending on the condition of the joint.[20] A hypomobile sternoclavicular joint may be correctly mobilized in several ways depending on its restrictions. To increase shoulder elevation, a caudal glide to the proximal clavicle can be used.[20,45]

Scapulothoracic Joint

Scapular muscles have been included in the rotator cuff repair protocol. However, some patients require more intense conditioning of these muscles. The scapula moves with concentric/eccentric motions. Patients with poor eccentric control of the scapular stabilizers demonstrate scapula winging on the return from full shoulder flexion. These same patients may have full ROM and normal movement during flexion. If muscle weakness is apparent, ensuring normal muscle strength around the scapulothoracic and glenohumeral joints is the goal. If the scapular muscles are weak and overstretched, scapular motion during arm elevation may result in excessive lateral gliding of the scapula.

The therapist can use various PNF techniques such as scapular slow reversal holds, rhythmic stabilization,

Table 4-6 The Shoulder Complex—Range and Axis of Motion

Joint Motion	Range (Degrees)	Axis of Motion
Sternoclavicular		
Rotation (counterclockwise)	0-50	Longitudinal axis of clavicle
Elevation	0-30	Oblique through
Depression	0-5	costoclavicular ligament
Protraction	0-15	Vertical through
Retraction	0-15	costoclavicular ligament
Glenohumeral		
Flexion	0-180	Coronal through
Hyperflexion	0-55	glenohumeral joint
Abduction	0-180	Sagittal through glenohumeral
Horizontal adduction	0-145	joint; vertical through
		glenohumeral joint
Internal rotation	0-90	Vertical axis through
External rotation	0-90	shaft of humerus
Acromioclavicular		
Winging of scapula	0-50	Vertical axis through
		acromioclavicular joint
Abduction of scapula	0-30	Anteroposterior axis
Inferior angle of scapula tilts away	0-30	Coronal axis
from chest wall		
Scapulothoracic		
Upward rotation	0-60	From 0°-30° near vertebral
		border on spine of scapula;
		from 30°-60° near acromial
		end of spine of scapula
Elevation	Translatory	No axis
Depression	Translatory	No axis
Protraction	Translatory	No axis
Retraction	Translatory	No axis

Material for this table was compiled from a number of references.[1,2,4,9,14,18,21] When conflicting information occurred, the most frequently cited numbers were used.

and timing for emphasis to intensify the dynamic control and kinesthesia of the scapulothoracic joint. Other recommended exercises are scapular protraction, retraction, elevation, and depression against manual resistance.[67]

Exercises that enhance dynamic control of the scapulothoracic musculature are encouraged.[67] These should be directed to the scapular rotator muscles (i.e., the serratus anterior, rhomboid, trapezius, levator scapula) to position the glenoid and coracoid appropriately for the humerus. Exercises that mimic the rowing motion and shoulder horizontal abduction are both excellent for all portions of the trapezius and for the levator scapulae and rhomboid muscles. Flexion and scaption (scapular plane elevation) exercises are valuable for most of the scapular muscles (see Fig. 4-4). In addition, shoulder shrugs and press-ups with a "plus" are essential exercises for the levator scapula, upper trapezius, serratus anterior, and pectoralis minor muscles.

Summary

The general guidelines described help guide therapists and provide treatment ideas. Rotator cuff repairs vary in size from small to massive. The condition of the torn tissue and the joints (AC and glenohumeral) varies. Along with these differences therapists must consider the patient's unique history, profile, and abilities. They must consider each case and choose the treatment ideas that will work best, constantly assessing the patient's responses. Therapists must always address the individual when deciding on a treatment plan.

Suggested Home Maintenance for the Postsurgical Patient

Older, more sedentary patients will progress more slowly than younger, more active patients. Some of the exercises suggested may be inappropriate for the older patient. The therapist can alter the home exercise prescription according to the individual's abilities, status, and needs.

Weeks 1-4

GOALS FOR THE PERIOD: Achieve control of pain and inflammation; increase ROM as tolerated.
1. Active cervical spine rotations
2. Upper trapezius (UT) stretches
3. Pendulum exercises
4. Begin submaximal isometrics at 3 weeks for shoulder flexion and internal rotation
5. Begin submaximal isometrics at 4 weeks for shoulder abduction and external rotation
6. Begin wand exercises when able

Weeks 5-7

1. Continue with previous exercises
2. Progress with wand exercises
3. Add active shoulder flexion in supine position when cleared by the surgeon
4. Perform self-mobilization to thoracic spine using tennis balls or foam roll
5. Massage scar area after incision has healed

Weeks 8-12

GOALS FOR THE PERIOD: Increase ROM, strength, and ability to perform functional movements.
1. Continue with wand exercises
2. Continue with active cervical ROM, UT stretches, and T/S mobilization as needed
3. Perform active shoulder flexion and abduction in the functional plane while facing a mirror; be sure to maintain voluntary humeral head depression
4. Initiate isotonic exercises when able to elevate arm without substitution patterns; initiate isotonic exercises for the following:
    a. Deltoid
    b. Supraspinatus
    c. Elbow flexors
    d. Scapular muscles
    e. Scaption exercises
5. Use tubing or Theraband for external and internal rotation while working with axillary roll
6. Do standing reverse rows using tubing or Theraband
7. Perform prone horizontal abduction in neutral position with external rotation of the humeral head
8. Do push-ups with a "plus" while standing and using a wall

Continued

❧ Suggested Home Maintenance for the Postsurgical Patient—cont'd

Weeks 13-16

GOALS FOR THE PERIOD: Increase ROM, strength, and endurance and begin transitioning into higher activity levels.
1. Continue with wand exercises
2. Continue with active ROM of the cervical spine, UT stretches, and T/S mobilizations as needed
3. Perform corner wall stretch for the anterior capsule
4. Use horizontal adduction stretch for the posterior capsule
5. Place hand behind back and stretch, using a towel for assistance
6. Continue and progress resistance with isotonic exercises
7. Continue and progress resistance with tubing and Theraband exercises
8. For appropriate patients (generally too difficult for elderly patients): do seated push-ups with a "plus" (see Fig. 4-11)
9. Perform prone horizontal abduction exercises with dumbbell

Weeks 17-21

1. Continue with previous stretches
2. Continue with PREs (isotonics)
3. Continue to progress with tubing and Theraband exercises
4. Begin interval sports program for athletes (see Appendix A)

Weeks 22-26

1. Continue stretches
2. Continue PREs
3. Progress with interval sports program

REFERENCES

1. Abrams JS: Special shoulder problems in the throwing athlete: pathology, diagnosis and nonoperative management, *Clin Sports Med* 10:839, 1991.
2. Anderson L et al: The effects of a Theraband exercise program on shoulder internal rotation strength, *Phys Ther* (suppl) 72(6):540, 1992.
3. Andrews JR, Kupferman SP, Dillman CJ: Labral tears in throwing and racquet sports, *Clin Sports Med* 10(4):901, 1991.
4. Ayoub E: Posture and the upper quarter. In Donatelli R, editor: *Physical therapy of the shoulder*, New York, 1987, Churchill Livingstone.
5. Baker CL, Liu SH: Comparison of open and arthroscopically assisted rotator cuff repairs, *Am J Sports Med* 23:99, 1995.
6. Baylis RW, Wolf EM: *Arthroscopic rotator cuff repair: clinical and arthroscopic second-look assessment,* presented at Annual Meeting of the Arthroscopy Association of North America, San Francisco, May 1995.
7. Bigliani LU et al: Operative treatment of failed repairs of the rotator cuff, *Am J Bone Joint Surg* 74A:1505, 1992.
8. Bigliani LU et al: Operative management of failed rotator cuff repairs, *Orthop Trans* 12:674, 1988.
9. Bigliani LU, Morrison DS, April EW: The morphology of the acromion and its relationship to rotator cuff tears, *Orthop Trans* 10:216, 1986.
10. Bigliani LU, Morrison D, April EW: The morphology of the acromion and its relationship to rotator cuff tears, *Orthop Trans* 10:228, 1986.
11. Blevins FT et al: Arthroscopic assisted rotator cuff repair: results using a mini-open deltoid splitting approach, *Arthroscopy* 12:50, 1996.
12. Brewster C, Moynes-Schwab D: Rehabilitation of the shoulder following rotator cuff injury or surgery, *JOSPT* 18(2):422, 1993.
13. Bross R et al: Optimal number of exercise bouts per week for isokinetic eccentric training of the rotator cuff musculature, *Wisc Phys Ther Assoc Newsletter* (Abstr) 21(5):18, 1991.

14. Brotzman BS: *Clinical orthopaedic rehabilitation*, St Louis, 1996, Mosby.

15. Burkhart S: Reconciling the paradox of rotator cuff repair versus debridement: a unified biomechanical rationale for treatment of rotator cuff tears, *Arthroscopy* 10(1):4, 1994.

16. Butler DS: *Mobilisation of the nervous system*, New York, 1991, Churchill Livingstone.

17. Calvert PT, Packer NP, Staker DJ: Arthrography of the shoulder after operative repair of the torn rotator cuff, *Br J Bone Joint Surg* 68:147, 1986.

18. Caspari RB, Thal R: A technique for arthroscopic subacromial decompression, *Arthroscopy* 8:23, 1992.

19. Codman EA, Akerson IB: The pathology associated with rupture of the supraspinatus tendon, *Am Surg* 93:348, 1931.

20. Corrigan B, Maitland GD: *Practical orthopaedic medicine*, London, 1987, Butterworth.

21. Craven WM: Traumatic avulsion tears of the rotator cuff. In Andrews JR, Wilk KE, editors: *The athlete's shoulder*, New York, 1994, Churchill Livingstone.

22. Cyriax J: *Textbook of orthopaedic medicine: diagnosis of soft tissue lesions*, vol 1, Baltimore, 1975, Williams and Wilkins.

23. Davies GJ, Dickoff-Hoffman S: Neuromuscular testing and rehabilitation of the shoulder complex, *JOSPT* 18(2):449, 1993.

24. de Palma AF: *Degenerative changes in the sternoclavicular and acromioclavicular joints in various decades*, Springfield, IL, 1957, Thomas.

25. Elvey R: *Treatment of conditions accompanied by signs of abnormal brachial plexus tension*, proceedings of the Manipulative Therapists Association of Australia, Neck and Shoulder Symposium, Queensland, Australia, 1983.

26. Esch JC et al: Arthroscopic subacromial decompression: results according to degree of rotator cuff tear, *Arthroscopy* 4:241, 1988.

27. Gartsman GM: Arthroscopic acromioplasty for lesions of the rotator cuff, *Am J Bone Joint Surg* 72:169, 1990.

28. Gerber C, Terrier F, Fane R: The role of the coracoid process in the chronic impingement syndrome, *Am J Bone Joint Surg* 67B:703, 1985.

29. Grieve G: Manual mobilizing techniques in degenerative arthrosis of the hip, Bulletin of the Orthopaedic Section, *APTA* 2(1):7, 1977.

30. Harryman DT, II, et al: Repairs of the rotator cuff: correlation of functional results with integrity of the cuff, *Am J Bone Joint Surg* 73:982, 1991.

31. Hawkins RJ, Misamore GW, Hobeika PE: Surgery for full-thickness rotator cuff tears, *Am J Bone Joint Surg* 67A:139, 1985.

32. Iannotti JP: Full thickness rotator cuff tears: factors affecting surgical outcome, *J Am Acad Ortho Surg* 2:87, 1994.

33. Iannotti JP et al: Prospective evaluation of rotator cuff repair, *J Shoulder Elbow Surg* 2:69, 1993.

34. Itoi E, Tabata S: Conservative treatment of rotator cuff tear, *Clin Orthop* 275:165, 1992.

35. Jenp NY et al: Activation of the rotator cuff in generating isometric shoulder rotation torque, *Am J Sports Med* 24(4):477, 1996.

36. Kapangi IA: *Physiology of joints*, vol 1, New York, 1970, Churchill Livingstone.

37. Kisner C, Colby LA: *Therapeutic exercise foundations and techniques*, Philadelphia, 1985, FA Davis Company.

38. Kopp S et al: Degenerative disease of the temporal mandibular, metatarso-phalangeal and sternoclavicular joints: an autopsy study, *Acta Odontol Scand* 23:34, 1976.

39. Kvitne RS, Jobe FW: The diagnosis and treatment of anterior instability in the throwing athlete, *Clin Orthop* 291:107, 1993.

40. Lazarus MD et al: Comparison of open and arthroscopic subacromial decompression, *J Shoulder Elbow Surg* 3:1, 1994.

41. Levy HJ, Uribe JW, Delaney LG: Arthroscopically-assisted rotator cuff repair. Preliminary results, *Arthroscopy* 6:55, 1990.

42. Lucas DB: Biomechanics of the shoulder joint, *Arch Surg* 107:425, 1973.

43. Lui SH: Arthroscopically-assisted rotator cuff repair, *Br J Bone Joint Surg* 76:592, 1994.

44. Lui SH, Baker CL: Arthroscopically-assisted rotator cuff repair: correlation of functional results with integrity of the cuff, *Arthroscopy* 10:54, 1991.

45. Maitland GD: *Peripheral joint manipulation*, ed 3, Newton, MA, 1991, Butterworth.

46. Maitland GD: *Vertebral manipulations*, ed 5, Newton, MA, 1986, Butterworth.

47. Moseley HF, Goldie I: The arterial pattern of the rotator cuff of the shoulder, *Br J Bone Joint Surg* 45:780, 1963.

48. Neer CS: Anterior acromioplasty for the chronic impingement syndrome in the shoulder: a preliminary report, *Am J Bone Joint Surg* 54:41, 1972.

49. Neer CS: Impingement lesions, *Clin Orthop* 173:70, 1983.

50. Neer CS, Welsh RP: The shoulder in sports, *Orthop Clin North Am* 8:583, 1977.

51. Nelson MC et al: Evaluation of the painful shoulder, *Am J Bone Joint Surg* (suppl) 73:707, 1991.

52. Neviaser RJ, Neviaser TJ, Neviaser JS: Concurrent rupture of the rotator cuff and anterior dislocation of the shoulder in the older patient, *Am J Bone Joint Surg* 70:1308, 1988.

53. Osternig LR et al: Differential responses to proprioceptive neuromuscular facilitation stretch techniques, *Med Sci Sports Exerc* 22(1):106, 1990.

54. Rathbun JB, Macnab I: The microvascular pattern of the rotator cuff, *Br J Bone Joint Surg* 45:540, 1970.

55. Rockwood CA, Jr, Williams GR: The shoulder impingement syndrome: management of surgical treatment failures, *Orthop Trans* 16:739, 1992.

56. Rothman RM, Parke WW: The vascular anatomy of the rotator cuff, *Clin Orthop* 41:176, 1965.

57. Roye KP, Grana WA, Yates CK: Arthroscopic subacromial decompression: two to seven year follow up, *Arthroscopy* 11:301, 1995.

58. Ryu RK: Arthroscopic subacromial decompression: a clinical review, *Arthroscopy* 8:141, 1992.

59. Seitz WH, Froimson AI, Shapiro JD: Chronic impingement syndrome: the role of ultrasonography and arthroscopic anterior acromioplasty, *Orthop Rev* 18:364, 1989.

60. Shields JR: *Manual of sports surgery,* New York, 1987, Springer-Verlag.

61. Stollsteimer GT, Savie FH, III: Arthroscopic rotator cuff repair: current indication, limitations, techniques and results. In Cannon WD, editor: *Instructional course lectures 47,* Rosemont, IL, 1998, American Academy of Orthopaedic Surgeons.

62. Tauro JC: Arthroscopic rotator cuff repair: analysis of technique and results at 2 year and 3 year follow-up, *Arthroscopy* 14(1):45, 1998.

63. Tibone JE et al: Shoulder impingement syndrome in athletes treated by anterior acromioplasty, *Clin Orthop* 134:140, 1985.

64. Trott PH: *Differential mechanical diagnosis of shoulder pain,* proceedings of the Manipulative Therapists Association of Australia, 1985.

65. Walch G et al: Impingement of the deep surface of the supraspinatus tendon on the posterosuperior glenoid rim: an arthroscopic study, *J Shoulder Elbow Surg* 1:238, 1992.

66. Weber S: *Arthroscopic vs. mini-open rotator cuff repairs. A prospective study,* presented at the 64th Annual American Academy of Orthopaedic Surgeons, San Francisco, 1997.

67. Wilk KE, Arrigo CA: An integral approach to upper extremity exercises, *Orthop Phys Ther Clin North Am* 9(2):337, 1992.

68. Wilk KE, Arrigo C: Current concepts in the rehabilitation of the athletic shoulder, *JOSPT* 18(1):365, 1993.

69. Wilk KE et al: Stretch-shortening drills for the upper extremity, theory and clinical application, *J Orthop Sports Phys Ther* 17(5):225, 1993.

70. Wiley AM: Arthroscopy for shoulder instability and a technique for arthroscopic repair, *Arthroscopy* 1:30, 1988.

Chapter 5

Extensor Brevis Release and Lateral Epicondylectomy

James Calandruccio
Kelly Akin
Kristen L. Griffith

A pathologic condition of the wrist extensor tendons at their origin on the elbow is commonly termed *lateral epicondylitis* or *tennis elbow*. However, the syndrome of lateral elbow pain is neither exclusively inflammatory nor always related to athletic activity.[15] The lack of inflammatory cells in the tissue removed from patients during surgical intervention makes the term *lateral epicondylitis* a misnomer. Moreover, many patients who have focal tenderness just distal and anterior to the lateral epicondyle and localized pain in the same region with wrist extension do not play tennis.

Surgical Indication and Considerations

Etiology

Injury to the extensor tendons at the elbow often can be attributed to repetitive trauma or overuse, leading to mechanical fatigue or biomechanical overload. Some literature reports the possibility of exostosis in the area of the extensor tendons or a degenerative process that causes pain at the lateral epicondyle.[7] Symptoms may be described as an ache at the elbow with sharp pain that infrequently radiates to the dorsal forearm and occasionally to the middle and ring fingers with attendant loss of grip.[18]

The most frequently involved tendon is that originating from the extensor carpi radialis brevis (ECRB). It is responsible for the static wrist extension required for certain tasks and stabilizes the wrist while grasping. Lesions can occur at the extensor digitorum communis, extensor carpi ulnaris, extensor digiti minimi, and supinator tendon. According to the current literature microtraumatic ECRB tendon tears may propagate to include the common extensors.[15] Plancher et al[15] report that gross tendon rupture is noted in a large number of patients at the time of surgical intervention.

Microtears can result from repeated sprains, repetitive forceful wrist extension and gripping, and suboptimal mechanics in hitting. Inadequate racquet size or improper tool grip size also can predispose to injury. Other factors that may influence the onset of symptoms are inadequate strength, endurance, and flexibility of the forearm musculature; changes in regular activity; increasing age; and hormonal imbalance in women.[18] The incidence is equal in men and women during the fourth and fifth decades, with 75% of all cases involving the dominant arm.[15] Among the older population, the insult is predominantly work-related, in contrast to the sports-related injuries seen in the younger population.

Lateral epicondylitis can be managed successfully nonsurgically in 90% of patients with a combination of activity modification, nonsteroidal antiinflammatory medication, functional and counter-force bracing, various therapeutic modalities, and injection therapy. A small percentage of patients with persistent and disabling symptoms require surgical intervention.[3] Lesions caused by overuse during job-related activities are more likely to require surgical intervention secondary to an inability to stop the aggravating activity.

Indications for surgery are individualized according to patient demands and activity level. The period of disability and previous conservative management must be considered before surgical management is chosen. There are no absolute indications for surgical intervention to treat lateral epicondylitis, and the clinician must exercise caution in cases in which secondary gain may be important.

The most important factors in considering surgical intervention are the intensity, frequency, and duration of disability caused by pain. Constant and unrelenting focal lateral elbow discomfort is not tolerated well by active individuals. Most patients treated surgically have symptoms for 1 year, but special consideration may be given to patients in whom other therapies have failed after 6 months of aggressive attempts. When symptoms are present for more than 12 months, they will rarely respond to further therapeutic management. Although cortisone injections are reserved for significant cases of tennis elbow, the failure of three or more injections to produce relief is another indication for surgery. These injections are usually delivered over a 6- to 12-month period.

Calcification around the lateral aspect of the elbow portends a less favorable outcome to conservative measures. Calcification seen on x-ray examination may occur in as many as 20% of cases and may indicate the need for surgical intervention before the 1-year period ends.

Surgical Procedure (Modified Nirschl Method)

Numerous surgical procedures to treat lateral epicondylitis have been described, and no single technique has been or will be adopted by all surgeons. The common denominator for all procedures, however, is the alleviation of traction on the diseased ECRB origin. Hypervascular granulation tissue is characteristically found on the undersurface of the ECRB attachment to

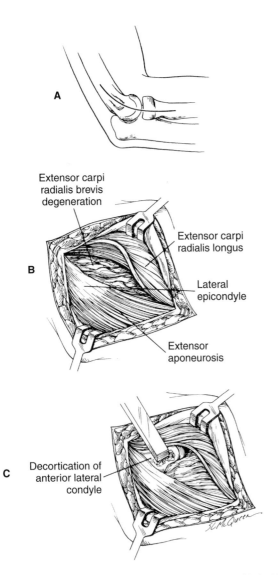

Fig. 5-1. Surgical technique for correction of tennis elbow. **A,** Skin incision, **B,** Identification of the origins of the extensor carpi radialis longus and extensor digitorum communis. **C,** Osteotome decortication. (Redrawn from Nirschl RP, Pettrone F: The surgical treatment of lateral epicondylitis, *J Bone Joint Surg* 61A:832, 1972. In Canale ST, editor: *Campbell's operative orthopedics,* St Louis, 1998, Mosby.)

the lateral epicondyle and appears as tan-gray degenerative regions. A limited approach that is commonly used consists of resection of the diseased section of the tendon and lateral epicondylectomy.

A 5-cm-long, gently curved incision is centered over the lateral epicondyle. The extensor fascia is identified through this opening (Fig. 5-1, *A*). The anterior edge of the ECRB tendon origin is clearly developed by elevating the posterior border of the extensor carpi radialis longus, which at this level is muscular and partially overrides the ECRB origin. The extensor digitorum communis origin partially obscures the deeper portion of the ECRB (Fig. 5-1, *B*). The ECRB portion of the conjoined tendon is elevated at the mid-portion of the lateral epicondyle, distally in line with the forearm axis toward the elbow joint. The abnormal-appearing ECRB tendon is sharply dissected from the normal-appearing Sharpey's fibers. The diseased tissue may appear fibrillated and discolored and can contain calcium deposits.

Occasionally the disease process also involves the extensor digitorum communis origin. There is no reason to enter the joint itself unless preoperative evaluation indicates an intra-articular process such as loose bodies, degenerative joint disease, effusion, and synovial thickening.

The lateral 0.5 cm of the lateral epicondyle is decorticated with a rongeur or osteotome, with the surgeon taking care not to enter the joint and damage the articular cartilage (Fig. 5-1, *C*). The ECRB is intimately associated with the annular ligament just proximal to the radial head, thereby limiting distal migration of the ECRB tendon. However, the remaining normal ECRB tendon may be sutured to the fascia or periosteum or attached with nonabsorbable sutures through drill holes in the epicondyle.

The extensor carpi radialis longus and extensor digitorum communis interval is closed with absorbable sutures. The skin incision may be closed with subcuticular nylon (4-0) sutures and adhesive strips.

Surgical Outcomes

According to Nirschl,[13,14] 85% of patients were able to return to all previous activities without pain. Pain that occurred during aggressive activities was noted in 12% of the cases observed, and no improvement was apparent in 3% of the cases. Reasons for failure include misdiagnosis or the concomitant diagnosis of entrapment of the posterior interosseous nerve, intra-articular disorders, or lateral elbow instability. Poor prognostic factors include poor initial response to cortisone injections, numerous previous cortisone injections, bilateral lateral epicondylitis, other concomitant associated disorders, and smoking.

Therapy Guidelines for Rehabilitation

Phase I

TIME: 1 to 14 days after surgery
GOALS: Achieve full range of motion (ROM) of adjacent joints, promote wound healing, control edema and pain, and increase active range of motion (AROM) of the elbow (Table 5-1)

After surgery, the therapist instructs the patient concerning the need to elevate the site to avoid edema and initiates gentle AROM exercises for the hand and shoulder. The patient is to remain immobilized in the postoperative splint with the elbow positioned at 90 degrees.

On the fifth day after surgery the postsurgical dressing and splint are removed and therapy is initiated to the elbow. In this phase the patient's wounds are kept clean and dry until the sutures are removed 10 to 14 days after surgery. After the operative site has been exposed, other forms of edema control can be used, including ice, pneumatic intermittent compression (performed at a 3:1 on/off ratio at a pressure of 50 mmHg), and high-voltage galvanic stimulation (HVGS). The recommended settings for the use of HVGS to prevent edema are negative polarity with continuous modulation at 100 intrapulse microseconds and intensity to the sensory level.[8] The patient also can be fitted with a light elastic compression wrap or stockinette (such as Coban or Tubi-Grip) to wear intermittently throughout the day and at night for continued edema control at home (Fig. 5-2). AROM exercises also are initiated for the elbow, forearm, and wrist after the postoperative dressing is removed.[11] Passive ROM (PROM) and joint mobilization of the elbow and forearm are contraindicated at this time.

Some surgeons prefer to keep the elbow immobilized in a removable posterior elbow splint until the second week after surgery. This splint is typically fabricated from a low-temperature plastic with the elbow positioned at 90 degrees; it is worn between exercise sessions and at night (Fig. 5-3).

Pain can be managed using HVGS at the same settings as those used for edema control; the physician also may prescribe oral medications.

The first postoperative visit is a good time to begin patient education regarding activity modification and proper mechanics during work- and sports-related activities. Patients should be taught to avoid forceful static grip, repetitive wrist extension, and resistive supination. The primary mode of lifting should be a bilateral underhanded or neutral forearm approach (Fig. 5-4).

During this initial phase the therapist should closely monitor the patient's reports of pain and tolerance to ROM exercises, noting any sympathetic changes that may lead to a complex pain syndrome. Signs and symptoms to be noted are as follows:

- Pain out of proportion to the stimulus
- Excessive edema
- Temperature and color changes
- Excessive joint stiffness

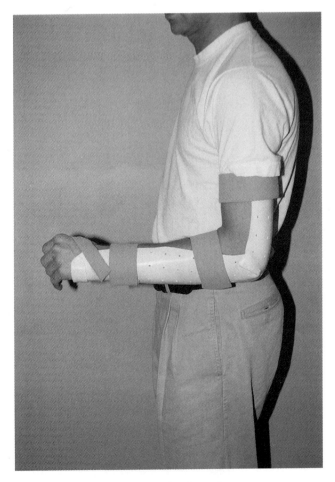

Fig. 5-3. Posterior elbow splint.

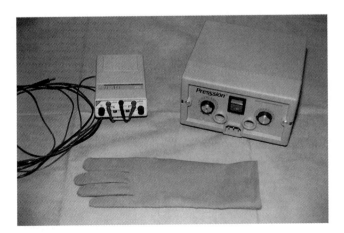

Fig. 5-2. Edema control. Portable HVGS unit, portable intermittent compression unit, and compressive garment (Isotoner glove).

Table 5-1   Extensor Brevis Release and Lateral Epicondylectomy

Rehabilitation Phase	Criteria to Progress to this Phase	Anticipated Impairments and Functional Limitations	Intervention	Goal	Rationale
Phase I Postoperative 1-2 weeks	Postoperative	• Postoperative pain • Postoperative edema • Limited upper extremity (UE) mobility • Unable to grasp and reach	• Monitoring of incision site • Instruction of client in activity modification • Cryotherapy • Pneumatic intermittent compression • HVGS • Elastic compression wrap or stockinette • Fabrication of removable splint • Passive range of motion (PROM)-AROM—Shoulder—all ranges, maintaining elbow in neutral position • AROM—Hand—Finger flexion/extension Wrist—flexion/extension Elbow (initiate after operative dressing is removed)—Flexion/ extension pronation/ supination	• Prevent infection • Decrease stress on surgical site • Decrease pain • Control and decrease edema • Protect surgical site • Maintain ROM of joints proximal and distal to the surgical site • Full AROM of neighboring joints • Elbow ROM to 60% (extension will be more limited)	• Prevention of postoperative complications • Decrease stress on the common extensor tendons • Pain control • Edema management • Prevent associated joint stiffness and dysfunction of neighboring joints and muscles • AROM to assist with pain control and promote edema management • Improved ROM of elbow (sutures are usually removed at 10 to 14 days)

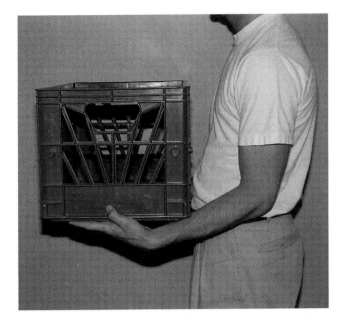

Fig. 5-4. Underhanded lifting technique.

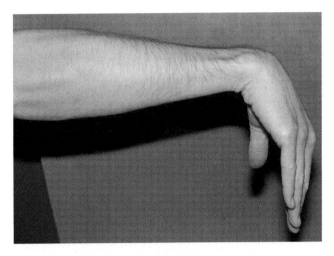

Fig. 5-5. Extreme wrist flexion with elbow extension.

Phase II

TIME: 15 days to 4 to 5 weeks after surgery
GOALS: Control edema and pain, achieve full elbow PROM, maintain full ROM of adjacent joints, and promote mobility of the scar tissue (Table 5-2)

After the immobilization phase, the therapist should initiate gentle AROM exercises for the patient's elbow three to four times each day.[9] During the first ROM phase the therapist should emphasize the importance of complying with the home exercise program as well as attending the regular therapy sessions.

ROM exercises to be included are as follows:
• Elbow extension and flexion
• Wrist extension and flexion
• Forearm supination and pronation

The patient should avoid positions that place maximal stress on the common extensor tendons such as elbow extension with extreme wrist flexion (Fig. 5-5).[18] To prevent re-injury, progressive resistive exercises also should be avoided at this time. Stanley and Tribuzi[18] recommend isometric exercises with the wrist in a neutral position or at no more than 30 degrees of extension or flexion in preparation for further resistive training.

As ROM progresses, the therapist should carefully monitor the patient's edema. The management of edema is specific to the patient and only one technique may be required. The following technique can be used for mild edema:
1. Ice and elevation for 10 minutes at the end of treatment
2. Compression wraps and stockinette
3. HVGS for 15 minutes

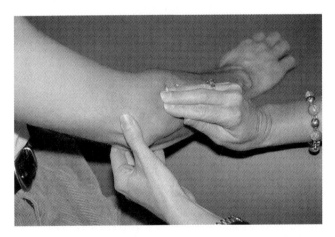

Fig. 5-6. Scar remodeling by manual massage technique.

Moderate edema is treated with the following:
1. Retrograde massage
2. Intermittent pneumatic compression with elevation
3. HVGS with elevation and ice for 20 to 30 minutes

After the sutures are removed and the incision has healed appropriately, scar management is needed. This includes both desensitization and scar remodeling. Because hypersensitivity can limit functional use, desensitization should begin during the patient's first therapy session after suture removal.[9] Scar remodeling consists of using massage (when appropriate) to help maintain mobility of the scar by freeing restrictive fibrous bands, increasing circulation, and allowing the pressure to flatten and smooth the scar site (Fig. 5-6).[9] The therapist also may consider using a silicone gel sheet or other silicone-based putty mix as a pad over the scar to assist in remodeling.

Table 5-2   Extensor Brevis Release and Lateral Epicondylectomy

Rehabilitation Phase	Criteria to Progress to this Phase	Anticipated Impairments and Functional Limitations	Intervention	Goal	Rationale
Phase II Postoperative 3-5 weeks	Incision well healed with no signs of infection Improving PROM of elbow No increase in pain or edema	• Continued pain and mild edema • Limited UE mobility • Unable to grasp and reach for functional use	• Continuation of edema and pain management techniques as in Phase I • Soft tissue massage • Retrograde massage with elevation • Scar desensitization after sutures are removed and incision is healed Silicon gel sheet for scar pad • PROM—Elbow flexion/extension (within pain tolerance) • Isometrics (with wrist in neutral position—between 30° flexion/extension) Wrist flexion/extension	• Intermittent pain • Manage edema • Encourage limited activity of daily living performance • Promote scar mobility and proper remodeling • Promote full elbow PROM • Encourage quality muscle contraction	• Management of edema and pain with progression to self-management • Improvement of soft tissue mobility • Use of compression to remodel scar • Promotion of normal joint arthrokinematics • Preparation of muscles for further resistive training

The therapist should instruct the patient to rub the sensitive area for 2 to 5 minutes three to four times daily with textures such as fur, yarn, rice, Styrofoam, or corn. Other useful textures include towels, clothing, dry beans, and rice.[9]

Patients will be limited to lifting no more than 10 pounds after surgery. On grip strength testing, patients typically demonstrate a 50% deficit when the operative hand is compared with the nonoperative one.

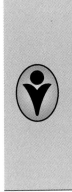

Q. Jim is 34 years old. Approximately 7 weeks ago he had an extensor brevis release and lateral epicondylectomy performed. He is anxious to recover quickly so he can play softball on the weekends. Mild resisted exercises were initiated 1 week ago, and Jim is performing them at home. His pain level has noticeably increased over the past 4 days. However, he can control the pain with ice and antiinflammatory medication. Should Jim's exercise program be altered? If so, how should it be altered?

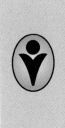

Q. Janet is a 35-year-old accountant. She had an extensor brevis releases and lateral epicondylectomy after various attempts at conservative treatment failed. At 7 weeks after surgery Janet's elbow extension ROM is −15 degrees. What type of treatment may be effective at this stage for increasing her elbow extension?

Phase III

TIME: Between 4 to 6 weeks to 6 months after surgery
GOALS: Control pain, maintain full elbow and forearm ROM, strengthen upper extremity, and regain normal forearm flexibility (Table 5-3)

Between 4 to 6 weeks after surgery the therapist should initiate a progressive strengthening program.[9] At this point in the rehabilitative process the patient should have full ROM of the hand, wrist, and elbow, and the focus should be on building strength and training for endurance with the goal of returning the patient to work or sports.

The goal of the strengthening program is to promote conditioning of the entire UE, particularly the forearm, to prevent re-injury caused by overstretching or overloading. To ensure that maximal strength-

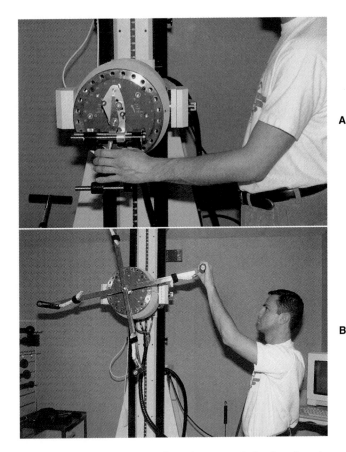

Fig. 5-7. A, Baltimore Therapeutic Equipment work simulator for grip strengthening. **B,** Simulated work activity.

ening is achieved, eccentric exercises are recommended for the extrinsic forearm muscles.[18] At this time it is appropriate to initiate extrinsic forearm stretching.

Each patient's conditioning program is formulated according to activity tolerance, previous activity level, and requirements for return to work or sports. If the patient can perform active exercises without pain, he or she is well enough to begin resistive and light work or sports-related activities using free weights and a work stimulator such as the Baltimore Therapeutic Equipment (BTE) or Lido (Fig. 5-7). The key is to continue educating the patient and training her or him to lift with the forearm in a neutral position and avoid postures that stress the extensor muscles.

The components of the program are as follows:
- Hand (grip and pinch) strengthening
- Forearm strengthening
- Upper arm strengthening
- Shoulder strengthening
- Endurance training

Normally a return to activity can be anticipated by the fourth month after surgery.[11]

Table 5-3 Extensor Brevis Release and Lateral Epicondylectomy

Rehabilitation Phase	Criteria to Progress to this Phase	Anticipated Impairments and Functional Limitations	Intervention	Goal	Rationale
Phase III Postoperative 6-24 weeks	PROM full and AROM near full Pain and edema controlled/self-managed No decrease in strength since last phase	• Minimal, intermittent pain and edema • Minimal mobility limitations in elbow • Unable to grasp and reach for functional use	• Continue pain and edema management as indicated • Patient education regarding activity modification and performance of activities with good mechanics • Progressive resistance exercises (PREs)—Putty exercises—finger pinch and grip • Isotonics—Shoulder (see Chapter 2) Elbow—flexion, extension, pronation, and supination Wrist—flexion, extension, radial and ulnar deviation • Work simulator (12-16 weeks) • Return to sport program (refer to Appendix A) (12-16 weeks)	• Self-manage pain • Prevent flare-up with progression of functional activities • Grip strength to 85% of uninvolved side • Symmetric strength of shoulder and scapula region • Wrist strength to within 80% • Return to previous activity/work level	• Avoidance of postures that place stress on the extensor musculature • Promotion of return to functional activities without flare of symptoms • Increased strength and endurance for return to work or sport • Strengthening of upper quarter to ensure optimal functional use of UE • Monitoring of wrist isotonics to ensure safe maximal strengthening • Simulation of work/sport loads in the clinic to train muscles to allow safe return to sport or work

A. Jim is aggravating his symptoms with the exercises. He also may be doing the home exercises too aggressively. The primary goal should be to alleviate pain and swelling. After pain and swelling are under control, gradual strengthening can be initiated in small doses with more rest periods than before. Treatment soreness should be minimal and controllable with the administration of ice packs. The amount of exercise and resistance should be gradually increased.

 A. The patient should be placed in a dynamic splint or in a static progressive splint at night to gain full extension.

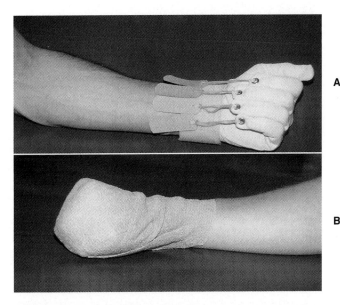

Fig. 5-8. A, Commercially available finger flexion glove for hand stiffness. B, Composite finger flexion using Coban.

Suggested Home Maintenance for the Postsurgical Patient

An exercise program has been outlined at the various phases. The home maintenance box on page 80 outlines the rehabilitation the patient is to follow. The physical therapist can use it in customizing a patient-specific program. Consideration of the patient's age, needs, and capabilities guides the rate of progression, intensity, and type of treatment provided.

Troubleshooting

Problems encountered after lateral epicondylectomy include pain, recurrence of symptoms, edema, inadequate ROM or stiffness, and scar expansion.

Increase in Pain Level or Recurrence of Symptoms

The therapist should carefully monitor the patient's pain level throughout the rehabilitation process. The Magill Pain Questionnaire can aid in monitoring changes in levels or characteristics of pain. Exercise progression should occur based on the patient's reports of pain. In some cases of severe pain, the physician may prescribe a transcutaneous electrical nerve stimulation (TENS) unit. If the pain persists or occurs at the end of the rehabilitative process, the therapist may consider the use of a counterforce brace to allow the patient to return to the previous level of activity.

Persistent Edema

Edema control involves ice, elevation, HVGS, pulsed ultrasound, compression wraps, retrograde massage, and lymphatic massage. Continuous passive motion machines have been used intermittently throughout the day and at night with some success to reduce edema. Decreasing the activity level or suspending the use of resistive exercises also may be necessary.

Inadequate ROM or Stiffness in Adjacent Areas

The most common mobility problem involves loss of full elbow extension. By 6 to 8 weeks after surgery, the therapist can talk to the surgeon about using static progressive or dynamic splints to improve extension. Static splinting is achieved by using custom-made low-temperature plastic material molded to the patient at the available end ROM and adjusted weekly. Dynamic splints are available commercially. For hand and finger stiffness, use of a flexion glove or composite flexion stretching with a Coban or elastic (Ace) wrap is usually successful (Fig. 5-8).

Increase in or Painful Scar

If the scar management techniques detailed earlier do not produce the desired result, additional methods include the following:
- Ultrasound
- Mechanical vibration
- Compressive dressings or garments to prevent scar adherence

Circumferential desensitization using fluidotherapy also may be considered.

❧ Suggested Home Maintenance for the Postsurgical Patient

Days 1-5

GOALS FOR THE PERIOD: Promote wound healing and control edema.
1. Elevation
2. Active range of motion (ROM) of hand and shoulder

Days 6-14

GOALS FOR THE PERIOD: Promote wound healing, control edema, and begin ROM.
1. Elevation
2. Compression wrap
3. Active range of motion (AROM) exercises for hand and shoulder
4. Gentle active flexion and extension of elbow
5. Gentle active supination and pronation of forearm

Day 15-Week 5

GOALS FOR THE PERIOD: Improve ROM, provide scar management, and control edema.
1. Scar massage
2. Desensitization
3. Use of scar pad
4. Compression wrap
5. AROM of hand, wrist, and shoulder
6. Gentle AROM of elbow and forearm

Weeks 6-18

GOALS FOR THE PERIOD: Strengthen muscles, increasing ROM if limited.
1. Scar management
2. Compression wrap for edema if needed
3. AROM and passive ROM of hand, wrist, elbow, forearm, and shoulder
4. Gentle progressive exercises of wrist, elbow, and forearm, including wrist curls, forearm rotation, and biceps and triceps strengthening

Months 4-6

GOAL FOR THE PERIOD: Return to activity.
1. Isotonic shoulder exercises as needed
2. Continue progressive exercises of the wrist, elbow, and forearm

REFERENCES

1. Brotzman SB: *Clinical orthopaedic rehabilitation,* St Louis, 1996, Mosby.
2. Brown M: The older athlete with tennis elbow. Rehabilitation considerations, *Clin Sports Med* 14:1, 1995.
3. Canale ST: *Campbell's operative orthopaedics,* ed 9, St Louis, 1998, Mosby.
4. Doran A et al: Tennis elbow. A clinicopathologic study of 22 cases followed for 2 years, *Acta Orthop Scand* 61:6, 1990.
5. Ernst E: Conservative therapy for tennis elbow, *Br J Clin Pract* 46:1, 1992.
6. Foley AE: Tennis elbow, *Am Fam Phys* 48:2, 1993.
7. Gellman H: Tennis elbow (lateral epicondylitis), *Orthop Clin North Am* 23:75, 1992.
8. Hayes KW: *Manual for physical agents,* ed 4, NJ, 1993, Appleton & Lange.
9. Hunter JM, Mackin EJ, Callahan AD: *Rehabilitation of the hand: surgery and therapy,* ed 4, St Louis, 1995, Mosby.
10. Morrey BF: *The elbow and its disorders,* ed 2, Philadelphia, 1993, WB Saunders.
11. Jobe FW, Ciccotti MG: Lateral and medial epicondylitis of the elbow, *J Am Acad Orthop Surg* 2:1, 1994.
12. Noteboom T et al: Tennis elbow: a review, *J Orthop Sports Phys Ther* 19:6, 1994.
13. Olliveierre CO, Nirschl RP: Tennis elbow. Current concepts of treatment and rehabilitation, *J Sports Med* 22:2, 1996.
14. Ollivierre CO, Nirschl RP, Pettroe FA: Resection and repair for medial tennis elbow: a prospective analysis, *J Sports Med* 23:2, 1995.
15. Plancher KD, Halbrecht J, Lourie GM: Medial and lateral epicondylitis in the athlete, *Clin Sports Med* 2:283, 1996.
16. Schnatz P, Steiner C: Tennis elbow: a biomechanical and therapeutic approach, *J Am Osteopath Assoc* 93(7):778, 1993.
17. Solveborn SA, Oelrud C: Radial epicondylalgia (tennis elbow): measurement of range of motion of the wrist and elbow, *J Orthop Sports Phys Ther* 22:4, 1996.
18. Stanley BG, Tribuzi SM: *Concepts in hand rehabilitation,* Philadelphia, 1992, FA Davis.
19. Verhaar J et al: Lateral extensor release for tennis elbow. A prospective long-term follow-up study, *J Bone Joint Surg Am* 75:7, 1993.
20. Weir S: Corticosteroid injections for tennis elbow, *J Fam Pract* 43:3, 1996.

Chapter 6

Reconstruction of the Ulnar Collateral Ligament with Ulnar Nerve Transposition

James Andrews
Wendy J. Hurd
Kevin E. Wilk

The ulnar collateral ligament (UCL) is the elbow's primary stabilizer to valgus stress within a functional range of motion (ROM). For the overhead-throwing athlete, throwing motions promote valgus stress at the elbow that exceeds the ultimate tensile strength of the UCL. Repetitive throwing motions produce cumulative microtraumatic damage and may eventually cause the ligament to overstretch and create symptomatic medial elbow instability. To correct this, both surgical intervention and a carefully coordinated rehabilitation program are required if the athlete is to return to full, pain-free function. This chapter describes the way the anatomy and biomechanics of the elbow can be applied to a scientifically based rehabilitation program for use after UCL reconstruction.

Surgical Indications and Considerations

Anatomy

Bony structures. The elbow joint has three articulations: the humeroulnar, humeroradial, and superior radioulnar joints. Collectively these joints may be classified as trochoginglymoid[21] and are enclosed by a single joint capsule.

The humeroulnar joint is a single-axis diarthrodial joint with 1 degree of freedom—flexion and extension. The bony structures of the joint include the distal humerus and proximal ulna (Fig. 6-1). The distal humerus flares to form the medial and lateral epicondyles, which are directly above the capitellum and trochlea, respectively. The medial epicondyle is much more prominent than the lateral epicondyle; the UCL and flexor-pronator muscle group attach to it (Fig. 6-2). The flat, irregular surface of the lateral epicondyle serves as the attachment site for the lateral collateral ligament and the supinator-extensor muscle groups. Just posterior to the medial epicondyle is the cubital tunnel, or ulnar groove, a key depression that protects

and houses the ulnar nerve. Immediately above the anterior articular surface of the humerus is a bony depression called the *coronoid fossa*. The olecranon process of the ulna glides into this concavity during flexion. The olecranon fossa, located on the posterior aspect of the humerus, accepts the large olecranon process during extension. The proximal ulna provides the major articulation of the elbow and is responsible for its inherent stability. The trochlear ridge is a bony projection running from the olecranon posteriorly to the coronoid process anteriorly. The trochlear notch is a concave surface located on either side of the trochlear ridge; it forms a close articulation with the humeral trochlea.

The proximal radius and distal lateral aspect of the humerus articulate to form the humeroradial joint, which is also a single-axis diarthrodial joint. Similar to the humeroulnar joint, the humeroradial joint contributes to flexion/extension movements by gliding around the coronal axis. However, the humeroradial articulation also pivots around a longitudinal axis with the superior radioulnar joint to perform rotational movements. The proximal radial head is mushroom-shaped,[7] with a central depression located above it. The radial head narrows distally to form the radial neck. The head and neck are not co-linear, with the shaft of the radius forming an angle of approximately 15 degrees. Further distal is the radial tuberosity, where the biceps tendon attaches. In the distal humerus the capitellum is almost spheroidal. A groove (the capitotrochlear groove) separates the capitellum from the trochlea. The rim of the radial head articulates with this groove throughout the arc of flexion and during pronation and supination.

The superior and inferior radioulnar joints function as single-axis diarthrodial joints that allow the elbow to pronate and supinate. Proximally, the convex medial rim of the radial head articulates with the concave radial ulnar notch. During supination and pronation the radial head rotates within a ring formed by the annu-

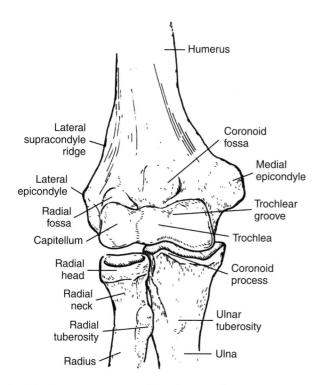

Fig. 6-1. The osseous anatomy of the elbow complex. (From Stoyan M, Wilk KE: The functional anatomy of the elbow, *J Orthop Sports Phys Ther* 17:279, 1993.)

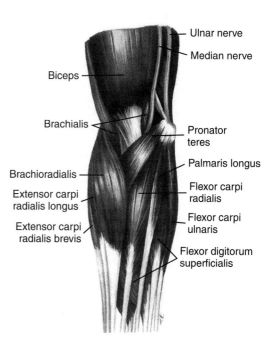

Fig. 6-2. The medial epicondyle serves as the attachment site for the UCL and flexor pronator group. (From Stoyan M, Wilk KE: The functional anatomy of the elbow, *J Orthop Sports Phys Ther* 17:279, 1993.)

lar ligament and radial ulnar notch. The shafts of the radius and ulna are connected by an interosseous membrane to form a syndesmosis. Distally the inferior radioulnar joint articulation is formed by the ulnar head with the radial ulnar notch. This joint is L-shaped and has an articular disc between the lower ends of the radius and ulna. During supination and pronation the ulnar notch and articular disc swing on the ulnar head.

Ligamentous structures. A single joint capsule surrounds the elbow joint and is lined by a synovial membrane. Specialized thickenings of the medial and lateral capsule form the collateral ligament complexes.

The UCL is traditionally described as having three portions: the anterior, posterior, and transverse bundles (Fig. 6-3).[7] The anterior bundle of the UCL is the strongest and most discrete component, coursing from the medial epicondyle to the sublime tubercle on the medial coronoid margin. The anterior bundle consists of two layers: a thickening within the capsular layers and an added complex superficial to the capsular layers.[23] The anatomic design of this ligament makes pathologic conditions in the central portion of the anterior bundle (as seen in a chronic, attenuated state) difficult to see during arthroscopic surgery. Functionally, the UCL is subdivided into two bands: the anterior band, which is tight in extension, and the posterior band, which is taut in flexion.[1] The anterior oblique

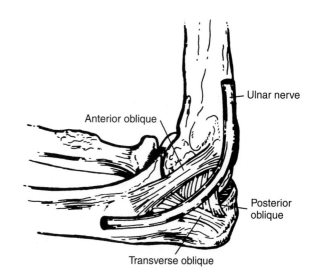

Fig. 6-3. The UCL complex of the elbow consists of three bundles: anterior, posterior, and transverse oblique. (From Stoyan M, Wilk KE: The functional anatomy of the elbow, *J Orthop Sports Phys Ther* 17:279, 1993.)

bundle of the UCL is the primary stabilizer to valgus stress at the elbow. Compromise of this structure causes gross instability in all elbow positions except full extension. The fan-shaped posterior bundle runs from the medial epicondyle to the middle margin of the trochlear notch. This band becomes especially taut in flexion after 60 degrees,[6,16] but sectioning the poste-

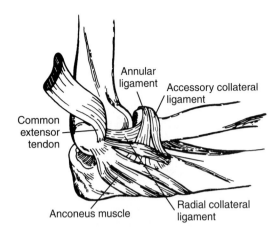

Annular ligament

Accessory collateral ligament

Common extensor tendon

Anconeus muscle

Radial collateral ligament

Fig. 6-4. The lateral collateral ligament complex of the elbow consists of the radial collateral ligament, annular ligament, and lateral UCL. (From Stoyan M, Wilk KE: The functional anatomy of the elbow, *J Orthop Sports Phys Ther* 17:279, 1993.)

rior oblique ligament does not significantly affect medial elbow stability.[20] The transverse ligament (also known as *Cooper's ligament*) has an ulnar-to-ulnar attachment and contributes minimally to elbow stability.[15]

The anatomy of the lateral collateral ligament complex can vary significantly.[15,17] Typically there are four components: the radial collateral ligament (RCL), annular ligament, lateral UCL, and accessory lateral collateral ligament (Fig. 6-4). The RCL originates from the lateral epicondyle and terminates on the annular ligament. It provides varus stability by maintaining close approximation of the humeral and radial articular surfaces.[15] The annular ligament is a strong band of tissue encompassing and stabilizing the radial head in the radial ulnar notch. The anterior part of this ligament becomes taut with extreme supination and the posterior portion with extreme pronation.[13] The lateral UCL originates at the mid-portion of the lateral epicondyle, passes over the annular ligament, and attaches to the tubercle of the supinator. This ligament is analogous to the anterior band of the UCL and is the primary lateral stabilizer of the elbow, preventing posterolateral rotary instability.[17] Finally, the accessory lateral collateral ligament extends proximally from the inferior margin of the annular ligament and attaches distally on the tubercle of the supinator crest. It further stabilizes the annular ligament during varus stress.[12,13,16]

Muscular structures. The musculature surrounding the elbow joint may be divided into four main groups:
1. The elbow flexors
2. The elbow extensors
3. The flexor-pronator group
4. The extensor supinator group

The *flexor group* is located anteriorly and comprises the biceps brachii, brachialis, and brachioradialis muscles. The biceps brachii acts both as a major elbow

flexor and as a supinator of the forearm (primarily with the elbow flexed), with a distal insertion at the radial tuberosity and bicipital aponeurosis, which attaches to the anterior capsule of the elbow. The brachioradialis originates at the proximal two-thirds of the lateral supracondylar ridge of the humerus and attaches distally at the base of the styloid process of the radius, giving it the greatest mechanical advantage of the elbow flexors. The cross-sectional area of the brachialis is the largest of the elbow flexors, but this has no mechanical advantage because it crosses so close to the axis of rotation. As the brachialis crosses the anterior capsule, some muscle fibers insert into the capsule and help retract the capsule during flexion.

The anconeus and triceps brachii perform *elbow extension* and are located posteriorly. The triceps brachii has three heads (long, lateral, and medial) proximally that converge distally to form a single insertion at the posterior olecranon. The much smaller anconeus originates at the posterior aspect of the lateral epicondyle and inserts on the dorsal surface of the proximal ulna. Besides extending the elbow, the anconeus may be a lateral joint stabilizer.

The *flexor-pronator muscles*, which all originate completely or in part at the medial epicondyle, include the pronator teres, flexor carpi radialis, palmaris longus, flexor carpi ulnaris, and flexor digitorum superficialis. The primary role of these muscles is in hand and wrist function, but they also act as elbow flexors and dynamically stabilize the medial aspect of the elbow.

Finally, the *extensor-supinator muscles* include the brachioradialis, extensor carpi radialis brevis and longus, supinator, extensor digitorum, extensor carpi ulnaris, and extensor digiti minimi. Each of these muscles originates near or directly onto the lateral epicondyle of the humerus and provides dynamic support over the lateral aspect of the elbow.

Neurologic structures. The relationship of neurologic structures coursing through the elbow to their surrounding features can be crucial to function, pathologic conditions, and treatment (Fig. 6-5).

The radial nerve descends anterior to the lateral epicondyle behind the brachioradialis and brachialis muscles. At the antecubital space the nerve divides into superficial and deep branches, with the superficial branch continuing distally in front of the lateral epicondyle and running under the brachioradialis muscle while on top of the supinator and pronator teres muscles. The deep branch pierces the supinator, travels around the posterolateral radial neck, and emerges distally 8 cm below the elbow joint to the terminal motor branches.

The median nerve follows a straight course into the medial aspect of the antecubital fossa, medial to the biceps tendon and brachial artery. From the antecubital fossa the median nerve continues under the bicipital

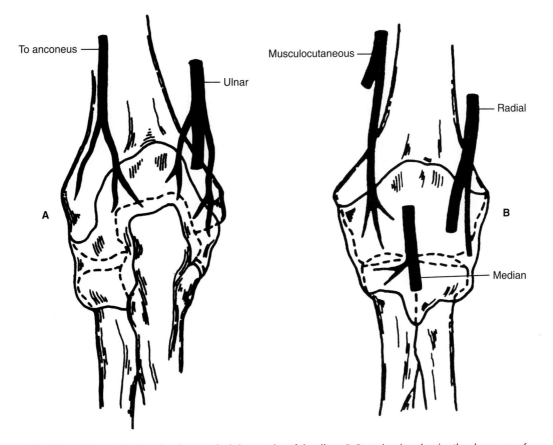

Fig. 6-5. A, Anterior view showing the neurologic innervation of the elbow. **B,** Posterior view showing the ulnar nerve of the elbow ligament. (From Stoyan M, Wilk KE: The functional anatomy of the elbow, *J Orthop Sports Phys Ther* 17:279, 1993.)

aponeurosis and usually passes between the two heads of the pronator teres, then travels below the flexor digitorum superficialis.

The musculocutaneous nerve innervates the major elbow flexors of the anterior brachium, then passes between the biceps and brachialis muscles to pierce the brachial fascia lateral to the biceps tendon. It continues distally to terminate as the lateral antebrachial cutaneous nerve, providing sensation over the lateral forearm.

Finally, the ulnar nerve travels anterior to posterior in the brachium through the arcade of Struthers. It then extends around the medial epicondyle and through the cubital tunnel. The cubital tunnel is the most frequent site for ulnar nerve injury; length changes in the medial ligament structures during elbow flexion can lead to significant reduction of the volume of the cubital tunnel, resulting in ulnar nerve compression.[8] This compression occurs as the cubital retinaculum, which forms a roof over the cubital tunnel, tightens with elbow flexion.[14] Absence of the cubital tunnel retinaculum has been associated with congenital ulnar nerve subluxation. After passing through the cubital tunnel, the ulnar nerve enters the forearm by traveling between the two heads of the flexor carpi ulnaris.

Etiology

Injury to the UCL and resultant medial elbow instability are secondary to valgus loads that exceed the ultimate tensile strength of the ligament. Although excessive valgus loads may be secondary to trauma, as with an elbow dislocation caused by a fall or playing a sport such as football or wrestling, the most common mechanisms of injury are associated with repetitive overhead activities, such as baseball, javelin throwing, tennis, swimming, and volleyball. The single largest patient population experiencing medial elbow instability is undoubtedly overhead throwers.[31] This is secondary to the tremendous forces imparted to the elbow joint during the overhead throwing motion.

The initiation of valgus stress occurs at the conclusion of the arm cocking stage. The thrower's shoulder is abducted, extended, and externally rotated about 130 degrees, with the elbow flexed at about 90 degrees. In transition from cocking to acceleration, the shoulder then internally rotates and the elbow flexes another 20 to 30 degrees; this further increases the valgus load on the medial elbow. As the arm continues to accelerate, the elbow extends from about 125 to 25 degrees of flexion at ball release.[18,28] Dillman et al[4] re-

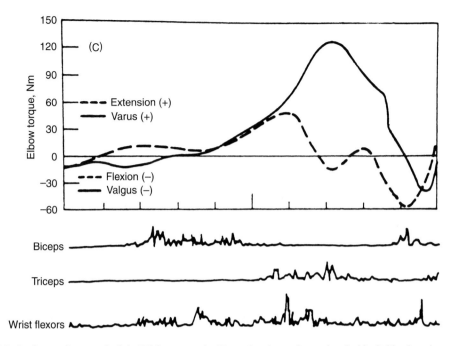

Fig. 6-6. Resting tensile strength of the UCL is measured at 33 nm, but demands associated with pitching have been measured at 35 nm. (From Werner SL et al: Biomechanics of the elbow during baseball pitching, *J Orthop Sports Phys Ther* 17:274, 1993.)

port that mean ultimate valgus torque measured from cadaveric testing was 33 NΣm (newton-meters) (Fig. 6-6). During analysis of the dynamic demands of the pitching motion, Fleisig et al[5] estimate that 35 NΣm of valgus torque is placed on the UCL. The flexor carpi ulnaris and flexor digitorum superficialis muscles are located directly over the anterior band of the UCL and assist in combating medial joint distraction forces during the throwing motion. With any increased load transmitted to the UCL—whether with improper mechanics, warm-up, or conditioning—the structural integrity of the primary medial stabilizer of the elbow may be compromised.

Injuries to the UCL are described as either *acute* or *chronic*. An acute rupture of the UCL is frequently associated with a "pop," a feeling of pain during late acceleration or at ball release; it is often accompanied by severe swelling. More commonly, chronic injuries to the ligament are seen in the overhead throwing athlete.[9] This occurs from the accumulated repetitive microtrauma of overloading the ligament with throwing, can result in symptomatic medial elbow instability,[3] and is often incorrectly diagnosed as flexor/pronator tendinitis. Accurate identification of medial instability is often difficult with clinical examination alone because laxity is only slightly increased. In addition, performing valgus laxity assessment is often difficult because of humeral rotation. Often magnetic resonance imaging (MRI) is used to confirm diagnosis. Timmerman et al[25] believe that use of saline-enhanced MRI improves

the results when a UCL tear is suspected. The authors of this chapter have found a typical leakage of contrast fluid around the ulnar insertion of the UCL when an undersurface tear is present, which has been called the *T-sign*.[25]

Surgical reconstruction of the UCL is indicated in athletes who have persistent medial elbow pain, cannot throw or participate in desired sports, show documented valgus laxity, and fail a 6-month conservative course of treatment.

Surgical Procedure

The goal of reconstruction is to restore the static stability of the anterior bundle of the UCL. The surgical procedure used at the authors' center by Dr. James Andrews is a modification of an earlier technique.

The presence or absence of the palmaris longus must be documented before surgery because it is the preferred donor tendon. If it is not present, alternate donor sites must be evaluated, including the contralateral palmar longus, the plantaris tendon, and the extensor tendon from the fourth toe.

Surgery to correct for valgus instability is initiated with a brief arthroscopic evaluation. The procedure itself begins with arthroscopic examination to assess the integrity of the intra-articular structures and valgus instability. After that is completed, a medial incision is made with subcutaneous ulnar nerve transposition. The incision is centered over the medial epicondyle and ex-

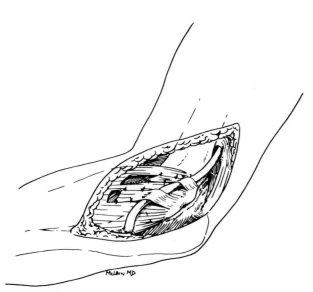

Fig. 6-7. To begin the reconstruction procedure, a medial incision is made in the elbow for UCL reconstruction and ulnar nerve transposition. (From Andrews JR et al: Open surgical procedures for injuries to the elbow in throwers, *Oper Tech Sports Med* 4(2):109, 1996.)

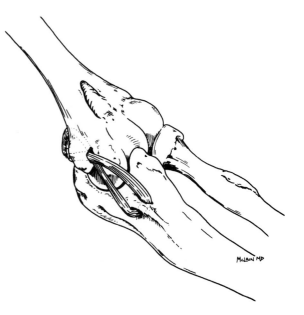

Fig. 6-8. Figure-eight reconstruction of the UCL using an autogenous graft. (From Andrews JR et al: Open surgical procedures for injuries to the elbow in throwers, *Oper Tech Sports Med* 4(2):109, 1996.)

tends about 3 cm proximally and distally (Fig. 6-7). The medial antebrachial cutaneous nerve is identified, preserved, and protected during the procedure to avoid neuroma development. After elevating the skin flaps to expose the deep fascia covering the flexor pronator muscles, the surgeon identifies the ulnar nerve. Anterior transposition of the ulnar nerve must be performed before the medial ligament complex is explored. To do so, the cubital tunnel is first incised to mobilize the nerve. Proximally, the mobilization continues to include the arcade of Struthers, and a portion of the intermuscular septum is excised to prevent impingement of the nerve as it is transposed anteriorly. Distally, the flexor carpi ulnaris is incised along the course of the nerve. The ulnar nerve is then transposed anteriorly and preserved throughout the remainder of the procedure.

To complete visualization of the UCL, the split in the flexor carpi ulnaris is followed down to the insertion of the anterior band of the UCL on the sublime tubercle of the ulna. Starting at the insertion of the ulna, the surgeon develops the interval between the UCL and flexor muscle mass, extending proximally to the medial epicondyle. The flexor muscles are then retracted anteriorly to provide full exposure to the ligament, at which point the pathologic condition can be assessed. In a complete rupture, the joint is exposed. If the external surface appears normal, a longitudinal incision is made in line with the fibers of the anterior bundle. This incision may reveal pathology, including tissue discoloration, fraying of the tissue, and detachment from the bony insertion on the ulna indicative of an undersurface tear, as described by Timmerman and Andrews.[24]

The remnants of the ligament are preserved and augmented with the tendon graft. After the donor tendon has been secured, muscle is stripped off the graft, the ends are trimmed, and a nonabsorbable suture is placed at each end with a locking stitch to help graft passage. Two drill holes are made at right angles just anterior and posterior to the sublime tubercle at the level of insertion of the anterior bundle. The drill holes are then connected with curettes and a towel clip. Proximally, two convergent tunnels are drilled to meet at the insertion of the ligament on the medial epicondyle. The graft is then passed through the ulna and crossed in a figure eight across the joint. Each end is then brought out through the two tunnels at the humerus end. If the graft is long enough, one end is passed through a second time. The graft tension is adjusted with the elbow in 30 degrees of flexion and by application of a varus stress. The graft is then secured with nonabsorbable 2-0 sutures over the medial epicondyle. The remaining ligament is sutured to the graft for added stability, and the flexor carpi ulnaris is loosely closed (Fig. 6-8).

Ulnar nerve transposition is now completed. An incision is made in the flexor pronator fascia, leaving attachments at the medial epicondyle; these flaps are about 3 cm long and 1 cm wide. Muscle is dissected away from the fascia, and the defect is closed to prevent herniation. The nerve is then transferred subcutaneously and anteriorly to lie under the fascial flaps. The flaps are reattached loosely to provide a sling to keep the nerve in position without compressing it. A drain is placed subcutaneously and the skin is closed with an absorbable 3-0 subcuticular suture.

Table 6-1   Ulnar Nerve Transposition

Rehabilitation Phase	Criteria to Progress to this Phase	Anticipated Impairments and Functional Limitations	Intervention	Goal	Rationale
Phase 1 Postoperative 1-3 weeks	Postoperative	• Postoperative pain • Postoperative edema • Arm immobilized in postoperative dressing • Limited elbow and wrist ROM • Limited upper extremity (UE) strength • Limited reach, grasp, and lift capacity of UE	• Posterior splint with elbow at 90° of flexion (see Fig. 6-9) • Remove splint at 2 weeks after surgery and place in a hinged elbow brace set at −30° extension and 100° flexion • At 3 weeks progress brace ROM to −15° extension and 110° flexion • Cryotherapy • Compression dressing • Isometrics—Submaximal Shoulder flexion, extension, abduction, and internal rotation At 2 weeks add wrist flexion and extension • Active ROM—Wrist flexion and extension	• Protect surgical site • Increase elbow ROM • Improve tolerance to elbow ROM • Control pain • Manage edema • Improve UE strength and muscle contraction • Improve active ROM of wrist	• Soft tissue healing without irritating surgical site • Hinged brace to avoid valgus stress • Gradual addition of stress to surgical site allowing ROM progression on a graduated basis • Self-management of pain and edema • Prevention of associated UE muscle atrophy without stressing UCL (avoiding external rotation) • Non-painful, safe strengthening of wrist musculature • Increase in available active ROM gradually as function and strength progress

Therapy Guidelines for Rehabilitation

Rehabilitation after UCL reconstruction should match the surgery used and meet the needs of the patient. The following guidelines are based on the procedure just described and are geared to the overhead-throwing athlete. The complete rehabilitation program is outlined in the Home Exercise Program.

Phase I

TIME: 1 to 3 weeks after surgery
GOALS: Decrease pain and inflammation, retard muscle atrophy, protect healing tissues (Table 6-1)

The therapist should place the elbow in a posterior splint at 90 degrees of flexion (Fig. 6-9), which allows initial healing of the UCL graft and soft tissue healing of the fascial slings for the transferred ulnar nerve.[29] Edema and pain are managed with frequent gripping exercises, cryotherapy, and a bulky dressing. The therapist initiates submaximal shoulder isometrics (except internal rotation, which promotes a valgus stress at the elbow) and active wrist ROM to prevent neuromuscular inhibition.

The therapist evaluates ulnar nerve function postoperatively and frequently throughout the rehabilitation process. Paresthesia and impaired motor function occur at rates as high as 31% with intramuscular ulnar nerve transposition. The procedure described in this chapter uses fascial slings to complete transposition of the nerve, so the chance of postoperative neurologic complications is extremely low, usually less than 3%. Compression wraps that are too tight and ill-fitting braces also may lead to transient ulnar nerve paresthesia and should be carefully assessed. The easiest way to treat an elbow flexion contracture is to prevent its development. Early ROM and frequent assessment are vital in the early rehabilitative process.

After 2 weeks the posterior splint is removed and the elbow placed in a hinged brace set at 30 to 100 degrees. At week 3 the ROM of the brace is increased to 15 to 110 degrees (Fig. 6-10). ROM is then advanced weekly by 5 degrees of extension and 10 degrees of flexion to week 6, when the patient should have full motion and no longer need the brace.

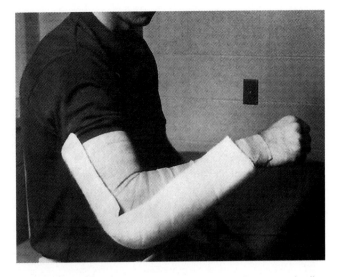

Fig. 6-9. A postoperative posterior elbow splint is used to protect healing tissues.

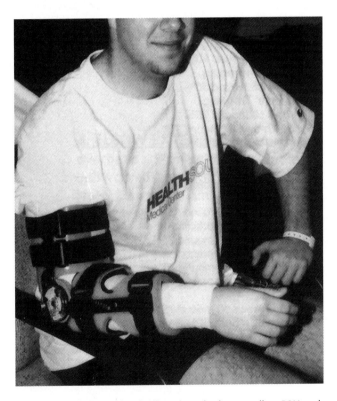

Fig. 6-10. The postoperative ROM brace is used to improve elbow ROM gradually while allowing soft tissue healing.

Q. David is a pitcher for a college baseball team. He complained of a painful and unstable medial elbow. Approximately 7 weeks ago he underwent reconstruction of the UCL with an ulnar nerve transposition. He is now performing some light isotonic exercises. What two muscles should the therapist target to enhance the stabilization of the medial elbow during a throwing motion?

Table 6-2   Ulnar Nerve Transposition

Rehabilitation Phase	Criteria to Progress to this Phase	Anticipated Impairments and Functional Limitations	Intervention	Goal	Rationale
Phase II Postoperative 4–8 weeks	• No sign of infection • No loss of ROM • No increase in pain	• Limited ROM • Limited UE strength • Limited reach, grasp, and lift capacity of UE • Pain	Continue exercises as in Phase I as indicated • Elbow brace set at −10° extension and 120° flexion Increase by 5° extension and 10° flexion per week • Isotonics (1–2 lb)—Wrist flexion, extension Forearm pronation, supination Elbow flexion, extension Rotator cuff exercises (Box 6-2) avoiding internal rotation After 6 weeks • Brace ROM set at 0°–130° • Active ROM—Elbow flexion, extension • Add shoulder internal rotation exercises • Progression of all exercises as indicated	• Elbow active ROM 0°–145° • Protect elbow from unprotected valgus force • Increase functional strength of UE • Improve tolerance to active ROM • Increase upper quarter strength • Increase lift tolerance	• Promotion of elbow ROM • Progression toward protected active ROM of elbow • Advancing of UE strength and ROM in preparation to restore previous level of functioning • Continued avoidance of valgus forces • By 6 weeks soft tissue healing should be stable enough to tolerate valgus stress • Attaining of full ROM • Objective progression of exercises

Phase II

TIME: 4 to 8 weeks after surgery
GOALS: Gradually increase ROM, heal tissues, restore muscular strength (Table 6-2)

The intermediate phase begins approximately at week 4. Advancement through the rehabilitation process is adjusted based on the response of the patient to surgery, tissue healing constraints, and a criterion-based progression. The patient should avoid external rotation movements until the sixth week.

Light wrist and elbow isotonics can be initiated later, as well as rotator cuff strengthening. The therapist should advance the resistance with isotonic exercises as the patient's strength improves.

Training the muscles in the way they are to perform with throwing is the focus. For example, the flexor carpi ulnaris and flexor digitorum superficialis muscles are located directly over the anterior band of the UCL and may contribute to dynamic stabilization of the medial elbow. Rhythmic stabilization drills in the throwing position assist in training these muscles in a similar manner. In addition, the elbow extensors act concentrically to accelerate the arm during the acceleration phase, whereas the elbow flexors act eccentrically to control the rapid rate of elbow extension during follow-through. Biasing the exercise selection appropriately for these muscle groups allows more effective strength training and provides neuromuscular training, allowing the muscles to function more efficiently when performing skilled movement patterns.

During this phase the therapist should pay careful attention to the patient's ROM. One of the most common complications after UCL reconstruction is development of an elbow flexion contracture and joint stiffness. In addition, flexion contracture is common in overhead-throwing athletes. Therefore early intervention and progressive motion and stretching exercises are important preventatives against elbow flexion contracture (Box 6-1).[30]

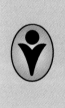 **A.** The focus should be on training the muscles in the way they are to perform during throwing. The flexor carpi ulnaris and the flexor digitorum superficialis muscles are located directly over the anterior band of the UCL and may contribute to dynamic stabilization of the medial elbow.

Phase III

TIME: 9 to 13 weeks after surgery
GOALS: Increase strength, power, and endurance, maintain full ROM, gradually add sports activities (Table 6-3)

Box 6-1   Stretching Program to Improve Elbow Motion

1. Passive warm-up (warm whirlpool) (7 to 10 minutes)
2. Active warm-up (upper body ergometer) (10 minutes)
3. Joint mobilization
   a. Distraction glides
   b. Posterior ulnar glide for upward elbow extension
   c. Mobilization of radial head
4. Low-load, long-duration stretching (12 to 15 minutes)
5. Manual proprioceptive neuromuscular facilitation (PNF) stretches using contract/relax technique
6. Passive stretching
7. Repeat process twice

Box 6-2   Thrower's Ten Program

1. Diagonal pattern D$_2$ flexion and extension
2. External and internal rotation strengthening
3. Shoulder abduction
4. Empty can
5. Prone horizontal abduction
6. Press-ups
7. Prone rowing
8. Push-ups
9. Elbow flexion and extension
10. Wrist extension and flexion
11. Forearm supinator and pronator

During this phase aggressive wrist, forearm, elbow, and shoulder strengthening are advanced with a Thrower's Ten Program (Box 6-2). The patient may begin light plyometric exercise when ROM and strength are normal. These drills are used to develop power and explosiveness with weighted balls, often incorporating the functional throwing position (Fig. 6-11). Manual proprioceptive neuromuscular facilitation (PNF) drills such as D$_2$ flexion/extension encourage strengthening in functional movement patterns and facilitate dynamic joint stabilization (Fig. 6-12). The stretch shortening plyometric neuromuscular drills simulate the throwing motion.

Phase IV

TIME: 14 to 26 weeks after surgery
GOALS: Increase strength, power, and endurance of upper extremity muscles, gradually return to sports activities (Table 6-4)

In this final phase the physical therapist should take care to return the patient to sports activities gradually; an interval sport program may help ensure that goal (Boxes 6-3 and 6-4). Other throwing programs

Text continued on p. 96

Table 6-3 Ulnar Nerve Transposition

Rehabilitation Phase	Criteria to Progress to this Phase	Anticipated Impairments and Functional Limitations	Intervention	Goal	Rationale
Phase III Postoperative 9–13 weeks	No increase in pain No loss of ROM Steady progression of elbow and wrist ROM	• Limited UE strength • Limited tolerance to reach, grasp, and lift activities	• Continue exercises as in Phases I and II • Progress with plyometric exercises • Isotonics—Progress wrist, elbow, and shoulder exercises • Initiate eccentric elbow flexion and extension exercises • Plyometrics—Incorporate functional throwing position (see Fig. 6-11) • Proprioceptive neuro-muscular facilitation (PNF) patterns (see Fig. 6-12) • Light sporting activities (golf, swimming) • Continue shoulder Throwers' Ten Program (see Box 6-2)	• Increase strength of UE • Increase muscular control of UE • Prepare for return to previous activities • Improve recruitment of UE musculature • Allow client to become pain free or self-manage with gradual return to activities • Strengthen UE with sport-specific activities	• Continuation of strengthening UE and progressing resistance • Training of muscles in movement patterns similar to overhead activities • Preparation of UE for accelerating and decelerating activities • Use of neuromuscular patterns to enhance functional strength and dynamic joint stabilization • Use of cross-training to vary stresses on UE • Specificity of training principle

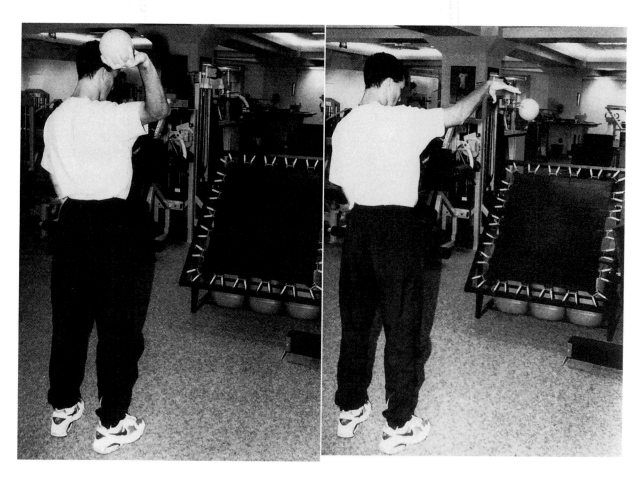

Fig. 6-11. Plyometric exercise drills develop power and explosiveness. The one-handed baseball throw to simulate throwing mechanics is shown.

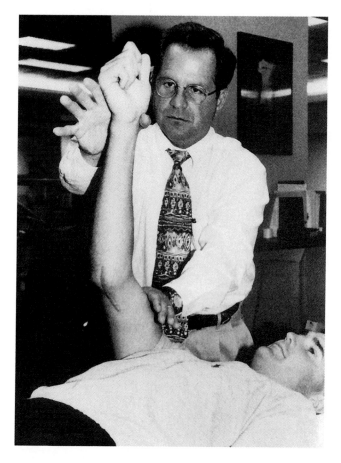

Fig. 6-12. Manual resistance PNF promotes strengthening in functional movement patterns and dynamic joint stabilization. This movement pattern is referred to as a *D₂ flexion/extension upper extremity pattern.*

Table 6-4 Ulnar Nerve Transposition

Rehabilitation Phase	Criteria to Progress to this Phase	Anticipated Impairments and Functional Limitations	Intervention	Goal	Rationale
Phase IV Postoperative 14-26 weeks	No increase in pain No loss of ROM No loss of strength	• Limited tolerance to repetitive overhead activities • Limited strength	• Initiate interval throwing program (see Boxes 6-3 and Box 6-4) • Continue strengthening as in Phases I through III • Return to competitive sports between 22 and 28 weeks	• Symmetric UE strength • Gradual return to unrestricted sport activity	• Normalization of UE strength to avoid reinjury with return to sport activities • Gradual progression to sport

Box 6-3   Interval Throwing Program Phase I

45' Phase

Step 1
- A. Warm-up throwing
- B. 45' (25 throws)
- C. Rest 15 minutes
- D. Warm-up throwing
- E. 45' (25 throws)

Step 2
- A. Warm-up throwing
- B. 45' (25 throws)
- C. Rest 10 minutes
- D. Warm-up throwing
- E. 45' (25 throws)
- F. Rest 10 minutes
- G. Warm-up throwing
- H. 45' (25 throws)

60' Phase

Step 3
- A. Warm-up throwing
- B. 60' (25 throws)
- C. Rest 15 minutes
- D. Warm-up throwing
- E. 60' (25 throws)

Step 4
- A. Warm-up throwing
- B. 60' (25 throws)
- C. Rest 10 minutes
- D. Warm-up throwing
- E. 60' (25 throws)
- F. Rest 10 minutes
- G. Warm-up throwing
- H. 60' (25 throws)

90' Phase

Step 5
- A. Warm-up throwing
- B. 90' (25 throws)
- C. Rest 15 minutes
- D. Warm-up throwing
- E. 90' (25 throws)

Step 6
- A. Warm-up throwing
- B. 90' (25 throws)
- C. Rest 10 minutes
- D. Warm-up throwing
- E. 90' (25 throws)
- F. Rest 10 minutes
- G. Warm-up throwing
- H. 90' (25 throws)

120' Phase

Step 7
- A. Warm-up throwing
- B. 120' (25 throws)
- C. Rest 15 minutes
- D. Warm-up throwing
- E. 120' (25 throws)

Step 8
- A. Warm-up throwing
- B. 120' (25 throws)
- C. Rest 10 minutes
- D. Warm-up throwing
- E. 120' (25 throws)
- F. Rest 10 minutes
- G. Warm-up throwing
- H. 120' (25 throws)

150' Phase

Step 9
- A. Warm-up throwing
- B. 150' (25 throws)
- C. Rest 15 minutes
- D. Warm-up throwing
- E. 150' (25 throws)

Step 10
- A. Warm-up throwing
- B. 150' (25 throws)
- C. Rest 10 minutes
- D. Warm-up throwing
- E. 150' (25 throws)
- F. Rest 10 minutes
- G. Warm-up throwing
- H. 150' (25 throws)

180' Phase

Step 11
- A. Warm-up throwing
- B. 180' (25 throws)
- C. Rest 15 minutes
- D. Warm-up throwing
- E. 180' (25 throws)

Step 12
- A. Warm-up throwing
- B. 180' (25 throws)
- C. Rest 10 minutes
- D. Warm-up throwing
- E. 180' (25 throws)
- F. Rest 10 minutes
- G. Warm-up throwing
- H. 180' (25 throws)

Step 13
- A. Warm-up throwing
- B. 180' (25 throws)
- C. Rest 10 minutes
- D. Warm-up throwing
- E. 180' (25 throws)
- F. Rest 10 minutes
- G. Warm-up throwing
- H. 180' (25 throws)

Box 6-4   Interval Throwing Program Phase II

Stage 1: Fastball only
Step 1: Interval throwing
    15 throws off mound at 50%
Step 2: Interval throwing
    30 throws off mound at 50%
Step 3: Interval throwing
    45 throws off mound at 50%
Step 4: Interval throwing
    60 throws off mound at 50%
Step 5: Interval throwing
    30 throws off mound at 75%
Step 6: 30 throws off mound at 75%
    45 throws off mound at 50%
Step 7: 45 throws off mound at 75%
    15 throws off mound at 50%
Step 8: 60 throws off mound at 75%

Stage 2: Fastball only
Step 9: 45 throws off mound at 75%
    15 throws in batting practice

Step 10: 45 throws off mound at 75%
    30 throws in batting practice
Step 11: 45 throws off mound at 75%
    45 throws in batting practice

Stage 3
Step 12: 30 throws off mound at 75% during warm-up
    15 throws off mound; 50% breaking balls
    45-60 throws in batting practice (fastball only)
Step 13: 30 throws off mound at 75%
    30 breaking balls at 75%
    30 throws in batting practice
Step 14: 30 throws off mound at 75%
    60-90 throws in batting practice; 25% breaking balls
Step 15: Simulated game, progressing by 15 throws per work-out (use interval throwing to 120' phase in Box 6-3 as warm-up). All throwing off the mound should be done in the presence of the pitching coach to stress proper throwing mechanics. Use speed gun to aid in effort control.

---

are described in Chapter 3 and Appendix A. An interval throwing program may be initiated for an overhead thrower about 4 to 5 months after surgery, with throwing off the mound usually occurring around 5 to 6 months after surgery.[30] The competitive overhead athlete should participate in a year-round conditioning program that consists of isotonic strengthening (see Box 6-2), plyometric and neuromuscular training, and a sport-specific training program. In addition, the athlete should continue flexibility exercises for the elbow, wrist, and hand. The interval throwing program emphasizes a proper warm-up, correct throwing mechanics, and a gradual progression of intensity. The therapist also must teach the athlete to "listen" to the arm: if pain is present, the patient should not advance the program prematurely.

Q. Cynthia is a professional volleyball player. She complains of pain on the medial side of the elbow of the arm she uses to serve the volleyball. She also has medial elbow instability. Cynthia underwent reconstruction of the UCL with ulnar nerve transposition 12 weeks ago. She still has a slight elbow flexion contracture. What are some techniques that may be effective in facilitating increased elbow extension?

Suggested Home Maintenance for the Postsurgical Patient

The home maintenance box on pages 98 and 99 as well as Boxes 6-1 through 6-4 review exercises that are commonly prescribed for the patient to perform at home. The exercises are progressed gradually to allow the tissue proper healing time, with the ultimate goal of full restoration of strength and ROM. The exercises are to be performed at home in conjunction with treatment sessions in the rehabilitation setting.

Troubleshooting

As already noted, the most common complication after UCL reconstruction is a flexion contracture or stiff joint. Factors that predispose the elbow joint to this loss of ROM include the following:
1. The intimate congruency of the elbow joint complex, especially the humeroulnar joint
2. The tightness of the elbow joint capsule
3. The tendency of the anterior capsule to scar and become adhesive[22]

Box 6-1 outlines a program found to be effective in combating flexion contractures of the elbow. It includes both passive and active warm-up, joint mobilizations, and manual stretching techniques. One of the most effective components to the stretching regimen is the low-load, long-duration stretching technique. The three most important components of this technique are duration of stretch (10 to 15 minutes), intensity of stretch

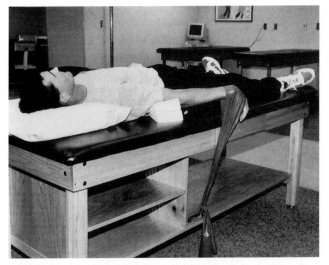

Fig. 6-13. A low-load, long-duration stretch is performed to improve elbow extension. A Theraband is secured at one end and wrapped around the patient's distal forearm.

(low to moderate), and frequency of stretch (five to six times daily) (Fig. 6-13).

This stretching technique may be enhanced by the use of other modalities such as moist hot packs or ultrasound. The rationale for the success of this technique is its ability to produce a plastic response within the collagen tissue, resulting in permanent elongation.[11,19,26,27]

If ROM complications persist, the therapist may want to prescribe a splint to be worn both day and night. A static splint holds the joint in a constant position, whereas a dynamic splint uses a spring to exert force and create a progressive stretch. Patients are encouraged to remove the splint daily for strengthening and stretching exercises.

During the aggressive stretching program the patient often experiences increased elbow soreness or pain. Pain control using cryotherapy, high-voltage galvanic stimulation, transcutaneous electrical nerve stimulation (TENS), and interferential current is highly effective.

Other complications include hand and grip weakness, ulnar neuropathy, rotator cuff tendonitis, and UCL failure. Intrinsic weakness of the hand may be avoided by initiating gripping exercises immediately after surgery and increasing intensity as rehabilitation progresses. Ulnar neuropathy generally develops immediately after surgery. Transposition of the ulnar nerve may cause sensory changes of the little finger and ulnar half of the ring finger. Motor deficits may include the inability to adduct the thumb, weakness of the finger abductor and adductors, adduction of the little finger, and weakness of the flexor carpi ulnaris. The most frequent patient complaint is paresthesia through the ulnar nerve sensory distribution, but this is usually transient and should resolve within 7 days.

Inactivity can lead to rapid deterioration of rotator cuff strength and a subsequent inability to stabilize the glenohumeral joint during the throwing motion. Integrating a Throwers' Ten program with the emphasis on rotator cuff strengthening several weeks before throwing greatly reduces the chances of developing tendonitis.

UCL failure is the most serious of all postoperative complications. Graft failure or poor bone quality with inadequate graft stabilization necessitates subsequent surgery or the cessation of overhead activities. Fortunately, with advanced surgical and rehabilitation techniques, successful outcomes are much more likely than failures. Andrews and Timmerman[2] found 78% of professional baseball players returning to their previous level of play after UCL reconstruction.

A. Some effective techniques include joint mobilizations, contract/relax techniques, and a low-load, long-duration stretching technique followed by passive and active ROM exercises. These techniques are listed in Box 6-1 and are effective with flexion contractures.

Suggested Home Maintenance for the Postsurgical Patient

Weeks 1-3

GOALS FOR THE PERIOD: Protect healing tissues, decrease pain and inflammation, and limit muscle atrophy

Week 1:
1. Posterior splint at 90 degree elbow flexion
2. Wrist assisted range of motion (ROM) extension and flexion
3. Elbow compression dressing (2 to 3 days)
4. Gripping exercises, wrist ROM, shoulder isometrics (except shoulder external rotation), biceps isometrics, others as indicated
5. Cryotherapy

Week 2:
1. Application of functional brace 30 to 100 degrees
2. Initiation of wrist isometrics
3. Initiation of elbow flexion and extension isometrics
4. Continuation of all exercises listed previously

Week 3:
1. Advance brace 15 to 110 degrees (gradually increase ROM; 5 degrees of extension and 10 degrees of flexion per week)

Weeks 4-8

GOALS FOR THE PERIOD: Gradually increase ROM, healing tissues, regain and improve muscle strength

Week 4:
1. Functional brace set (10 to 120 degrees)
2. Begin light resistance exercises for arm (1 lb), wrist curls, extensions, pronation and supination, and elbow extension and flexion
3. Progress shoulder program, emphasizing rotator cuff strengthening (avoid external rotation until sixth week)

Week 5:
Continue as for week 4

Weeks 6-8:
1. Functional brace set (0 to 130 degrees); assisted ROM (0 to 145 degrees) without brace
2. Progress elbow strengthening exercises
3. Initiate shoulder external rotation strengthening
4. Progress shoulder program

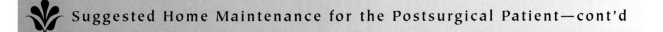

Suggested Home Maintenance for the Postsurgical Patient—cont'd

Weeks 9-13

GOALS FOR THE PERIOD: Increase strength, power, and endurance, maintain full elbow ROM, gradually begin sports activities

Week 9:
1. Initiate eccentric elbow flexion and extension
2. Continue isotonic program for forearm and wrist
3. Continue shoulder program (Throwers' Ten Program)
4. Begin manual resistance diagonal patterns

Week 10:
Continue as for week 9

Week 11:
1. Continue all exercises listed previously
2. Initiate plyometric exercise program
3. Begin light sports activities (e.g., golf, swimming)

Weeks 12-13:
Continue as for week 11

Weeks 14-26

GOALS FOR THE PERIOD: Continue to increase strength, power, and endurance of upper extremity muscles, gradually return to sports activities

Week 14:
1. Initiate interval throwing program (phase I)
2. Continue strengthening program
3. Emphasize elbow and wrist strengthening and flexibility exercises

Weeks 15-21:
Continue with program

Weeks 22-26:
Return to competitive sports as appropriate

REFERENCES

1. Andrews JR: *Ulnar collateral ligament injuries of the elbow in throwers*, presented at the Injuries in Baseball Course, Birmingham, AL, Jan. 28, 1990.

2. Andrews JR, Timmerman LA: Outcome of elbow surgery in professional baseball players, *Am J Sports Med* 23(4):407, 1995.

3. Conway JE et al: Medial instability of the elbow in throwing athletes, *Am J Bone Joint Surg* 74:67, 1992.

4. Dillman C, Smutz P, Werner S: Valgus extension overload in baseball pitching, *Med Sci Sports Exer* 23:S135, 1991.

5. Fleisig GS et al: Kinetics of baseball pitching with implications about injury mechanisms, *Am J Sports Med* 23(2):233, 1995.

6. Warwick R, Williams PL: *Gray's anatomy, descriptive and applied*, ed 35, Philadelphia, 1980, WB Saunders.

7. Guerra JJ, Timmerman LA: Clinical anatomy, histology, and pathomechanics of the elbow in sports, *Sports Med Arthrosc Rev* 3(3):160, 1995.

8. Jobe FW, Fanton GS: Nerve injuries. In Morrey BF, editor: *The elbow and its disorders*, Philadelphia, 1985, WB Saunders.

9. Jobe FW, Kvitne RS: Elbow instability of the athlete, *Instr Course Lect* 40:17, 1991.

10. Jobe FW, Stark H, Lombardo SJ: Reconstruction of the ulnar collateral ligament in athletes, *J Bone Joint Surg* 68:1150, 1986.

11. Kottke FJ, Pauley DL, Ptak RA: The rationale for prolonged stretching for correction of shortening of connective tissue, *Arch Phys Med Rehab* 47:345, 1968.

12. Martin BJ: The oblique of the forearm, *J Anat* 52:609, 1958.

13. Martin BJ: The annular ligament of the superior radioulnar joint, *J Anat* 52:473, 1958.

14. Morrey BF: Anatomy and kinematics of the elbow. In Tullos HS, editor: *American Academy of Orthopaedic Surgeons instructional course lectures 40*, St Louis, 1991, Mosby.

15. Morrey BF: Anatomy of the elbow joint. In Morrey BF, editor: *The elbow and its disorders*, Philadelphia, 1993, WB Saunders.

16. Morrey BF, An RN: Articular and ligamentous contributions to the stability of the elbow joint, *Am J Sports Med* 11:315, 1983.

17. O'Driscoll SW, Bell DF, Morrey BF: Posterolateral rotary instability of the elbow, *Am J Bone Joint Surg* 73:440, 1991.

18. Pappas A, Zawack RM, Sullivan TJ: Biomechanics of baseball pitching: a preliminary report, *Am J Sports Med* 13(4):216, 1985.

19. Sapega AA et al: Biophysical factors in range of motion exercise, *Arch Phys Med Rehab* 57:122, 1976.

20. Schums GH et al: Biomechanics of elbow stability: role of the medial collateral ligament, *Clin Orthop* 146:42, 1980.

21. Steindler A: *Kinesiology of the human body*, Springfield, IL, 1955, Charles C. Thomas.

22. Timmerman LA, Andrews JR: Arthroscopic treatment of posttraumatic elbow pain and stiffness, *Am J Sports Med* 22(2):230, 1994.

23. Timmerman LA, Andrews JR: Histology and arthroscopic anatomy of the ulnar collateral ligament of the elbow, *Am J Sports Med* 22(5):667, 1994.

24. Timmerman LA, Andrews JR: Undersurface tear of the ulnar collateral ligament in baseball players: a newly recognized lesion, *Am J Sports Med* 22(1):33, 1994.

25. Timmerman LA, Schwartz ML, Andrews JR: Preoperative evaluation of the ulnar collateral ligament by magnetic resonance imaging and computed tomography arthrography, *Am J Sports Med* 22(1):26, 1994.

26. Warren CB, Lehman JF, Koblanski JN: Elongation of cat-tail tendon: effect of load and temperature, *Arch Phys Med Rehab* 52:465, 1971.

27. Warren CG, Lehman JF, Koblanski JN: Heat and stretch procedures: an evaluation using cat-tail tendon, *Arch Phys Med Rehab* 57:122, 1976.

28. Werner SL, Fleisig GS, Dillman CJ: Biomechanics of the elbow during baseball pitching, *J Orthop Sports Phys Ther* 17:274, 1993.

29. Wilk KE, Arrigo CA, Andrews JR: Rehabilitation of the elbow in the throwing athlete, *J Orthop Sports Phys Ther* 17:305, 1993.

30. Wilk KE et al: Rehabilitation following elbow surgery in the throwing athlete, *Op Tech in Sports Med* 4(2):69, 1996.

31. Wilk KE, Azar FM, Andrews JR: Conservative and operative rehabilitation of the elbow in sports, *Sports Med Arthrosc Rev* 3:237, 1995.

Chapter 7

Carpal Tunnel Syndrome: Postoperative Management

Benjamin M. Maser
Christina M. Clark
David Girard

Carpal tunnel syndrome (CTS) should be termed the industrial problem of the nineties. It results from compression of the median nerve as it crosses the wrist and is characterized by numbness, tingling, pain, and weakness in the hand. The symptoms of CTS can range from mild to severe. They may have far-reaching effects on a person's job, hobbies, and activities of daily living (ADLs).[21]

CTS is the most common entrapment neuropathy of the upper extremity. Paget described the complex of symptoms caused by median nerve entrapment at the wrist in 1854, and Moersch gave the syndrome its name in 1938. Brain, Wright, and Wilkerson described the first series of carpal tunnel releases by division of the transverse carpal ligament in 1947. Since that time a number of variations of this procedure have been developed, all of which involve division of the transverse carpal ligament.[12]

A survey[34] in the United States indicated the prevalence of self-reported CTS at approximately 1.6% in the adult (working and non-working) population. CTS affects people during their most productive years. Its prevalence peaks between the ages of 35 and 44 years for both men and women. Women appear to be affected more often than men.

The Bureau of Labor Statistics tracks CTS under repetitive motion injuries. In 1994, 40.8% of 92,576 repetitive motion injuries were CTS cases.[8] These data demonstrate the importance of clinicians fully understanding the prevention and treatment of CTS.

Surgical Indications and Considerations

Etiology

CTS can be classified into two categories: acute and chronic. Acute CTS is associated with a traumatic event such as blunt trauma to the wrist, wrist fracture, and burns. These traumas produce a sudden and sustained increase in interstitial pressure within the carpal tunnel, resulting in a median nerve conduction block from intracompartmental and intraneural ischemia. This form of CTS is a medical emergency and requires an immediate carpal tunnel decompression.

Chronic CTS is the result of an insidious rise of the interstitial pressure in the carpal tunnel and is classified as early, intermediate, or advanced. Patients with early CTS experience mild, intermittent symptoms that have been present less than 1 year. Intermediate CTS is characterized by more constant symptoms, including numbness and paresthesia with little or no atrophy of the thenar muscles. Surgery performed at this time uncovers a nerve that has undergone chronic changes, including epineural and intrafascicular edema. If decompression is performed at this time, the neural changes are frequently reversible. Advanced CTS is characterized by progressive paresthesia, atrophy of the thenar muscles, and pinch and grip weakness. Even after a successful surgical decompression, the chronic changes in the median nerve may be permanent.[20]

CTS can affect anyone. It is often seen in patients who perform repetitive activities in their work or hobbies. It can be associated with a number of other disease processes, including thyroid disease and diabetes, and also with various anatomic anomalies such as a persistent median artery.[12,15] Tumors of the wrist can precipitate CTS as the lesion occupies space within the carpal canal.[11] Wrist trauma can cause CTS because of the resulting edema and hematoma surrounding the median nerve. Pregnancy can precipitate CTS by causing edema around the structures traversing the carpal canal. During pregnancy the symptoms of CTS tend to occur in the last trimester, secondary to fluid retention; the condition usually resolves within 6 to 12 weeks after surgery.[20]

The diagnosis of CTS can usually be made based on a thorough history and careful physical examination. In cases in which the diagnosis is uncertain, electro-diagnostic studies can be helpful in either confirming or ruling out the disorder.[32]

In general, patients who are diagnosed with CTS are initially treated without surgery. Nonsteroidal antiinflammatory medications can reduce inflammation within the carpal canal. In some patients, local injection of steroid medication into the carpal canal can significantly reduce or even eliminate the symptoms of median nerve compression. Splinting the patient's wrist can be very helpful in controlling nighttime pain symptoms. The wrist is splinted in a neutral position that maximizes the carpal tunnel space[31] and minimizes the carpal tunnel pressure.[38] The splint is chosen based on the patient's needs and comfort. The metal stay of a prefabricated wrist splint is easily replaced with a custom-molded thermoplastic stay to position the wrist in neutral. All patients should sleep in their splints. Patients who have constant or activity-induced paresthesia should wear their splints during the day.[31] Postoperative night splinting is continued only when the patient has persistent nighttime paresthesia or numbness. When such conservative measures fail to resolve symptoms, surgery is indicated.

Classic CTS symptoms include the following:

1. Sensory changes in the hand
2. Pain
3. Weakness in pinch and grip
4. Clumsiness of the hand

Sensory changes are commonly the first symptoms noted. The patient reports paresthesia and numbness of the digits served by the sensory branches of the median nerve and in the tips of the thumb, index finger, middle finger, and radial half of the ring finger.

The onset of pain is most often the primary reason a person with CTS seeks medical attention. The pain associated with CTS tends to begin in the latter aspects of the early and intermediate stages. The patient complains of an intermittent, vague, dull aching in the wrist or forearm. Less common is pain radiating to the elbow and even the shoulder. Night pain is a common complaint most likely caused by congestion of the venous system during sleep.[5] Neurologic muscle weakness associated with CTS occurs late in the disease process. Atrophy is first noted in the abductor pollicis brevis. In advanced cases atrophy of the full thenar musculature may be seen. The unlucky patient with symptoms progressed to this state is at high risk for permanent nerve damage and may require a tendon transfer to substitute for the loss of the opponens pollicis muscle.

The clinician must be able to visualize the anatomic structures that make up the carpal tunnel. The carpal canal is bounded by the transverse carpal ligament volarly, the scaphoid tuberosity and the trapezium radially, the hook of the hamate and the pisiform ulnarly, and the volar radiocarpal ligament and volar ligamentous extensions between the carpal bones dorsally.[12,30] The carpal canal is traversed by the median nerve, the four flexor digitorum profundus tendons, the four flexor digitorum superficialis tendons, and the flexor pollicis longus tendon. Any condition that causes enlargement of the contents of the carpal canal (such as inflammation or edema) or occupies space within the canal (such as a tumor or hematoma) compresses the median nerve. This occurs because the structures that make up the carpal canal are relatively inelastic, and do not expand as the contents of the canal enlarge. The resulting pressure compromises circulation within the substance of the nerve, leading to nerve ischemia, which in turn leads to the symptoms and signs seen in CTS.

Surgical Procedure

Surgery to relieve CTS involves division of the transverse carpal ligament with resulting decompression of the median nerve. The standard approach to the transverse carpal ligament is through an open incision on the palm. It also can be divided with an endoscope, which is inserted at the level of the distal wrist crease.[1] The open approach is the most commonly used and is described here.

The patient is positioned supine on the operating table. The hand is anesthetized using either local anesthesia (Fig. 7-1), intravenous regional anesthesia (e.g., Bier block), or an axillary regional nerve block. Occasionally general anesthesia is used. The procedure is performed under tourniquet control, which allows excellent visualization of the nerve. After sterile preparation, an incision is made on the palm. This incision is designed to run between the palmar sensory branches of the median and ulnar nerves, which corresponds to the axis of the ring finger ray. The incision is kept proximal to the level of the superficial vascular arch of the hand to avoid damage to this structure. Proximally, the incision crosses the distal wrist crease in a zigzag fashion, just ulnar to the ulnar border of the palmaris longus tendon (Fig. 7-2). The incision is made sharply and deepened through the subcutaneous tissue of the palm and the palmar fascia, thereby exposing the transverse carpal ligament (Fig. 7-3). The ligament is then divided sharply under direct visualization, with the surgeon taking care to avoid damage to the underlying median nerve and tendons. After the ligament is divided, the nerve is carefully examined (Fig. 7-4). The wound is then irrigated with saline and the incision closed by reapproximating the skin edges with interrupted monofilament nonabsorbable sutures (Fig. 7-5). Sterile dressings are placed over the incision, and a wrist splint is applied with the wrist in slight extension, leaving the metacarpal-phalangeal and interphalangeal joints free.

The splint is left in place for approximately 10 days, after which it is taken off and the sutures are removed. Patients are instructed in any necessary local wound care, which is usually minimal, and encouraged to resume use of the hand gradually.

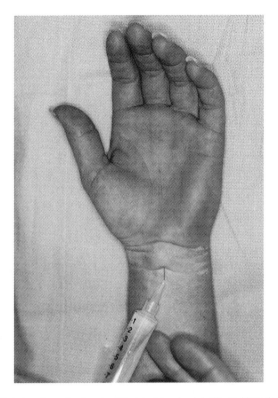

Fig. 7-1. Local anesthesia using 1% plain lidocaine is infiltrated into the operative area through a 25-gauge needle.

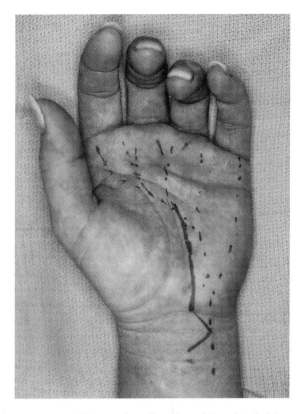

Fig. 7-2. Exposure of the carpal canal is performed through an incision represented by the *solid line*. *Dashed lines* represent the course of the ulnar artery and its branches (common digital and proper digital arteries) that must be preserved during exposure.

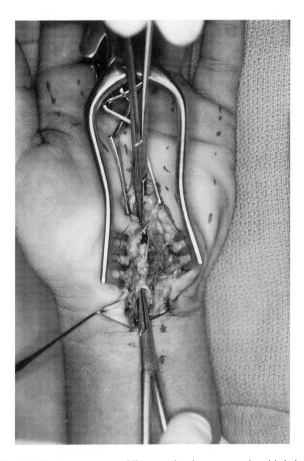

Fig. 7-3. The transverse carpal ligament has been exposed and is being tented proximally and distally by hemostats.

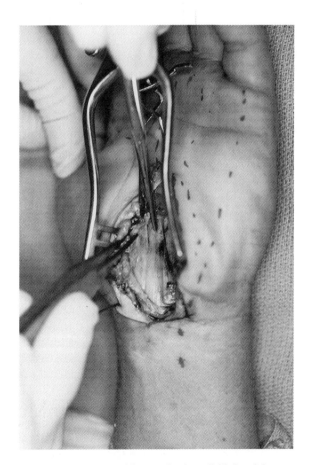

Fig. 7-4. The transverse carpal ligament has been divided, and the contents of the underlying carpal canal are exposed. The median nerve is demonstrated at the tip of the dissecting scissors.

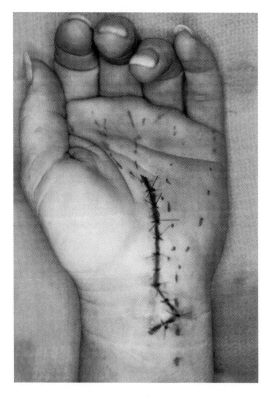

Fig. 7-5. Skin closure is achieved with the use of simple interrupted monofilament nonabsorbable suture.

Therapy Guidelines for Rehabilitation

Postoperative Rehabilitation

The frequency and duration of treatment is highly variable after a carpal tunnel release. All patients referred to therapy are instructed in a home exercise and ergonomic program appropriate to the phase of recovery and their individual needs.

In general, patients tend to do quite well after carpal tunnel release. However, because the extent of the damage to the median nerve cannot fully be known before surgery, predicting the exact outcome of carpal tunnel release is difficult. Patients with mild to moderate symptoms can expect full recovery of sensation and resolution of the numbness and tingling caused by entrapment of the nerve. Patients with more advanced disease who have significant sensibility loss and muscle weakness usually achieve significant improvement of their condition. Patients with muscle atrophy can expect a halt to progression of muscle wasting and in some cases can regain muscle mass.

Patients must understand that they may have some element of incisional pain after surgery, which can last as long as 3 to 6 months. They also must be informed that they will temporarily lose some strength in the hand, which usually improves after 3 to 6 months.

Postoperative Evaluation

A comprehensive evaluation after carpal tunnel release includes the following:
- Patient history
- Subjective pain report
- Finger dexterity assessment
- Edema measurement
- Grip and pinch measurements
- Manual muscle testing
- Active range of motion (AROM) measurements
- Sensibility testing
- Wound and scar assessment
- Nerve tension testing
- Documentation of the patient's previous and present functional status

The patient's history is obtained by patient interview. Information to be noted in the history includes age, gender, hand dominance, etiology of CTS, type and date of the carpal tunnel release, occupation, avocational interests, onset and description of symptoms before surgery, and notes regarding whether symptoms were unilateral or bilateral.

The patient is asked to quantify the pain on a scale from 0 (representing no pain) to 10 (indicating severe pain requiring medical attention). The patient is asked to rate the pain both at rest and with use. The quality of the patient's pain is obtained by documenting the descriptive terms the patient uses when discussing the symptoms.[17]

Finger dexterity is generally evaluated on a nine—hole peg test. The nine-hole pegboard is positioned on the table with the end containing the pegs on the same side as the hand being tested. The score is recorded as the total time in seconds to put the nine pegs into the board one at a time and remove the pegs one at a time for the dominant and nondominant hand. A comparison of the time required for the patient's postoperative hand is made with the hand that was not operated on or with the norms established in 1985 by Mathiowetz et al.[26]

Edema of the hand is recorded either by volumetric or circumferential measurements. If edema is profuse throughout the hand, volumetric measurements are preferred provided that stitches have been removed and the patient has no open wounds. The volumetric assessment should be administered following the American Society of Hand Therapists (ASHT) guidelines: the thumb should be oriented toward the spout of the volumeter and the hand lowered into the volumeter so the web space between the middle and ring fingers rests on the bar. The displaced water is measured in milliliters and recorded for both hands.[18] If edema is minimal or the stitches have not yet been removed, circumferential measurements recorded in centimeters should be obtained at the distal wrist crease and the distal palmar crease.

Grip strength is recorded using a dynamometer with the handle positioned at the second setting[2,3] per American Society of Surgery of the Hand (ASSH) and ASHT guidelines. If the patient is seen before day 21 after surgery, grip strength testing may be deferred. To perform a grip test the patient should be "seated with the shoulder adducted and neutrally rotated, elbow flexed to 90 degrees, forearm in neutral position" and unsupported.[13,14] The therapist may support the dynamometer to prevent dropping. However, the dynamometer should not be allowed to rest on the table. The therapist should document three grip measurements alternating the right and left hands[24] unless repetitive grasping of the dynamometer would increase the discomfort in the patient's hand. Several authors have published normal values for grip strength. However, because of the high standard deviation[9] and inconsistencies in the studies "comparison of grip scores to the contralateral extremity or longitudinal comparison to earlier values for each patient is recommended by ASSH and ASHT."[3,14,25]

Two types of pinch are recorded using a pinch meter. Finger positioning for three-point pinch is performed with the index and middle finger on the top of the pinch meter and the thumb on the bottom. Lateral pinch positioning is performed with the pinch meter held between the radial side of the index finger and the thumb on the top of the meter. Early forceful pinch is contraindicated and may be deferred until 3 weeks after surgery.

Manual muscle testing is performed after the hand is assessed for obvious atrophy of the thenar eminence. The "abductor pollicis brevis is the muscle of choice for clinical assessment because it is superficial, solely innervated by the median nerve, and the earliest affected."[23,29]

AROM measurements are obtained using a goniometer for the wrist and forearm. Individual finger AROM measurements may not be necessary when motion limitations are minimal. A global measurement of finger flexibility is obtained by measuring composite finger flexion to the distal palmar crease (DPC). The distance from the middle of the fingertips to the DPC is measured in centimeters for each finger. Functional thumb opposition is recorded as the ability to oppose the thumb to each fingertip as well as the ability to touch the thumb to the base of the small finger. The therapist should record any inability in centimeters. To prevent bowstringing (i.e., subluxing of the flexor tendons through the healing transverse carpal ligament) wrist flexion measurements should be deferred until 3 weeks after surgery.

"Sensibility testing is the evaluation of the ability to feel or perceive a stimulus applied to an area."[33] Sensibility assessment is completed using the Semmes-Weinstein Pressure Esthesiometer Kit (a five-filament kit is adequate). This type of sensory test is a pressure threshold test. The patient is seated comfortably for testing with the forearm supinated and the hand supported on a towel roll. The therapist should occlude the patient's vision during the test and instruct the patient to report when a finger is stimulated and which finger feels the stimulus. The volar fingertips and thumb pulp are tested starting with the 2.83 monofilament. "Each monofilament is applied perpendicular to the skin for 1.5 seconds and lifted for 1.5 seconds."[33] The therapist should apply monofilaments 2.83 and 3.61 three times to the same spot and apply monofilaments 4.31 through 6.65 once. The lowest numbered monofilament felt for each digit should be recorded on the evaluation form.[33] Full hand mapping is rarely required after a carpal tunnel release. "Two point discrimination values are most often normal in CTS, and if they are abnormal it indicates advanced disease."[16] The therapist should complete two-point discrimination testing if the patient demonstrates significant deficits on the Semmes-Weinstein Monofilament Test. Two point discrimination is an innervation density test.[16] The difference between the pressure threshold test and an innervation density test is the sensitivity of the pressure threshold test to gradual loss or improvement in nerve function versus an all-or-none response on an innervation density test. The difference can be explained by the comparison of a light bulb having a dimmer switch versus being on or off. Tinel's testing is helpful in evaluating a patient before surgery. However, the authors of this chapter do not recommend Tinel's testing after surgery to avoid aggravating an irritable healing nerve.

The surgical incision or scar is evaluated for its stage of healing. The therapist should document whether the scar is raised or flat, tough or soft, mobile or adherent. The color of the scar also is noted. Upper limb tension testing of the median nerve is appropriate to determine whether the patient has restrictions in nerve gliding.

The patient's present functional status is documented in the areas of grooming, dressing, bathing, cooking, home care, work, avocational activities, and driving. The patient is re-evaluated monthly or before returning to the doctor.

Phase I: The Inflammatory Phase

TIME: Weeks 1-6
GOALS: Decrease pain, manage edema, improve AROM of upper extremity, initiate self-management and patient education

Treatment of the patient after carpal tunnel release is based on the phases of wound healing. Phase I (inflammatory phase) is from the day of surgery through day 21 after surgery[4] (Table 7-1).

Table 7-1   Carpal Tunnel Release

Rehabilitation Phase	Criteria to Progress to this Phase	Anticipated Impairments and Functional Limitations	Intervention	Goal	Rationale

Phase Ia Postoperative 1-10 days	Postoperative	• Edema
		• Pain
		• Limited ROM of upper extremity (UE)
		• Limited functional use of UE
			• Instruct on surgical site protection and monitor for drainage
			• Elevate and ice hand and wrist
			• AROM—
			  Shoulder—all ranges
			  Elbow—all ranges
			  Forearm—pronation, supination
			  Fingers—tendon gliding
			  thumb AROM all ranges
				• Prevent infection and postoperative complications
				• Manage edema
				• Decrease pain
				• Full AROM of shoulder, elbow, forearm
				• Increase AROM of fingers within limits of postoperative dressing
					• Catch infection early to prevent further complications
					• Begin to have patient self-manage edema and pain
					• Restore ROM to prepare UE for functional use
					• Limit scar adhesions to tendons and nerves

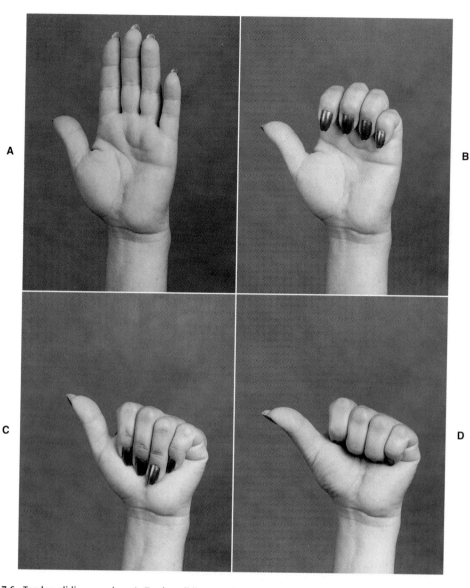

Fig. 7-6. Tendon gliding exercises. **A,** Tendon gliding exercises are initiated in full finger extension. The patient then completes ten repetitions in the hook fist (**B**), straight fist (**C**), and full fist (**D**) to maximize differential tendon gliding and full excursion of the tendons through the carpal tunnel. (From Wehbe M: Tendon gliding exercises, *Am J Occup Ther* 41:164, 1987.)

Postoperative care of the patient in Phase I is divided into pre- (Ia) and post- (Ib) suture removal. During Phase Ia a postoperative dressing is usually worn for 7 to 10 days after surgery. The patient should be instructed to elevate the hand above the heart and ice frequently to help decrease edema. Exercises during Phase Ia consist of AROM to the shoulder, elbow, and digits. The patient is instructed in tendon gliding exercises (Fig. 7-6) to prevent adhesion of the tendons and nerves through the carpal tunnel and decrease edema.[37] AROM exercises are performed three times per day for ten repetitions each. The patient at this time will most likely not require a formal therapy program, and after instruction can perform exercises as a home program.

Phase Ib begins when the sutures are removed and the patient is referred for formal therapy (Table 7-2). Modalities are used to decrease pain, co-contraction

Q. Yvonne is a 48-year-old grocery checker who has been diagnosed with intermediate CTS; she has constant numbness and paresthesia but no thenar atrophy. She had surgery 3 weeks ago for a carpal tunnel release and the edema is persistent. What are some treatment techniques that may be helpful for decreasing edema at this point?

Table 7-2 Carpal Tunnel Release

Rehabilitation Phase	Criteria to Progress to this Phase	Anticipated Impairments and Functional Limitations	Intervention	Goal	Rationale
Phase Ib Postoperative 11-21 days	No signs of infection Sutures removed	• Edema • Pain • Limited functional use of UE • Limited AROM of hand and wrist • Limited strength of hand and wrist • Scar sensitivity, adhesions, and thickening • Persistent paresthesia, especially at night • Limited hand function • Limited patient knowledge of neutral wrist positioning	• Hot pack • Electrical stimulation • Ultrasound, phonophoresis • Iontophoresis • Cryotherapy • Retrograde massage • Isometrics—Wrist—flexion, extension • AROM—Progress exercises as indicated and add Wrist—extension, radial deviation, and ulnar deviation • AROM—Progressive resistance exercises (PREs)—Paper crunches Rice gripping • Wrist splint worn at night as needed • Scar desensitization: gentle manual massage, mini-vibrator massage, add different textures • Mobilization of the median nerve • Use of wrist splint as night as needed • Instruct patient in the following: • Proper use of hand protection while performing self-care • Neutral wrist positioning • Nerve gliding techniques • Fabricate scar conformer	• Decrease postoperative pain by 50% • Manage edema • Increase strength and facilitate gross grasp and wrist stabilization • Full AROM of shoulder, elbow, and forearm • AROM of Wrist—Extension 45° Radial deviation 20° Ulnar deviation 30° Thumb—Opposition to tip of small finger Finger—Flexion to 1 cm of DPC • Decrease sensitivity of scar • Increase mobility of scar • Decrease scar adhesion to flexor tendons, skin, and median nerve • Decrease paresthesia • Promote independent self-care • Maintain neutral wrist position during exercises • Encourage self-management of exercise program • Fatten and or soften scar	• Modalities to manage edema and decrease pain; help in preparation for stretching and strengthening • Massage to facilitate lymphatic return • Increased wrist stabilization strength • Promote full return of UE AROM, continuation of tendon gliding exercises to decrease scar adhesion • *Wrist flexion exercises are contraindicated until 21 days after surgery to prevent bowstringing of tendons* • Strengthening and improvement of endurance of wrist and hand while maintaining neutral position • Encouragement of wrist extension with finger flexion • Neutral position to minimize pressure on median nerve • Organized sensory input normalizes sensory interpretation • Early motion organizes collagen development in scar and limits scar from restricting median nerve • Neutral position is optimal for minimizing pressure on the median nerve • Initiation of self-management • Minimizing of development of pillar pain • Incorporation of neutral position during exercises and ADLs to prevent complications • Pressure applied over a scar organizes collagen

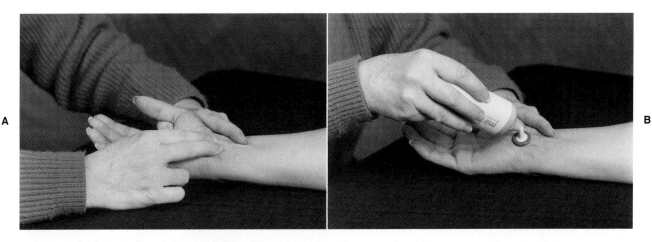

Fig. 7-7. Scar massage is initiated using manual techniques to decrease scar adhesion to the underlying tissues (**A**) and progressed with a mini-vibrator (**B**).

of muscles, and edema. Modalities also are used to increase elasticity of tissues and promote tissue healing.[35]

Moist heat by itself or in conjunction with transcutaneous electrical stimulation (TENS) or interferential current is used for pain control before exercise. Severe pain is rare, but patients experiencing it may consider renting a home unit for a few weeks. The modalities of phonophoresis,[27] iontophoresis,[35] and high voltage galvanic stimulation[35] (HVGS) are helpful in reducing the local swelling and pain experienced by patients after carpal tunnel release. Phonophoresis using a 3-MHz head[27] is performed over the closed healing incision and the thenar and hypothenar eminences. The ultrasound intensity is set between .30 and .50 w/cm^2 for 5 minutes.

Iontophoresis is the modality of choice for decreasing local edema about the incision site.[35] However, the incision must be completely healed and able to tolerate the stimulation.

Cryotherapy administered after exercises for 10 minutes may be helpful for managing edema and pain. Light retrograde massage also may facilitate lymphatic return. Patients with persistent edema may benefit from wearing a compression glove in conjunction with other edema-controlling modalities. The glove should be worn almost continuously at first and then worn only at night as edema decreases. Splinting the wrist in a neutral position may be beneficial for patients experiencing moderate to severe surgical discomfort or persistent paresthesia.

The therapist should initiate scar desensitization when the surgical incision is closed. The desensitization process is initiated gently and can be performed in many ways. These methods include manual self-massage of the scar or the use of a mini-vibrator, gripping of different textured particles, and rubbing the scar with different textures such as a towel.[36] Scar massage is initiated with minimal force, and the force is increased as the incision increases in tensile strength (Fig. 7-7). Scar massage is done for 1 to 3 minutes five times per day. Performing scar massage with the mini-vibrator can be especially helpful for patients with bilateral involvement.

Limiting the development of scar adhesion to tendons, skin, and nerves is another important aspect of scar management in the patient after carpal tunnel release surgery. Tendon gliding exercises are continued to move the flexor tendons differentially in the carpal tunnel. Nerve gliding techniques are helpful in maintaining mobility of the median nerve after a carpal tunnel release.[4] The patient's initial home program for median nerve gliding begins with the arm held at the side of the body, the elbow extended, and the forearm and wrist in neutral position. The patient is instructed to extend the wrist from a neutral position in a pumping action for three sets of four repetitions, three times per day. The patient should be cautioned not to be overzealous with these exercises and to inform the therapist if symptoms increase.

When the incision is fully closed, a scar conformer can be fabricated from silicone elastomers[4] or cut from silicone gel sheets (Fig. 7-8). Because the scar conformer works by applying pressure over the scar, it needs to be held firmly in place. The therapist should use a self-adherent wrap such as Coban to secure the conformer over the scar. The patient should be instructed not to wrap the scar conformer too tightly with the Coban because tight wrapping will cause edema and pain in the hand. An explanation should be given to the patient regarding the purpose and importance of wearing the scar conformer properly at night for at least 3 months. The patient should wash the scar conformer daily to prevent skin irritation and replace the scar conformer if it becomes worn or soiled. The patient should observe the skin closely for signs

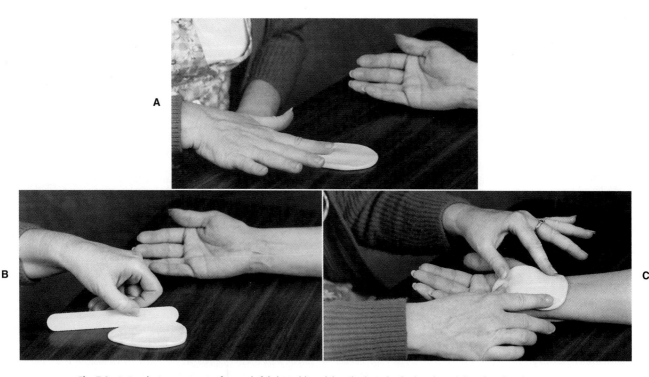

Fig. 7-8. A, An elastomer scar conformer is fabricated by mixing the base in the hands and then forming the scar conformer on the table to ensure a smooth back. **B,** A tongue depressor is used to shape the edges while the scar conformer partially sets up. **C,** The scar conformer is molded to the patient just before setting up is completed.

of skin maceration or heat rash. If these problems occur, the patient should stop using the scar conformer and inform the therapist. Skin maceration and heat rash may be controlled by decreasing the amount of wear time or placing a light gauze or tissue between the scar conformer and the skin.

The exercises given in Phase Ia are continued and wrist exercises are added. Wrist AROM exercises should be limited to extension, radial deviation, and ulnar deviation. Flexion of the wrist is avoided until 21 days after surgery to prevent bowstringing of the flexor tendons through the healing carpal ligament.

Paper crunches and rice gripping are two beneficial activities to facilitate the development of gross grasp, maintain a neutral wrist position, and increase finger and wrist extensor endurance. Fig. 7-9 provides instructions for the paper crunch exercise. Rice gripping is beneficial for scar site desensitization and encouragement of wrist extension with finger flexion. The exercise is performed with the patient standing at a table with the container of rice stabilized on the table. The patient grasps the rice while extending the wrist and releases it into the same container. Wrist flexion is avoided in this phase. Grasping endurance is built up to 3 minutes and is continued as a home exercise two times per day.

The therapist should then initiate isometric strengthening exercises for wrist extension and flexion. Wrist isometrics are performed in a neutral wrist position.[19] The patient applies enough resistance with the oppo-

site hand to create a muscle contraction, which is held for 5 seconds without increasing pain. Isometric exercises should be performed for five repetitions three times per day. The exercises can be progressed by increasing resistance and repetitions. Instruction on ways to maintain a neutral wrist position during functional

A. Light retrograde massage may facilitate lymphatic return. Patients with persistent edema may benefit from wearing a compression glove in conjunction with other edema-controlling modalities. Initially the glove should be worn almost continuously. As the edema decreases, the patient only needs to wear the glove at night.

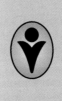

Q. Yvonne tends to heal quickly after having surgery. In fact, she had difficulty regaining full knee ROM after knee surgery because adhesions quickly formed around the joint. Limiting the development of scar adhesions also is important in the patient who has had a CTR. What are some problematic areas Yvonne may have after her CTR? What types of treatment can be used to limit scar adhesions in this area?

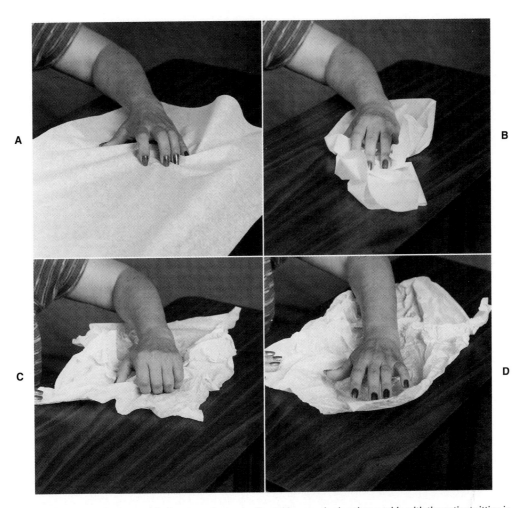

Fig. 7-9. Paper crunches. **A,** A 22-inch square of examination table paper is placed on a table with the patient sitting in a straight-back chair, elbow at about 90 degrees and the wrist positioned in neutral. **B,** The patient starts at one corner of the paper and crumples it into a ball using the involved hand. **C,** The patient then stabilizes the paper with the uninvolved hand and makes a fist with the involved hand with the forearm and wrist in neutral 2 inches above the paper. **D,** The patient rapidly extends the digits, pushing the paper open while maintaining a neutral wrist position. The process of fisting and extending the digits is repeated until the paper is opened fully. The paper crunches are progressed from one to three repetitions per session as the patient tolerates.

use of the hand is emphasized with paper crunch activity and isometric strengthening exercises. This education is further emphasized with ergonomic instruction in Phase II.

The patient should be encouraged to use the affected hand for self-care while avoiding wrist flexion, forceful repetitive grip, and lifting more than 3 pounds. Tasks that require forceful grip such as vacuuming, handling wet laundry, putting fitted sheets on the bed, yard work, tool use, lifting, and pushing should be avoided for 6 to 8 weeks to allow healing.

Phase II: The Proliferation Phase

TIME: Weeks 4-6
GOALS: Complete self-management of symptoms and home maintenance program, return to full-time work activities

Phase II focuses primarily on strengthening and education (Table 7-3). It begins on day 22 after surgery and continues until day 42 (6 weeks after surgery). Phase Ib modalities are continued for edema and pain control. Moist heat is continued before exercises. Scar desensitization is continued with scar massage, and the patient may progress to use of a larger vibrator for desensitization. Texture desensitization techniques are continued, especially as part of the home program. Use of a gel shell to pad the sensitive palm may increase comfort for performing self-care and light home care. Tendon gliding and nerve gliding exercises and scar massage are continued to decrease scar adhesions. The pressure used for scar massage is increased in intensity for manual massage. Use of the scar conformer is continued at night to soften and flatten the scar.

The patient can add active wrist flexion exercises after 21 days with the expectation of full wrist flexion

Table 7-3   Carpal Tunnel Release

Rehabilitation Phase	Criteria to Progress to this Phase	Anticipated Impairments and Functional Limitations	Intervention	Goal	Rationale

Phase II Postoperative 4-6 weeks	Pain controlled
	No loss of ROM
	No loss of strength
	Well-healed incision
		• Mild edema
		• Mild pain
		• Limited AROM of wrist, fingers, and thumb
		• Scar sensitivity
		• Scar adhesion
		• Scar raised or thickened
		• Limited UE strength
		• Limited ability to perform light ADLs involving gripping and twisting
		• Limited knowledge of proper work environment organization (ergonomics)
		• Limited tolerance to repetitive finger and hand use
			Continuation of modalities as indicated from Phases Ib
			Continuation of the following:
			• Scar desensitization techniques
			• Retrograde massage
			• AROM and PREs
			• Scar conformer at night
			• Progress firmness of manual scar massage and use larger vibrator to massage scar
			Add the following:
			• PROM (stretches)—Pectoralis
			Composite motions of the following:
			1. Wrist flexion forearm pronation, and elbow extension
			2. Wrist extension, forearm pronation and elbow extension
				As in Tables 7-1 and 7-2
				• Resolve edema in fingers
				• Decrease pain by 70%
				• Decrease sensitivity of scar and increase scar mobility
				• Decrease scar adhesion to flexor tendons, skin, and median nerve
				• Increase tolerance of UE to reaching away from body
				• AROM of wrist—
				  Extension 60°
				  Radial deviation 25°
				  Ulnar deviation 35°
				• Make a full fist to DPC
				• Thumb to DPC at base of small finger
				• Grip strength 30%-50% of uninvolved hand
				• Wrist strength 80%-90%
				• Proximal strength greater than 85%
				• Lift and carry 3-5 lb with involved hand
					As in Tables 7-1 and 7-2
					• Decrease reliance on modalities and increase patient's ability to self-manage edema and pain
					• Continuation of exercises as indicated to allow progression of program as tolerated by patient
					• Scar should now be able to handle increased mobilization techniques
					• UE stretches to elongate muscle tendon units for increased function
					• Healing of transverse carpal ligament is adequate to prevent bowstringing of the flexor tendons
					• *Monitor triggering of one or more digits, stop gripping exercises and treat per physician's orders*

3. Wrist extension, forearm supination, and elbow extension

- AROM—Wrist flexion
- Putty exercises (light resistive putty)—
  - Finger pinch
  - Finger grip
- Isotonics—
  Upper quarter exercises as in Table 4-3 (using 1- or 2-pound weights)
  Wrist (weight well)—Flexion, extension (begin with 0-2 lb and progress as indicated)
  Forearm—Pronation supination (progress as indicated)
- Patient education regarding body mechanics, joint protection, and modification of ADLs using adaptive equipment (grip assistive devices)
- Ergonomic evaluation
- Work simulated exercises, emphasizing neutral position of the wrists and pacing tasks; may need handwriting re-training

- Independence with ADLs using assistive devices as necessary and limiting exposure to heavy grasping activities
- Organize work environment to decrease potential for reinjury and maximize efficiency
- Work simulation for 10 minutes, alternating tasks

- Upper quarter strengthening as a functional unit
- Initiate exercises with low repetitions to prevent development of tenosynovitis and pillar pain
- Use appropriate assistive device to prevent reinjury and increase independence with ADLs; avoiding heavier gripping activities such as vacuuming, laundry, and yard work; use forearms to carry versus finger grip (groceries in paper bags versus plastic)
- Promote self-management of symptoms and prevent reinjury in the work environment
- Prepare for return to work

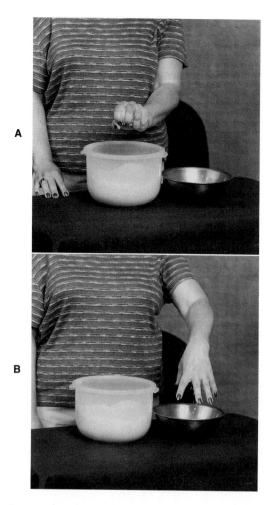

Fig. 7-10. A, Rice gripping is initiated by grasping the rice and extending the wrist. **B,** During phase II the patient is allowed to flex the wrist while transferring the rice into a separate bowl.

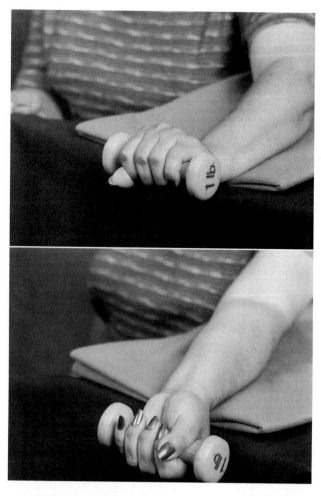

Fig. 7-11. PREs are important to strengthen the wrist extensor (**A**) and flexor (**B**) musculature. The table is padded with a towel to prevent excessive pressure on the median and ulnar nerves.

by the end of the sixth week after surgery. Rice gripping (Fig. 7-10) and paper crunches are continued. However, the patient transfers the rice to a second container, focusing on wrist extension when gripping the rice and wrist flexion when dropping the rice into the second container.

Full upper extremity stretching exercises are added at this time. Upper extremity stretches include composite motions of (1) wrist flexion, forearm pronation, and elbow extension; (2) wrist extension, forearm pronation, and elbow extension; and (3) wrist extension, forearm supination, and elbow extension.[28]

Resistive gripping and pinching exercises with light resistive putty may be started 28 days after surgery. Initially, putty exercises should be limited to 3-minute sessions two times per day. Putty exercises must be comfortably tolerated before moving to more resistive putty. Clinically the authors of this chapter have noted that the overuse of repetitive gripping with putty increases the chance of developing pillar pain. Pillar pain is described as pain in the thenar or hypothenar eminence and is distinguished from local

scar tenderness.[6,7,22] The therapist should instruct the patient that the maximum use of putty is two times a day for 5 minutes and tell him or her to stop using the putty and notify the therapist if the pain increases significantly.

Wrist isometric exercises are continued along with the initiation of grip isometric exercises. Grip isometric exercises can be performed by squeezing a towel roll in the hand. Light progressive resistance exercises (PREs) are added when pain is controlled. PREs are added for both wrist extension and flexion (Fig. 7-11).[19] Resistance should begin at $\frac{1}{2}$ to 1 pound and progressed to 3 pounds as the patient tolerates. *The abductor pollicis longus and the extensor pollicis brevis are prone to tenosynovitis at the first dorsal extensor compartment so specific strengthening in radial deviation is not done.*

Wrist and grip strengthening are progressed to using a weight well or computerized work simulator (Fig. 7-12). The patient starts on the weight well with no weight or on the work simulator at minimal torque and progresses as tolerated.

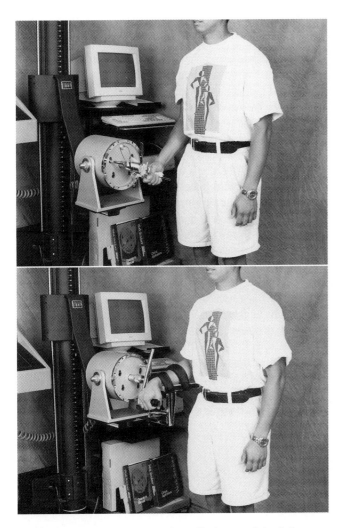

Fig. 7-12. Computerized equipment is an effective way of simulating many work tasks and strengthening muscles; it requires a relatively small area in the clinic.

Proximal muscle strengthening of the forearm, elbow, shoulder, and shoulder girdle are started on day 28 after surgery. Forearm rotation can be strengthened using a 16-oz hammer held with the elbow flexed at 90 degrees and stabilized against the side of the body. The therapist should ask the patient to rotate the forearm from the neutral position into supination and then return to neutral. After completing the desired repetitions, the patient repeats the exercise into pronation. Simply moving the hammerhead away from the hand to increase or toward the hand to decrease resistance can change the resistance of the exercise. Biceps curls and elbow extension exercises can be performed with dumbbells beginning at 1 or 2 lb and progressing as the patient tolerates. Shoulder and shoulder girdle exercises beginning with 1 to 2 lb are important and are performed for flexion, abduction, internal and external rotation, and scapular retraction. The patient should be monitored closely during the advancement of the proximal strengthening program to prevent the develop-

ment of other cumulative trauma disorders such as shoulder impingement syndrome, lateral epicondylitis, or de Quervain's syndrome.

Treatment of the patient after carpal tunnel release surgery also must include instruction on ergonomic principles, proper posture, and body mechanics for lifting to prevent recurrence of CTS or the development of other repetitive stress injuries. Instruction should include general topics for all patients and job-specific teaching for those returning to highly repetitive or heavy labor jobs.

Ergonomic recommendations. Patients with jobs involving computers should be instructed in workstation setup. A good chair is important. An ergonomic chair should include (1) an adjustable height, (2) a proper seat depth (two to three fingers' clearance from the front edge of the seat pan of the chair to the back of the knees), and (3) an adjustable back height with lumbar support.[10] The keyboard should be placed directly in front of the patient and the height of the chair adjusted so the patient's elbows are flexed to 90 degrees or a little less with wrists in a neutral position over the keyboard. A keyboard tray may need to be added to the desk to achieve proper positioning. A footrest is used for patients whose feet do not reach the floor after the chair height is properly adjusted. Using ergonomic keyboards or negatively tilting the keyboard also may be useful for maintaining a neutral wrist position. When a wrist rest is used, the patient should be instructed not to press on it during typing but to use it to support the upper extremities when scanning the monitor screen. The monitor should be positioned with the top at eye level and approximately 18 in away from the patient.[28] When typing from text the patient should position the work next to the monitor and at the same height and use a monitor stand to decrease cervical and shoulder strain. He or she also should position the mouse at the same height as the keyboard and within forearm length. The therapist should try as many ergonomic adjustments as possible in the clinic and encourage the patient to evaluate other options at a local computer store and pick items that are most comfortable for their individual work stations.

Patients in highly repetitive jobs (such as assembly workers) or those involved in heavy labor present other problems. Patients in these fields are constantly using their wrists and hands for turning screwdrivers, using wrenches, swinging hammers, and using power equipment. These activities generate high torque, pressure, and vibration on the carpal tunnel. Therefore they should be instructed to perform their job tasks using a neutral wrist position. Various ergonomic tools or a change to a power tool may assist the patient with achieving the most ergonomically correct position. Patients may be encouraged to go to their local hardware store to evaluate tools for comfort and applicability to their work. The use of work splints and anti-vibration gloves also may provide benefits by decreasing pain, providing support, and decreasing hypersensitivity. The patient should wear the gloves only when performing heavy or highly repetitive tasks.

Patients with sedentary jobs are usually discharged to a home program by the end of phase II. Heavy laborers generally progress to phase III at 6 to 8 weeks after surgery, where more emphasis is placed on increasing strength, endurance, and return to work activities.

 **A.** Limiting the development of scar adhesion to tendons, skin, and nerves is another important aspect of scar management in the patient after carpal tunnel release surgery. Tendon gliding exercises are continued to move the flexor tendons differentially in the carpal tunnel. Nerve gliding techniques are helpful in maintaining mobility of the median nerve after a carpal tunnel release.

Phase III: The Remodeling and Maturation Phase

Phase III begins at 43 days (6 weeks) after surgery and ends when the scar is mature (Table 7-4). This phase can last for a year or longer. The patient is normally discharged by day 84 (after 12 weeks). The types of patients who progress to phase III are heavy laborers, construction workers, mechanics, and assembly workers. These patients should be able to progress from local heating modalities such as hot packs to aerobic exercise using a bicycle, treadmill, or upper extremity ergometer. The stretching program and scar management program from phase II is continued. Scar massage also continues, with the patient wearing the scar conformer until the scar color is no longer reddened. Scar maturation can take as long as 1 year. Phase II strengthening exercises should be continued and progressed as tolerated. Large muscle group exercises using gym equipment or free weights are appropriate at this time for general body conditioning.

Work activity simulation is an important aspect of the phase III therapy protocol. These activities can include a using pipe tree or assembly boards and learning lifting and carrying techniques. The use of work simulation equipment can be helpful for strength-

---

Table 7-4   Carpal Tunnel Release

Rehabilitation Phase	Criteria to Progress to this Phase	Anticipated Impairments and Functional Limitations	Intervention	Goal	Rationale
Phase III Postoperative 6-12 weeks	Patients need to perform job that requires heavy lifting	• Limited UE and grip strength • Limited UE and grip endurance	Continuation of exercises and stretches in Phases I and II as indicated • Progress UE strengthening exercises, emphasizing endurance for return to work activities • Functional capacity evaluation • Work simulated activities	Decrease number of exercises and stretches • Adequate strength to return to work activities full time • Self-management of symptoms	• Increase efficiency of home exercises in self-management of condition • Promote muscle balance of UE • Assess potential to return to work • Initiate appropriate program (work hardening, work conditioning, or supervised gym program)

ening and simulation of specific work activities (see Fig. 7-12).

Clearly, CTS affects patients physically, financially, and psychologically. Comprehensive management of the patient recovering from surgery for CTS optimizes the potential to return to ADLs, work, and avocational activities.

Suggested Home Maintenance for the Postsurgical Patient

The home maintenance box on pages 117 to 118 outlines the shoulder rehabilitation the patient is to follow. The physical therapist can use it in customizing a patient-specific program.

❧ Suggested Home Maintenance for the Postsurgical Patient

Days 1-10

GOALS FOR THE PERIOD: Decrease pain, manage edema, improve AROM of upper extremity, initiate self-management and patient education
1. Protect incision
2. Elevate the hand above the heart
3. Ice frequently
4. AROM exercises for shoulder, elbow, forearm, and thumb
5. Tendon gliding exercises

Days 11-21

GOALS FOR THE PERIOD: Decrease pain, manage edema, improve AROM of upper extremity, initiate self-management and patient education
1. Moist heat
2. Retrograde massage when incision has closed
3. Scar massage when incision has closed
4. Continue tendon gliding exercises
5. Nerve-gliding exercises
6. Continue AROM exercises for shoulder, elbow, forearm, and thumb
7. Add AROM exercises for wrist extension, radial deviation, and ulnar deviation (avoid wrist flexion)
8. Paper crunches
9. Rice gripping (into same container)
10. Isometric exercises for wrist extension and flexion
11. Use scar conformer at night
12. Use splint at night as needed to control persistent paresthesia
13. Ice as necessary

Days 22-42

GOALS FOR THE PERIOD: Decrease pain, manage edema, improve AROM of upper extremity, initiate self-management and patient education
1. Continue all previous exercises and modalities as indicated
2. Add wrist flexion AROM
3. Rice gripping (transferring rice to a second container)
4. Add upper extremity stretching exercises
   a. Wrist flexion, forearm pronation, and elbow extension
   b. Wrist extension, forearm pronation, and elbow extension
   c. Wrist extension, forearm supination, and elbow extension
5. Add putty gripping and pinching exercises with light resistive putty (only two times a day for 5 minutes)

Continued

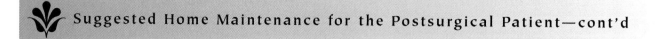

Suggested Home Maintenance for the Postsurgical Patient—cont'd

Days 22-42—cont'd

6. Add grip isometric exercises by squeezing a towel roll
7. Add PREs for wrist extension and flexion with $1/2$ to 1 lb
8. Add PREs for shoulder girdle, shoulder, elbow with 1 to 2 lb
9. Add forearm strengthening using a 16-oz hammer
10. Continue to use scar conformer at night
11. Practice ergonomic principles

Days 43-84

GOALS FOR THE PERIOD: Complete self-management of symptoms and home maintenance program, return to full-time work activities
1. Aerobic warm-up exercise using a bicycle or treadmill
2. Continue previous exercises as indicated, progressing intensity and duration as indicated

REFERENCES

1. Agee J et al: Endoscopic release of the carpal tunnel: a randomized prospective multicenter study, *J Hand Surg* 17A:987, 1992.

2. American Society for Surgery of the Hand: *The hand: examination and diagnosis,* Aurora, CO, 1978, The Society.

3. American Society for Surgery of the Hand: *The hand: examination and diagnosis,* ed 2, New York, 1983, Churchill Livingstone.

4. Baxter-Petralia PL: Therapist's management of carpal tunnel syndrome. In Hunter JM et al, editors: *Rehabilitation of the hand: surgery and therapy,* ed 3, St Louis, 1990, Mosby.

5. Beckenbaugh RD: Carpal tunnel syndrome. In Cooney WP, Linsscheid RL, Dobyns JH, editors: *The wrist: diagnosis and operative treatment,* St Louis, 1998, Mosby.

6. Brown RA et al: Carpal tunnel release: a prospective, randomized assessment of open and endoscopic methods, *J Bone Joint Surg* 75A:1265, 1993.

7. Buchanan RT et al: Method, education and therapy of carpal tunnel patients, *Hand Surg Quarterly,* Summer 1995.

8. Bureau of Labor Statistics: *Survey of occupation injuries and illness in 1994,* Washington, DC, 1996, US Department of Labor.

9. Crosby C, Wehbe M, Mawr M: Hand strength: normative values, *J Hand Surg* 19A:665, 1994.

10. Donkin S: *Sitting on the job, how to survive the stresses of sitting down to work—a practical handbook,* Boston, 1989, Houghton Mifflin.

11. Evangelisti S, Reale V: Fibroma of tendon sheath as a cause of carpal tunnel syndrome, *J Hand Surg* 17A:1026, 1992.

12. Eversmann WW, Jr: Entrapment and compression neuropathies. In Green DP, editor: *Operative hand surgery,* ed 3, New York, 1993, Churchill Livingstone.

13. Fess EE, Morgan C: *Clinical assessment recommendations,* Indianapolis, 1981, American Society of Hand Therapists.

14. Fess EE: Grip strength. In American Society of Hand Therapists, editors: *Clinical assessment recommendations,* ed 2, Chicago, 1992, The Society.

15. Frymoyer J, Bland J: Carpal tunnel syndrome in patients with myxedematous arthropathy, *J Bone Joint Surg* 55A:78, 1973.

16. Gelbrman R et al: Sensibility testing in peripheral-nerve compression syndromes, an experimental study in humans, *J Bone Joint Surg* 65A(5):632, 1983.

17. Gretchen L, Jezek S: Pain assessment. In American Society of Hand Therapists, editors: *Clinical assessment recommendations,* ed 2, Chicago, 1992, The Society.

18. Jaffe R, Farney-Mokris S: Edema. In American Society of Hand Therapists, editors: *Clinical assessment recommendations,* ed 2, Chicago, 1992, The Society.

19. Kasch M: Therapists evaluation and treatment of upper extremity cumulative trauma disorders. In Hunter JM, Mackin EJ, Callahan AD, editors: *Rehabilitation of the hand: surgery and therapy,* ed 4, St Louis, 1995, Mosby.

20. Kerwin G, Williams CS, Seilier JG, III: The pathophysiology of carpal tunnel syndrome, *Hand Clin* 12(2):243, 1996.

21. Louise DS et al: Carpal tunnel syndrome in the work place, *Hand Clin* 12(2):305, 1996.

22. Ludlow KS et al: Pillar pain as a postoperative complication of carpal tunnel release: a review of the literature, *J Hand Ther* 10(4):277, 1997.

23. MacDermid J: Accuracy of clinical tests used in the detection of carpal tunnel syndrome: a literature review, *J Hand Ther* 4(4):169, 1991.

24. Macmermid J et al: Interrater reliability of pinch and grip strength measurements in patients with cumulative trauma disorders, *J Hand Ther* 7(1):10, 1984.

25. Mathiowetz V et al: Grip and pinch strength: normative data for adults, *Arch Phys Med Rehabil* 66:69, 1985.

26. Mathiowetz V et al: Adult norms for the nine hole peg test of finger dexterity, *Occup Ther J Res* 5:24, 1985.

27. Michlovitz SL: Use of ultrasound in upper extremity rehabilitation. In Hunter JM, Mackin EJ, Callahan AD, editors: *Rehabilitation of the hand: surgery and therapy*, ed 4, St Louis, 1995, Mosby.

28. Pascarelli E, Quilter D: *Repetitive strain injury, a computer user's guide*, New York, 1994, John Wiley & Sons.

29. Phalen G S: The carpal tunnel syndrome: seventeen years experience in diagnosis and treatment of six hundred and fifty-four, *J Bone Joint Surg* 48:211, 1966.

30. Robbins H: Anatomical study of the median nerve in the carpal tunnel and etiologies of the carpal tunnel syndrome, *J Bone Joint Surg* 45A:953, 1963.

31. Sailer SM: The role of splinting and rehabilitation in the treatment of carpal and cubital tunnel syndromes, *Hand Clin* 12(2):223, 1996.

32. Spindler H, Dellon A: Nerve conduction studies and sensibility testing in carpal tunnel syndrome, *J Hand Surg* 7:260, 1982.

33. Stone J: Sensibility. In American Society of Hand Therapists, editors: *Clinical assessment recommendations*, ed 2, Chicago, 1992, The Society.

34. Tanaka S et al: Prevalence and work-relatedness of self-reported carpal tunnel syndrome among U.S. workers: analysis of the occupational health supplement data of 1988 National Health Interview Survey, *Am J Industr Med* 27:451, 1995.

35. Taylor Mullins PA: Use of therapeutic modalities in upper extremity rehabilitation. In Hunter JM, Mackin EJ, Callahan AD, editors: *Rehabilitation of the hand: surgery and therapy*, ed 4, St Louis, 1995, Mosby.

36. Waylett-Rendall J: Desensitization of the traumatized hand. In Hunter JM, Mackin EJ, Callahan AD, editors: *Rehabilitation of the hand: surgery and therapy*, ed 4, St Louis, 1995, Mosby.

37. Wehbe M: Tendon gliding exercises, *Am J Occup Ther* 41:164, 1987.

38. Weiss ND et al: Position of the wrist associated with the lowest carpal-tunnel pressure: implications for splint design, *J Bone Joint Surg* 77A(11):1695, 1995.

PART TWO

Spine

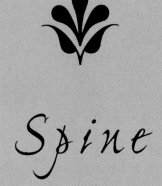

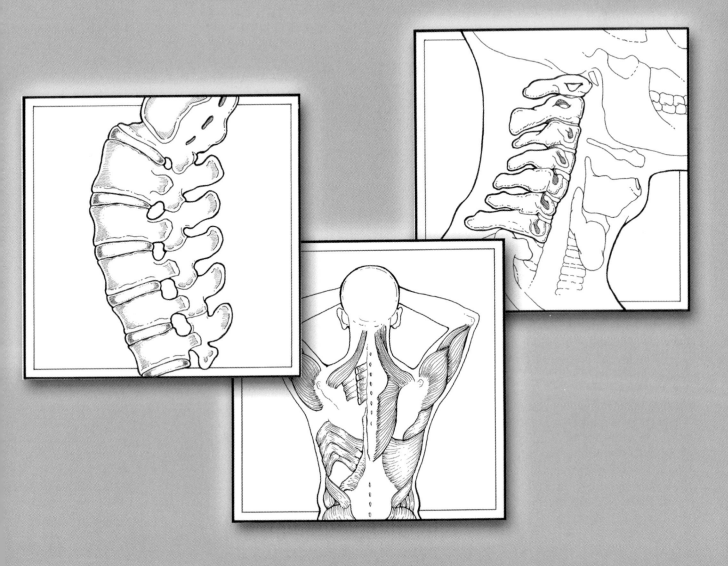

Chapter 8

Lumbar Microdiscectomy and Rehabilitation

Rick B. Delamarter
James Coyle
David Pakozdi

Lumbar disc herniation and the acute radicular syndrome that occasionally ensues are common occurrences. About 35% of patients with lumbar disc herniation develop true sciatica. However, not all lumbar disc herniations produce symptoms. In patients younger than 60 years, 20% to 35% of lumbar disc herniations are asymptomatic.[2,3] Also, 90% of those with their first episode of sciatica improve with conservative care.

Surgical Indications and Considerations

In patients with radicular symptoms, surgery may be considered if certain criteria are met (Box 8-1). A clearly defined lesion that anatomically corresponds with the clinical nerve root level should be evident on magnetic resonance imaging (MRI).[27]

Etiology

Despite the prevalent misconception that most lumbar disc herniations result from a single event or trauma, Kirkaldy-Willis[19] has stated that microtrauma, primarily from repetitive lumbar flexion and rotation movements, leads to a degenerative cascade that frequently results in a herniated nucleus pulposus (see Table 9-1). Adams and Hutton[1] provide additional evidence for the gradual process of posterior disc herniation.

The clinical presentation of lumbar disc herniation varies because of the level, size, and position of the herniation. However, common signs and symptom patterns do exist. About 80% of the population experience significant low back pain during herniation. In addition, the pain may radiate into the lower extremity along the anatomic distribution of the affected nerve root. Neural compression or irritation may precipitate motor weakness, reduced reflexes, and sensory loss. The lumbar lordosis may be reduced, and a compensatory lateral shift of the trunk frequently occurs. The pain can be quite severe, limiting all upright activities. About 90% of all lumbar disc herniations occur at the L4-L5 and L5-S1 levels, so the L5 and S1 nerve roots are the most involved. The straight leg raise test (at less than 30 degrees) and crossed straight leg raise test are sensitive mechanical tests for lumbar disc herniation.

Conservative treatment varies, although the evidence favors a kinetic management approach (an extension program[29] followed by dynamic muscular stabilization[45] with progressive activity resumption). Traction, manual therapy techniques, electrotherapeutic modalities, and physical agents are usually used to support the functional restoration program. Pharmacologic intervention also varies and typically consists of appropriate analgesics, nonsteroidal antiinflammatory agents, and occasionally muscle relaxants. Oral corticosteroids and epidural steroids can be employed.

Box 8-1 Indications for Lumbar Discectomy

Strong Indications for Surgical Intervention

1. Bladder and bowel involvement (cauda equina syndrome)
2. Progressive neurologic deficit

Relative Indications for Surgical Intervention

1. Failure to respond to an active conservative treatment regimen of at least 6 weeks
2. Severe, incapacitating pain that eludes all forms of medicinal and physical pain control
3. Recurrent episodes of sciatica
4. Significant neurologic deficit with significant positive straight leg raise test

---

Surgical Procedure

Discectomy via laminectomy is gradually being replaced by lumbar microdiscectomy as the standard of care for the surgical treatment of lumbar disc herniation. Although microscopic surgery for lumbar disc disease is a technique that has evolved over the past 20 years, its use and acceptance are steadily increasing. Clinical outcomes at follow-up are in the 85% to 90% good to excellent range.[27]

Other minimally invasive surgical techniques addressing lumbar disc herniation include percutaneous and endoscopic discectomy. The clinical efficacy of these techniques is somewhat controversial because they only apply to certain types and positions of herniations. Moreover, their ability to match the clinical outcomes obtained with microdiscectomy has not been demonstrated in widespread use.

The goals of postoperative rehabilitation after spinal surgery are well served by the surgical techniques employed in microdiscectomy. These goals are focused on early patient return to maximal functional status and include reduction of pain frequency and intensity; limitation of scar tissue formation and maintenance of dural mobility; and rehabilitation of lumbar paraspinal muscles to maximize strength, flexibility, and conditioning and prevent recurrence of injury. To these ends, microdiscectomy offers advantages over the traditional laminectomy and discectomy by combining a smaller surgical exposure with far superior visualization of the operating field. This less invasive surgical approach results in decreased perioperative bleeding and hematoma formation and less paraspinal muscle denervation and fibrosis. Improved visualization of the operating field allows for more precision in surgical technique, better nerve decompression, less chance of iatrogenic injury, and a reduction in the amount of peridural scar tissue formed postoperatively. Patients who undergo microdiscectomy typically have less postoperative pain and morbidity and a shorter hospital stay. The length of postoperative hospitalization after microdiscectomy typically ranges from 6 to 36 hours.

Guidelines for Surgery

The guidelines applicable to surgical decision making for microdiscectomy are the same as those employed for a traditional discectomy. They include proper patient selection, as well as a complete history and physical examination. The patient's symptoms and neurologic signs should correlate closely with findings of nerve root impingement seen on MRI. In many cases nerve root impingement results from a combination of disc herniation and stenosis caused by facet hypertrophy or ligamentum flavum thickening. Other causes of nerve root impingement include far lateral disc herniation, synovial cyst formation caused by facet arthritis, and foraminal stenosis secondary to facet hypertrophy. When an MRI cannot be obtained, evidence of nerve root impingement may be seen on a computed tomographic (CT) myelogram.

A decision for surgery using the microdiscectomy technique should incorporate a precise understanding of the location and extent of pathology causing nerve root compression. This allows the surgeon to formulate a specific surgical plan before surgery that includes the level of approach and extent of decompression of lamina, ligamentum flavum, and facets.

The primary goal of a microdiscectomy is not to remove a portion of the disc, but rather to decompress the involved nerve root or roots while minimizing scar tissue formation and avoiding iatrogenic nerve damage and decompression that may biomechanically destabilize the spinal column. The surgical technique employed depends on the location and type of disc herniation. Disc herniations may be subligamentous or extruded and sequestered. The position of the disc herniation may be central and intraannular, pericentric within the spinal canal, intraforaminal, or extraforaminal. Extruded fragments may migrate caudally or cephalad with respect to the disc space of origin.

Instruments

Microdiscectomy requires a set of surgical instruments that are in general smaller, lighter, and more precise than standard spinal instruments. An operating microscope that provides a global view of the operating field is a necessity. The microscope is covered with a sterile drape and must be configured and balanced to allow the operating surgeon to adjust position in all planes easily. Focal length and magnification power also should be adjustable, with magnification typically ranging from 2× to 7× power. The microscope uses a high-intensity light source and may have video monitor and photographic capability. The operating microscope allows the surgeon to maintain a stereoptic, three-dimensional view of the operating field through surgical incisions smaller than 30 mm, something not possible with surgical magnification loupes. Additionally, the surgeon's assistant is afforded the same unobstructed view of the operating field (Fig. 8-1).

A surgical retractor is used to expose the surgical site after the initial incision has been made and the surgical approach established. The ideal retractor has a low profile and provides good visibility to the surgical site with no soft tissue obstruction of the wound. At the same time, it should be designed to be atraumatic to soft tissues. One such retractor is the McCullough frame retractor (Fig. 8-2).

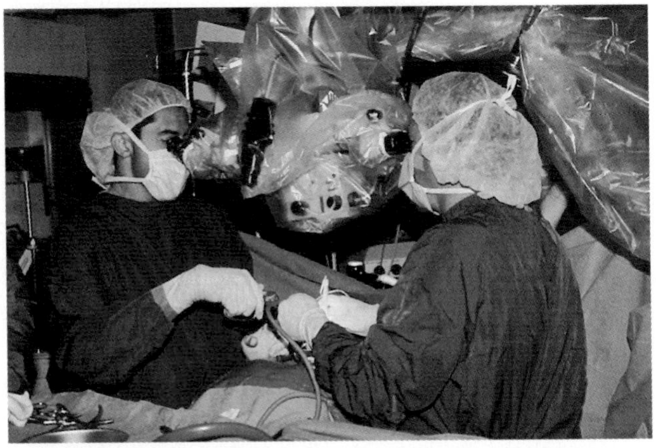

Fig. 8-1. A surgeon and an assistant surgeon using the operative microscope with a high intensity light source and microscopic magnification. The two surgeons can work hand-in-hand with unobstructed view of the operative field.

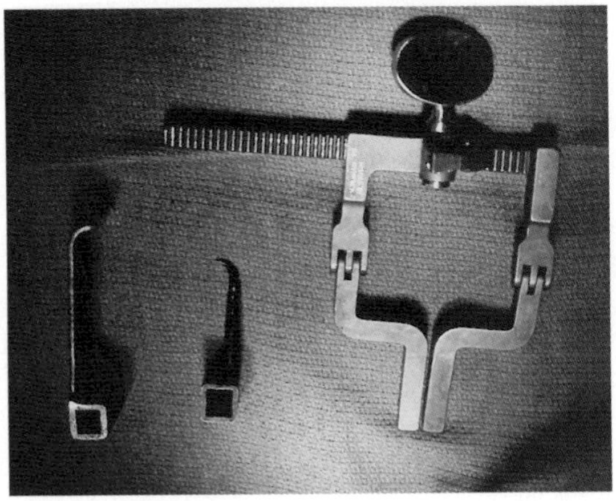

Fig. 8-2. The McCullough microdiscectomy retractor is a small retractor that provides atraumatic retraction of the soft tissues and excellent visualization of the surgical site.

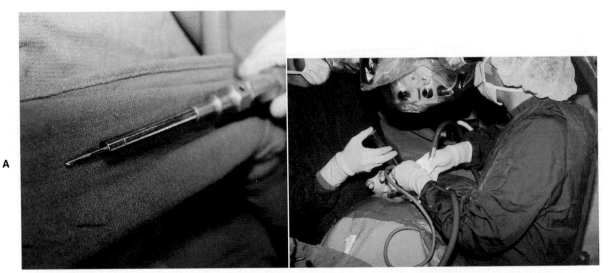

A   B

Fig. 8-3. **A,** This Midas AM-8 high-speed burr provides well-controlled removal of the bony lamina. **B,** Intraoperative photograph showing a microdiscectomy in progress. Note the Midas-Rex AM-8 high-speed drill in the surgeon's right hand. The microscope facilitates the use of microsurgical instruments in the 1-inch incision.

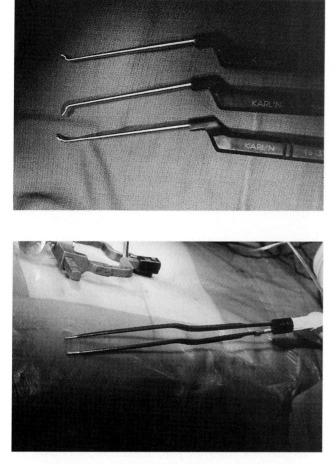

Fig. 8-4. These microcurettes, in various sizes and angulations, allow easy removal of soft tissue, including the ligamentum flavum, from the lamina and median wall of the facet joint. The angled handles keep the surgeon's hand out of the operative field.

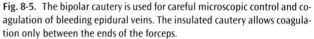

Fig. 8-5. The bipolar cautery is used for careful microscopic control and coagulation of bleeding epidural veins. The insulated cautery allows coagulation only between the ends of the forceps.

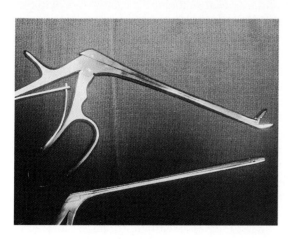

Fig. 8-6. These small pituitary forceps come in various sizes and angulations and allow easy removal of the herniated nucleus pulposus, including fragments from the spinal canal and inside the disc space.

A Cobb periosteal elevator is used to dissect and elevate the paraspinous muscle off the spinous process and lamina. Removal of a portion of the lamina (laminotomy) and other bony tissue is accomplished with a high-speed burr or drill such as the Midas-Rex AM-8 dissector (Fig. 8-3). In addition, Kerrison rongeurs are used to under-bite the lamina and facets and accomplish the necessary laminotomy and foraminotomy. Microcurettes of various sizes and angulations facilitate removal of the ligamentum flavum from the undersurface of the lamina and the medial wall of the superior facet (Fig. 8-4). A nerve root retractor is used to displace the dura and nerve structures medially, exposing the disc space. Bipolar electrocautery provides an electrical current for coagulation of bleeding epidural veins (Fig. 8-5). A No. 11 blade scalpel is used to incise the annulus and gain access to the disc space. Pituitary forceps of various sizes and angulations are used to extract disc fragments (Fig. 8-6).

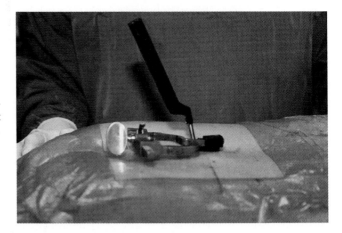

Fig. 8-7. An intraoperative example of a localizing curette. Note the Mc-Cullough spinal retractor and the angled curette at the appropriate disc space. An x-ray film is then taken to identify the appropriate operative level.

Surgical Technique

After induction of anesthesia, the patient is placed on the operating table in either the prone or kneeling prone position. A Wilson frame provides for decompression of abdominal contents, which in turn reduces pressure on the plexus of epidural veins within the spinal canal and results in decreased intraoperative bleeding. The frame also maintains the lumbar spine in flexion, thus widening the interspace between each lamina and reducing the amount of lamina that must be removed to gain access to the spinal canal.

After the patient is placed on the operating table the operative field is prepared and draped in a sterile manner. The incision site is initially determined through palpation of the spinous processes and posterior superior iliac spines. A spinal needle or curette may be placed at the appropriate level and a lateral x-ray film obtained to ascertain the correct operative level (Fig. 8-7).

For a single-level discectomy, a skin incision about 3 cm long is made slightly lateral to midline on the operative side. The lumbodorsal fascia is exposed and sharply incised lateral to the midline with a curvilinear incision extending from the spinous process above to the one below. At this point the paraspinal muscles are elevated subperiosteally with a Cobb elevator. For a single-level discectomy the exposure is confined to the interspace at the level of the herniation.

After the laminae are exposed (Fig. 8-8, *A*), the McCullough retractor is placed in the incision and opened. The operating microscope, sterilely draped, is brought into the operating field. Under direct visualization with the microscope the Midas-Rex Am-8 dissector is used to remove a portion of the inferior aspect of the lamina and then remove 1 to 2 mm of the medial edge of the superior facet (Fig. 8-8, *B*).

A forward-angled curette is used to reflect the ligamentum flavum off the undersurface of the cephalad lamina and the medial wall of the superior facet. The ligamentum flavum may be retracted medially to expose the spinal canal. Alternatively, it may be excised if it is thickened and contributing to nerve root or dural compression. Excision of the ligamentum flavum affords better exposure of the nerve root and disc space, whereas a ligamentum-sparing approach results in less peridural scarring postoperatively.

After the spinal canal is exposed, the dura is retracted medially along with the traversing nerve root. The surgeon uses the medial wall of the pedicle as a landmark because the nerve root is medial to the pedicle and the disc space is superior to it. Retraction of the dura typically exposes most centrally and paracentrically located disc herniations (Fig. 8-8, *C*). After cauterization of the overlying epidural veins, the disc protrusion can be seen. Frequently the nucleus has herniated through the annulus, making an annulotomy unnecessary. If the annulus is intact, an annulotomy may be accomplished with a No. 11 blade scalpel, with the surgeon carefully protecting the nerve root and dura. All extruded disc material, as well as any unstable disc fragments within the disc space, are removed with a combination of pituitary forceps and curettes. The disc space is then irrigated with saline solution through a long angiocatheter to flush out any residual disc fragments.

Before completing the microdiscectomy, the surgeon palpates above and below the nerve root and anterior to the dura to ascertain that no disc fragments are retained. The nerve root should be freely mobile and free from residual compression. Meticulous hemostasis is obtained, and, after irrigation of the wound, the incision is closed using absorbable polyglycolate interrupted sutures for the lumbodorsal fascia and subcutaneous layers. A running subcuticular closure is used for the most superficial layer. A local anesthetic may

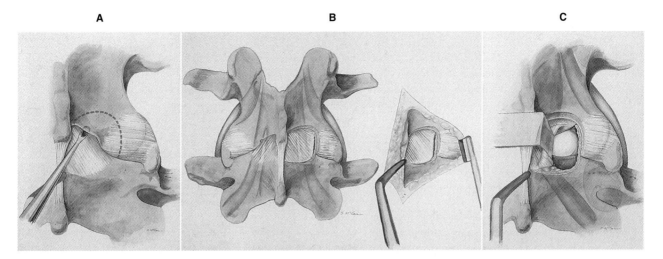

Fig. 8-8. A, Early step of a microdiscectomy showing the exposure of the upper and lower lamina. The *dotted line* shows the minimal bone to be removed with the Midas AM-8 burr and the curette freeing the ligamentum flavum. **B,** After the minimal bone has been removed, the ligamentum is well visualized. The outline of the nerve root can be seen directly below the ligamentum flavum. **C,** Retraction of the ligamentum flavum, dura, and nerve root, showing the disc herniation. At this point the disc is excised with a #11 blade and removed with the pituitary forceps. Note the atraumatic appearance and minimal exposure of neural structures.

be injected around the incision at the discretion of the surgeon. Steri-Strips and a sterile dressing are applied to the wound.

Immediately after surgery the patient is maintained at bed rest for several hours. Patients should be able to walk, void spontaneously, and take oral fluids before discharge. Patients are typically discharged to home on the day of surgery or within 23 hours.

Therapy Guidelines for Rehabilitation

Postoperative spine rehabilitation allows for a safer and faster return to functional activities. The early return to *appropriate* activities has been encouraged after surgeries of the extremities for many years. The same approach should be applied to the spine. Careful instruction and frequent reevaluation enable a therapist to progress the patient's functional activities to premorbid levels safely. The therapist should apply a functionally appropriate and suitably aggressive postoperative protocol to the patient recovering from lumbar microdiscectomy.

Lumbar disc herniations can do more than compromise the nerve root. Compensatory movement patterns, altered mechanics of the motion segment, and muscle splinting may result in misleading referred pain patterns (e.g., myofascial trigger points). Furthermore, the literature suggests that abnormal changes in paraspinal muscle activity occur after a herniated nucleus pulposus.[10,31] Triano and Schultz[52] found a

high correlation between the absence of the flexion-relaxation phenomenon (i.e., the relaxation of the lumbar paraspinal muscles at terminal flexion in standing) and poor results on the Oswestry Pain Disability Scale (Box 8-2).

Microdiscectomy is designed to decompress neural tissues by removing the disc material that is causing the neurologic signs and symptoms not alleviated through aggressive conservative care.[27] Surgery *cannot* correct poor posture and body mechanics, nor can it relieve myofascial pain syndromes or remedy faulty motor patterns of synergistic activity accompanying muscle substitution that exist in many patients with low back pain. Additionally, Hides, Richardson, and Jull[12] have found that the lumbar multifidi, a primary segmental stabilizer, do not spontaneously recover after low back pain, so it is doubtful that they will spontaneously recover after the trauma of spine surgery. The loss of these crucial active segmental stabilizers may lead to recurrent lumbar pain syndromes. To avoid this and aid the patient's rehabilitation after spinal surgery, the therapist must tirelessly question and reassess, using a problem-solving approach.

The following guidelines are not intended to be a substitute for sound clinical reasoning. Rather it is a guideline for the successful postoperative rehabilitation of patients after lumbar microdiscectomy. The primary goals after a lumbar microdiscectomy are the reduction of pain, prevention of recurrent herniation,

Box 8-2   Oswestry Low Back Pain Disability Questionnaire

This questionnaire has been designed to give your physical therapist information as to how your back pain has affected your ability to manage in everyday life. Please answer every question by marking the *one* box that applies. We realize you may consider that two of the statements in any one section relate to you, but please just mark the box that most closely describes your problem.

Name: _____   Date: _____   Initial   Interim   Discharge

1) Pain Intensity
   - ☐ I can tolerate the pain I have without having to use pain killers.
   - ☐ My pain is bad, but I manage without taking pain killers.
   - ☐ Pain killers give me complete relief from my pain.
   - ☐ Pain killers give me moderate relief from my pain.
   - ☐ Pain killers give me very little relief from my pain.
   - ☐ Pain killers have no effect on my pain, and I do not use them.

2) Personal Care
   - ☐ I can look after myself normally without causing extra pain.
   - ☐ I can look after myself normally, but it causes extra pain.
   - ☐ It is painful to look after myself, and I am slow and careful.
   - ☐ I need some help, but I manage most of my personal care.
   - ☐ I need help everyday in most aspects of self-care.
   - ☐ I do not get dressed, wash with difficulty, and stay in bed.

3) Lifting
   - ☐ I can lift heavy objects without causing extra pain.
   - ☐ I can lift heavy objects, but it gives me extra pain.
   - ☐ Pain prevents me from lifting heavy weights off the floor, but I can manage light to medium objects if they are conveniently positioned.
   - ☐ I can lift only very light objects.
   - ☐ I cannot lift anything at all.

4) Walking
   - ☐ Pain does not prevent me from walking any distance.
   - ☐ Pain prevents me from walking more than 1 mile.
   - ☐ Pain prevents me from walking more than ½ mile.
   - ☐ Pain prevents me from walking more than ¼ mile.
   - ☐ I can only walk using a cane or crutches.
   - ☐ I am in bed most of the time and have to crawl to the toilet.

5) Sitting
   - ☐ I can sit in any chair as long as I like.
   - ☐ I can sit only in my favorite chair as long as I like.
   - ☐ Pain prevents me from sitting more than 1 hour.
   - ☐ Pain prevents me from sitting more than ½ hour.
   - ☐ Pain prevents me from sitting more than 10 minutes.
   - ☐ Pain prevents me from sitting at all.

6) Standing
   - ☐ I can stand as long as I want without extra pain.
   - ☐ I call stand as long as I want, but it gives me extra pain.
   - ☐ Pain prevents me from standing more than 1 hour.
   - ☐ Pain prevents me from standing more than ½ hour.
   - ☐ Pain prevents me from standing more than 10 minutes.
   - ☐ Pain prevents me from standing at all.

7) Sleeping
   - ☐ Pain does not prevent me from sleeping well.
   - ☐ I can sleep well only by taking medication for sleep.
   - ☐ Even when I take medication, I have less than 6 hours' sleep.
   - ☐ Even when I take medication, I have less than 4 hours' sleep.
   - ☐ Even when I take medication, I have less than 2 hours' sleep.
   - ☐ Pain prevents me from sleeping at all.

8) Sex Life
   - ☐ My sex life is normal and gives me no extra pain.
   - ☐ My sex life is normal but causes some extra pain.
   - ☐ My sex life is nearly normal but is very painful.
   - ☐ My sex life is severely restricted by pain.
   - ☐ My sex life is nearly absent because of pain.
   - ☐ Pain prevents any sex life at all.

9) Social Life
   - ☐ My social life is normal and gives me no extra pain.
   - ☐ My social life is normal but increases the degree of pain.
   - ☐ Pain has no significant effect on my social life apart from limiting my more energetic interests, such as dancing, etc.
   - ☐ Pain has restricted my social life, and I do not go out as often.
   - ☐ Pain has restricted my social life to my home.
   - ☐ I have no social life because of pain.

10) Traveling
   - ☐ I can travel anywhere without extra pain.
   - ☐ I can travel anywhere, but it gives me extra pain.
   - ☐ Pain is bad, but I manage journeys over 2 hours.
   - ☐ Pain restricts me to journeys of less than 1 hour.
   - ☐ Pain restricts me to short, necessary journeys of less than ½ hour.
   - ☐ Pain prevents me from traveling except to the doctor or hospital.

maintenance of dural mobility, improvement of function, and early return to appropriate activities. Each patient's program must be individualized to attain these goals for the following reasons:

1. Patients have slightly different pathoanatomic abnormalities and surgical procedures.
2. Patients experience different levels of strength, flexibility, and conditioning after surgery.
3. Patients' goals vary.
4. Patients have varying psychosocial factors.
5. Patients possess different levels of kinesthetic-proprioceptive coordination that affect their rate of motor learning.

Each patient must therefore receive care in accordance with individual needs. To this end the guidelines should be *progressed as tolerated,* and the therapist should *not* try to keep the patient "on schedule." Increasing lower extremity symptoms, progressive neurologic deficit, and incapacitating pain are obvious "red flags" that require prompt reevaluation. Although the therapist must not ignore pain, an acceptable level of discomfort is reasonable if the patient is increasing functional activities and progressing in the program as anticipated. Pain should be monitored in three parameters, with the therapist carefully noting the pain pattern (e.g., left lateral thigh to knee), observing the frequency (e.g., constant, intermittent, rare), and having the patient rate the intensity (0 to 10). This allows close tracking of changes in pain with exercise and activity so the program can be progressed or modified accordingly.

Finally, any successful spinal rehabilitation program must not ignore psychosocial factors that negatively affect the program. It has been suggested that the greatest indicator for postoperative results is preoperative psychologic testing, not MRI or clinical signs.[48] Additionally, patients who have active litigation or worker's compensation claims have been shown to return to activity later than patients who do not.[39] These factors must be considered in evaluating patients, progressing exercise programs, and assessing clinical results.

Q. Rick is 41 years old. He has had progressing back pain episodes over the past 2 years. An MRI shows a herniated disc at L4-L5. Rick also has intermittent complaints of left radicular leg pain. He had microdiscectomy surgery 2 weeks ago and has come to outpatient physical therapy for evaluation and treatment. How should a spinal evaluation be altered to assess a patient who has recently had microdiscectomy surgery?

Phase I: The Protective Phase

TIME: Weeks 1 to 3
GOALS: Protect the surgical site to promote wound healing, maintain nerve root mobility, reduce pain and inflammation, educate patient to minimize fear and apprehension, and establish consistently good body mechanics for safe and independent self-care (Table 8-1)

The first postoperative week typically consists of protective rest, progressive ambulation, and appropriately limited activities. Activity tolerance is the result of progressive activity, not rest. The patient should be encouraged to walk at a comfortable pace for short distances several times a day. Patients are usually allowed to shower 7 days after surgery depending on wound healing. Driving is usually not allowed for 1 to 2 weeks, although this may be extended if the right lower extremity is significantly compromised. Typically patients can return to office-level work within 1 week. Because the patient in phase I has difficulty tolerating sustained positioning, he or she may require support during driving, sitting, and lying postures. Patients may have significant incisional pain, especially with flexion movements. *The therapist must avoid all loaded lumbar flexion in patients in phases I and II.* The patient can apply cold packs to the surgical site for 20 to 30 minutes several times a day to help control pain, muscle spasm, and swelling.

The therapist may begin outpatient physical therapy as soon as the patient can comfortably come to the clinic, usually in the second or third week. Treatment begins only after the patient is evaluated to ascertain the following:

- A thorough history of the condition, including previous treatments or surgeries and time out of work
- The present pain pattern (intensity and frequency) plus activities or postures that alter these symptoms
- The status of the wound site
- Anthropometric data and postural assessment
- Limited mechanical testing (standing motion testing and end-of-range movements are not assessed until after the fifth week postoperatively)
- Neurologic status (examination to include neural tension testing)

The therapist must take care during the initial evaluation to avoid any testing that may injure an already compromised patient. The authors of this chapter typically include Waddell signs[55] to help delineate nonorganic physical signs (Box 8-3). The mechanical examination must be very limited in the phase I and phase II patient. It is intended to elicit symptomatic and mechanical responses that suggest mechanical problems and so dictate the treatment course. Because weight-bearing motion testing and end-of-range movements are typically not performed until after the fifth week postoperatively, the therapist uses responses to posi-

Table 8-1 Microdiscectomy

Rehabilitation Phase	Criteria to Progress to this Phase	Anticipated Impairments and Functional Limitations	Intervention	Goal	Rationale

Phase I Postoperative 1-3 weeks	Postoperative	• Edema
		• Pain
		• Limited tolerance to transfers
		• Limited tolerance to sustained positions
		• Limited activities of daily living (ADLs)
		• Limited nerve mobility
		• Limited lower extremity (LE) range of motion (ROM)
		• Limited trunk and LE strength
		• Limited mobility of neighboring regions
		• Limited walking
		• Limited cardiovascular endurance
			• Cryotherapy
			• Electrical stimulation
			• Supportive corset or brace as indicated
			• Body mechanics training–Maintenance of lumbar lordosis and avoidance of trunk flexion with the following:
			  1. Sitting and driving (supported as appropriate)
			  2. Sleeping (supported as necessary, avoiding fetal position)
			  3. Standing and walking (limit based on symptoms)
			  4. Transfers, supine—Sit-stand, in and out of car, and floor to stand
			  5. Self-care
			  6. Lifting (avoid)
			  7. Bending using "hip hinging" and "neutral spine" method
			• Supine dural stretch
			• Prone dural stretch
			• Passive range of motion (PROM) stretches—
				• Manage edema
				• Control pain
				• Decrease pain with upright postures
				• Prevent complications and reinjury
				• Good understanding of and use of proper body mechanics
				• Sit up to 20 minutes
				• Resume driving after 2 weeks
				• Improve sleep patterns
				• Use "log roll" technique with transfers
				• Independent with self-care
				• Improve nerve mobility
				• Prevent adhesions that limit nerve mobility
				• Restore ROM to LE
				• Improve mobility of restricted joints
				• Increase tolerance to walking level surfaces for 30 minutes
					• Promote self-management of edema and pain
					• Provide abdominal support and decompression
					• Initiate education to prepare patient for independence with ADLs, avoiding reinjury
					• Maintain lordosis and avoid flexion postures to avoid excessive elongation tension on surgical site
					• Promote protective rest and resumption of limited activities
					• Transfer while avoiding unnecessary stress on surgical site
					• Avoid lifting to prevent risk of reinjury
					• Decrease stress on surgical site
					• Prevent nerve fibrosis and dural adhesions
					• Improve LE flexibility to decrease stress on the lumbar spine
					• Avoid irritating sciatic nerve

Hip
  Flexion (knee bent)
  Straight leg raise (SLR) gently
  External rotation
Standing
  Gastrocnemius-soleus

- Joint mobilization of hip and thoracic spine as indicated
- Progressive walking program on treadmill or flat surfaces
- Begin progressive exercise program (unloaded positions only)
- Pelvic rocks
- Supine "pelvic rocks" (mid-range lumbar flexion AROM)
- Side-lying "pelvic rocks" (mid-range lumbar lateral flexion)
- Quadruped pelvic rocks (mid-range lumbar AROM)
- Prone "pelvic rocks" (mid-range lumbar extension AROM)
- Supine abdominal bracing (isolated transverse abdominis contraction)
- Supine abdominal bracing with arms behind head, progressed to alternating arm raises
- Prone abdominal bracing with alternating arm raises, progressed to bilateral arm raises
- Partial squatting to 60°

- Establish a healthy environment for the disc
- Good neutral control of lumbar spine while supine and prone
- Increased lower extremity strength

- Maintain and improve proximal and distal mobility to reduce stress on the surgical site
- Prepare patient to resume ADLs and promote good cardiovascular conditioning
- Controlled lumbar movements are beneficial after microdiscectomy secondary to hydrostatic changes of the disc promote vascularity
- Increase strength of trunk musculature to stabilize and protect the spine from injury
- Increase tolerance to upright postures
- Help with maintaining good body mechanics

Box 8-3   The Waddell Signs

1. Superficial tenderness to light touch in the lumbar region or widespread tenderness to deep palpation in nonanatomic distributions
2. Increased symptoms with simulated axial loading or simulated rotation tests
3. Inconsistent supine and sitting straight leg raising tests
4. Regional weakness or sensory abnormalities that are not myotomal or dermatomal
5. Physical overreaction or disproportionate verbalization during assessment

---

tioning and mid-range movements in prone, supine, and side-lying positions to determine mechanical problems in the initial weeks. Hip muscle strength testing should be postponed in the early stages of healing to prevent stressing inflamed lumbosacral tissues. Neural tension testing is an integral part of the lumbar evaluation. Therefore the therapist should have the patient perform the straight leg raise, Cram's test, femoral nerve stretch test (prone knee flexion), and supine dural stretch and do the appropriate measuring, recording, and comparison with the opposite limb. Slump testing should not be performed until after the fourth or fifth week postoperatively. A good understanding of soft tissue healing rates, spinal mechanics, and the specific surgical procedure helps avoid needless soft tissue trauma. For further evaluation of the patient's physical limitations and guidance toward appropriate functional training, the therapist can use the Modified Low Back Pain Oswestry Questionnaire[16] (see Box 8-2) or the Roland-Morris Functional Disability Questionnaire.[44] These are easily administered and helpful. The therapist should document the patient's perceived disability status before treatment and at predetermined intervals to monitor functional progress and determine the appropriate direction of functional training exercises.

After evaluation the therapist thoroughly explains the existing problems and the treatment plan to the patient. Therapist and patient should work together to reach mutual agreement on realistic goals. Patient education is crucial to achieving positive results because the patient ultimately treats himself or herself several hours each day with a home exercise program and self-treatment techniques. *Furthermore, avoiding reinjury is perhaps the single most important postoperative factor responsible for a rapid progression in the program and ultimately full recovery.* Through thorough patient education, a safe and relatively rapid return to activities can occur. The physical therapist educates

the patient regarding proper postures, home exercises, self-care techniques, and body mechanics for the safe performance of activities of daily living (ADLs). Proper postures and body mechanics are crucial during the postoperative healing phase. Ideally the therapist should instruct the patient before surgery, but if this does not occur, the first postoperative task is to teach the patient correct postures and body mechanics.

Proper postures. The physical therapist teaches the patient to maintain normal lumbar lordosis. Patients should avoid lumbar flexion in standing or sitting because intradiscal pressures are increased and excessive shear forces occur. Intolerance to prolonged postures are typical in phase I, and frequent movement breaks are recommended. The therapist also should investigate the ergonomics of the patient's workstation to avoid potential problems.

SITTING AND DRIVING
- Caution the patient to never slouch while sitting.
- Instruct the patient in the use of a lumbar roll or similar device to maintain lordosis during sitting and driving.
- Advise the patient to try to always sit on firm, straight-back chairs and never sit on soft sofas or chairs.
- Caution the patient to avoid all backless seating. If the patient eventually will need to sit in bleachers or similar backless seating, recommend a Nada-Chair (Nada Concepts Inc., Minneapolis, MN) or a similar device that supports the lumbar spine during this type of sitting.
- Encourage frequent movement breaks. Instruct the patient to avoid sitting longer than 20 minutes at a time for the first 2 weeks. This increases in subsequent weeks, depending on tolerance to pain.
- Allow patients to return to driving for short periods after about 1 to 2 weeks. Remind the patient that safety is a priority for them—not a convenience.

SLEEPING
- Teach the patient to sleep in supported supine, supported side-lying, or supported prone three-quarter lying with the spine straight (see Figures 9-7, A to C). Instruct the patient to avoid sleeping in the fetal position because of the prolonged lumbar flexion. Have the patient avoid unsupported prone three-quarter lying positions because of the rotational component.
- Caution the patient to avoid lying on soft mattresses or sofas.

STANDING AND WALKING
- Advise patients to limit standing at the kitchen sink or bathroom counter to short periods and avoid bending at the waist.

- Encourage the patient to maintain lumbar lordosis during standing and walking while performing an abdominal brace.

Body mechanics. To allow the patient to progress rapidly, the therapist should do everything possible to avoid reinjury. Minor setbacks may delay progression of the program, and a major setback may be irreparable. The therapist should pay close attention to the patient's movements. Patients may say they understand correct mechanics but display incorrect movement patterns. Frequent and critical observation allows the therapist to evaluate the patient's spinal mechanics and determine whether the patient has integrated the correct postures and mechanics. A checklist of basic functional movements (i.e., rising from lying, rising from sitting, sitting in neutral, reaching overhead, bending to knee level) is helpful to record the performance of these skills and whether they require cues to complete the task.

TRANSFERS
- Teach the patient to move correctly from supine to sitting (see Fig. 9-4), from standing to lying on the floor (see Fig. 9-6), and from sitting to standing (see Fig. 9-5). Rolling in bed as a unit and rising from bed must be performed correctly. Also, give instruction on entering and exiting a car.
- All twisting motions are prohibited. Instruct them to move their feet to turn instead.

DRESSING
- Instruct the patient in the correct way to put on pants, socks, and shoes in the supine position. Slip-on shoes are the easiest to handle in the first 2 weeks. Tying shoes can later be performed safely by putting the foot on a stool or chair.

HYGIENE
- Showering can begin after the second week. Have the patient shave her legs in the standing position, with the foot on the tub or shower seat, avoiding lumbar flexion.

LIFTING
- Although correct lifting techniques should be taught early on (see Fig. 9-11), instruct patients to try to avoid all lifting in phase I. "Swoop lifting" is usually a safe and well-tolerated technique for light lifting in phase II. It is performed by making a long stride forward to the kneeling position (lunge) and then reaching to lift a light object. The exercise is then performed in reverse.

BENDING
- Advise the patient to avoid all bending at the waist. Lumbar flexion with loading is arguably the most hazardous movement in the first two phases. The interdiscal pressures are significantly increased, and tension on the healing posterior annulus compounds the problem. Prolonged or repetitive bending is especially injurious.[11]

- Occasionally limited bending is necessary. Teach the patient the correct way to bend and instruct him or her to avoid lumbar flexion while bending. The patient can safely bend by simultaneously flexing at the knees and hips ("hinge at the hips") while maintaining a neutral spine and an abdominal brace. This is easy to teach by placing a 4-foot wood pole (1 to 2 inches in diameter) along the spine with contact at the thoracic and sacral regions (see Fig. 9-9). By flexing slowly at the hips and knees while maintaining a neutral spine position and viewing themselves in a mirror, patients can practice this important movement.

Occasionally, patients with low back pain possess poor kinesthetic-proprioceptive coordination. A simple technique to improve the patient's sense of lumbar movement and position involves the use of tape. First the therapist places the patient on all fours and has him or her assume a neutral spine position. The therapist places a 12 to 18 cm long piece of tape on the paraspinals parallel to the spine (Fig. 8-9), while avoiding placing the tape directly over the incision site. The therapist then asks the patient to make small movements into flexion and extension, always returning to neutral. The additional feedback from the tape pulling or wrinkling will assist the patient in learning spinal proprioception. Various postures can then be tried, including kneeling, side-lying, sitting, and standing, with small motions of the lumbar spine while in each position. The patient then progresses to functional movements (e.g., transfers, walking, bending).

Exercise. *Dural stretching* (i.e., mobilization of the nervous system, neurodynamic exercise, nerve root gliding, neural tension exercises) should begin as soon as possible in the first week. The preoperative neural compromise and the postoperative inflammation in and around the epidural space contribute to neural fibrosis and dural adhesions. They are occasionally problematic and are easily preventable. An excellent presentation of neural mobilization principles and techniques can be found in Butler.[5]

TECHNIQUE
- Supine dural stretching (lower lumbar neural mobilization): Have the patient lie supine on a firm surface with both knees extended. While the patient holds the back of the thigh with both hands, he or she slowly extends the knee with the ankle dorsiflexed to the point of stretch. He or she then slowly flexes and relaxes the limb. Any symptoms and the maximal amount of knee extension attained should be recorded to monitor progress.
- Prone dural stretching (upper lumbar neural mobilization): Have the patient lie prone on a firm surface with both knees extended. Initially the patient may use a pillow under the abdomen

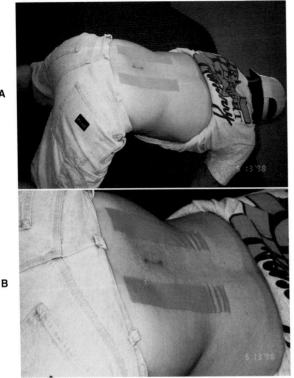

A

B

Fig. 8-9. Patient assumes a quadruped position while the therapist places a 12- to 18-cm strip of tape on the paraspinals adjacent to the spine. The therapist should take care to avoid the incision site. **A,** Appearance of tape in squatting position. **B,** Close-up view of tape with return to standing position.

for comfort if needed. Have the patient slowly flex the knee to the point of stretch, then slowly extend the knee and relax. Make sure the patient maintains the abdominal brace throughout the exercise to stabilize the lumbar spine. Alternate legs.

Dural stretching should be done several times a day. The therapist must caution the patient that this exercise may provoke neural symptoms and that he or she must allow the pain or tingling to resolve to baseline levels before beginning the next repetition. The patient should not overstretch the neural tissues. As with any exercise, self-mobilization of the nervous system at home is inappropriate until a positive response has been established from repeated movements in the clinic. The dural stretches are progressed as tolerated to include other components of the affected nerve (e.g., ankle dorsiflexion, hip internal rotation). Eventually (in phase III) the patient can perform neural stretches while sitting ("sitting slump stretch").

The early initiation of a progressive spinal stabilization program is crucial to the eventual tolerance of more strenuous functional activities and sports skills. Because the lumbar spine is inherently unstable around the neu-

tral zone, the trunk musculature must be sufficiently strong and coordinated to stabilize and protect the spine from injury.[36] The stabilization program progresses from unloaded spinal positions to partially loaded and eventually fully loaded functional training. The posterior pelvic tilt exercise is the *least* desirable exercise to obtain active lumbar stability.[42,43] The transversus abdominis must be isolated from the remaining abdominal musculature because it has consistently been shown to be active before the other abdominal muscles or the primary movers during limb motions, regardless of direction.[14,63] In addition, the transversus abdominis can become dysfunctional in patients with low back pain.[14] Therefore the transversus abdominis possesses a superior ability to stabilize the lumbar spine actively and locally. Although the more superficial abdominal muscles (the obliques) are important in lumbar stability, they are trained later in the program for their rotational contribution to limit lateral shear and torsional stresses and create trunk rotation. Early in phase II the lumbar multifidi are isolated and trained because of their ability to stabilize segmentally.[29] Eventually a co-contraction of transversus abdominis and multifidus (abdominal bracing) is performed during all exercises and functional activities. All the exercises should focus on control and technique and be progressed as tolerated to improve endurance of these primary stabilizers.

The physical therapist should instruct the patient in the *neutral spine* concept and help the patient find the neutral spine position in various postures. The patient can then be taught to *control the transverse abdominus* with electromyographic (EMG) biofeedback or pressure biofeedback (Stabilizer Inc., Chattanooga, TN) in several positions (e.g., supine, all fours, prone). After that the patient can progress the postures to include sitting and standing and increase the duration of the contractions to 60 seconds.

Based on the information obtained in the history, the responses to various positions, and the limited clinical testing performed during the initial evaluation, the therapist determines which midrange lumbar movements are tolerated and are indicated for exercise. Correct and controlled lumbar movements are beneficial to the patient after microdiscectomy because hydrostatic changes of the disc promote improved vascularity.[15,53] To this end the therapist teaches "pelvic rocks" in pain-free positions (e.g., all fours, prone). A pelvic rock is a repetitive and continuous pelvic tilt from an anterior to a posterior position. A bias toward lumbar extension is typical in the patient who has undergone microdiscectomy because lumbar extension reduces tangential stress posteriorly. A flexion bias is usually not recommended because the surgical entry is into the posterior disc and flexion positions tend to create stress to this area and tension on the incision. A healthy respect for soft tissue healing periods is essential.

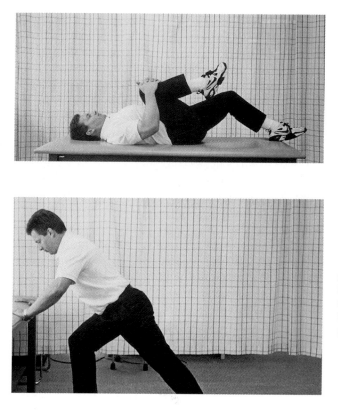

Fig. 8-10. Hip flexion is very important. When stretching the gluteals, the patient should pull the thigh toward the belly rather than toward the nose. This patient is attempting to increase the hip flexion angle rather than draw the pelvis into a posterior tilt.

Fig. 8-11. Gastrocnemius-soleus stretching. While keeping the foot and heel of the back leg on the floor, the patient shifts the weight forward to the front leg. A stretch should be felt in the calf area. The patient should maintain the spine in neutral with an abdominal brace as the weight is shifted toward the front foot and keep the supporting thigh directly below in the frontal plane.

The therapist instructs the patient in most of the following exercises in phase I, but he or she should not prescribe any exercise or position for the home program until repeated trials in the clinic have proven painless. Stabilization, flexibility, coordination, and spinal mobility exercises are included in an attempt to address all parameters. The exercise sequence is important and should be considered by the physical therapist when adding exercises. Good technique and control of movement are essential. *No exercise should increase the pain pattern or cause lingering pain.* Clearly some muscular soreness may accompany the program, but this should be well tolerated and transient. The typical patient should be able to *contract the transversus abdominis* for 60 seconds in various positions within approximately 1 week after the initial visit.

The following exercises are taught in phase I:

1. Abdominal bracing on all fours (isolated transverse abdominis contraction and lumbar multifidus co-contraction) progressed to quadruped abdominal bracing with alternate arm raises
2. Quadruped "pelvic rocks" (i.e., midrange lumbar active range of motion [AROM])
3. Supine dural stretching (or prone dural stretching for upper lumbar disorders)
4. Supine abdominal bracing (isolated transverse abdominis contraction and lumbar multifidus co-contraction)
5. Supine "pelvic rocks" (i.e., midrange lumbar flexion active range of motion)
6. Supine abdominal bracing with arms behind head progressed to abdominal bracing with alternating arm raises
7. Supine gluteal, hip external rotator, and hamstring stretches to correct myofascial limitations; actively holding neutral spine during these low-load, long-hold exercises is important (Fig. 8-10)
8. Side-lying "pelvic rocks" (i.e., midrange lumbar lateral flexion AROM)
9. Prone "pelvic rocks" (i.e., midrange lumbar extension AROM)
10. Prone abdominal bracing with alternate arm raises progressed to prone abdominal bracing with bilateral arm raises
11. Gastrocnemius-soleus stretching in standing position (Fig. 8-11)
12. Partial squats to 60 degrees of knee flexion while maintaining neutral spine with abdominal bracing

Spinal mobilization. Spinal mobilization of the lumbar spine is rarely used in phase I or II. Mobilization of the hips or thoracic spine may be needed and is best addressed on an individual basis. When progress is poor with active movements and deemed secondary to a hypomobile segment, mobilization to restore lumbar movement may be necessary in phase II. In phase

III, mobilization can play an important role and is used frequently to reduce pain during specific lumbar motions, especially at end of range. A review of Maitland,[24] Mulligan,[33] and Paris[38] may assist in clinical reasoning.

Cardiovascular conditioning. Cardiovascular conditioning is an important part of the rehabilitation program and is beneficial both for patients recovering from lumbar microdiscectomy and those with chronic low back pain.[25] In addition, endurance training of the lower extremity musculature improves tolerance to prolonged standing and walking. When lower extremity muscles fatigue, poor body mechanics soon follow. Aerobic training is typically performed by progressive walking (on a treadmill or outdoors without hills), stationary cycling (on recumbent or upright bikes with the patient paying close attention to the maintenance of lordosis and avoidance of hip sway), or swimming (initially only the freestyle stroke with avoidance of "craning" during the breathing phase). Craning is suboccipital extension with rotation (occipito-atlantal [OA] to atlanto-axial [AA]) or cervical extension with rotation (C2 to C7). Swimming and aqua-therapy are usually delayed until the second or third week after surgery to ensure complete wound healing and sufficient lumbar stabilization. The physical therapist must caution patients never to jump or dive into the water, but rather use the ladder or steps. Aquatic therapy for postoperative lumbar rehabilitation is not covered in this chapter, but Watkins and Buhler[59] present a good source for the interested clinician.

The therapist determines the patient's training heart rate and adheres to this guideline during all conditioning exercises. Patients who have no prior history of aerobic exercise or who are very deconditioned must progress slowly and be carefully monitored. Aerobic conditioning in phase I (with focus on correct postures and mechanics) may include walking, stationary cycling, and water exercises. Patients should avoid stair climbers and cross-country skiing machines until phase II, when adequate trunk stability is usually attained. In addition, rowing, running, and in-line skating should be avoided until phase III, when significant active lumbar stability has been achieved.

The progression of cardiovascular training is highly variable and depends on the patient's prior level of conditioning and present goals. He or she can usually begin with 5- to 10-minute bouts and progress at 5-minute intervals up to 30 or 60 minutes. The therapist must pay careful attention to patient position because correct postures deteriorate as fatigue increases. Neurologic weakness of the hip flexors or abductors, quadriceps, hamstrings, ankle dorsiflexors, and plantar flexors significantly alters gait and requires modification of the aerobic program to avoid abnormal mechanical stress.

Modalities. In general, the use of passive treatment techniques alone should be avoided, but occasionally they may be necessary to augment the functional restoration program. The therapist should use pain control modalities only as needed to support the exercise program. Cryotherapy and interferential stimulation applied to the low back for 15 to 20 minutes after an exercise session are helpful. Some therapists may prefer electric myo-stimulation (EMS), microstimulation, or transcutaneous electrical nerve stimulation (TENS) for muscle spasm reduction and pain control. However, EMS that is delivered too intensely in the first several weeks after surgery may unwittingly jeopardize the healing paraspinal muscle tissue and should therefore be used judiciously. The patient's posture during modalities is always important and varies depending on positional tolerance. Supported prone lying or supported supine lying (see Fig. 9-7, *A* and *C*) is usually quite comfortable in this phase.

Wound care. Along with the patient's history, the inspection of the incision site during the initial evaluation helps determine whether extra measures are needed. Any signs of infection are a "red flag" that requires prompt medical intervention. Some patients desire "invisible" scars, while others are much less concerned. Because patients scar differently the therapist should monitor their progress and offer solutions to excessive scarring or scar stretching. A compression taping technique can be used to limit hypertrophic scar formation and reduce surgical scar widening. First the therapist folds a 10 × 6 cm Neoprene pad in half and secures it with a 2-inch wide elastic tape (Elastikon Tape, Johnson & Johnson, New Brunswick, New Jersey) (Fig. 8-12). The pad is then

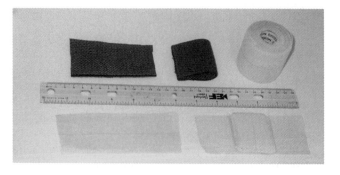

Fig. 8-12. Materials to manufacture compression patch (10- × 6-cm Neoprene pad, 2-inch elastic tape).

affixed horizontally over the closed wound (Figs. 8-13 and 8-14) to provide both compression and approximation of the surgical scar. The patient wears the compression patch constantly for 6 to 10 weeks, removing it only to bathe. It should not be applied until the wound site is completely healed (about 2 weeks).

A. Mechanical testing should be limited (standing motion testing and end-of-range movements are not assessed until 5 weeks after surgery). Hip muscle strength testing should be postponed in the early stages of healing to prevent stressing inflamed lumbosacral tissues. Slump testing is not performed until much later. A good understanding of soft tissue healing rates, spinal mechanics, and the specific surgical procedure helps avoid needless soft tissue trauma.

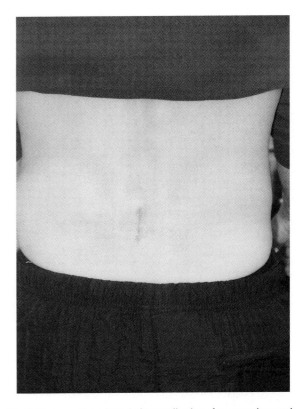

Fig. 8-13. Inspection of scar before application of compression patch.

Q. Verlyn is a 40-year-old woman. She had microdiscectomy surgery for the L5 disk 6 weeks ago. Back pain is minimal. Lower extremity flexibility and strength is gradually improving. Trunk strength also is progressing. She is now seeing a physical therapist for treatment. Previous treatments have included modalities for pain control, lower extremity flexibility exercises, trunk and general strengthening, cardiovascular conditioning, and body mechanics. Verlyn is concerned about the intermittent radicular pain in her right leg. Prolonged sitting, walking, or standing aggravates her right leg. She reports reproduction of calf pain with hamstring stretching. What treatment technique should be used to decrease calf pain frequency and intensity?

Phase II: The Functional Recovery Phase

TIME: Weeks 4-6
GOALS: Understand neutral spine concept, improve cardiovascular condition, increase trunk strength to 80%, increase soft tissue mobility and lower extremity flexibility and strength, maintain nerve root mobility (Table 8-2)

As surgical site pain diminishes and active spinal stability improves, the physical therapist can increase the patient's program of functional activities and exercise. The patient in phase II should have complete wound healing, although some tenderness and paraspinal spasm may persist. Neural tension signs should

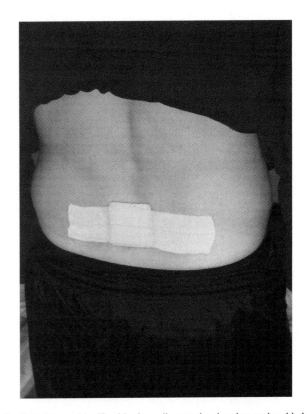

Fig. 8-14. The pad is affixed horizontally over the closed wound and held in place by 2-inch elastic tape.

Table 8-2   Microdiscectomy

Rehabilitation Phase	Criteria to Progress to this Phase	Anticipated Impairments and Functional Limitations	Intervention	Goal	Rationale
Phase II Postoperative 4-6 weeks	• No signs of infection • No increase in pain Gradual increase in tolerance to activity Demonstration of good knowledge of body mechanics Performance of self-care with minimal modifications	• Pain • Limited nerve mobility • Limited trunk strength • Limited scar mobility • Limited soft tissue mobility • Limited tolerance to ADLs and sustained postures • Limited trunk stability and strength in numerous postures • Limited mobility of lumbar spine soft tissues • Poor recruitment of paraspinal muscles • Limited LE ROM • Limited cardiovascular endurance	• Continue as in Phase I and progress cardiovascular activities as appropriate • Self-nerve mobilization using a belt to enhance the stretch • Isometrics with AROM— Supine • Abdominal bracing with alternate straightleg raises; progressed to "cycling" and "dying bug" when appropriate • Partial sit-ups with added rotation for obliques when appropriate Prone • Abdominal bracing with SLR (extension): begin with single leg and progress to double leg • On-elbows lying, progress to partial press-ups • AROM with isometrics— All fours— • Abdominal bracing with single leg raise, progress to opposite arm and leg raises Standing— • Abdominal bracing with squats to 60°, progress to 90° for 2-3 minutes Sitting on Swiss Ball— • Abdominal bracing with hip flexion, arm flexion, and combinations of opposite arm and leg • Electromyographic training of lumbar spine multifidus muscles • PROM (stretches), then add iliopsoas and quadriceps • Soft tissue massage (STM)	• Cardiovascular exercise 20 minutes • Minimal to no neural tension signs • Trunk strength 80% • Use of "neutral spine" concepts in a variety of positions • Avoidance of lumbar spine extension while performing hip extension • Partial press-ups without pain • Good neutral control of lumbar spine in a variety of postures • Increased strength of LEs • Improved sitting tolerance • Isolated contraction of lumbar spine paraspinal muscles • Increased LE flexibility • Increased soft tissue mobility	• Improve cardiovascular fitness • Restore neural gliding mechanics • Prevent neural fibrosis and dural adhesions • Strengthen trunk musculature via "neutral spine" concepts • Perform exercises in midrange of lumbopelvic mobility • Stabilize and strengthen trunk while moving extremities, progressing from passive prepositioning to dynamic stabilization • Restore full extension in non-weight-bearing position • Strengthen paraspinals and abdominals in a neutral position • Promote maintenance of a "neutral spine" in an upright posture to improve tolerance to compression positions • Increase tolerance to upright postures • Use biofeedback to improve recruitment of paraspinals • Improve flexibility of LEs to decrease stress on the spine • Improve myofascial interface and restore soft tissue mobility

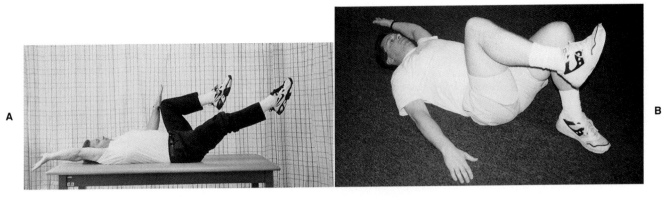

Fig. 8-15. Dying bug. This exercise teaches the patient to control extension and side-bending at the same time. The patient starts with the hands touching the knees directly over the hips and then extends the same-side arm and leg slowly and deliberately. The physical therapist monitors the patient for side-bending or extension. This exercise can be modified by moving the arms and legs in smaller increments.

be negative, but neurodynamic testing may reveal limitations. The patient should be gaining tolerance to functional activities and be able to perform all self-care with minor modifications. The patient's tolerance to aerobic exercise also should be improving. Correct body mechanics and postures should be maintained as functional activity increases. Patients should have confidence in their ability to stabilize the lumbar spine actively in all loaded positions. Pain-free lumbar AROM should be increasing to end-of-range strain only, although terminal flexion may still provoke pain. The patient should continue to avoid loaded lumbar flexion. Through brief reevaluations in each treatment session, the therapist collects additional lumbar motion data. For example, if prone pelvic rocks are well tolerated, the patient's positional tolerance to elbow lying and partial extension in lying can be assessed safely. The therapist should avoid standing motion testing and sitting testing except for the most conditioned patients who are doing very well.

Exercise. The therapist should instruct the patient in the correct way to contract and control the *lumbar multifidus* with *EMG biofeedback*. Special attention to the training of this important segmental stabilizer is essential.[61] Retraction of the paraspinal muscles during surgery can denervate the multifidus muscle.[49a] Fortunately, lumbar microdiscectomy requires a minimal wound opening, so this complication is lessened. The patient should perform abdominal bracing (holding neutral spine with a co-contraction of the transverse abdominis and multifidus) in supine, prone, and all fours positions, progressing to transition movements. Ultimately, the co-contraction is used to stabilize the lumbar spine during all ADLs. The therapist can progress the patient's mid-range lumbar movements and spinal stabilization program as tolerated, using

Swiss ball exercises to improve balance and dynamic lumbar stabilization during sitting. The patient should continue to avoid axial loading during end-range lumbar flexion or lateral flexion movements. As the patient shows control and tolerance, the exercise level may be increased. Pain during exercise typically requires correction of the technique or exercise modification. In addition, muscle groups that may have been weakened by neurologic compromise (such as hip abductors, quadriceps, ankle plantar flexors, or dorsiflexors) must be strengthened. The slow twitch fibers are most involved and are easily fatigued. The longer that neural compression and inflammation have been present, the longer the period before regeneration occurs. Careful attention to back-protected positions during strengthening exercises is crucial to avoiding reinjury.

TYPICAL PHASE II EXERCISES

1. Supine abdominal bracing with alternate straight leg raises, progressed to abdominal bracing with unsupported lower extremity extension (i.e., "cycling"), progressed to abdominal bracing with unsupported upper and lower extremity extension (i.e., "dying bug") (Fig. 8-15)
2. Supine dural stretching, progressed to incorporate a belt or towel around the foot to enhance the stretch
3. Supine partial sit-ups, progressed to partial sit-ups with rotation to facilitate oblique strengthening (Fig. 8-16)
4. Double leg bridging, progressed to single leg bridging and then to single leg bridging with opposite knee straight (Fig. 8-17)
5. Prone elbow lying, progressed to partial press-ups
6. Prone abdominal bracing with single leg raises, progressed to prone double leg raises
7. Standing repetitive squats to 60 degrees, progressed to 90 degrees for 2 to 3 minutes

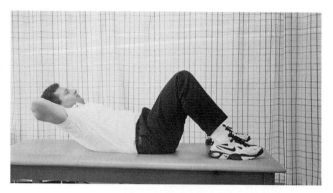

Fig. 8-16. Partial sit-ups are done in many positions. The important point is that the spine must remain in neutral, the abdominals must remain contracted throughout the exercise, and eccentric control must be emphasized. The lift is of the chest, not the head. Legs can be in extended position to bias lumbar extension.

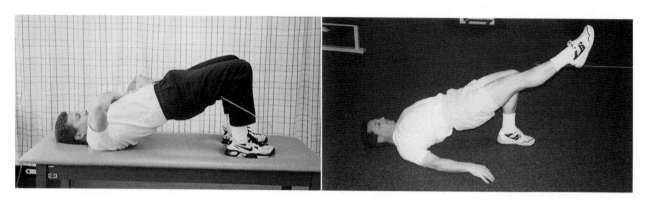

Fig. 8-17. Bridging. This exercise teaches the patient to brace the spine first, then lift the trunk as a unit. Note that the patient is moving in and out of a hip hinge. The emphasis is on coordinating the trunk and hip muscles.

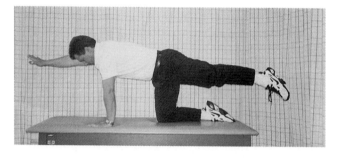

Fig. 8-18. From the quadruped position, teach the patient to keep the hands under the shoulders and knees under the hips. Extend the opposite arm and leg.

8. Abdominal bracing on all fours with single leg raise, progressed to opposite arm and leg raises (Fig. 8-18)
9. Balance board training on both limbs, progressed in duration
10. Isolated strengthening of neurologically compromised muscles
11. Swiss ball sitting exercise progression (in neutral spine with abdominal brace)
12. Stretching of the quadriceps, gluteals, hip external rotators, iliopsoas, hamstrings, and calves as required to correct myofascial limitations (see Fig. 8-11 and Figs. 8-19 to 8-22)

Soft tissue mobilization. Scarring of myofascial elements with collagen cross-fibers or fibrofatty tissue limits muscle broadening during contraction and connective tissue elasticity during movement.[9] Muscle spasm and protective guarding of the gluteals and low back musculature may persist. Soft tissue mobilization of the lumbar paraspinals and buttock musculature is frequently needed to improve muscle function and reduce spasm. The physical therapist must exercise care when performing soft tissue mobilization to the paraspinals before the third or fourth week after surgery because the tissue healing is incomplete. The mechanical and re-

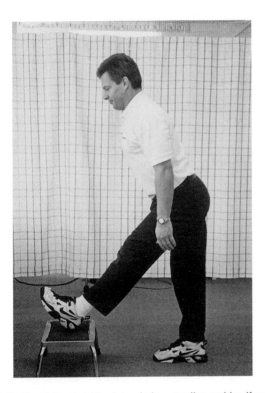

Fig. 8-19. Hamstring stretching is taught in a standing position if possible so the patient can work on contralateral hip stability as well as trunk control while stretching. The patient can work the foot up and down while maintaining the stretch to increase the nerve-gliding component. A slight bend in the knee with more hip hinge will move the stretch up from the musculotendinous junction into the muscle belly.

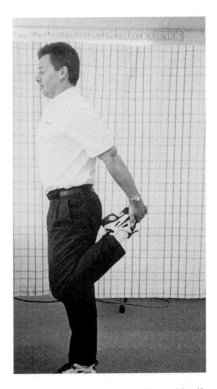

Fig. 8-20. Quadriceps stretch is taught in standing position if possible to develop trunk control against an extension moment. If the patient does not have sufficient range of motion, modify the stretch by placing the foot on a table. Abdominal control prevents lumbar extension.

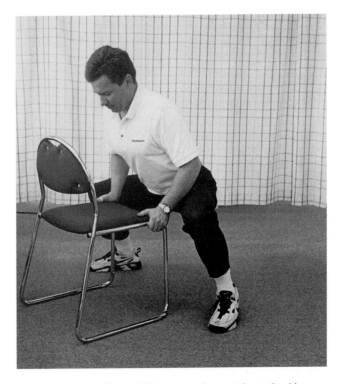

Fig. 8-21. Gracilis stretch is important for squatting to the side.

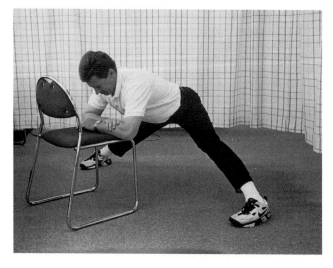

Fig. 8-22. Adductor flexibility is important for squatting. The patient can vary the trunk angle, or apply pressure to the inner knee to increase the stretch.

flexive effects of soft tissue mobilization are well suited for patients recovering from microdiscectomy, and certain techniques are particularly beneficial before paraspinal strengthening (e.g., side-lying paraspinal pull from midline). Careful questioning and soft tissue examination will uncover gluteal trigger points that can cause buttock or lower extremity pain patterns.[51] These myofascial pain syndromes are not uncommon preoperatively and may linger postoperatively. With appropriate treatment they can be relieved so that the functional restoration program may progress. Scar massage to release adherent soft tissue also may be needed.

Spinal mobilization. Spinal mobilization using non-thrust maneuvers may be beneficial for patients in phase II if they do not have protective muscle spasm, bone disease of the spine, or hypermobile or irritable adjacent motion segments. Muscle energy techniques are usually well tolerated and best suited for phase II. Thrust maneuvers (grade V or high-velocity manipulations) are not indicated.

Cardiovascular conditioning. The physical therapist should continue to progress the cardiovascular program in intensity and duration of aerobic training. The use of cross-country ski machines, stair climbers, and swimming for aerobic exercise is allowed if sufficient trunk stability has been achieved. Patients should avoid rowing and in-line skating until phase III. Running is not recommended until after the twelfth week after surgery because of the degree of spinal stabilization required and the repetitive axial loading sustained by the disc.

Modalities. The therapist and patient should use modalities only as needed to support the exercise program. Cryotherapy and interferential stimulation to the low back after exercise may be beneficial.

Phase III: The Resistive Training Phase

TIME: Weeks 7-11
GOALS: Ensure patient is independent in self-care and ADLs with minimal alterations, increase tolerance to activities, progress return to previous level of function (Table 8-3)

 A. Verlyn tested positive for adverse neural tension in the right leg. After several treatments of mobilization to the nervous system, complaints of pain decreased significantly in intensity and frequency.

The patient in phase III should consistently perform correct body mechanics and postures without prompting and should tolerate almost all functional activities. Prolonged positioning (e.g., unsupported sitting) may still provoke low back pain, but this should be easily relieved with change of position or simple stretching exercises. Soft tissue healing at this stage is largely complete, although some surgical site tenderness may still be present. All self-care and ADLs should be performed confidently and painlessly with minimal modifications. Patients in phase III should have good tolerance to mid-range lumbar movements and sufficient spinal stabilization to perform spinal movements in loaded positions.

The resumption of lifting activities must be progressive and occur with careful instruction (see Fig. 9-11, *A* and *B*). Because approximately half of all worker's compensation claims for low back injury result from lifting objects, this patient group needs proportionally more instruction and functional training.

Because soft tissue healing is nearly complete by phase III, more extensive mechanical testing can be performed to ascertain tolerance to various lumbar movements as well as the end range sensation. Standing motion testing (without overpressure) and seated testing can be performed safely on most patients after 6 weeks. The outcome of the movement testing determines to a great extent the treatment and exercise progression. Neural tension signs should be negative unless scarring has occurred. Occasionally some neurologic signs and symptoms persist into the third phase, but with monitoring and calm encouragement the physical therapist can reassure affected patients that these symptoms will subside with continued neural stretching and time.

Researchers[52] and clinicians note that flexibility, strength (stability), and coordination return at different rates after injury. During spinal rehabilitation, flex-

Table 8-3 Microdiscectomy

Rehabilitation Phase	Criteria to Progress to this Phase	Anticipated Impairments and Functional Limitations	Intervention	Goal	Rationale

Phase III Postoperative 7-11 weeks	No increase in pain
	No loss in mobility or function
	Good knowledge of "neutral spine" concepts during a variety of positions
		• Limited stability of trunk in challenging positions
		• Not totally independent with self-care
		• Limited tolerance to prolonged positions
			• Continuation of interventions from phases I and II as appropriate
			• Progressive resistance exercises (PREs)
			• Isotonics
			• Progressive lifting training using the following:
			  Change of position
			  Rotational and overhead activities
			  Balance boards
			• Cardiovascular exercise, walking progressed to running (after 12 weeks), stationary bike, or cross-country skiing (after 8 weeks)
			• Sport- and activity-specific drills when appropriate (see criteria on p. 145)
			• Functional capacity evaluation after 10 to 12 weeks
				• Weaning from interventions that are no longer of benefit
				• Consistent use of good body mechanics
				• Independent self-care
				• Independence with ADLs with minimal modifications
				• Increased tolerance to physically demanding activities
				• Return to previous level of activity as appropriate
					• Promote self-management of condition
					• Use of pain easing techniques to relieve symptoms from prolonged positions
					• Prevent reinjury
					• Prepare for discharge
					• Promote continuation of good cardiovascular fitness as indicated
					• Gradually progress to previous activities
					• Evaluate the ability to return to previous function

A   B   C

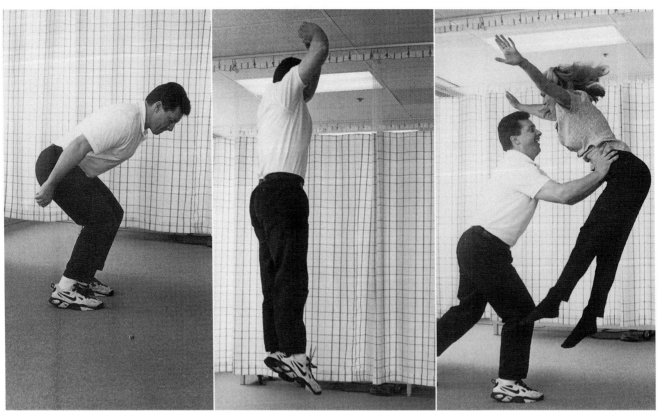

Fig. 8-23. **A,** Landing from a jump is invariably more difficult for jumping athletes. It is imperative that they learn to land in a hip hinge position and be trained to absorb as much shock as possible eccentrically through the hips, knees, and ankles, before it reaches the spine. Plyometric drills are helpful. **B,** While in the air with the arms overhead, train the jumping athlete to perform a brace with the transverse abdominals to prevent extraosseous lumbar motion. When blocking a ball with the arms overhead (as in volleyball), they should brace more intensely to resist the impact of the ball. Medicine ball drills are helpful. **C,** In some contact sports the athlete will be hit while in the air (e.g., basketball, football). For a frontal impact the athlete should give way at the hips; for a hit from an angle, he or she should learn to pivot away from the blow. Drills such as those shown here with progressively more difficult blows are helpful to train this specialized skill.

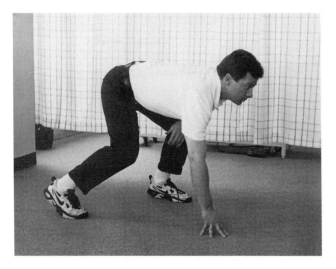

Fig. 8-24. A three-point stance is frequently used in football. It is essentially an exaggerated hip hinge. Adequate hip flexibility is essential, as well as pre-action abdominal bracing.

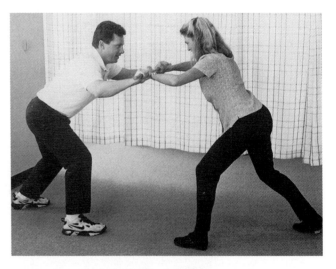

Fig. 8-25. In rugby and football, an athlete is frequently required to prevent someone from running around him or her. Stick drills such as this can teach a patient to adapt quickly to changing forces, while maintaining a neutral spine with an abdominal brace.

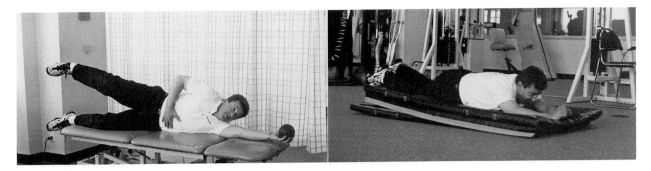

Fig. 8-26. When diving for a ball (as in baseball, volleyball), an athlete is taught to go low to the ground, stay horizontal, and land as a unit. A significant abdominal brace is required.

ibility should precede strength, proximal strength should precede distal strength, and strength should precede coordination. This culminates in the more rapid and fluid functional movements seen in uninjured persons. The physical therapist must be sure to consider the sequence of return of these various elements, the existing limitations uncovered during mechanical testing, and the patient's realistic goals when planning the progression of the exercise program.

Exercise. Functional training exercises (i.e., sports-specific drills and work-hardening activities) typically begin in phase III. Pre-set goals determine the kinetic activities that are to be the focus of rehabilitation. The therapist closely supervises the progression of these activities, paying careful attention to the quality of spinal mechanics and lumbar stabilization. Functional training is focused on trunk movements that simulate activities to which the patient will return. Sports-specific training (Figs. 8-23 through 8-26) can begin if the patient has achieved sufficient active lumbar stability and spinal mobility in fully loaded positions as well as adequate myofascial flexibility and conditioning. The therapist can use proprioceptive training with balance boards and Swiss balls. Initially athletes who take part in running and jumping activities are most safely trained with unloading devices (e.g., Vigor Equipment Inc. Stevensville, MI) during supervised treadmill running or jump training. These patients are typically well conditioned before surgery and have progressed postoperatively without setbacks.

Golfers need to be trained to hold the neutral spine dynamically during all five phases of the swing. The physical therapist can incorporate specific strength, flexibility, and balance exercises to achieve a safe and mechanically sound golf swing.[59]

Work-hardening activities for medium to heavy work classifications typically begin at 8 weeks and include lift training from 25 to 50 lb (see Fig. 9-11). Workers in these fields need special attention with regard to materials handling and should have a functional capacity evaluation 10 to 12 weeks after surgery to determine appropriate return-to-work status.

The exercise program progresses in intensity and difficulty to include rotational trunk stability, overhead activities, and balance training using a balance board. Training the patient in diagonal patterns in loaded positions better simulates real-life situations. A new stabilization exercise for patients in phase III challenges the obliques and transverse abdominals with minimal stress to passive tissues.[51] McGill refers to this exercise as "isometric side-support" on knees or on feet (depending on the degree of difficulty). Therapist should prescribe this exercise for home performance only after proving patient tolerance during clinic sessions.

The spinal mobility program attempts to restore painless and full lumbosacral ROM. The physical therapist should prescribe appropriate exercises and incorporate mobilization to achieve full and pain-free lumbar ROM and continue the stretching exercises needed to attain normal myofascial flexibility.

Soft tissue mobilization. Soft tissue mobilization should continue as needed to ensure a pliable surgical scar, proper gluteal and paraspinal muscle function, and soft tissue extensibility.

Spinal mobilization. Spinal mobilization should be used when necessary to restore motion at hypomobile segments and reduce pain associated with movement. Because the restoration of normal spinal motion is a primary goal, the therapist must identify and correct aberrant arthrokinematics. The expanded mechanical testing in phase III will reveal limitations or provoke symptoms that require attention. Maitland,[24] Mulligan,[33] and Paris[38] can be reviewed to assist in clinical reasoning.

Cardiovascular conditioning. Cardiovascular conditioning should continue to progress in intensity and duration. The patient's aerobic fitness program is determined by the ultimate activity goals. A typical sedentary office worker obviously does not train as intensely as a professional athlete. However, the therapist should not underestimate the aerobic demands placed on a manual laborer and should encourage appropriate endurance exercises.

Aerobic conditioning (focusing on correct postures and mechanics) may include treadmill walking, stationary cycling, the use of cross-country ski machines and stair climbers, swimming, and skating (in-line or on ice). Patients who have had previous experience with rowing may resume this exercise. Attention to proper stroke form is important, and modification to maintain lordosis may be necessary. Patients should not start a running program until after the twelfth week postoperatively because of the high compressive and repetitive axial loads at heel strike. A walk-run program should be initially implemented on a treadmill, with the therapist supervising and analyzing gait. When the patient does resume running, it should be in the morning hours when the disc is maximally hydrated.[60]

Modalities. Cryotherapy may still be beneficial after intensive training sessions. Myostimulation, TENS, microcurrent, interferential stimulation, and other modalities are seldom necessary.

Discharge planning. When the anticipated goals and desired outcomes have been attained, the patient is discharged with a home and/or club exercise program. The exercise program is to be maintained indefinitely. As always, the postsurgical patient should try to return to premorbid activity levels. Because goals vary dramatically among patients, some may require sub-

stantially more training than others such as overhead lift training, plyometric jump training, or sport-specific skill training. A reasonable level of tolerance to strenuous work activities or recreational sports should be attained before these higher activity level patients are discharged.

The comprehensive lumbar evaluation performed in phase III reveals any limitations in motion, weaknesses, neural restrictions, and painful movements that still need to be addressed. The physical therapist can obtain additional information from computerized testing devices[52] (e.g., the Lumbar Motion Monitor, Chattanooga Group Inc., TN) that provide objective data on lumbar motion speed, acceleration and deceleration, and degree of ROM. Other testing equipment such as computerized isokinetic machines determines objective trunk strength values at various speeds of lumbar ROM. This information can be helpful in guiding the therapist to choose appropriate exercises to remedy any weaknesses or limitations, especially in more physically active patients.

Most patients recovering from lumbar microdiscectomy progress uneventfully if properly educated and carefully rehabilitated. The physical therapist can facilitate the systematic training program to achieve a safe and rapid return of function by applying clinical knowledge and manual skills.

Suggested Home Maintenance for the Postsurgical Patient

The home maintenance box on pages 147 to 148 outlines rehabilitation guidelines the patient may follow. The home maintenance program is customized to the individual patient. Patients may progress at different rates depending on age, previous level of function, goals, nerve and tissue conditions, and rate of healing.

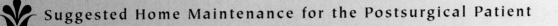

Suggested Home Maintenance for the Postsurgical Patient

Week 1

GOALS FOR THE WEEK: Protect the surgical site to promote wound healing, maintain nerve root mobility, reduce pain and inflammation, educate patient to minimize fear and apprehension, and establish consistently good body mechanics for safe and independent self-care

1. Protect the incision site.
2. Begin gentle nerve root gliding.
3. Maintain lumbar lordosis and correct body mechanics.
4. Avoid holding positions for prolonged periods and avoid all lumbar flexion.
5. Walk daily with a gradual increase in the duration and speed.
6. Use ice as needed for discomfort.

Weeks 2-3

GOALS FOR THE PERIOD: Protect the surgical site to promote wound healing, maintain nerve root mobility, reduce pain and inflammation, educate patient to minimize fear and apprehension, and establish consistently good body mechanics for safe and independent self-care

1. Progress walking program to 20 to 30 minutes.
2. Maintain nerve root mobility.
3. Begin progressive exercise program (unloaded positions only):
   a. Pelvic rocks in quadruped and prone positions
   b. Abdominal bracing in several positions
   c. Supported "dying bug" (when appropriate)
   d. Elbow lying to partial extension in lying
   e. Prone alternating arm raises
   f. Partial squatting (to 60 degrees)
   g. Gentle stretching of hamstrings, calves, gluteals, hip adductors, and rotators as needed
4. Maintain proper postures and body mechanics.
5. Practice isolated contractions of transverse abdominal muscles used frequently during daily activities.
6. Begin scar compressive taping as needed.
7. Use ice as needed for discomfort.

Weeks 4-6

GOALS FOR THE PERIOD: Understand neutral spin concept, improve cardiovascular condition, increase trunk strength to 80%, increase soft tissue mobility and lower extremity flexibility and strength

1. Maintain nerve root mobility.
2. Progress exercise program (partially loaded positions):
   a. Partial press-ups to full press-ups
   b. Prone alternating leg raises to prone double leg raises
   c. Unsupported "dying bug"
   d. Double-leg bridging progressing to single-leg bridging
   e. Partial sit-ups with rotation
   f. Side-lying double leg raises
   g. All fours arm-leg raises
   h. Repetitive squatting (starting at 60 degrees and progressing to 90 degrees)
3. Strengthen neurologically compromised muscles as needed (e.g., hip abductors, ankle dorsiflexors, plantar flexors, evertors).
4. Gentle stretching of hamstrings, calves, quadriceps, gluteals, hip adductors, and rotators as needed.

Continued

❧ Suggested Home Maintenance for the Postsurgical Patient—cont'd

Weeks 4-6—cont'd

5. Progress aerobic conditioning (walking, swimming, cycling) to 30 to 60 minutes.
6. Practice co-contractions of transverse abdominal muscles and multifidus frequently during daily activities.
7. Use ice as needed for discomfort.
8. Massage the scar as needed.
9. Continue compressive scar care as needed.

Weeks 7-11

GOALS FOR THE PERIOD: Ensure patient is independent in self-care and ADLs with minimal alterations, increase tolerance to activities, progress return to previous level of function
1. Progress exercise program (loaded positions):
    a. Press-ups
    b. Prone "Superman" (simultaneous arm/leg raises)
    c. "Dying bug" with weights
    d. Single leg bridging with weights
    e. Partial sit-ups with rotation
    f. Side-lying double leg raises with weights
    g. Isometric side support on elbow and knees progressed to feet
    h. All fours arm/leg raises with weights
    i. Standing rotary-torso with resistive tubing
    j. Repetitive squatting (to 90 degrees)
2. Begin functional training exercises (sports- and work-specific activities) at end of phase if able.
3. Continue lower extremity myofascial stretching as needed.
4. Continue strengthening neurologically compromised muscles.
5. Develop and segue into final home and/or club exercise program.

REFERENCES

1. Adams MA, Hutton WC: *Gradual disc prolapse,* Spine 10:524, 1985.
2. Beattie P: The relationship between symptoms and abnormal magnetic resonance images of lumbar intervertebral disks, *Phys Ther* 76:601, 1996.
3. Boden SD et al: Abnormal magnetic-resonance scans of the lumbar spine in asymptomatic patients. A prospective investigation, *J Bone Joint Surg* 72:403, 1990.
4. Brinkmann P: Injury of the annulus fibrosus and disc protrusions: an in vitro investigation of human lumbar discs, *Spine* 11:149, 1986.
5. Butler DS: *Mobilisation of the nervous system,* Melbourne, 1991, Churchill Livingstone.
6. Cottingham JT, Maitland J: A three-paradigm treatment model using soft tissue mobilization and guided movement-awareness techniques for a patient with chronic low back pain: a case study, *J Orthop Sports Ther* 26(3):155, 1997.

7. Goald HJ: Microlumbar discectomy, *Spine* 3(2):183, 1978.
8. Graves JE et al: Effect of training frequency and specificity on isometric lumbar extension strength, *Spine* 15(6):505, 1990.
9. Groslin AJ, Cantu R: *Myofascial manipulation: theory and clinical management,* New York, 1989, Forum Medicum.
10. Haig A et al: Prospective evidence for changes in paraspinal muscle activity after herniated nucleus pulposus, *Spine* 17(7):926, 1993.
11. Hickey DS, Hukins DWL: Relation between the structure of the annulus fibrosus and function and failure of the intervertebral disc, *Spine* 5(2):106, 1980.
12. Hides JA, Richardson CA, Jull GA: Multifidus inhibition in acute low back pain: recovery is not spontaneous, *MPAA Conference Proceedings* p. 57, 1995.
13. Hides JA et al: Evidence of lumbar multifidus muscle wasting ipsilateral to symptoms in patients with acute/subacute low back pain, *Spine* 19(2):165, 1994.

14. Hodges PW, Richardson CA: Contraction of the abdominal muscles associated with movement of the lower limb, *Phys Ther* 77:132, 1997.

15. Holm S, Nachemson A: Variations in the nutrition of the canine intervertebral disc induced by motion, *Spine* 8(8):866, 1983.

16. Hudson-Cook N, Tomes-Nicholson K, Breen A: A revised Oswestry disability questionnaire. In Roland MO, Jenner JR, editors: *Back pain: new approaches to rehabilitation and education*, New York, 1989, Manchester University Press.

17. Johannsen F et al: Exercises for chronic low back pain: a clinical trial, *J Orthop Sports Ther* 22(2):52, 1995.

18. Karas R et al: The relationship between nonorganic signs and centralization of symptoms in the prediction of return to work for patients with low back pain, *Phys Ther* 77(4):354, 1997.

19. Kirkaldy-Willis WH, Burton, CV: *Managing low back pain*, ed 3, New York, 1992, Churchill Livingstone.

20. Kuslich SD, Ulstrom CL, Michael CJ: The tissue origin of low back pain and sciatica, *Orthop Clin North Am* 22(2):181, 1991.

21. Lee HWM: Progressive muscle synergy and synchronization in movement petters: an approach to the treatment of dynamic lumbar instability, *J Manual Manip Ther* 2(4):133, 1994.

22. Lindgren K-A et al: Exercise therapy effects on functional radiographic findings and segmental electromyographic activity in lumbar spine instability, *Arch Phys Med Rehabil* 74:933, 1993.

23. Dai LY et al: The effect of flexion-extension motion of the lumbar spine on the capacity of the spinal canal, *Spine* 14(5):523, 1989.

24. Maitland GD: *Vertebral manipulation*, ed 5, London, 1986, Butterworths.

25. Manniche C et al: Intensive dynamic back exercises with or without hyperextension in chronic back pain after surgery for lumbar disc protrusion, *Spine* 18(5):560, 1993.

26. Marras WS et al: Quantification and classification of low back disorders on trunk motion, *Eur J Phys Med Rehab* 3:218, 1993.

27. McCulloch JH: Microdiscectomy: the gold standard for minimally invasive disc surgery, *Spine: State of the Art Rev* 11(2):373, 1997.

28. McGill SM: Distribution of tissue loads in the low back during a variety of daily and rehabilitation tasks, *J Rehabil Res Dev* 34(4):448, 1997.

29. McKenzie RA: *The lumbar spine*, Waikanae, New Zealand, 1981, Spinal Publications.

30. Moffroid M et al: Some endurance measures in persons with chronic low back pain, *J Orthop Sports Ther* 20(2):81, 1994.

31. Moreland J et al: Interrater reliability of six tests of trunk muscle function and endurance, *J Orthop Sports Ther* 26(4):200, 1997.

32. Mow VC, Holmes MH, Lai WM: Fluid transport and mechanical properties of articular cartilage: a review, *J Biomechanics* 17(5):377, 1984.

33. Mulligan BR: *Manual therapy "NAGS", "SNAGS", "MWMS" etc*, ed 3, New Zealand, 1995, Plane View Services.

34. Nagata CB, Tsujii Y: Manual therapy rounds, *J Manual Manip Ther* 5(2):87, 1997.

35. Ng JK-F, Richardson CA, Jull GA: Electromyographic amplitude and frequency changes in the iliocostalis lumborum and multifidus muscles during a trunk holding test, *Phys Ther* 77(9):954, 1997.

36. Panjabi MM: The stabilizing system of the spine. Part I, function, dysfunction adaptation and enhancement, *J Spinal Dis* 5:383, 1992.

37. Panjabi MM et al: On the understanding of clinical instability, *Spine* 19(23):2642, 1994.

38. Paris SV: Mobilization of the spine, *Phys Ther* 49:988, 1979.

39. Peterson M, Wilson J: Job satisfaction and perceptions of health, *J Occup Environ Med* 38(9):891, 1996.

40. Rantanen J et al: The lumbar multifidus muscle five years after surgery for a lumbar intervertebral disc herniation, *Spine* 18(5):568, 1993.

41. Richardson C et al: Techniques for active lumbar stabilisation for spinal protection: a pilot study, *Austral Physiother* 38(2):105, 1992.

42. Richardson C, Toppenberg R, Jull G: An initial evaluation of eight abdominal exercises for their ability to provide stabilisation for the lumbar spine, *Austral Physiother* 36(1):6, 1990.

43. Richardson CA, Jull GA: Muscle control-pain control. What exercises would you prescribe? *Manual Ther* 1:2, 1995.

44. Roland M, Morris R: A study of the natural history of back pain, part 1: the development of a reliable and sensitive measure of disability in low-back pain, *Spine* 8:141, 1983.

45. Saal JA: Dynamic muscular stabilization in the nonoperative treatment of lumbar pain syndromes, *Orthop Rev* 19(8):691, 1990.

46. Scalzitti DA: Screening for psychological factors in patients with low back problems: Waddell's nonorganic signs, *Phys Ther* 77(3):306, 1997.

47. Schofferman J et al: Childhood psychological trauma correlates with unsuccessful lumbar spine surgery, *Spine* 17(6):138, 1992.

48. Schofferman J et al: Childhood psychological trauma and chronic refractory low-back pain, *Clin J Pain* 9(4):260, 1993.

49. Sihvonen T, Partanen J: Segmental hypermobility in lumbar spine and entrapment of dorsal rami, *Electromyogr Clin Neurophysiol* 30:175, 1990.

49a. Sihvonen T et al: Local denervation atrophy of paraspinal muscles in postoperative failed back syndrome, *Spine* 18:575, 1993.

50. Spengler DM et al: Elective discectomy for herniation of a lumbar disc, *J Bone Joint Surg* 72:230, 1990.

51. Travell JG, Simmon DG: *Myofascial pain and dysfunction: the trigger point manual*, vol 1 (1983), vol 2 (1992), Baltimore, William & Wilkins.

52. Triano JJ, Schultz AB: Correlation of objective measures of trunk motion and muscle function with low-back disability ratings, *Spine* 12(6):561, 1987.

53. Urban JPG et al: Nutrition of the intervertebral disc, *Clin Orthop Related Res* 170:296, 1982.

54. Vucetic N, Maattanen H, Svensson O: Pain and pathology in lumbar disc hernia, *Clin Orthop Related Res* 320:65, 1995.

55. Waddell G et al: Non-organic physical signs in low-back pain, *Spine* 5:117, 1980.

56. Waddell G: A new clinical model for the treatment of low-back pain, *Spine* 12(7):632, 1987.

57. Waddell G: Evaluation of results in lumbar spine surgery. Clinical outcomes measures—assessment of severity, *Acta Orthop Scand Suppl* 251:134, 1993.

58. Walker ML et al: Relationships between lumbar lordosis, pelvic tilt, and abdominal performance, *Phys Ther* 67(4):512, 1987.

59. Watkins RG, Dillin WH: Lumbar spine injury in the athlete, *Clin Sports Med* 9(2):419, 1990.

60. White T, Malone T: Effects of running on intervertebral disc height, *J Orthop Sports Phys Ther* 12:410, 1990.

61. Wilke HJ et al: Stability increase of the lumbar spine with different muscle groups, *Spine* 20(2):192, 1995.

62. Williams CA, Singh M: Dynamic trunk strength of Canadian football players, soccer players, and middle to long distance runners, *J Orthop Sports Phys Ther* 25(1):271, 1997.

63. Wohlfahrt D, Jull G, Richardson C: The relationship between the dynamic and static function of abdominal muscles, *Austral Physiother* 39(1):9, 1993.

Chapter 9

Lumbar Spine Fusion

Paul Slosar
Jessie Scott

In the early 1900s two surgeons began performing lumbar fusions. Dr. Russell Hibbs and Dr. Fred Albee pioneered the posterior approaches for arthrodesis.[1,9] Over the subsequent decades, many surgeons improved fusion techniques, with extension of the fusion laterally to incorporate the transverse processes and the sacral ala.[3,6,27,31] The patient's autogenous iliac crest is the standard source of bone graft material.[7,8] A rapid evolution has occurred in the development and use of spinal fixation devices. Although tracing the historical evolution of these devices is beyond the scope of this chapter, they can simply be categorized as anterior or posterior fixation devices. The most common and most controversial are the pedicle screw and rod/plate systems. Anterior fixation devices include screw and rod/plate systems, as well as the recently introduced interbody cages. This chapter describes the indications for elective lumbar fusions and discusses the various methods of arthrodesis.

Surgical Indications and Considerations

In the elective patient population, most indications for lumbar arthrodesis are based on the presence of severe, disabling back or leg pain. Posttraumatic cases of segmental instability or potential neurologic injury also may require fusions, but this chapter focuses on patients with degenerative spinal pathology.

Patients with low back pain experience symptoms resulting from tissue aggravation during the degenerative cascade.[29] Trauma or overuse causes the disc wall to begin to develop microtears; this eventually results in a loss of disc height that alters the alignment of the facet joints. This may lead to pain, with accompanying spasm and guarding. The joints begin to develop synovitis, articular cartilage degeneration, and adhesions. This alters the spinal motion mechanics at that segment, further stressing the annulus of the disc and accelerating the degenerative process of the facet. Increased wearing of the cartilage and hypermobility of the facet also occur. The superior and inferior facet surfaces begin to enlarge. As the joint becomes more disrupted, normal motion at that segment becomes impossible. The disc begins to undergo greater strain. The disc wall weakens further, begins to bulge, and can eventually frankly herniate. The disc continues to lose fluid and height, causing narrowing of the neural foramen, or foraminal stenosis. This process is outlined in Table 9-1.

Patients with severe back pain that is refractory to conservative care may be candidates for surgical evaluation. Conservative care should include a rigorous attempt at exercise-based dynamic stabilization training, therapeutic injections, and medications. Surgical treatment should only be discussed with the patient after a firm diagnosis has been made.

Diagnostic Tests

Spinal radiographs show osteophytes and segmental disc space narrowing in patients with degenerative spondylosis. A defect in the pars interarticularis is seen in patients with spondylolysis. Anterolisthesis, or a forward slippage of one vertebra on the next, is the hallmark radiographic finding in spondylolisthesis. Instability or excessive motion on flexion/extension films, although rare in degenerative lumbar conditions, can occasionally be observed.

Computed tomography (CT) reliably evaluates the bone or spondylosis compression against the nerves. Computer-enhanced reformatted CT images are as effective in evaluating spinal stenosis as myelography. CT scanning is more sensitive than magnetic resonance imaging (MRI) in the evaluation of bony stenosis, whereas MRI gives useful information about the health of the discs and nerves. Combining the two imaging modalities gives a very accurate, thorough picture of the lumbar spinal pathoanatomy.

Provocative discography is an essential diagnostic tool in the work-up of patents with painful degenerative lumbar disc disease. Unfortunately, the practitioner cannot examine the disc directly as a knee or hand can be observed. The lumbar discs are deep within the abdominal cavity and do not have true dermatomal pain patterns in axial discogenic cases. Overlapping sclerodermal referred pain patterns in the lumbar spine make the localization of the true pain generator difficult. Discography has evolved as a test to examine the lumbar discs morphologically and, most importantly, provocatively. On injection into the disc, the patient

Table 9-1   The Degenerative Cascade

	Damage at Each Stage		
Structure	**Stage 1: Dysfunction**	**Stage 2: Instability**	**Stage 3: Stability**
Intervertebral disc	• Circumferential tears • Inflammatory exudates and irritation	• Radial tears • Loss of disc height • Internal disruption • Disc bulges and herniations	• Loss of proteoglycans and water, fibrotic resorption • Sclerosis and eventual bony ankylosis
Facet joints	• Synovitis • Minor cartilage degeneration	• Laxity of joint capsule • Moderate cartilage degeneration	• Significant bony overgrowth • Grossly degenerated cartilage • Hypomobility
Muscles	• Spasm, guarding	• Chronic shortening and fibrosis	• Further shortening and fibrosis
Neural foramen	• Unaffected	• Narrowed through annular bulges • Disc narrowing • Bony overgrowth	• Significant stenosis • Disc narrowing

must communicate to the discographer if that disc is concordantly painful. Many degenerative discs are either not painful or discordantly painful. This information is essential for the surgeon and the patient contemplating lumbar arthrodesis.

Diagnosis

Among patients undergoing elective lumbar arthrodesis, painful degenerative disc disease is the most prevalent diagnosis. Confirmatory diagnostic testing often includes MRI scanning and discography. Overlap occurs among patients who have had previous surgery and have a diagnosis of "failed back surgery syndrome," a nonspecific diagnosis. Before surgery is contemplated, every effort must be made to arrive at a diagnosis that specifically isolates the source of pain.

Patients often have numerous diagnoses, each of which may be valid. For example, a 45-year-old man who had a laminotomy performed 5 years ago for a herniated nucleus pulposus comes to his physician complaining of 50% low back pain and 50% right leg pain and numbness. Diagnostic imaging is significant for L4-L5 segmental degeneration with osteophytes and narrowing of the disc space. A multiplanar CT scan reveals moderate spondylosis (bone spurs) with stenosis along the right neural foramen. Discography is concordant with pain reproduction at the L4-L5 disc. The appropriate diagnoses include painful degenerative disc disease, lumbar spondylosis with stenosis, and post-laminectomy syndrome.

The absolute requisite for a successful lumbar surgery outcome is matching concordant patient symptoms with the appropriate surgical procedure. Patients who cannot manage their pain with conservative measures and have demonstrable, concordant pathology on diagnostic testing may benefit from lumbar arthrodesis.

Types of Fusions

Instrumentation Versus Non-Instrumentation

The goal of a lumbar arthrodesis is the successful union of two or more vertebra. Controversy exists over the most efficient way to achieve this result. Instrumentation can be used to immobilize the moving segments while the fusion becomes solid. One of the original and most popular systems is the Harrington hook/rod construct. Although this *distraction*-type fixation immobilizes the spine in certain planes, it causes a loss of physiologic lordosis, or a "flat-back syndrome," in many patients.

Today, most spine surgeons use pedicle screw constructs to immobilize the vertebrae rigidly while preserving the normal lumbar lordosis[9] (Fig. 9-1). Typically, external orthosis bracing is not needed in these cases. As well-controlled studies emerge, data support the use of internal fixation for fusion.[10] Most studies support the use of pedicle screw fixation to obtain a more reliable bony union, although complication rates tend to be higher with these devices as well.[11,12]

Some surgeons do not routinely use pedicle screws for arthrodesis. In most of these situations (when pedi-

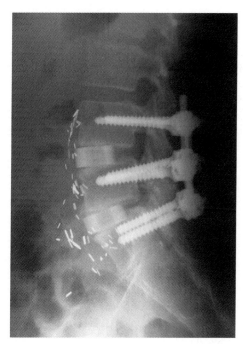

Fig. 9-1. Pedicle screw instrumentation in a circumferential lumbar fusion.

cle screws are used) the patient must wear a lumbar orthosis for an extended period postoperatively. To immobilize the L5-S1 motion segment effectively, an orthosis with a thigh-cuff extension must be applied. Patients with non-instrumented fusions may take an extensive amount of time to stabilize and become comfortable in their rehabilitation. Conversely, most patients with internal fixation become mobile and independent more rapidly, making early rehabilitation more predictable.

Posterior Fusion

Posterolateral lumbar fusion. Different surgeons use different techniques to perform a lumbar fusion. The traditional approach is through a midline posterior incision. If necessary the surgeon performs a laminectomy/laminotomy to address the pertinent pathology. Most surgeons perform a posterolateral fusion, which means that the transverse processes, pars interarticularis, and, if needed, the sacral alae are decorticated. The patient's own iliac crest bone graft is harvested and morselized. The bone graft is then placed on the decorticated surfaces, forming a fusion bed contiguous with all the surfaces to be fused. Pedicle screws and rods or plates may be placed to immobilize the motion segments rigidly and augment the formation of a solid union.

The problems with a posterolateral fusion are both mechanical and physiologic. The fusion is attempting to form at a mechanical disadvantage because of tension. Bone heals more reliably under protected phys-

iologic loads of compression, not tension. Also, the available area for the bone union to occur is limited to the remaining posterolateral bone surfaces. After extensive decompression of the neural elements (laminectomy), the available fusion area is reduced and often poorly vascularized. These local factors reduce the likelihood of a successful arthrodesis. Nicotine use negatively influences the formation of posterolateral lumbar fusions.

Finally, the usual source of pain in these patients is the disc itself, hence the term discogenic. In routine cases of posterolateral fusions the disc is not radically resected. Biomechanical studies have shown that people bear load through the middle and posterior thirds of the disc. Several reports describe a persistently painful disc under a solid posterior fusion.[32] As surgeons recognized the biomechanical and physiologic aspects of the discs, they began performing interbody fusions.[33]

Interbody fusion

POSTERIOR LUMBAR INTERBODY FUSION. Interbody fusions evolved to address many of the drawbacks of traditional posterolateral fusions. Radical excision of the disc and anterior column support with rigid bone grafting are performed. The available area for successful bone union is greatly increased by using the interbody space.

Using a posterior lumbar approach, a surgeon performs a posterior lumbar interbody fusion (PLIF). After a wide laminectomy the posterior two thirds of the disc is resected and an interbody tricortical strut is placed into the evacuated disc space. This provides anterior interbody stability through a posterior approach. PLIF is a technically demanding procedure associated with a higher incidence of postsurgical nerve injuries.

ANTERIOR LUMBAR INTERBODY FUSION. Because the risks associated with PLIF were too great for routine use, many surgeons moved to anterior lumbar interbody fusion (ALIF). Using the same principles of disc excision and interbody bone grafting, many surgeons achieved excellent results. However, ALIF alone cannot withstand the forces across the grafts, so many collapse or do not fuse. Surgeons who perform ALIF have learned to protect the grafts with posterior instrumentation, leading to a predictable fusion rate and good clinical results.

From a technical standpoint anterior lumbar surgery is most easily and safely accomplished through a retroperitoneal approach. After the anterior disc is exposed, it is relatively simple to perform a discectomy and insert the bone graft of the surgeon's choice. Posterior fusion and instrumentation can be placed through a separate posterior approach on either the same day or in a staged procedure. A circumferential fusion is accomplished in this manner (see Fig. 9-1).

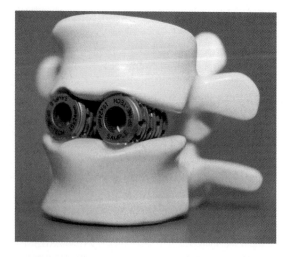

Fig. 9-2. BAK interbody cage device (Sulzer Spine-Tech, Minneapolis, Minnesota).

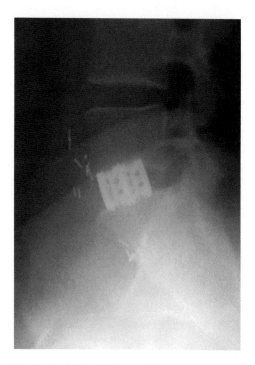

Fig. 9-3. Lumbar fusion with the BAK interbody cage (SpineTech).

CAGES. Recent technologic advances have been made in interbody cages. Essentially, these devices are hollow cylinders made of titanium, carbon, or bone (Fig. 9-2). They are filled with autogenous bone graft and inserted between the vertebral bodies. The cages usually have threads along the outside edges that afford very rigid immediate fixation. This has dramatically reduced the need for posterior fixation. Research is moving rapidly to find a reliable substitute for the autogenous bone graft, most likely with the use of bone-morphogenic protein. If medical advances could eliminate the need to harvest bone from the patient's iliac crest, cage technology would certainly represent a minimally invasive spinal fusion (Fig. 9-3).

Most surgeons implant these devices through an anterior approach, with some using laparoscopic-assisted anterior surgery. This can potentially reduce the length of stay in hospital but can produce a slightly higher complication rate.

Most patients begin physical therapy between 6 weeks and 3 months after surgery. *Extension-biased exercises should be avoided during the first 6 months of the postoperative recovery phase.*

Surgical Procedure

The most common lumbar fusion is the posterolateral fusion. The patient is placed in a knee-chest position, which allows the abdomen to hang free. This decompresses the lumbar epidural veins and minimizes bleeding. A skin incision is made over the operative levels, and the paraspinal muscles are stripped off the posterior elements (spinous process, lamina, and transverse processes). Deep retractors hold back the muscles to allow the surgeons to expose the bone for fusion. Using small curettes or a high-speed burr, the surgeon decorticates the dorsal aspect of the transverse processes and facet joints in preparation for the bone graft placement. Through a separate fascial incision the surgeon harvests the necessary amount of cortical and cancellous bone graft from the posterior iliac crest. This bone graft material is then carefully placed in the recipient site.

If screws are used to augment the fusion, a pilot hole is made over the entry site of the pedicle with a burr. Usually probes are placed in the pedicles and a radiograph is taken to confirm the position of the pedicle probes. After confirmation, the pedicles are tapped and appropriate length screws are placed into the pedicles. Again, an intraoperative radiograph is taken to confirm the position of the screws. The rods or plates are connected to the screws, and lordosis is preserved in the construct. The wound is usually irrigated with an antibiotic solution to minimize the chance of infection and closed over a deep suction drain. The drain is removed when the postsurgical drainage is minimal. Patients are mobilized out of bed as tolerated on the first or second day after surgery.

Therapy Guidelines for Rehabilitation

An understanding of the specific procedure performed is essential for safe rehabilitation. Before beginning a rehabilitation program, the therapist must know whether the patient has had a fusion with or without instrumentation. Patients who were operated on with instrumentation can generally be progressed more aggressively in the first phase of rehabilitation. Patients who were operated on without instrumentation require more time for the bony fusion to take place. Generally a callus should form within 6 to 8 weeks; the surgeon monitors this by x-ray and usually does not refer for therapy before a callus has formed. The therapist also must know the surgical approach and the levels fused. After a motion segment is fused, increased stress is placed on the levels above and below the fusion. This creates risk for acceleration of the degenerative cascade at the adjacent levels. Obviously the more levels that have been fused, the greater the stress placed on the remaining segments. When the fusion includes the L5-S1 motion segment, abnormal forces are then translated to the sacroiliac joints. To minimize these forces, the therapist must be sure that normal motion exists at all remaining segments, including the thoracic spine and lower extremities.

During a posterior fusion, the multifidi are retracted from the spine. This partially tears the dorsal divisions of the spinal nerves, resulting in partial denervation of the multifidi.[29] If an anterior fusion also has been performed, a midline skin incision will be apparent and the abdominal muscular incision is lateral. The incision passes through the obliques, also partially denervating them. For this reason the therapist should teach the patient the proper way to recruit the abdominal muscles and watch for any substitution patterns.

Description of Rehabilitation and Rationale for Using Instrumentation

Opinion about the degree of rehabilitation needed after spinal surgery ranges from the optimistic view that no rehabilitation is needed to others who argue for aggressive exercise- and education-based programs. This chapter is written from the point of view that the patient is not merely recovering from surgery but from a breakdown in the spine exacerbated by predisposing factors such as stiffness and poor muscle tone, movement habits, and proprioception.

The following guidelines are not intended to substitute for sound clinical reasoning but rather serve as a foundation on which a trained physical therapist can base the rehabilitation of a patient after spinal fusion. It is assumed that the therapist will know the basics of spinal evaluation and will monitor the patient for symptoms that require prompt reevaluation.

Q. Tom is 50 years old. He had a lumbar fusion at L4-L5 and L5-S1 3 weeks ago. He is now in therapy. The physical therapist gives Tom an exercise to facilitate nerve root gliding. The patient asks "What is the significance of this exercise?". What should the therapist tell the patient?

Phase I

TIME: Days 1-5
GOALS: Patient education about daily movements, nerve mobilization, and home care principles (Table 9-2)

Inpatient phase. Most patients remain in the hospital for several days after fusion surgery. Physical therapy management during this phase consists of teaching patients the proper way to get in and out of bed, dress and undress, and walk (perhaps with a walker for the first 1 or 2 days). The therapist also can teach basic and simple nerve mobilization for the involved level and principles for using ice at home. Patients should leave the hospital with an understanding of the home care required until they begin their outpatient physical therapy. If the physician requests bracing of any kind, the patient should understand the way to get in and out of the brace and when to wear it. Patients will be given instructions from their physician to avoid driving, prolonged sitting, lifting, bending, and twisting. The physical therapist should reinforce this information and teach patients the way to avoid these activities by hip hinging or pivoting. This information should be provided in written form because many patients may be medicated or overwhelmed from the recent surgery and therefore have difficulty recalling or applying what they have just been taught. Most patients are referred for physical therapy 5 weeks after their discharge from the hospital.

Phase II

TIME: Weeks 6-10
GOALS: Increased activity, tissue modeling, stabilization, and reconditioning (Table 9-3)

During phase II patients gradually increase their activity level. While taking account of soft tissue healing, the physical therapist can safely begin to influence the direction of tissue modeling through carefully applied stress. Patients should begin to approximate normal activities while the therapist controls the intensity of movement and exercise.

Patients progressing to the latter portion of phase II increase the intensity of the stabilization program begun in the earlier stages of the phase. They may increase repetitions and level of difficulty. Patients should do 20 minutes of cardiovascular exercise daily and add stabilization exercises for the lumbar paraspinal muscles and the upper back. They can begin a light weight training program, avoiding exercises that load the lumbar spine. Patients should no longer require assistance with most daily activities. (Common restrictions are no lifting greater than 10 pounds and no overhead lifting.) Examples of exercises for this phase are listed in the following sections.

Table 9-2   Lumbar Fusion and Laminectomy

Rehabilitation Phase	Criteria to Progress to this Phase	Anticipated Impairments and Functional Limitations	Intervention	Goal	Rationale
Phase I Postoperative 1-5 days	Postoperative (inpatient)	• Pain • Limited bed mobility • Limited self-care • Limited activities of daily living (ADLs) • Limited tolerance to prolonged postures (sit/stand) • Limited tolerance to walking	Inpatient care • Bed mobility training Log roll technique with supine–sit–stand • ADL training with assistive devices as necessary (dressing, bathroom transfers) • Body mechanics training • Gait training, with walker if necessary	• Independent with the following: 1. Bed mobility 2. Don/doff clothing, and corset if indicated 3. Transfers 4. Gait, using assistive device as appropriate • Demonstrate appropriate body mechanics with self-care and basic ADLs	• Promote restoration of independent function • Use log roll to avoid placing stress on the surgical site • Emphasize walking to improve tolerance to upright postures • Use proper body mechanics to avoid reinjury

Table 9-3   Lumbar Fusion and Laminectomy

Rehabilitation Phase	Criteria to Progress to this Phase	Anticipated Impairments and Functional Limitations	Intervention	Goal	Rationale

Phase II Postoperative 6–10 weeks	• Outpatient candidate
	• No signs of infection
	• Cleared by physician to begin therapy
		• Pain limited with ADLs
		• Limited nerve root mobility
		• Limited trunk stability
		• Limited mobility of regions adjacent to surgical site
			• Cryotherapy
			• Relative rest
			• Review of body mechanics training
			• Nerve mobilization
			• Passive range of motion—
			• Lower extremity stretches—
			  Hip flexors (gently initiate after 8 weeks with physician approval)
			  Gluteals
			  Hip rotators
			  Quadriceps
			  Hamstrings
			  Calf
			• Isometrics with active range of motion—Abdominal bracing with squats, transfers, and gait
			• Spinal stabilization exercises—
			  Bridging
			  Dying bug (after 8 weeks, with physician approval)
			  Quadruped
			  Superman (after 8 weeks, with physician approval)
			• Walking program—emphasize "tiny steps" after 8 weeks (with physician approval)
			• Joint mobilization to thoracic spine
			• Soft tissue massage after incision is closed
			• Patient education
			• UBE and/or brisk walking
				• Control pain
				• Protect surgical site
				• Improve or maintain nerve root mobility
				• Improve flexibility of lower extremity musculature
				• Improve trunk stability strength
				• Improve walking tolerance
				• Improve mobility of thoracic spine as indicated
				• Decrease patient apprehension
				• Improve cardiovascular conditioning
					• Self-manage pain
					• Prevent reinjury
					• Perform ADLs without adding increased stress to the lumbar spine
					• Prevent neural adhesions
					• Improve mobility of lower extremities to decrease stress on the lumbar spine
					• Initiate trunk stabilization while performing ADLs to decrease potential for reinjury
					• Perform cardiovascular conditioning and "tiny steps" to avoid excessive lumbar spine movement during gait
					• Improve mobility of thoracic spine to decrease stress on the lumbar spine
					• Improve mobility of soft tissue
					• Reduce volitional muscle guarding
					• Perform cardiovascular conditioning

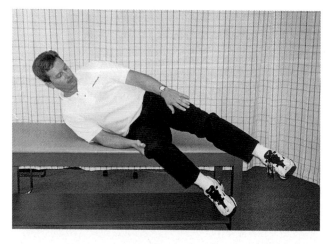

Fig. 9-4. To rise from a lying position, the patient begins with an abdominal brace to maintain a neutral spine and rolls to the edge of the bed as a unit. The patient then pivots off the elbow while throwing the legs to the ground. This momentum makes an otherwise difficult movement easier. To avoid twisting the trunk, the patient should reach toward the top foot with the top arm.

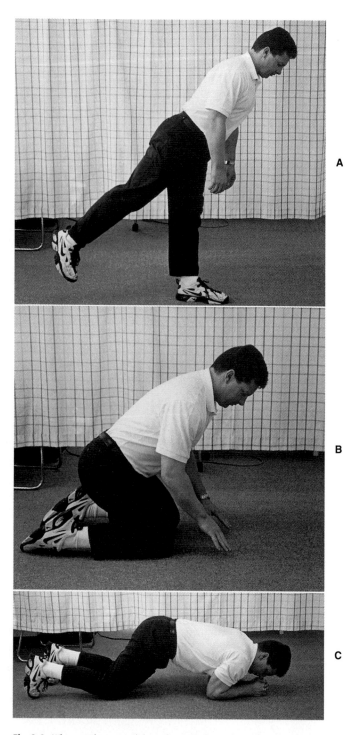

A

B

C

Fig. 9-6. When getting up and down from the floor, the patient moves from a single leg hip hinge (**A**) through a reverse lunge position to double kneeling (**B**). Next, the patient hinges the hips from double kneeling to about 45 degrees. Another balance point occurs here (**C**). From this balance point, the patient rocks forward onto the elbows and rolls as a unit onto the side. To avoid uncontrolled extension the stomach should never touch the ground. The process is reversed to rise from the ground.

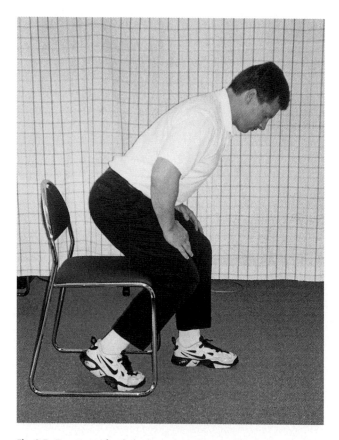

Fig. 9-5. To get out of a chair, the patient places one foot under the chair, hinges the hip, and then raises off the thigh. The hips should be the first to leave the chair and the last to land. The patient should *not* attempt to keep the back vertical, merely straight. To get into the chair the process is reversed. If no room is available to get the foot under the chair, such as in a couch, the patient pivots on the hips until perpendicular to the chair. This offsets the feet and allows for easier rising.

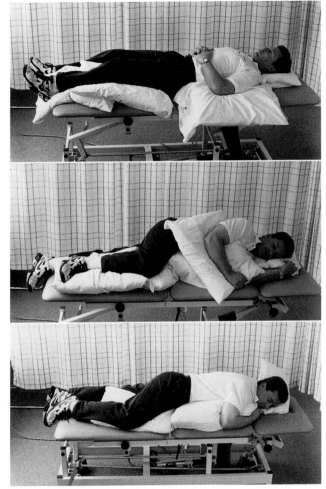

Fig. 9-7. A, Supported supine lying. Patients generally prefer to have the whole leg supported rather than just the knees. Any unsupported area becomes uncomfortable and causes the patient to shift and wake. The shoulders also should be supported in whatever degree of protraction exists. Any soft tissue subjected to prolonged stretch eventually becomes uncomfortable. **B,** Supported side-lying. The patient needs enough pillows to support the upper extremities. A body pillow frequently works well. The patient should pull the support directly into the upper thigh and chest and then roll slightly onto it; he or she should not lie on the same side all night. **C,** Three-quarter prone lying is the most popular position. It is similar to supported side-lying, except that the patient rolls one quarter turn more. A wedge-shaped pillow minimizes cervical strain in this position.

Evaluation. Before initiating treatment the therapist should assess the physical problems that can be addressed in therapy such as strength, body mechanics, range of motion, and neuromuscular control; the therapist can then establish goals for treatment. This evaluation should include range of motion for the thoracic spine and lower extremities but *not* of the lumbar spine. A complete neurologic examination should be performed to establish a baseline and should include neural tension testing. The therapist can perform strength testing for the lower extremities with the exception of testing hip flexor strength. He or she also can check the patient's ability to stabilize or brace the lumbar spine isometri-

cally, which is a test of the patient's ability to recruit the trunk muscles to control the spine. The patient's spontaneous body mechanics and the way the patient responds to the challenge of daily activities should be assessed. The goals of phase II are as follows:

- Consistently good body mechanics for activities of daily living (ADLs)
- Protection of the surgical site from infection and mechanical stress
- Maintenance of nerve root mobility at the involved levels
- Control of pain and inflammation
- Minimizing of patient fear and apprehension
- Beginning of a stabilization/reconditioning program
- Maintenance of scar and soft tissue mobility
- Treatment for restrictions of thoracic motion and motion at the hip and lower extremity
- Education to minimize sitting time and maximize walking time

Body mechanics training. If body mechanics training was provided preoperatively, it should be reviewed after surgery. If body mechanics training is new to the patient, the therapist should go through the entire program, which is as follows:

- In and out of bed (Fig. 9-4)
- In and out of a chair (Fig. 9-5)
- Up and down from the floor (Fig. 9-6)
- Lying postures (Fig. 9-7)
- Sitting (Fig. 9-8)
- Standing
- Dressing
- Bending (Fig. 9-9)
- Reaching
- Pushing and pulling (Fig. 9-10)
- Lifting (Fig. 9-11)
- Carrying (Fig. 9-12)

Patients must perform these activities to get dressed, use the bathroom, travel to doctor's appointments, and shop for and prepare meals. A patient who can do these activities without stressing the surgical site will heal faster and with less discomfort. Patients can accomplish all these tasks without lumbar motion if they move their hips rather than the spine. Instead of flexing the lumbar spine, they can "hip hinge" (see Fig. 9-9). Rather than twist in the lumbar spine, they can pivot on another body part (knees, elbows, hips). When teaching a hip hinge, the physical therapist should point out that the hips should move *back* rather than *down*. After surgery, patients tend to guard and move cautiously. Showing them the way to use their momentum safely in many maneuvers makes the postoperative transition easier. For example, getting out of bed requires less of an abdominal brace if the legs are moved quickly to the floor, transferring the momentum to the torso (see Fig. 9-4). Outpatient physical therapy begins at this point.

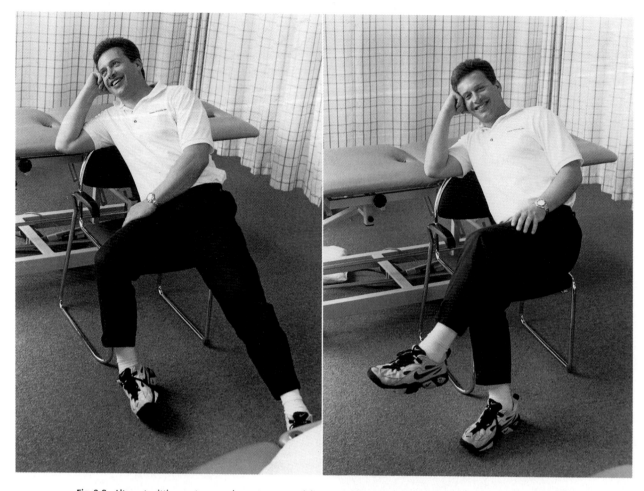

Fig. 9-8. Alternate sitting postures are important to teach because patients will want to change sitting postures frequently. As long as a neutral spine position is maintained, the variations are limitless. These positions successfully take the weight off the left pelvis, thereby relieving pressure on the piriformis and sensitive sciatic notch.

Fig. 9-9. Hip hinging is flexing the hips and knees while maintaining a neutral spine. A dowel can be helpful for patients with difficulty perceiving spinal motion. The spine should *not* be kept vertical, but merely straight. This is one of the essential motions patients use to perform functional activities. Hip hinging also can be done on one leg as in Fig. 9-6, *A*. This is especially useful when getting up and down from the ground. The position shown is a balance point that patients should learn because it requires little or no effort to maintain. Patients should attempt to move from one balance point to another.

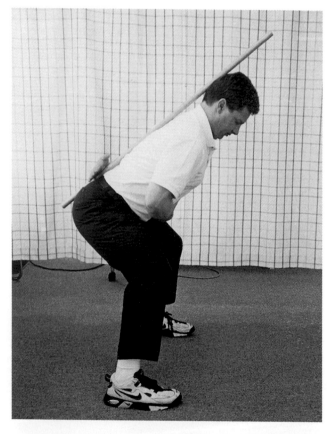

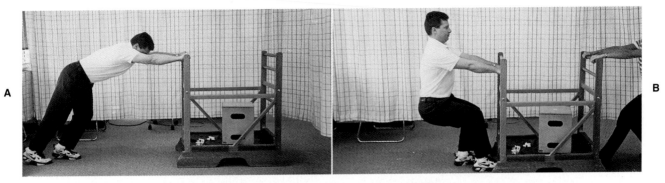

Fig. 9-10. A, To push an object, the patient leans into it with a hip hinge until the body weight begins to move it forward. The heavier the object, the more the patient needs to line the shoulders up behind the hands. Arms can be bent or straight. The patient should take tiny steps because if the feet move anterior to the hips, a lumbar flexion moment will occur. **B,** To pull an object, the patient leans back, maintaining neutral position, until the body weight begins to move the object. The heavier the object, the more the patient needs to flex at the hips and knees. The patient should take tiny steps and hold the upper body erect because the weight tends to pull the body into flexion.

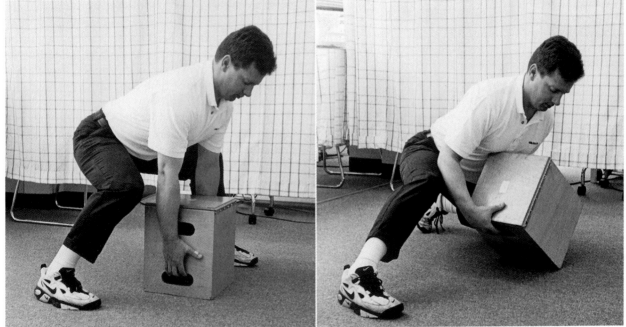

Fig. 9-11. A, Lifting from a hip hinge position. The spine remains straight but not vertical. This method works for conveniently placed objects. **B,** To lift a less conveniently placed object safely, the patient goes down onto one knee, then hinges the hips and tilts the object to its maximal height. The patient then locks the object to the chest, reverses the hip hinge, and places the object on the thigh. As the patient stands up, the thigh lifts the majority of the weight.

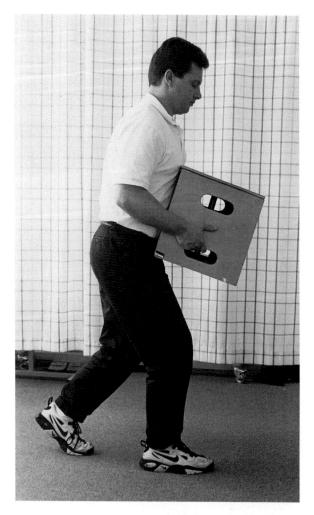

Fig. 9-12. Slight knee flexion reduces the tendency toward lumbar extension while the patient carries objects. It may feel "funny" at first, but with continued practice this flexion becomes simple.

NERVE ROOT GLIDING. Patients should extend the knee while lying supine with the spine in a neutral position and the hip flexed to a 90-degree angle. When tension is encountered, the therapist helps the patient work the knee gently back and forth, gradually increasing the range of motion. This stretch may cause increased symptoms during the stretch, which should resolve immediately on relaxing. Education should be provided to the patient regarding expected and adverse reactions to neural gliding. Any lingering symptom is reason to halt the stretch until the therapist can reassess the problem.

Local inflammation occurs after lumbar spine surgery. Because the body forms scar tissue in response to inflammation, the nerve root can become adherent to the neural foramen or lose elasticity. It is theorized that a nerve root that is kept moving within its sheath cannot develop adhesions.[4,7,19,21] Patients with nonirritable chronic leg symptoms tend to respond well to nerve tension stretching. However, the patient must keep the spine stabilized while moving the leg.

DECREASING PAIN AND INFLAMMATION. Patients should use ice packs for about 20 minutes three or four times per day to help control pain and swelling. Patients can be taught to alternate rest periods with periods of light activity because sustained postures increase pain and swelling. The therapist may apply modalities in the clinic to control pain after therapy. Ultrasound should *not* be applied over a healing bony fusion. Patients with severe pain problems can try using a home transcutaneous electrical nerve stimulation (TENS) unit.

If patients know they can control their pain level, they are less fearful of trying activities that may cause a pain flare-up or those that have been painful in the past. They will rely less on inactivity and medication to control pain. Keeping the inflammation to a minimum is important to minimize scarring. The therapist should spend some time initially discovering the patient's fears and alleviating those that are groundless. Not everything has to be accomplished during the first visit. Greater progress will occur in the long run if the therapist initially allays patient fears and teaches the patient ways to control pain. Patients who are sensitive to load bearing through the spine should take frequent short unloading rests throughout the day. Those who cannot tolerate any one position for a length of time can learn to make a circuit of their activities, frequently changing tasks. Patients with specific position intolerance benefit from learning ways to avoid that position while doing daily activities. Lumbar rolls are not recommended during this phase because most patients cannot tolerate pressure on the incision site after surgery.

PATIENT EDUCATION. Patients should understand the expected postoperative course of events, particularly concerning postoperative pain. Increasing leg pain is not a good sign, even if low back pain diminishes; conversely, decreasing leg symptoms is a good sign, even if low back pain is increasing. Less leg pain is consistent with less neurologic involvement, whereas the low back is expected to be sore because of the incision and altered facet mechanics.[16] Incisional pain can be expected to decrease gradually over 6 to 8 weeks. As patients begin to return to normal activities, an associated increase in muscle soreness frequently occurs. The sooner they recondition themselves, the better they will feel. Patients should be aware that their bodies will be adapting to and remodeling from the surgery for as long as 1 to 2 years. Symptoms often shift and change during that time. The therapist should teach patients to manage flare-ups using ice, rest, and resumption of previous activities within 1 or 2 days.

Patients are generally very fearful after lumbar spine surgery. Anxiety causes increased muscular tension and therefore discomfort. Patients also may be afraid to move, thinking they will somehow ruin the surgical results. Patients can better tolerate flare-ups and vari-

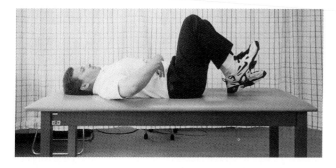

Fig. 9-13. Abdominal brace with tiny steps. The patient creates an abdominal brace by pulling in and up with the abdominals. It is important to remember to move the abdominals without moving the spine. While maintaining the brace the patient slowly takes the weight off one foot, only unweighting the foot as much as possible without allowing the hips to rotate or the spine to extend. Eventually the patient should be able to lift the foot an inch off the ground. The patient then alternates feet.

ations in their symptoms if they expect them and have been instructed in self-management of these flare-ups. Patients are generally less apprehensive if the therapist is not apprehensive. Most people recover well and should start with that expectation. If the patient appears to be developing neuropathic pain, nerve root signs, symptoms from a new level, or any other complications, the therapist should note the symptoms calmly and convey the information to the treating surgeon for advice without conveying anxiety to the patient.

STABILIZATION AND RECONDITIONING. The physical therapist should teach patients the following stabilization and reconditioning exercises:
- Abdominal bracing
- Squats (Fig. 8-21)
- Walking
- "Tiny steps," or lower abdominal biased, supported stabilization can be initiated after 8 weeks, with physician approval (Fig. 9-13)
- Cardiovascular reconditioning (using stair climber, brisk walking, and pool exercises when the incision is closed)

Abdominal bracing and "tiny steps" are good exercises to begin strengthening the trunk. Patients should perform squats and walking for leg strengthening and conditioning, cardiovascular exercises for cardiovascular conditioning, and overall endurance training for good health.

MAINTAINING SCAR AND SOFT TISSUE MOBILITY. The therapist should use soft tissue techniques to maintain good scar and soft tissue mobility without disrupting the healing of these tissues. Scar tissue tends to contract while healing. This can create a "tight" scar that restricts mobility.[5]

ASSESSMENT AND TREATMENT FOR RESTRICTIONS OF THORACIC AND HIP MOBILITY. The following steps will help ease restrictions of the thoracic spine and hip:
- Manual therapy for thoracic motion restrictions

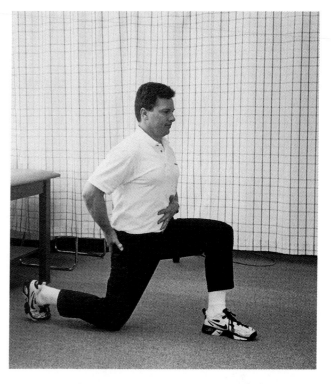

Fig. 9-14. Hip flexor stretch. The patient kneels on one leg with the other leg in front, braces the spine with the abdominals, and gradually begins to shift weight forward to the front foot. The patient should feel a stretch in the groin area of the kneeling leg. The spine should not be extended.

- Lower extremity stretches for soft tissue restrictions
- Hamstring stretches (Fig. 8-19)
- Hip flexor stretches (Fig. 9-14)
- Quadriceps stretches (Fig. 8-20)
- Lumbar flexion stretch (Fig. 9-15)—when initiating this stretch the therapist must not be overly aggressive, obtaining ROM at the expense of compromising the fusion site; Fig. 9-15 demonstrates an ideal ending position for this stretch, which may take several months to obtain
- Up and down from the floor (Fig. 9-16)
- Hip rotator stretches (Fig. 9-17)

The loss of motion caused by the spinal fusion places additional demands for motion on the adjacent segments. One of the most stressful motions in the lumbar spine is rotation, which causes a shearing effect across the disc. The thoracic spine is designed to rotate. Free and easy rotation of the thoracic spine allows this motion to take place in a spinal region better designed to perform this motion. The hip joint is a large ball-and-socket joint with free motion in all planes. This joint can compensate for the lack of motion in the lumbar spine and should remain as flexible as possible. Physical therapists can teach patients to use two tennis balls taped together to form a fulcrum that can lie over a segment of the thoracic spine and localize mo-

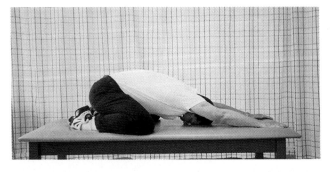

Fig. 9-15. Lumbar flexion stretch. Occasionally when the patient has been working the spinal extensor muscles hard, these muscles may get sore and tight. From an all-fours position, the patient can gradually spread the knees and sit back on the heels, allowing the spine to relax and stretch.

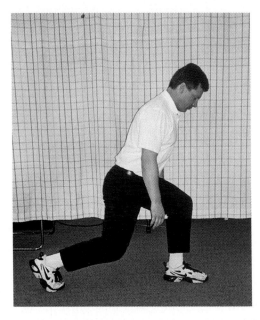

Fig. 9-16. Up and down from the floor. This photo shows the midpoint of getting up or down from the floor.

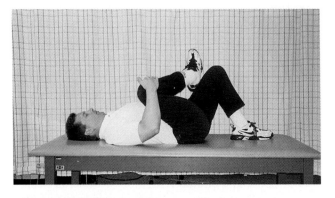

Fig. 9-17. Hip rotator stretch. While lying on the back, the patient crosses the ankle of one leg over the knee of the other leg. The stretch is performed by pulling the knee and ankle toward the chest. The patient should feel a stretch deep in the back of the hip.

tion to the segment above, thus maintaining good segmental mobility of the thoracic spine at home. This can be done in a standing or later (when appropriate) in a semi-reclined position, but the patient should keep the tennis balls a safe distance away from the fusion site.

Stretching throughout phase II should be very gentle and only pushed to the point the patient can brace to prevent lumbar motion. Because these muscles attach directly to the lumbar spine or pelvis, the patient should review the principles of stretching. To stretch a muscle, one end must be fixed by something while the other end is pulled away from the fixed end. If patients are not stabilizing the spine while stretching the hips, they will invariably pull on the lumbar spine, jeopardizing the fusion. All stretching should involve stabilizing one area while pulling against it with another. Iliopsoas stretching is initiated in a later phase. The aggressiveness of any hip stretching is dictated by the patient's ability to control the spine while stretching. Also, any stretches that pull on the lumbar spine or healing soft tissues should be avoided until adequate healing has occurred.

Examples of exercises initiated in the later stages of phase II include the following:

- Bridging (Fig. 8-17)
- Dying bug (Fig. 8-15)
- Squats (Fig. 8-21)
- Quadruped with arm and leg raise (Fig. 8-18)
- Heel lifts
- Superman (avoiding lumbar extension)
- Lateral pulls (light resistance)
- Seated upright rowing machine
- Scapular depression (avoid resisting more than 40% of body weight)
- Push-ups
- Stair climber
- UBE
- Brisk walking

A callus is forming at this stage, and patients are expected to tolerate slowly increasing their activity level and returning to normal activities. What the therapist is attempting to develop at this stage is not so much muscle power as kinesthetic sense for the muscles and their role in protecting the spine. Therefore the proper form of each exercise should be emphasized. Muscles learn to do what they are taught. The physical therapist should ensure that the patient is bracing *inward* with the abdominals. If the patient has trouble moving the abdominals without moving the spine, he or she should get on all fours, find a neutral position for the spine, keep it there, and practice dropping and lifting the stomach without moving the spine. The lifted contractions felt in this position form the brace that is needed to stabilize the spine. The patient can then return to a supine position and practice. When the patient can do this properly, he or she should be able to palpate a contraction of the obliques and lower abdominals as well as the upper rectus.

Patients generally find they have much less endurance with this brace and need to concentrate to maintain it. This brace is used to prevent spinal motion throughout all activities, so patients must learn to grade the contraction. Often they will attempt to give an "all-or-nothing" brace, but they should attempt to brace only as strongly as needed to prevent the spine from moving. Some activities are easy and some are difficult. For example, the amount of strength required to hold up a feather differs significantly from that used to hold a 5-pound weight, and the body automatically adjusts the degree of contraction of the hand muscles to fit the load.

A. Local inflammation occurs after lumbar spine surgery. The body forms scar tissue in response to inflammation. The nerve root may become restricted from the scar tissue as it exits through an opening called the *intervertebral foramen*. Because of the inflammatory process the nerve also can lose elasticity within itself. Therefore by performing movements that move the nerve within its covering (sheath), the nerve root will not develop adhesions or may free itself from adhesions, which can cause pain, numbness, tingling, and other symptoms.

Q. Lindsey is 38 years old. She had a lumbar fusion at L4-L5 7 weeks ago. She tells her physical therapist that her back pain has been increasing over the past 7 to 10 days. Lindsey has complied with all instructions and restrictions. The physical therapist reviews her chart and exercise program. Over the past 2 weeks Lindsey has begun doing squats and using the treadmill and the upper body ergometer (UBE) for cardiovascular exercise. She has been stretching her hamstrings, hip flexors, quadriceps, and calf muscles. She also has been doing trunk stabilization exercises in the prone, supine, and quadruped positions. Lindsey also has been strengthening her upper body with biceps curls, seated military presses, and push-ups. Which of these exercises may be aggravating her condition and why?

Phase III

TIME: Weeks 11-19
GOALS: Return to work, advance of exercise program, specific skills program, weight program (Table 9-4)

During phase III, patients whose jobs are sedentary or light often begin to return to work, although often on a modified schedule or to modified duties. They begin to establish a routine home maintenance program.

Body mechanics are becoming a habit. The exercise program is advancing and approaching its final version. Pain is minimal. Add partial and diagonal sit-ups. Patients should do these without any lumbar rotation or flexion. The early development of these muscles in their role as spinal stabilizers rather than spinal movers is a crucial component of this phase. After 12 weeks, dips can be added as appropriate. Trunk stabilization exercises begun in phase II are progressed to include more repetitions or to increase in difficulty. Isotonic exercises using weights also may be increased with repetitions or resistance.

At this phase the physical therapist is helping to recondition the patient to the expected level of function, while protecting the spine. The body adapts to the stresses placed on it. The therapist applies stress carefully to the body, in doses that the spine can tolerate, to increase the body's ability to withstand stress. While putting the patient through a conditioning program, he or she should monitor closely for the ability to make a brace that prevents rather than creates motion and modify the program according to the patient's sensitivities. Load-sensitive patients need to avoid overhead lifting for a longer time and should be taught ways to unload the spine while exercising; they may do better in a pool. Patients with a poor tolerance for any one position do better on a circuit-training program. Exercises should simulate as closely as possible the tasks the patient expects to do.

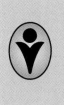

A. Hip flexor stretches should not be initiated until later, when sufficient healing has occurred at the surgical repair area. The iliopsoas originates at the T12-L5 vertebra and intervertebral discs. Also, exercises such as the military press that load the lumbar spine should be avoided. Finally, all exercises should be executed correctly.

Phase IV

TIME: 20 weeks-1 year
GOALS: Restore pre-injury status, continue home program of conditioning and stabilization (Table 9-5)

During phase IV the body finishes remodeling and adapting to the changes induced during and after surgery. Patients should be fully restored to their pre-injury level of function and be independent in caring for the spine. The same programs they have been following in therapy now become home programs of cardiovascular conditioning, stabilization exercises, and hip and thoracic spine stretching. They have a good grasp of body mechanics for everything they need to

Table 9-4 Lumbar Fusion and Laminectomy

Rehabilitation Phase	Criteria to Progress to this Phase	Anticipated Impairments and Functional Limitations	Intervention	Goal	Rationale
Phase III Postoperative 11–19 weeks	No increase in pain Improved tolerance to upright postures	• Mild pain • Limited tolerance to upright positions (sit/stand) • Limited trunk, lower extremity, and upper extremity strength	Continue intervention from phase II as indicated • Partial sit-ups (no diagonal movement) • Isometrics with active range of motion—Abdominal bracing with the following: Bridging "Dying bug" Quadruped with arm and leg raise Heel lifts Supermans (avoiding lumbar spine extension) Scapular depressions Push-ups • Progressive resistance exercises— Lateral pull-downs Seated upright/Rows Triceps dips • Cardiovascular conditioning Stair stepper UBE Brisk walking	• Independent with most ADLs • Increased trunk and extremity strength • Maintenance of neutral spine while performing strengthening exercises • Performance of 20 minutes of cardiovascular exercise daily	• Promote return to independent lifestyle • Develop kinesthetic sense for the muscles and their role in protecting the spine • Improve the ability to brace the spine and maintain a neutral position • Increase strength of trunk and extremities to avoid excess stress on the spine • Start weight training to begin hypertrophy of associate musculature • Promote good cardiovascular fitness

Table 9-5   Lumbar Fusion and Laminectomy

Rehabilitation Phase	Criteria to Progress to this Phase	Anticipated Impairments and Functional Limitations	Intervention	Goal	Rationale
Phase IV Postoperative 20 weeks–1 year	No increase in pain No loss in functional status Patient has decreased reliance on formal therapy Clearance from physician for progression to phase IV	• Limited trunk and extremity strength • Limited tolerance to sustained postures • Mild pain associated with activities • Limited with lifting and carrying	• Continue exercises from previous phases as indicated • Advance exercises with regard to repetitions and weight • For appropriate patients, initiate running, cutting, and jumping progression. This would not be indicated in a majority of lumbar fusion patients. • Specific activity drills related to home, work, or sport environment • Functional capacity evaluation • Continue progression of interventions in phases II through IV • Progress home exercises • Continue patient education with regard to activity modification and performance with assistive device	• Return to work • Increase trunk and extremity strength • Increase muscular endurance • Prepare to return to more strenuous activities • Return to previous level of activity as appropriate • Discharge patient to self-management of flare-ups • Improve trunk strength to previous levels of functioning	• Patients with sedentary jobs should be able to resume their schedule • Continue reconditioning to an expected level of function while protecting the spine • Carefully apply stress to the body in tolerable doses to increase the spine's ability to withstand stress • Evaluate the ability to return to previous function • Because patients with lumbar spine fusion may continue to have problems with joints above and below the fusion site, continuation of some level of maintenance must be emphasized • Fusion patients must also maintain constant body awareness, always using proper body mechanics

do. The exercise program has been well outlined in earlier phases. Patients should be able to problem solve unusual situations to determine correct mechanics and manage mild flare-ups independently, knowing which symptoms require professional help.

The bone continues to remodel and adapt to the fusion for as long as 1 year. Patients with fusions frequently develop problems at the level above or below the fusion. For both of these reasons the patient should learn that spinal care is now a lifetime habit and must be maintained with regular exercise and good mechanics during all daily activities (not just those the patient perceives as stressful). Some patients who enjoy exercise prefer extensive exercise programs, but many patients like to keep a minimal program for maintenance. The best home program is one the patient actually does. A realistic home program provides the best chance of consistent follow-through.

Patients returning to a more strenuous job or sports are developing the extra degree of strength and skill to do so. They begin agility drills specific to their sport or job, such as running, cutting, and jumping (Figs. 8-23 to 8-26). A more comprehensive weight program is established, again geared to the specific activity faced by the patient. The program may require a greater focus on power, endurance, or skill, depending on the activity. Patients should work on maintaining control of a neutral spine during job- or sport-specific challenges during this phase, and *the physical therapist should obtain the clearance of the surgeon to begin working on these higher-level activities*. The patient

must demonstrate good trunk strength and control and good lower extremity strength and flexibility before initiating agility drills.

A certain number of patients can be expected to stop progressing at any stage of rehabilitation. The physical therapist should notify the physician if a patient stops making measurable progress at any stage and if possible provide a reason for the lack of progress. Is the patient pain-inhibited? Is he or she not making a consistent effort? If the physician determines that no further medical treatment is indicated, possible recommendations include a functional capacity evaluation, work conditioning or work hardening, or a pain management program. Although all therapists would like to relieve pain, some suffering is beyond the ability of current medical science to remove. This is a difficult concept and patients can be unwilling to accept it. Therapists should make every effort to help patients accept this reality and learn to care for themselves without seeking constant medical intervention. Most people can manage chronic pain and maintain a high functional level despite the pain.

Suggested Home Maintenance for the Postsurgical Patient

An exercise program has been outlined at the various phases. The home maintenance box on pages 168 to 169 outlines the rehabilitation the patient may follow. The physical therapist can use it in customizing a patient-specific program.

❦ Suggested Home Maintenance for the Postsurgical Patient

Days 1-5

GOALS FOR THE PERIOD: Educate patient about simple movements, teach nerve mobilization and home care principles
1. Gentle nerve gliding
2. Walking daily as tolerated (should slowly increase in time and speed)
3. Consistent use of proper body mechanics
4. Icing as needed
5. Protection of incision

Weeks 6-10

GOALS FOR THE PERIOD: Educate patient about simple movements, teach nerve mobilization and home care principles
1. Progress walking tolerance to 20 to 30 minutes
2. Begin low-level, isometric stabilization
   a. Abdominal bracing
   b. Gluteal squeezes
   c. Heel lifts

Weeks 6-10—cont'd

    d. Ankle pumps to heel lifts
    e. Wall slides (to approximately 135 degrees of knee flexion)
3. Reinforce body mechanics
4. Continue nerve gliding
5. Begin stretching the hips and legs, bracing the spine in neutral
    a. Hamstrings
    b. Quadriceps
    c. Gluteals
    d. Calves (gastrocnemius and soleus)
    e. Adductors
    f. Piriformis
    g. Hip flexors (initiate after 8 weeks, with physician approval)

Weeks 11-19

GOALS FOR THE PERIOD: Increase activity, emphasize tissue modeling, stabilization, reconditioning, weight programs, and return to work
1. Progress walking tolerance to 30 to 60 minutes daily
2. Increase aggressiveness of stabilization program slowly and to the patient's tolerance
    a. Partial and diagonal sit-ups (*no* lumbar motion)
    b. Bridging
    c. Dying bug
    d. Squats (to 90 degrees of knee flexion)
    e. Quadruped
    f. Heel lifts
    g. Superman (*no* lumbar extension)
    h. Push-ups
3. Continue to maintain nerve root mobility
4. After 11 weeks the patient can use the seated upright rowing machine
5. After 12 weeks the patient may add the following exercises:
    a. Latissimus pulls
    b. Scapular depressions
    c. Dips
6. Continue cardiovascular training using the following:
    a. Stair climber
    b. Brisk walking

Week 20 and Beyond

GOALS FOR THE PERIOD: Restore pre-injury status, continue home program of conditioning and stabilization
1. Progress stabilization program to the level required by the patient's activity level
2. Continue to work on hip and leg flexibility
3. Develop a gym program for independent maintenance of strength, using the following:
    a. Cardiovascular exercise
    b. Stabilization exercises
    c. Latissimus pulls
    d. Seated rowing
    e. Scapular depression
    f. Inclined leg press
    g. Stretches for hips and legs
4. Begin sport- or work-specific activity

REFERENCES

1. Albee FH: A report of bone transplantation and osteoplasty in the treatment of Pott's disease of the spine, *NY Med J* 95:469, 1912.
2. Biemborn D, Morrissey M: A review of the literature related to trunk muscle performance, *Spine* 13(6):655, 1988.
3. Bourcher HH: A method of spinal fusion, *J Bone Joint Surg* 41B:248, 1959.
4. Butler SD: *Mobilization of the nervous system,* ed 4, Melbourne, 1994, Churchill Livingstone.
5. Cyriax J: *Textbook of orthopedic medicine: diagnosis of soft tissue lesions,* vol 1, ed 6, Baltimore, 1975, Williams and Wilkins.
6. Gibson A: A modified technique for spinal fusion, *Surg Gynecol Obstet* 53:365, 1931.
7. Grabiner M, Koh T, Ghazawi AF: Decoupling of bilateral paraspinal excitation in subjects with low back pain, *Spine* 17(10):1219, 1992.
8. Hasue M: Pain and the nerve root, *Spine* 18(14):2053, 1993.
9. Hibbs RA: An operation for Pott's disease of the spine, *JAMA* 59:133, 1912.
10. Hides JA, Jull GA: *Multifidus inhibition in acute low back pain: recovery is not spontaneous,* MPAA Conference Proceedings, Department of Physical Therapy, Brisbane, Queensland, 1995, University of Queensland.
11. Kawaguchi Y, Matsui H, Tsuji H: Back muscle injury after posterior lumbar spine surgery, *Spine* 19:2598, 1994.
12. Kirkaldy-Willis WH, Burton CV: *Managing low back pain,* ed 3, New York, 1992, Churchill Livingstone.
13. Knapp DR, Jones ET: Use of cortical cancellous allograft for posterior fusion, *Clin Orthop* 229:99, 1988.
14. Lonstein JE: Use of bank bone for spinal fusions, *Proc Scoliosis Res Soc* 1984.
15. Lorenz M et al: A comparison of single level fusions with and without hardware, *Spine* 16(8)[suppl]:455, 1991.
16. McKenzie RA: *The lumbar spine, mechanical diagnosis and therapy,* Upper Hutt, New Zealand, 1990, Wright and Carman Limited.
17. O'Sullivan P, Twomey L, Allison G: Dysfunction of the neuromuscular system in the presence of low back pain-implications for physical therapy management, *J Man Manip Ther* 5(1):20, 1997.
18. Panjabi M: The stabilizing system of the spine. Part II, neutral zone and instability hypothesis, *J Spinal Dis* 5:390, 1992.
19. Rantanen J et al: The stabilizing system of the spine. Part II. Neutral zone and instability hypothesis, *J Spinal Disord* 5(4):390, 1992.
20. Richardson CA, Jull GA: Concepts of assessment and rehabilitation for active lumbar stability. In Boyling, Palastanga N, editors: *Grieves modern manual therapy,* ed 2, Edinburgh, Churchill Livingstone.
21. Shacklock M: Neurodynamics, *Physiother* 81(1):9, 1995.
22. Sihvonen T et al: Local denervation atrophy of paraspinal muscles in postoperative failed back syndrome, *Spine* 18:575, 1993.
23. Smith SA et al: Straight leg raising: anatomical effects on the spinal nerve root with and without fusion, *Spine* 18(8):992, 1993.
24. Steffee A et al: Segmental spine plates with pedicle screw fixation: a new internal fixation device for disorders of the lumbar and thoracolumbar spine, *Clin Orthop* 203:203, 1986.
25. Trammell TR et al: Luque interpeduncular segmental fixation of the lumbosacral spine, *Orthop Rev* 20:57, 1991.
26. Waddell G: A new clinical model for the treatment of low back pain, *Spine* 12(7):633, 1987.
27. Watkins MB: Posterolateral bone-grafting for fusion of the lumbar and lumbosacral spine, *J Bone Joint Surg* 41A:388, 1959.
28. West JL, Bradford DS, Ogilvie JW: Results of spinal arthrodesis with pedicle screw-plate fixation, *J Bone Joint Surg* 73A:1179, 1991.
29. White AH, Schofferman JA: *Spine care: diagnosis and conservative treatment,* vol 1, St Louis, 1995, Mosby.
30. White A: *Spine* 18:575, 1994.
31. Wiltse LL et al: The paraspinalis splitting approach to the lumbar spine, *J Bone Joint Surg* 50A:919, 1968.
32. Weatherly CR, Prickett CF, O'Brien JP: Discogenic pain persisting despite solid posterior fusion, *J Bone Joint Surg Br* 68(1):142, 1986.
33. Crock HV: Anterior lumbar interbody fusion: indications for its use and notes on surgical technique, *Clin Orthop* 165:157, 1982.

PART THREE

Lower Extremity

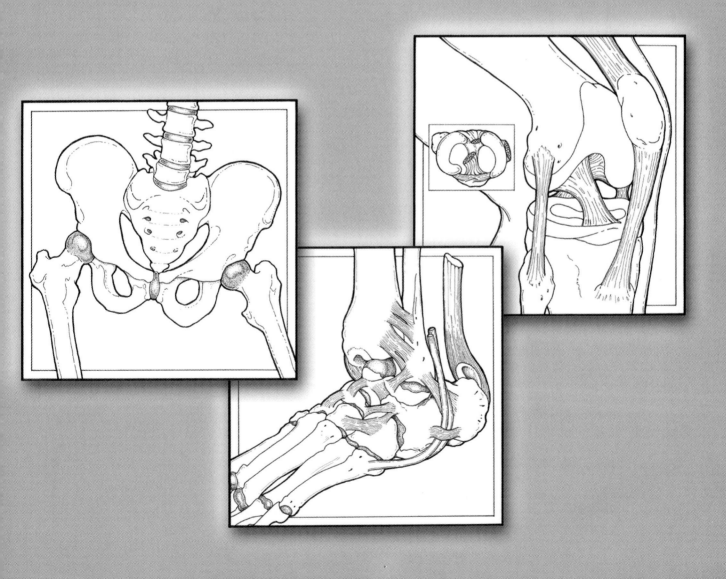

Chapter 10

Total Hip Replacement

Edward Pratt
Patricia A. Gray

Each year in the United States approximately 80,000 to 130,000 patients undergo total hip replacement[10] (THR) procedure hoping to eradicate persistent pain, increase their range of motion (ROM), and improve their functional status. The majority of these people have tried and failed to find relief from their symptoms with conservative medical intervention.

Surgical Indications and Considerations

THR is used to correct intractable damage resulting from osteoarthritis, rheumatoid arthritis, avascular necrosis, and the abnormal muscle tone caused by cerebral palsy.[8] Nonelective THR procedures are performed for fractures in which open reduction internal fixation (ORIF) is deemed inappropriate.

Contraindications for THR surgery include inadequate bone mass, inadequate periarticular support, serious medical risk factors, signs of infection, and lack of patient motivation to observe precautions and follow through with rehabilitation. Surgery also is contraindicated if it is unlikely to increase the patient's functional level.[8]

The prostheses used currently have a projected life span of less than 20 years. Therefore candidates for THR are usually older than 60 years. Younger patients may elect this surgery when their functional status is severely compromised and pain becomes intolerable. In the case of a fracture, younger patients are treated with an ORIF whenever practical. Given the projected lifespan of current prostheses, younger THR candidates may require a revision surgery later in life.

THR predictably improves function and reduces pain in virtually all patients with disabling disease. Patient satisfaction (with a rating of *very good* or *excellent*) regarding pain relief and improvement of function has been measured as high as 98% at 2 years after THR. The long-term survivability rate has been reported as high as 87.3% to 96.5% at 15 years.[9,29,30]

Surgical Procedures

In its essence THR consists of two parts. First, the remaining arthritic bone and articular cartilage is reamed from the acetabular cup and a new metal cup with a polyethylene plastic inner liner is press fit into place. Second, the arthritic femoral head is removed and replaced by a femoral head/stem component that is secured into the medullary canal of the proximal femur (Figs. 10-1 through 10-3).

Several aspects of the procedure greatly affect the course of postoperative rehabilitation. First, two approaches are commonly used, each with its own risks and advantages. Second, controversy still exists as to whether it is better to cement or press fit the femoral stem into position.[3,15] Noncemented implants tend to be more expensive and technically demanding to implant; however, they are easier to revise when they fail. As yet it is not clear which technique produces the most durable hip replacement. However, it is generally accepted that noncemented implants are best suited for younger, more active patients and more complicated revisions.[18] Recently, resurfacing arthroplasty has been recommended for young patients with avascular necrosis because it preserves bone for later conversion to THR if necessary because of implant failure or pain. Many surgeons believe that noncemented femoral components should not have weight borne on them for 6 weeks, whereas cemented femoral components can support weight immediately after surgery. This has been contested recently, and many surgeons now allow patients with noncemented hips to bear weight from the outset.[28] Both approaches have in common the creation of instability around the hip during the early postoperative period. The release of muscle, bone, and joint capsule during accessing of the joint renders the hip vulnerable to dislocation at its extreme ranges of motion. Patient education of "hip precautions" becomes extremely important during early convalescence and is alluded to later in this chapter. Controversy remains as to which approach provides the lowest postoperative dislocation rate, the shortest operative time, and the least blood loss.[19] Because of problems with trochanteric nonunion and long-term abductor weakness, the original transtrochanteric approach (in which the greater trochanter or the gluteus medius is completely released) is used most often today in revision surgery. Its main advantage lies in an excellent view of the proximal femoral shaft. The two exposures discussed in the following paragraphs are the

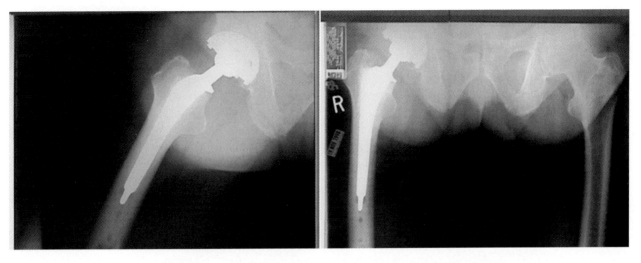

Fig. 10-1. Hybrid cemented total hip arthroplasty (Biomet Integral Design, Warsaw, IN).

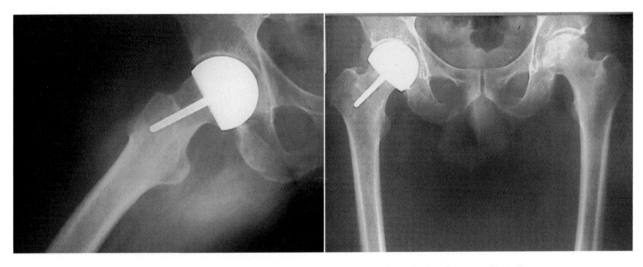

Fig. 10-2. Resurfacing arthroplasty for avascular necrosis (Wright Medical Design, Memphis, TN).

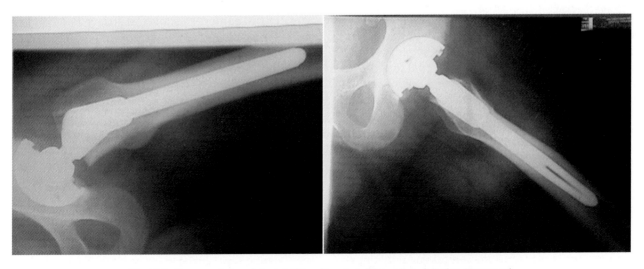

Fig. 10-3. Noncemented modular total hip arthroplasty (Biomet Impact Design, Warsaw, IN).

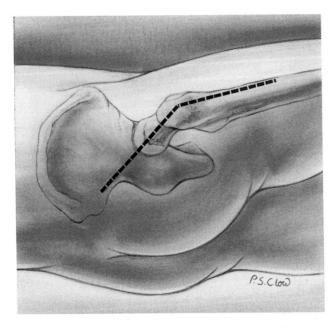

Fig. 10-4. The incision for a posterior approach is centered over the greater trochanter, the distal limb being straight and the proximal limb curved posteriorly. (From Cameron HU: *The technique of total hip arthroplasty,* St Louis, 1992, Mosby.)

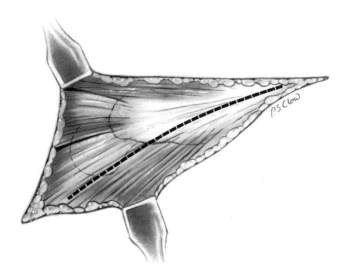

Fig. 10-5. The fascia lata is split in line with the skin incision, and the gluteus maximus is split proximally. (From Cameron HU: *The technique of total hip arthroplasty,* St Louis, 1992, Mosby.)

posterolateral approach (Gibson) and the anterolateral approach (Watson-Jones).

Posterolateral Approach

The posterolateral approach accesses the hip in the interval between the gluteus maximus and medius. The capsule and short external rotators are released and the hip is dislocated posteriorly. In extremely large or contracted patients the surgeon must occasionally release the gluteus maximus and even the adductor magnus at their femoral insertions to translate the proximal femur anteriorly, gaining acetabular exposure. This exposure places traction on the gluteus maximus, medius, and tensor fascia lata. Care must be taken not to place traction on the sciatic nerve or the superior gluteal nerve and artery, which may cause nerve palsy. Repair of the posterior capsule and short external rotators remains controversial, although several recent reports suggest decreased rates of posterior dislocation and heterotopic bone formation when this is done. The posterolateral approach is the author's personal preference for THR because it preserves the gluteus medius and minimus, as well as the vastus lateralis, making rehabilitation of these muscle groups easier. It also provides for a quicker normalization of gait in the postoperative period, although this is personal surgeon preference and may be disputed by surgeons who prefer the anterolateral approach.

The patient is placed in the lateral decubitus position with the affected hip up. The entire limb is washed, prepared, and surgically draped. The incision is begun 4 to 5 inches superior and medial to the top of the greater trochanter (Fig. 10-4). The line of incision runs down to the greater trochanter, then 3 or 4 inches along the course of the posterior femur. The skin and subcutaneous tissues are incised and the deep fascia is exposed and divided in line with the skin incision (Fig. 10-5). After mobilizing the fascia, the surgeon inserts a large, self-retaining retractor to hold the fascia apart. The sciatic nerve is then either exposed or palpated to ensure that it is not being stretched or traumatized (Fig. 10-6). The posterior border of the gluteus medius is identified, as well as the interval between the gluteus minimus and piriformis as they pass into the posterior greater trochanter. This interval is developed and a retractor placed around the medius and minimus as they are pulled anteriorly. The remainder of the posterior structures are released from the posterior femoral neck and intertrochanteric line, including the piriformis, obturator internus, superior and inferior gemelli, and the superior half of the quadratus femoris (Fig. 10-7). The surgeon releases the posterior hip capsule with the short external rotators, allowing them to retract together (Fig. 10-8). This decreased dissection around the crucial nervous plane under the inferior border of the piriformis leaves a stronger posterior cuff of tissue to repair at the end of the procedure. The limb is next measured for its length between the ilium and greater trochanter, and the hip is posteriorly dislocated. A reciprocating saw is used to cut through the femoral neck, and the arthritic femoral head is delivered from the

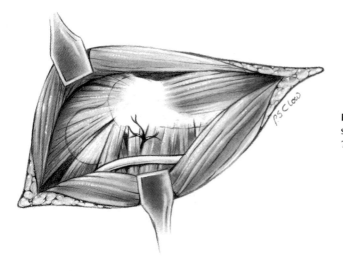

Fig. 10-6. The short external rotators are exposed by blunt dissection. The sciatic nerve lies superficial to the external rotators. (From Cameron HU: *The technique of total hip arthroplasty*, St Louis, 1992, Mosby.)

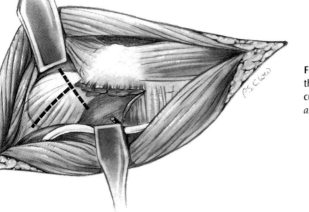

Fig. 10-7. The short external rotators are divided. When the upper part of the quadratus is released, brisk bleeding usually ensues from the medial circumflex femoral artery. (From Cameron HU: *The technique of total hip arthroplasty*, St Louis, 1992, Mosby.)

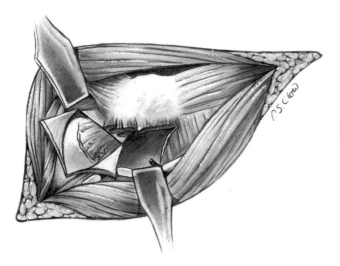

Fig. 10-8. Retraction now exposes the hip joint capsule. (From Cameron HU: *The technique of total hip arthroplasty*, St Louis, 1992, Mosby.)

field. The hip annulus is débrided sharply, and a minimal anterior capsulotomy is performed to help mobilize the proximal femur. As mentioned previously, the surgeon must sometimes go back and release the gluteus maximus, adductor longus, and occasionally even the adductor magnus from the proximal femur so that it can be translated anteriorly. A cobra retractor is placed under the femur and over the front edge of the acetabulum, allowing the femur to be levered anteriorly out of the way of the acetabulum. The acetabulum is then reamed and the acetabular component inserted.

Femoral preparation is begun by placing a large retractor under the femur and levering it out of the wound. The surgeon then reams the femoral shaft, increasing the reamer size each pass by 2 mm until good bony contact is made. The intertrochanteric area is then broached or rasped in the same manner until good proximal fill of the femur is obtained. A provisional head is applied and the joint is placed back together and ranged to check for stability and length. At this stage a stable hip should allow 80 to 90 degrees of flexion, 60 to 80 degrees of internal rotation, and 20 to 30 degrees of external rotation while being held in neutral abduction. After this the surgeon press fits or cements the implant in place and begins closure. Many surgeons prefer repair of the capsule and short external rotators as a single cuff of tissue held by large #2 nonabsorbable sutures through drill holes in the bone. The gluteus maximus and hip adductors are repaired if they were released, and the deep fascia is repaired again with nonabsorbable suture. After closure of subcutaneous tissue and skin the patient is placed in a triangular-shaped pillow that holds the hip in approximately 30 degrees of abduction. The pillow straps should not be tightened to the point that they compress the common peroneal nerve.

Rehabilitation begins as soon as the patient is coherent. Ankle pumps, quadriceps sets, and leg lifts help reestablish the distal venous circulation, minimizing the risk of thromboembolic disease and helping with postoperative edema. Standing, sitting, and walking can be started on the first day after surgery if hip precautions are followed carefully.

Anterolateral Approach

The anterolateral approach has been popularized by Smith-Peterson[24] as providing better visibility without the risk of posterior dislocation associated with the posterolateral approach. It avoids the need for postoperative abduction pillows and can allow the patient greater freedom of movement during the initial postoperative period because hip precautions become less crucial. Because of the reported decreased incidence of posterior dislocation, the anterolateral approach is sometimes preferred in patients who have suffered strokes or those who have cerebral palsy and therefore have a significant muscle imbalance or spasticity that induces flexion and internal rotation of the hip. This approach has been associated with a greater incidence of heterotopic bone formation, greater blood loss, and longer operative times. However, individual surgical expertise seems to have a greater influence on these variables than the exposure chosen.[21,27]

The anterolateral approach uses the interval between the gluteus medius and tensor fascia lata. Both of these muscles are innervated by the superior gluteal nerve near the ilium. Injury to this nerve can result in a partial or complete abductor paralysis that can vary from a temporary neurapraxia to complete and permanent paralysis. Also, the femoral nerve can be injured through overretraction of soft tissues in the front of the hip, leaving significant quadriceps weakness. This approach preserves the short external rotators of the hip and prevents direct exposure of the sciatic nerve. The tissues violated include the gluteus medius and minimus, the tensor fascia lata, the vastus lateralis, the referred head of the rectus femoris, the anterior hip capsule, and the iliopsoas tendon.

The patient is placed in the lateral decubitus position with the affected hip up (Fig. 10-9, *A*). A lateral incision is made with a slight anterior curvature in its proximal aspect. After dividing the subcutaneous tissue, the surgeon incises the lateral fascia and finds and develops the interval between the gluteus medius and the tensor fascia lata (Figs. 10-9, *B*, and 10-10). The surgeon must be careful not to extend the incision too far proximally or the investing nerve of both muscles (the superior gluteal nerve) can be injured, resulting in paralysis of the tensor. The vastus lateralis origin is often dissected off its vastus ridge origin to access the anterior hip capsule fully. The capsule is then bluntly released from the front of the femoral neck to gain access to the hip joint itself (Fig. 10-11). The last deep layer of exposure requires the release of the anterior aspect of the gluteus medius off the greater trochanter and the reflection of the rectus femoris off the anterior acetabulum (Fig. 10-12). The gluteus release can be done either through the tendon or through trochanteric osteotomy, although trochanteric osteotomy has fallen out of favor to some extent because of the incidence of nonunion. After the gluteus release the hip can be dislocated anteriorly and joint replacement begun much as in the posterolateral approach.

External rotation and flexion must be avoided postoperatively to prevent dislocation. Hip range of motion precautions remain important, especially during the first 6 weeks. Normalization of gait via abductor and quadriceps strengthening remains the focus during early rehabilitation. Pool exercise appears to be extremely helpful in this regard.

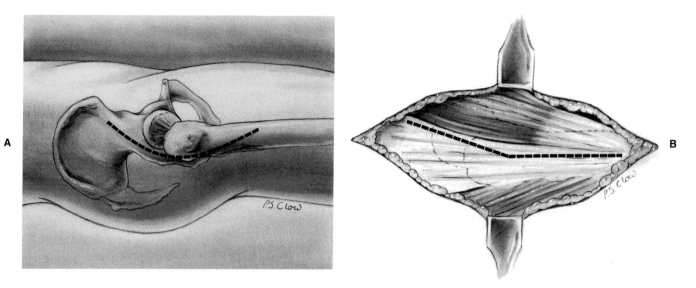

Fig. 10-9. A, The skin incision is roughly C-shaped and centered over the back of the greater trochanter. **B,** The fascia lata is divided over the summit of the greater trochanter. (From Cameron HU: *The technique of total hip arthroplasty,* St Louis, 1992, Mosby.)

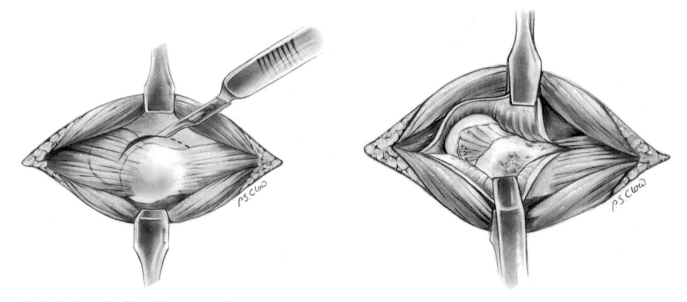

Fig. 10-10. The anterior fibers of the gluteus medius are released from the greater trochanter. The muscle incision is not extended proximally. (From Cameron HU: *The technique of total hip arthroplasty,* St Louis, 1992, Mosby.)

Fig. 10-11. An anterior capsulectomy is carried out with a blunt Homan retractor above and below the femoral neck and a medium Homan retractor placed on the pelvic brim. (From Cameron HU: *The technique of total hip arthroplasty,* St Louis, 1992, Mosby.)

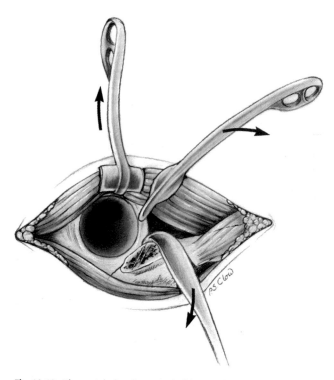

Fig. 10-12. The acetabulum is exposed with a medium Homan retractor on the pelvic brim, a long sharp Homan retractor inferiorly, and a bent Homan retractor posteriorly levering down on the stump of the femoral neck. (From Cameron HU: *The technique of total hip arthroplasty,* St Louis, 1992, Mosby.)

Generally, a walker or crutches is required for 3 weeks after THR. A cane is used for an additional 3 weeks before unassisted walking is allowed. This varies depending on the age and preoperative condition of the patient. Driving and a return to sedentary activities may be allowed at 3 weeks, and some of the hip precautions can be relaxed at 6 weeks. Improvement in strength and ROM can be expected for as long as 6 months with a motivated patient.

Therapy Guidelines for Rehabilitation

No hard and fast rules exist for the progression of rehabilitation after THR, but the following text can be used as a guideline. Flexibility on the part of the therapist is essential because medical centers and individual surgeons may impose their own protocols after THR.

The therapist's role is crucial at the postsurgical stage of recovery. Santavista's[22] study showed that the majority of patients recovering from THR report receiving most of their information regarding the recovery phase from physical therapists. Patients depend on their therapists for encouragement and advice. They should be prepared by their therapists to anticipate a unique recovery progression. Comparisons with other patients should be avoided. The early setting of patient expectations toward independence and wellness

plays a major role in shorter hospital stays and convalescence times.

Phase I: Preoperative Training Session

TIME: Days 1-2
GOALS: Educate patient regarding precautions with transfers and movements, help patient become independent in exercises for postoperative phases

Many institutions have initiated preoperative THR training sessions to increase patient confidence and reduce the length of the hospital stay. These sessions may take place in the physical therapy department or in the patient's home through a home care agency's physical therapist. Educational videos are becoming popular as an adjunct tool.

The preoperative session generally includes an assessment of the patient's strength (including upper extremity potential), ROM, neurologic status, vital signs, endurance, functional level, and safety awareness. Any existing edema, contractures, and leg length discrepancies should be noted at this time, as well as the patient's scar healing ability.[20] If the evaluation takes place in the patient's home, the status of stairways, equipment needs, and safety adaptations (such as moving furniture and electrical cords) should be evaluated.

Instruction in THR precautions should begin during the preoperative session and be repeated throughout the rehabilitation process. The posterolateral approach to THR requires precaution instructions that prohibit flexion of the hip past 90 degrees, adduction past the body's midline, and internal rotation of the hip. After an anterolateral THR the patient should observe these precautions and avoid external rotation (especially with flexion). A review of proper body mechanics for safe functional mobility at home along with appropriate postoperative sleeping and sitting positions should accompany the precautions training.

The therapist must teach transitional movements for safe transfer techniques. The proper use of assistive devices such as walkers and crutches according to the patient's projected weight-bearing status follows. A non–weight-bearing order may be given if the prosthesis is noncemented. Strict adherence to ROM and weight-bearing precautions should be emphasized throughout the entire rehabilitation process.

Postoperative exercises can be taught at this time. These exercises may include the following:
- Ankle pumps (Fig. 10-13)
- Quadriceps sets
- Gluteal sets
- Active hip and knee flexion (heel slides) while maintaining hip ROM within the physician's recommended guidelines for the surgical technique performed

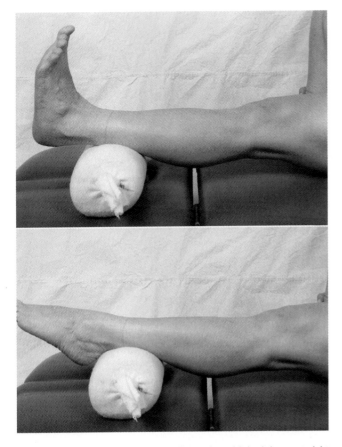

Fig. 10-13. Ankle pumps. The patient lies supine with both knees straight and pumps the feet up and down as far as possible.

- Isometric hip abduction
- Active hip abduction

The patient should not perform hip abduction if a trochanteric osteotomy was performed.

Dislocation of the THR prosthesis is possible if inappropriate stresses are placed on the new joint. Because the surgical cement is dry and attains its greatest strength within 10 to 20 minutes of its application, it is not a factor in dislocation. *The danger is largely a result of compromised integrity of the hip's joint capsule caused by surgical disruption. This information may assist in motivating the patient to adhere to precautions and the strengthening program.*

Traditional THR exercise programs have become controversial in recent years. The contact pressures on the hip joint during specific activities have been measured and compared with pressures on the hip during gait. Although some practitioners dispute the methodology used, the results of these studies have caused many to question the prescription of some of the standard THR exercises.

Enloe's consensus group eliminated the straight leg raise from their "ideal" THR rehabilitation plan because Strickland et al[26] found that it created greater stresses than the amount incurred at the hip during

normal unsupported gait.[4] Lewis states that "straight leg raises may be beneficial, but should be initiated once the patient has regained partial or full weight bearing."[13] Gilbert believes that straight leg raises are unnecessary and may cause dislocation; he warns therapists against using them.[5]

Strickland found that active hip flexion and isometric hip extension produced the greatest stresses on the joint. Based on these findings, Lewis and the consensus group recommend performing gluteal sets at submaximal levels of contraction to avoid the possibility of dislocation.

The Givens-Heiss et al study found that a maximal isometric hip abduction contraction generated greater peak pressures than both the straight leg raise and unsupported gait.[6] The Krebs study also found that maximal contraction during exercise generated greater pressures at the hip than did gait.[11] Lewis recommends that isometric hip abduction be done at submaximal levels based on the results of these studies and suggests slow, supine hip abduction as an alternative.[13]

Q. Sabrina had a noncemented total hip replacement 3 days ago. She is touchdown weight bearing (TDWB) with a walker but continues to place a moderate amount of weight on her affected lower extremity. Because she has difficulty maintaining TDWB during gait, what can be done to help her?

Phase IIa: Hospital Phase

TIME: Days 1-2
GOALS: Prevent complications, increase muscle contraction and control of involved leg, help patient sit for 30 minutes, continuously reinforce THR precautions

Day of surgery. Postoperative physical therapy (Table 10-1) may begin on the day of surgery when the patient regains consciousness. The patient will be resting in the supine position, wearing thromboembolic disease (TED) hose with the legs abducted and strapped to a triangular foam cushion. The therapist is expected to check the tightness of the cushion straps around the legs to avoid damage to peripheral nerves.

Pulmonary hygiene exercises typically begin immediately after awakening. The patient's lower extremity exercise program also may be initiated at this point with ankle pumps, quadriceps sets, and gluteal sets. Heel booties used to prevent bedsores can be removed for these exercises.

Patients may be groggy and unable to remember the THR precautions at this point and therefore a review is in order. Some benefit from a sign placed by the bed

Table 10-1 Total Hip Replacement

Rehabilitation Phase	Criteria to Progress to this Phase	Anticipated Impairments and Functional Limitations	Intervention	Goal	Rationale
Phase IIa Postoperative 1-2 days	Postoperative (Inpatient) No signs of infection Medically stable	• Pain • Immobilized postoperatively in bed with abduction pillow • Limited respiratory exchange	• Adjust abduction pillow ankle straps • Order foot cradle • Provide patient education regarding total hip precautions • Isometrics— Quadriceps sets Gluteal sets • Active range of motion (AROM)—Ankle pumps • Encourage use of cough and incentive spirometer On the second postoperative day, begin the following: • Bed mobility training • Transfer training • Gait training (weight bearing per physician's orders) as appropriate	• Avoid the following: Peripheral nerve damage Heel ulcers Dislocations of prosthesis Pooling of fluid in legs Fluid build-up in lungs • Improve volitional control of involved leg • Initiate mobility training • Sit up in chair 30 minutes • Maintain precautions while performing mobility activities	• Decrease strap pressure on legs • Decrease prolonged, unchecked pressure against heels • Prevent excessive stresses on hip • Promote distal venous circulation • Initiate muscle contractions • Prevent respiratory complications • Reinforce precautions to avoid complications • Prepare patient to perform transfers independently • Use assistive device during ambulation for safety and protection of hip

that lists the ROM precautions or from a knee immobilizer placed on the affected leg to reduce the possibility of making dangerous movements.

Repositioning of the patient every 2 hours with the abductor pillow in place is essential at this stage. Foot cradles are often attached to the foot of the bed to avoid internal rotation of the operated hip and prevent the heel sores that may develop as a result of pressure from the blankets. The majority of medical centers assign these functions to the nursing staff and begin physical therapy intervention on the first day after surgery. Changes in vascularity to the limb as well as neurologic status should be monitored closely by all personnel rendering care to the patient.

Postoperative day one. Acute care physical therapy sessions vary in frequency from one to three times per day and from 5 to 7 days per week depending on the medical center's protocol.[4] The therapist proceeds after being informed as to the surgical approach used, special precautions, and the patient's weight-bearing status. Assessment and treatment are conducted at the patient's bedside. The patient is situated as described previously.

The THR precautions should be repeated at this time. The patient must observe these precautions until the scheduled follow-up visit with the orthopedist 6 weeks later. The surgeon decides then whether to relax or continue precautions for another 6 weeks. The physical therapist can initiate ankle pumps (see Fig. 10-13), quadriceps sets, and gluteal sets if the patient did not begin them on the day of surgery. Ankle circles are not indicated because the patient may inadvertently rotate the affected extremity while performing the exercise. As stated previously, submaximal contraction of the muscles is recommended. Bilateral upper extremity exercises also begin at this time. Lower extremity exercises should be repeated ten times every hour.[4] However, many patients may not meet this expectation.

The therapist begins transfer training by assisting the patient in moving safely from a supine to a sitting position and then from sitting to a standing position while observing precautions. Frequently patients are in a great deal of pain and very anxious and therefore require encouragement. The physical therapist should allot a considerable amount of time for this task and emphasize the use of the upper extremities in shifting weight. The patient must avoid pivoting on the affected leg.

Surgeons usually allow patients to transfer to an appropriate bedside chair and sit up as tolerated, which is rarely more than 30 to 60 minutes. The therapist then supervises their return to bed. If a patient is not complaining of excessive pain, fatigue, or dizziness, gait training may begin on the first postoperative day. More frequently gait training begins on day two.

Postoperative day two. Treatment on the second postoperative day includes a review of the previous day's activities. The patient should be able to maintain hip ROM within the physician's recommended guidelines for the surgical technique performed.

The physical therapist expands the exercise program to include heel slides and isometric or active assistive hip abduction. Short arc quadriceps sets may require active assistance at this time. Again, submaximal force is recommended for isometric hip abduction. Active assistance from the therapist may be necessary for some exercises at first. The use of verbal cues such as "point the moving knee or big toe toward the ceiling" to avoid rotation of the leg also may be helpful.

Gait training usually begins during this session. The patient's assistive device is adjusted to its correct height before instruction and practice in its use is given. Most older patients are issued a front-wheeled walker. Younger patients may be issued crutches and instructed in the three-point crutch pattern. Patients who have undergone bilateral THR are instructed in the four-point crutch pattern.

The weight-bearing status after a noncemented THR depends on the surgeon's discretion. The patient may be ordered not to bear weight on the affected extremity for several weeks. Most patients with cemented prostheses are instructed to bear weight as tolerated.

Some complex surgeries may require more caution. Concepts such as toe touch weight bearing (TTWB) or partial weight bearing (PWB) are difficult for the patient to grasp at first. If the postoperative order calls for only TTWB, taping a "cracker" to the sole of the patient's affected forefoot may be helpful. Stepping onto a bathroom scale with the affected extremity helps the PWB patient (through visual cues) to determine the appropriate amount of pressure (usually 50% of body weight or less) to be put on that leg. Patients who still experience difficulty may benefit from practicing weight shifting on the parallel bars before using a walker.

Patients who have undergone THR frequently walk with the affected leg in abduction. They should be encouraged to normalize their gait pattern early in the recovery phase. Although no maximal distance has been dictated, some facilities encourage the patient to walk a specific minimum distance. The patient's short-term goal is to meet the discharge criteria, which typically demand walking on a level surface for 100 feet.

Phase IIb

TIME: Days 3-7
GOALS: Promote transfers and gait independence (using assistive devices as indicated), continuously reinforce THR precautions, discharge to home

Table 10-2   Total Hip Replacement

Rehabilitation Phase	Criteria to Progress to this Phase	Anticipated Impairments and Functional Limitations	Intervention	Goal	Rationale

Phase IIb Postoperative 3–7 days	• Good tolerance to phase IIa
	• No signs of infection
	• No significant increase in pain
	• Medically stable
	• Gradual improvement in tolerance to inpatient program
		• Limited bed mobility
		• Limited transfers
		• Limited gait
		• Limited understanding of postoperative precautions
			• Continue interventions from phase IIa with progression of activity as tolerated
			  • AROM—
			    Heel slides
			    Hip abduction (if able; otherwise do active assisted hip abduction)
			    Terminal knee extension
			    Upper extremity exercises
			  • Bed mobility training
			  • Transfer training; initiate car transfers when appropriate
			  • Gait training; initiate stair training when indicated ("up with good, down with bad")
			  • Evaluation of equipment needs at home
			  • Caregiver training
				• Maintain postoperative precautions
				• Improve involved lower extremity AROM within boundaries of precautions
				• Improve arm strength
				• Become independent with transfers
				• Become independent with gait using appropriate assistive device
				• Promote carry over of precautions at home
					• Prevent prosthesis dislocation
					• Restore volitional control of involved lower extremity
					• Prepare arms to assist during transfers and gait
					• Emphasize restoration of independence with self-care activities (bed mobility, transfers)
					• Promote independence with activities of daily living (ADLs)
					• Ambulate safely and decrease stress on the involved lower extremity
					• Ensure patient and caregiver safety (reinforce precautions) and prevent falls

Postoperative day three (until discharge). Patients are often moved from the acute care section to a rehabilitation center or skilled nursing facility on day three (Table 10-2). Some patients (usually those who are younger and more fit) may be discharged to home care at this time. Treatment at the rehabilitation center is conducted in the physical therapy gym.

Stair training generally begins on day three. A step-to gait pattern (involved leg not to pass ahead or in front of the uninvolved leg) with minimal weight bearing on the affected leg is taught for ambulation on even surfaces; on steps or stairs the patient leads upstairs with the unaffected leg and downstairs with the affected leg. Patients should become comfortable climbing the number of stairs demanded by the home situation. If the patient is not comfortable with the stairs, arrangements can be made for the patient to live on the ground floor.

Refinement of the skills learned on previous days continues daily at the rehabilitation center until the time of discharge. By the discharge date, family members or other caregivers must be trained to assist the patient safely whenever necessary.

Common discharge criteria for THR are as follows:
- The patient is able to demonstrate and state the THR precautions.
- The patient is able to demonstrate independence with transfers.
- The patient is able to demonstrate independence with the exercise program.
- The patient is able to demonstrate independence with gait on level surfaces to 100 feet.
- The patient is able to demonstrate independence on stairs.

Written instructions with illustrations pertaining to these criteria are included in a discharge packet for home use.

Patients are typically discharged between the fifth and tenth days after surgery. Zavadak et al[31] found that independence in functional activities required the following number of physical therapy sessions:

Supine to sit	8.1
Sit to stand	5.5
Ambulate to 100 feet	8.1
Independent on stairs	9.5

However, the therapist's expectations should not be unduly influenced by a statistical average. Munin et al[16] found that fewer than 40% of patients who undergo THR are independent in performing basic tasks at the time of discharge from the rehabilitation center. Approximately 80% of patients were at the supervision level of performance. Advanced age, solitary living conditions, and an increased number of comorbid conditions were the factors that predicted the duration of a patient's treatment stay.[17]

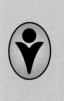

A. A "cracker" can be taped to the sole of the patient's forefoot. If the patient still has difficulty maintaining touch-down weight bearing, she should try using a thick-soled shoe only on the affected leg. If the patient is PWB, say 50%, a scale can be used to give feedback regarding how it feels to bear 50% of the weight on the lower extremity.

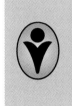

Q. Before having severe hip pain, Tracy was biking 20 to 30 miles a day, 4 days a week. She also competed in bicycle races and worked out in the gym with light weights three times a week. Should Tracy participate in a long-term exercise program after having a THR if it does not contradict the surgeon's orders? Why?

Phase III: Return to Home

TIME: Weeks 1-6
GOALS: Increase patient independence with gait and transfers (community appropriate), evaluate safety of home, plan return of patient to work or previous activities as indicated (Table 10-3)

Home care phase. Physical therapy home assessment usually occurs within 24 hours after hospital discharge. The elements to be assessed are those listed in the preoperative section, with the addition of the status of the surgical incision. The number of visits authorized by the patient's insurance company may limit the goals set by the therapist. Medicare coverage at this stage is restricted to patients who are homebound or severely limited in their ability to go out. The hope is that the patient will not be homebound at the time of home care discharge. Most patients are no longer homebound within 2 to 3 weeks.

Because managed care insurance has placed constraints on the number of nursing visits allowed, physical therapists are now being trained to remove staples, traditionally a nursing function. Staple removal normally occurs on the twelfth to fourteenth day after surgery.

Frequently patients still feel insecure after hospital discharge and appreciate safety advice regarding appropriate sitting and sleeping positions, what furniture must be moved or adjusted in height, and other safety issues such as slippery rugs or strung-out electrical cords. A review of the home exercise program and precautions is in order as well. Closed kinetic chain exercises (with involved leg firmly planted on the

Table 10-3 Total Hip Replacement

Rehabilitation Phase	Criteria to Progress to this Phase	Anticipated Impairments and Functional Limitations	Intervention	Goal	Rationale
Phase III Postoperative 1–6 weeks	• Discharged from hospital or other care center • No loss of ROM • No increase in pain • Need to restore further independence	• Limited tolerance to transfers • Limited tolerance to gait • Limited cardiovascular endurance and strength of involved lower extremity	• Continuation and progression of phase II interventions • Home evaluation for safety • Patient education review of precautions with performance of bed mobility transfers • Gait training on level surfaces, uneven surfaces, and stairs • Closed chain exercises (mini-squats, step-up, heel raises) • Pool therapy • Cross-country ski machine (with physician approval) • Treadmill • Straight-leg raises • Hip abduction	• Improve patient independence • Prevent falls • Prevent complications • Promote safety and independence with community ambulation • Improve lower extremity strength • Return to former employment or previous hobbies as indicated	• Promote restoration of independent function • Avoid potential for falls • Avoid prosthesis dislocation • Promote safety with ambulation on all types of surfaces • Improve tolerance of involved lower extremity to single-limb balance activities • Regain cardiovascular conditioning • Resume all ADLs and community activities

ground or on exercise equipment) such as heel raises and mini-squats can be incorporated into the home program. Cautious stretching may be warranted to stretch tight Achilles tendons in the standing position. Exercise equipment already in the patient's home may be added to the existing program if it can be used safely. Shoes often adapt in shape to the stresses imposed by an abnormal gait pattern and may encourage a return to the old pattern if worn after THR surgery. The patient's old misshaped shoes should be replaced if possible.

The patient progresses from the use of a front-wheeled walker or crutches to a single-point cane. This transition usually occurs 3 to 4 weeks after surgery. Occasionally a four-point cane is used as an interim device. Use of the cane is often discontinued after 3 to 4 more weeks. The patient should progress to walking safely with a normalized gait on level and sloped surfaces, jagged sidewalks, curbs, and stairs before discharge.

Enough strength may have been recovered to allow step-over-step stair climbing during the home phase. The patient should practice stepping up onto books or other household items that provide a stable, shallow rise at first. A modified lunge with the affected extremity placed on the step is another helpful pre-step exercise.

Patients are allowed to drive 3 to 4 weeks after surgery at the orthopedist's discretion. Permission may be given sooner depending on the patient's lifestyle requirements and rate of progress. The therapist may need to supervise the patient in getting on and off a bus or in and out of a car. A clean plastic trash bag placed over the seat of a car provides a surface that allows the patient to glide-pivot around more easily.

Outpatient clinic. Physical therapy intervention usually ends with the home care phase. A few patients with physically demanding lifestyles may require additional strength and endurance training. Some patients are referred to the clinic because of lingering gait problems. Others may be referred because they did not meet home care status requirements at the time of hospital discharge. The outpatient therapist should check with the surgeon for the status of precautions and activity level before designing an aggressive exercise program.

Exercises begun in the home or hospital can be expanded on in the clinic. Pool exercise is recommended after THR, as are stationary bicycling and simulated cross-country skiing with permission from the surgeon. As in home care the goals at this stage depend on the number of visits authorized by the patient's insurance company. Quick independence with a home exercise program should be encouraged.

After rehabilitation intervention. The surgeon determines the return-to-work date. Some patients may require job modification, and others may not be allowed to return to their previous jobs. Heavy manual labor is not permitted after THR surgery and vocational counseling may be indicated.[16] High-impact sports should be avoided after THR, especially running, water-skiing, football, basketball, handball, karate, soccer, and racquetball.[2] The sports most recommended are sailing, swimming, scuba, cycling, and golf. Tennis is not recommended, but doubles tennis is considered less stressful than singles.[14]

Sexual activity after an uncomplicated THR may resume in approximately 1 to 2 months with the surgeon's approval. Studies have shown that most patients feel uncomfortable asking for this type of information. Women tend to prefer the supine position or side-lying on the unoperated side. Men prefer the supine position. The patient is advised to take the more passive role for the first few weeks. The prone position may be resumed in 2 to 3 months after surgery.[25]

Patient compliance with home exercise programs is often questionable after the first few weeks and especially after discharge from therapy services. No agreement seems to exist among surgeons as to how long exercise programs should be continued. The surgeon may release the patient from the home exercise program at his or her discretion.

Sheh's study[23] states that flexion showed the slowest rate of recovery in diseased hips. Persistence of weakness was noted in all patients for at least 2 years after hip surgery despite the return of normal stride and phasic activity of muscles. Gluteus maximus or minimus weakness can result in aching near the hip during endurance activities. Sheh states that muscular weakness reduces the protection of the implant fixation surfaces during endurance activities. This may contribute to higher loosening rates reported in active patients.[23] Therefore therapists may want to encourage long-term continuation of exercise programs if this does not contradict the surgeon's orders.

A. Sheh[23] states that muscular weakness reduces the protection of the implant fixation surfaces during endurance activities. This may contribute to higher loosening rates reported in active patients. Therefore Tracy and other active patients should continue on a long-term exercise program to maintain good muscular strength around the hip.

Troubleshooting

The THR procedure has been refined to the point that patient progress is now fairly certain and predictable.

However, most complications call for a referral back to the surgeon. Examples include the following:

- Thigh pain with walking that clears quickly with sitting down, possibly indicating intermittent claudication
- A positive Trendelenburg sign that does not resolve with treatment, possibly caused by damage to gluteal innervation
- Severe rubor and swelling at the surgical site with accompanying fever, possibly indicating a wound infection
- Unexplained swelling of the limb that does not dissipate with elevation, possibly indicating thromboembolic disease
- General systemic effects, possibly indicating an allergy to the implant materials (rare), postoperative anemia, pulmonary embolus, or other medical complications
- Persistent, severe pain (even referred medial knee pain, unexplained limb shortening or extreme rotation, or pain with rotation of the limb), possibly resulting from dislocation of the prosthesis, heterotopic ossification, or a fracture of the adjacent bone or reflex sympathetic dystrophy

Other problems that arise may be the responsibility of the surgeon, but the therapist can take palliative measures to assist the patient. Many times the therapist is the first to see a developing complication, making identification and good communication with the surgeon extremely important. Leg length discrepancy is an example. The patient can continue gait training with a temporary shoe insert or with shoes of different heel heights. The surgeon may later prescribe a permanent orthotic. Persistent edema may be treated with medication. Patients should be advised to elevate their legs, rest more often, wear TED hose, pump their ankles, and apply ice to a swollen area. Pain flare-ups in nonaffected areas of the body are usually managed with medication. Possible side effects of the medication include nausea, constipation, and hypertension. The therapist can assist in pain reduction with modalities, exercises, and positioning. Significant abnormalities should always be reported to the surgeon.

Conclusion

A rapid, substantial improvement in quality of life follows THR surgery. Better physical function, sleep, emotional behavior, social interaction, and recreation are usually experienced in the first few months. At 2 years after surgery patients who had undergone THR reported greater satisfaction with their results than they had predicted in their best preoperative hypothetical scenario.[12]

❦ **Suggested Home Maintenance for the Postsurgical Patient**

Days 1-2 (in hospital)

GOALS FOR THE PERIOD: Protect healing tissues, prevent postoperative complications, improve volitional control of involved lower extremity
Isometric Exercises
1. Gluteal sets
2. Quadriceps sets
AROM Exercises
3. Ankle pumps

Days 3-7 (in hospital)

GOALS FOR THE PERIOD: improve lower and upper extremity strength
AROM Exercises
1. Heel slides
2. Hip abduction
3. Terminal knee extension
Resistive Exercises
4. Resisted shoulder internal and external rotation with Theraband
5. Shoulder depressions and triceps dips while seated

❧ **Suggested Home Maintenance for the Postsurgical Patient—cont'd**

Weeks 1-6 (after discharge to home setting or as appropriate in interim setting)

GOALS FOR THE PERIOD: Improve strength and balance of lower extremities, promote return to activities and hobbies as indicated

1. Closed-chain exercises (progression to gym equipment and inclined sled)
2. Pool therapy
3. Treadmill (as part of gym program)

REFERENCES

1. Cameron HU: *The technique of total hip arthroplasty*, St Louis, 1992, Mosby.
2. Chandler HP et al: Total hip replacement in patients under thirty years old, *J Bone Joint Surg* 63A:1426, 1981.
3. Engh CA, Glassman AH, Suthers KE: The case for porous-coated hip implants: the femoral side, *Clin Orthop* 261:63, 1990.
4. Enloe LJ et al: Total hip and knee replacement programs: a report using consensus, *J Orthop Sports Phys Ther* 23(1):3, 1996.
5. Gilbert R: Personal communication, June 10, 1998.
6. Givens-Heiss DL et al: In vivo acetabular contact pressures during rehabilitation. Part II: postacute phase, *Phys Ther* 72(10):700, 1992.
7. Hoppenfeld S, deBoer P, Thomas HA: *Exposures in orthopedics: the anatomic approach*, Philadelphia, 1984, JB Lippincott.
8. Hicks JE, Gerber LH: Rehabilitation of the patient with arthritis and connective tissue disease. In DeLisa JA, editor: *Rehabilitation medicine: principles and practices*, Philadelphia, 1988, JB Lippincott.
9. Kavanagh BF et al: Charnley total hip arthroplasty with cement: fifteen year results, *J Bone Joint Surg* 71A:1496, 1989.
10. Katz JM et al: Differences between men and women undergoing major orthopedic surgery for degenerative arthritis, *Arth Rheum* 37:687, 1994.
11. Krebs D et al: Exercise and gait effects on in vivo hip contact pressures, *Phys Ther* 71(4):301, 1991.
12. Laupacis A et al: The effect of elective total hip replacement on health-related quality of life, *J Bone Joint Surg* 75A(11):1619, 1993.
13. Lewis C, Knortz K: Total hip replacements, *Phys Ther Forum* May 20, 1994.
14. McGrorey BJ, Stewart MJ, Sim FH: Participation in sports after hip and knee arthroplasty: a review of the literature and survey of surgical preferences, *Mayo Clin Proc* 70B:202, 1995.
15. Mulroy RD, Jr, Harris WH: The effect of improved cementing techniques on component loosening in total hip replacement: an 11-year radiographic review, *J Bone Joint Surg* 72B:757, 1990.
16. Munin M et al: Rehabilitation. In Callaghan J, Rosenberg A, Rubash H, editors: *The adult hip*, Philadelphia, 1998, Lippincott-Raven.
17. Munin MC et al: Predicting discharge outcome after elective hip and knee arthroplasty, *Am J Phys Med Rehabil* 74:294, 1995.
18. American Academy of Orthopaedic Surgeons: *Orthopedic knowledge update 3*, Rosemont, IL, 1987, the Academy.
19. American Academy of Orthopaedic Surgeons: *Orthopedic knowledge update 4: home study syllabus*, Rosemont, IL, 1992, the Academy.
20. Petty W: *Total joint replacement*, Philadelphia, 1991, WB Saunders.
21. Roberts JM et al: A comparison of the posterolateral and anterolateral approaches to total hip arthroplasty, *Clin Orthop* 187:205, 1984.
22. Santavista N et al: Teaching of patients undergoing total hip replacement surgery, *Int J Nurs Stud* 31(2):135, 1994.
23. Sheh C et al: Muscle recovery and the hip joint after total hip replacement, *Clin Orthop* 302:115, 1994.
24. Smith-Peterson MN: A new supra acetabular subperiosteal approach to the hip, *Am J Orthop Surg* 15:592, 1917.
25. Stern FH et al: Sexual function after total hip arthroplasty, *Clin Orthop* 269:228, 1991.
26. Strickland EM et al: In vivo acetabular contact pressures during rehabilitation. Part I: acute phase, *Phys Ther* 72(10):691, 1992.
27. Vicar AJ, Coleman CR: A comparison of the anterolateral, transtrochanteric, and posterior surgical approaches in primary total hip arthroplasty, *Clin Orthop* 188:152, 1994.
28. Whitesides L: Personal communication, 1993, Total Hip Conference, St Louis.
29. Wickland I, Romanus B: A comparison of quality of life before and after arthroplasty in patients who had arthrosis of the hip joint, *J Bone Joint Surg* 73A:765, 1991.
30. Wroblewski BM: Fifteen twenty-one year results of Charnley low friction arthroplasty, *Clin Orthop* 261:63, 1990.
31. Zavadak KH et al: Variability in attainment of functional milestones during the acute care admission after total hip replacement, *J Rheumatol* 22:482, 1995.

Chapter 11

Open Reduction and Internal Fixation of the Hip

Edward Pratt
Mayra Saborio Amiran
Patricia A. Gray

Hip fractures are the most common bony injuries requiring surgical intervention in the United States. The estimated annual expense for the treatment of these patients has been estimated as high as $7.3 billion. Because of the steadily aging population and increasing incidence of osteoporosis, the number of hip fractures is expected to increase from 275,000 per year in the late 1987 to more than 500,000 by the year 2040.[1]

Surgical Indications and Considerations

Numerous classification systems have been devised to describe hip fractures. However, in the context of surgical exposure, soft tissue injury, and rehabilitation potential, they can be simplified into five main categories:
1. Nondisplaced or minimally displaced femoral neck fractures
2. Displaced femoral neck fractures
3. Stable intertrochanteric fractures
4. Unstable intertrochanteric fractures
5. Subtrochanteric fractures

Virtually all categories of patients with these fractures demonstrate superior outcomes with surgical intervention and early mobilization.[2] This is true regardless of age, gender, or co-morbidities, with the rare exception of an incomplete or impacted femoral neck fracture in a nonambulatory or extremely ill individual. The expected postoperative stability is directly proportional to the severity of the injury, the quality or density of the bone to be repaired, and the technical expertise of the surgeon.

A successful outcome also is profoundly affected by the patient's overall pre-injury physical and mental condition. Patients with major cardiopulmonary afflictions, obesity, poor upper body strength, osteoporosis, or dementia in its various forms are at increased risk in the treatment of hip fractures. Overall mortality rates of 20% after 1 year, 50% at 3 years, 60% at 6 years, and 77% after 10 years have been reported.[9]

The traditional goal of rehabilitation has been to restore the patient to the level of function that existed before the injury. In the majority of cases this is not realistic. Only 20% to 35% of patients regain their pre-injury level of independence. Some 15% to 40% require institutionalized care for more than a year after surgery. Many—50% to 83%—require devices to assist with ambulation.[14] Rehabilitation goals must be individualized, with the therapist taking into account all co-morbidities, fracture severity, and motivational level of the patient, all of which demonstrate a wide spectrum of disease severity and potential for recovery.

Surgical Procedures

Nondisplaced or Minimally Displaced Femoral Neck Fractures

Nondisplaced or minimally displaced femoral neck fractures represent the least severe injuries in the spectrum of hip fractures. They are stable and can bear the full weight of the patient immediately after surgery. Moreover, they require no limitations on range of motion (ROM) or exertion in the immediate postoperative period. The preferred surgical procedure is a fluoroscopically aided placement of cannulated 6.5-mm screws through a limited or percutaneous lateral approach. This approach violates the skin, subcutaneous fat, deep fascia of the fascia lata, and fascia and muscle fibers of the vastus lateralis. Typically the joint capsule is distended by blood, creating some limitation in hip ROM and pain. No major nerves or vessels are at risk in this approach.

The patient is brought to the operating room and anesthesia is induced. The patient is positioned supine on a fracture table capable of distracting and manipulating the affected limb. After satisfactory position of the fracture fragments is verified with an image intensifier, surgery is begun.

A 2-cm incision is made along the lateral femur in line with the fractured femoral neck. A guide pin is then placed percutaneously through the lateral musculature at or about the level of the lesser trochanter. The pin is

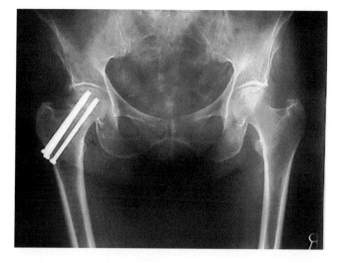

Fig. 11-1. AP x-ray film of the pelvis showing proper placement of three cannulated screws across a minimally displaced subcapital femoral neck fracture.

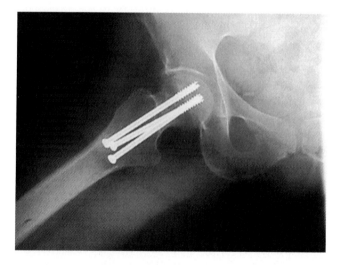

Fig. 11-2. Lateral view of the case illustrated in Fig. 11-1.

introduced up the femoral neck and across the fracture into the subchondral bone of the femoral head. After two to four guide pins have been placed, the outer cortex is drilled with a cannulated drill and cannulated screws are introduced over the guide pins (Figs. 11-1 and 11-2). The soft tissues are repaired and a dressing is applied. Femoral neck fractures that occur more toward the base of the femoral neck require fixation that is able to resist the bending moment between femoral neck and shaft. These are treated similar to intertrochanteric fractures and the operative procedure is described in that section.

Displaced Femoral Neck Fractures

Femoral neck fractures in which the femoral head has been separated widely from the neck do not heal if re-

duced and fixed by screws or pins. In these fractures the vascular supply to the femoral head (specifically the medial and lateral femoral circumflex arteries) are often severed. In younger patients it is still desirable to attempt fixation despite the high rate of nonunion and osteonecrosis. When open reduction is attempted the anterolateral exposure of Watson-Jones is preferred because it preserves the blood supply to the femoral head, which enters through the posteroinferior femoral neck. This approach is discussed in the section on total hip replacement. Most elderly patients are best treated by bipolar, endoprosthetic, or total hip replacement procedures using a posterolateral approach.

The posterolateral approach involves violation of the skin; subcutaneous tissue; fascia lata; gluteus maximus; and short external rotators of the hip, including the piriformis, obturator internus, gemelli, and quadratus femoris. The capsule is incised posteriorly and often released anteriorly. Traction is applied on the gluteus maximus, gluteus medius, and gluteus minimus throughout the procedure. Nerves and vessels at risk include the sciatic nerve, the superior gluteal nerve, the inferior gluteal nerve, and their accompanying vessels. Although the psoas is left alone, it is often inflamed and can scar down and across the anterior hip capsule if adequate postoperative mobilization is not encouraged. Generally incisions are healed by 2 weeks, deep soft tissue healing is well advanced by 6 weeks, and full bony healing is expected at 12 weeks.

The patient is anesthetized and placed in the lateral decubitus position with the injured hip up (see Fig. 10-4). The torso is stabilized and the hip and affected leg are draped to move freely. The initial incision is centered over the greater trochanter and taken distally 3 inches along the femoral shaft, then proximally and medially 4 inches along the course of the fibers of the gluteus maximus. The deep fascia is incised over the greater trochanter and carried distally along the same line as the skin incision, exposing the origin of the vastus lateralis without violating it. The surgeon digitally palpates the interval between the gluteus maximus and tensor fascia lata proximally, then extends the deep incision in this interval. A large, self retaining retractor is then positioned to hold the deep fascia apart. The greater trochanteric bursa is incised to expose the short external rotators. The interval between the piriformis, gluteus medius, and gluteus minimus is identified and the glutei are retracted anteriorly. Carefully the short external rotators are taken off the posterior femoral neck along the posterior hip capsule as a single cuff of tissue for later repair. Alternatively the capsule can be released separately with a T incision. Generally the surgeon must release the piriformis, gemelli, obturator internus, and half of the quadratus to expose the femoral neck to the level of the lesser trochanter. The hip is then flexed and internally rotated to bring the fracture into view. A saw is used to cut the femoral neck smoothly at the proper level, and the femoral head is retrieved from the acetabulum. The acetabulum is examined and bone fragments are removed along with the ligamentum teres. After exposure is completed the prosthesis is installed. It is often inserted in 15 to 20 degrees more anteversion than was present with the biologic hip to minimize the risk of dislocation. This occasionally limits external rotation after surgery but usually not enough to create a functional impairment.

Closure is somewhat more controversial. The author prefers to repair the capsule and short external rotators with large #2 nonabsorbable suture through drill holes in the greater trochanter and intertrochanteric line. This limits the formation of heterotopic bone, decreases the incidence of postoperative dislocation, and improves proprioception during rehabilitation. The deep fascia is then repaired, followed by the subcutaneous tissue and skin.

The initial postoperative rehabilitation is predicated on early mobilization to prevent morbidities associated with recumbency such as deep venous thrombosis, atelectasis, pneumonia, decubiti, and loss of muscle strength and joint mobility. Full weight bearing (FWB) is encouraged. After arthrotomy each patient must be educated and drilled regarding potentially dangerous hip positions that can lead to dislocation. The risk inherent in the posterolateral approach is greatest with hip flexion greater than 90 degrees and internal rotation and/or adduction across the midline. Patients with prosthetic hips should be instructed to follow their hip precautions religiously for the first 6 weeks after surgery, at which time the soft tissue has regained most of its tensile strength. Even then they are at greater risk of dislocation than they were before surgery. The next major emphasis of rehabilitation is the regaining of abductor strength. The combination of traction on the abductor tendons, occasional traction neurapraxia on the superior gluteal nerve, and an often shortened abductor lever arm leads to a Trendelenburg gait. Until abductor strength returns, secondary joint pain can often develop on the spine, knees, and contralateral hip because of the added stresses of shifting the center of gravity to and fro during ambulation.

Intertrochanteric Hip Fractures

Intertrochanteric hip fractures tend to be the most technically challenging. The intertrochanteric region joins the femoral shaft and neck at an angle of about 130 degrees. The angular moment created by weight bearing (WB) is great here, and often WB in the initial postoperative period is not feasible. Morbidity tends to be higher after these fractures owing to significant comminution of bone and the resultant inadequate stabilization provided by the internal fixation. These pa-

tients often must remain at touch down weight bearing (TDWB) or non-weight bearing (NWB) until fracture healing is demonstrated. The most important prognosticator in this subset of patients is the evaluation of fracture stability (i.e., the tendency of the fracture to collapse or angulate under physiologic loads after surgery). Fractures with an intact posteromedial cortex and those at the base of the femoral neck are stable. These fractures tolerate limited WB in the initial postoperative period without shifting. Patients with these fractures are best treated by placing a sliding compression hip screw device in an anatomically aligned fracture.

The best surgical approach for the unstable fracture is controversial. Suggested approaches include hip screw devices with or without medial displacement, third-generation intermedullary reconstruction nail fixation, and calcar replacement endoprostheses. The surgical exposure for placement of a calcar replacement prosthesis is as described under the use of endoprostheses for displaced femoral neck fractures. The exposure and morbidity involved in the placement of an intermedullary nail are discussed in the section on subtrochanteric fractures. The exposure for placement of a dynamic compression hip screw is the same regardless of whether a stable or unstable fracture is being addressed. Typically a long lateral approach is used. This approach violates the skin, subcutaneous tissue, fascia lata, vastus lateralis fascia, and muscle belly. Generally in unstable fractures the lesser trochanter and inserting psoas tendon are left free, limiting hip flexion strength in the initial postoperative period.

Controversy exists as to whether it is better to align unstable fractures anatomically with a highly angled 145 to 150 degree compression plate and allow it to collapse into stability under physiologic loads or to perform a "medical displacement" osteotomy to obtain good posteromedial cortical abutment and stability during surgery (Fig. 11-3).

Both methods can lead to stability or instability and therefore each case must be discussed with the surgeon to ascertain the degree of stability obtained and the amount of WB permitted. Also, both methods shorten the distance between the insertion of the hip abductors in the greater trochanter and the center of rotation of the hip, creating a mechanical disadvantage for the abductors. This can lead to Trendelenburg gait, which must be overcome during the postoperative rehabilitation period.

The patient is placed supine on a fracture table with the afflicted limb in the traction boot. Care is taken to place the correct rotation on the distal limb to prevent malalignment. Reduction is carried out under an image intensifier until satisfactory reduction is achieved. Occasionally a satisfactory preoperative reduction is not possible because of posterior sag of the bony frag-

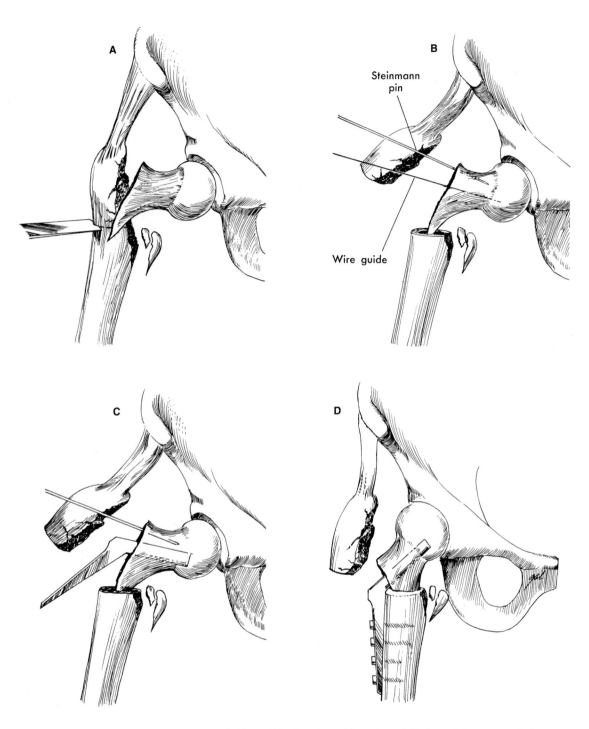

Fig. 11-3. Diamon and Hughston method of internal fixation of unstable trochanteric fractures. **A,** Transverse osteotomy of the lateral shaft. **B,** Insertion of a guide pin with a Steinmann pin for control of fragment. **C,** Insertion of nail in the proximal fragment. **D,** Fixation of the side plate to the shaft. (From Hughston JC: Intertrochanteric fractures of the hip, *Orthop Clin North Am* 5(3):585, 1974.)

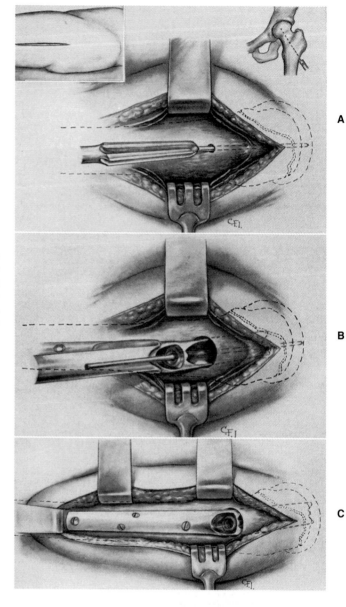

A

B

C

Fig. 11-4. Internal fixation of a trochanteric fracture. **A,** A guide pin is inserted and its position and that of the fracture are checked by roentgenograms. A cannulated Henderson reamer, placed over the guide pin, is used to make a hole through the lateral cortex. *Left insert,* skin incision; *right insert,* proper position of guide pin in anteroposterior view. **B,** A Jewett nail is inserted over the guide pin. **C,** The plate part of the Jewett nail has been fixed to the femoral shaft with screws.

Fig. 11-5. Unstable intertrochanteric fracture of the hip treated with a four-hole compression screw device. The lesser trochanter is often left floating, which can lead to weakness.

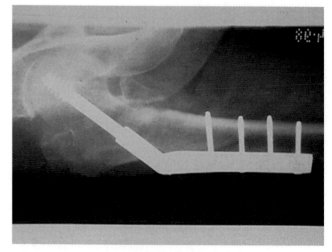

ments and further reduction must be done manually. After the limb has been prepared and draped a lateral incision is made from the level of the greater trochanter distally approximately 7 inches depending on the length of plate to be used. The incision is developed in the same line through skin, subcutaneous fat, and fascia lata. At this point the fascia of the vastus lateralis is followed posteriorly to its origin in the linea aspera. By incising it here the surgeon limits the amount of muscle denervated by the exposure and protects the main muscle mass from damage. The surgeon accesses the lateral cortex of the femoral shaft and places a retractor to maintain anterior retraction of the vastus lateralis, exposing the lateral femoral shaft. After exposure is completed, placement of the fixation device is begun (Fig. 11-4). Closure involves interrupted repair of the fascia of the vastus lateralis, fascia lata, subcutaneous tissue, and skin.

The dynamic compression screw device was not designed to hold the head and neck segment firmly (Fig. 11-5). Rather it allows the ambient muscle forces across the hip joint to pull the fracture fragments together until good bony resistance is encountered. In many comminuted osteoporotic fractures the ability of the screw device to contract is exceeded before good cortical abutment is obtained between the fracture fragments. In such cases WB must be curtailed until bony healing ensues or the screw will "cut out" and all stabilization will be lost. Again, the skin is healed by 2 weeks, the deep fascia and soft tissues are healed by 6 weeks, and good bony healing is expected by 12 weeks. In elderly osteoporotic patients with severely comminuted fractures, bony healing can sometimes be delayed for as long as 4 to 6 months. In patients with obviously unstable fractures WB should be delayed until good bony healing is demonstrated on x-ray films. The resultant collapse can often leave a limb significantly shorter. Leg length should be checked after healing and a lift provided if appropriate.

Subtrochanteric Hip Fractures

The use of advanced intermedullary nailing techniques has revolutionized the treatment of subtrochanteric fractures. Traditionally, these fractures have been difficult to fix because of the extreme angular force centered in this region, the muscular deforming forces, and the minimal bony interface between the two fragments available for healing (Fig. 11-6).

Moreover, the bone in this region is more cortical in character, with a poorer blood supply and less osteogenic activity than in the intertrochanteric region. The use of a sliding compression screw device has yielded a higher implant failure and nonunion rate than in other regions. The femur can be stabilized with a static locked intermedullary nail without exposing the fracture or disturbing its periosteal blood supply. The

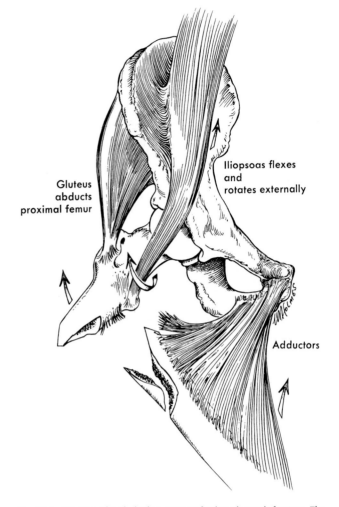

Fig. 11-6. Diagram of pathologic anatomy of subtrochanteric fracture. The proximal fragment is flexed, abducted, and externally rotated, whereas the femoral shaft is shortened and adducted. (From Froimson AI: Treatment of comminuted subtrochanteric fractures of the femur, *Surg Gynecol Obstet* 131(3):465, 1970.)

two preferred methods of fixation for patients with these fractures are a routine lateral approach for the placement of an extended compression screw device and the placement of a static locked intermedullary nail. The exposure for the lateral compression plate is discussed in the section on intertrochanteric fractures and deviates only in that the exposure must be taken more distally, causing more damage to the fascia lata and the vastus lateralis. Although this design stabilizes the fracture, WB usually must be delayed, soft tissue exposure is extensive, and healing is often delayed because of destruction of periosteal blood supply around the fracture.

The more limited exposure for a static locked or reconstruction nail runs more proximally through the abductors, with a second stab incision for the interlocking screws at the level of the greater or lesser trochanter and a third stab incision laterally along the supra-

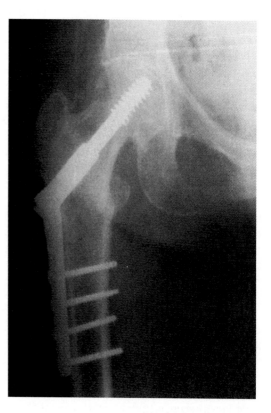

Fig. 11-7. A subtrochanteric fracture of the femur fixed with Richards compression screw-plate device. (From Crenshaw AH: *Campbell's operative orthopaedics,* vol 3, ed 7, St Louis, 1987, Mosby.)

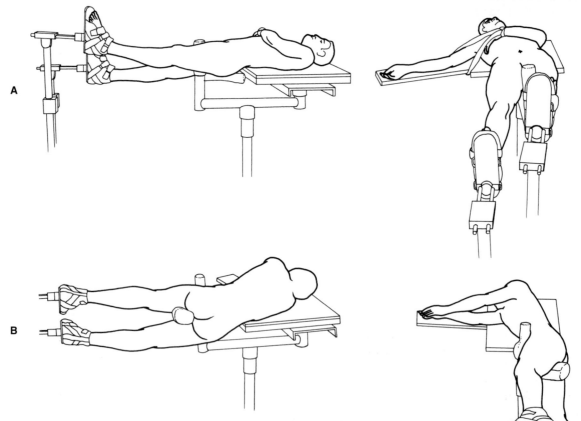

Fig. 11-8. Russell-Taylor interlocking nail technique. **A,** Patient in supine position. **B,** Patient in lateral decubitus position. (From Crenshaw AH: *Campbell's operative orthopaedics,* vol 3, ed 7, St Louis, 1987, Mosby.)

condylar femur. The newer reconstruction nails run the more proximal interlocking screws from the lateral femoral cortex (at the level of the lesser trochanter), across and through the prefabricated holes in the nail in the intermedullary canal. The nails then run up the femoral neck, ending in the hard bone of the subarticular femoral head. The distal interlocking screws pass lateral to medial through the lateral cortex of the femur, nail, and finally through the medial femoral cortex. This design effectively neutralizes deforming forces across the subtrochanteric femur, allowing FWB from the outset (Fig. 11-7).

The patient is placed supine on a fracture table with both legs inserted into traction boots. Traction is applied over a perineal post. The legs are positioned with the involved leg adducted across the midline and slightly flexed at the hip. The uninvolved leg is abducted and extended at the hip, lying adjacent to the operative leg (Fig. 11-8). An incision is started at a point 1 inch proximal to the greater trochanter (Fig. 11-9). It is developed proximally and slightly medially 3 inches. The surgeon then extends the incision through the skin and subcutaneous tissue to the fascia of the gluteus medius, which is divided for about 2 inches in line with the skin incision and the fibers of the gluteus medius. Using a small guide pin and fluoroscopy the surgeon makes a small entry point at the base of the superior posterior femoral area, the *piriformis fossa*. The guide pin is passed down the femoral shaft 6 inches or so and a cannulated reamer placed over the guide pin to enlarge the entry hole and begin the reaming process. The initial guide pin is replaced by a larger ball-tip guide that is run down across the fracture and down the intermedullary canal to the intercondylar notch. After this the canal is reamed with flexible reamers in progressively larger sizes until good cortical fit is obtained. After over-reaming a millimeter or two the surgeon carefully inserts the nail across the fracture under fluoroscopic guidance and then inserts the interlocking screws. The screws at the proximal end of the nail are aimed with the use of a special jig that attaches to the proximal end of the nail (Fig. 11-10). They are inserted percutaneously through the deep fascia and vastus lateralis. The distal screws are usually placed freehand, again percutaneously, using the image to visualize the holes in the nail passing through the iliotibial band and vastus lateralis. Closure consists of repairing the deep fascia, subcutaneous tissue, and skin.

Rehabilitation efforts during the initial postoperative period should consist of regaining control of the proximal hip musculature. Good functional quadriceps contraction and the ability to lift and maneuver the hip against gravity are prerequisites to adequate ambulation. Because of the strength of the fixation, patients can begin full WB immediately after intermedullary reconstruction nailing. Healing normally requires 3 months (Fig. 11-11); nail removal should not be considered before 18 to 24 months.

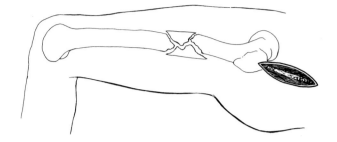

Fig. 11-9. Skin incision at the greater trochanter. (From Crenshaw AH: *Campbell's operative orthopaedics*, vol 3, ed 7, St Louis, 1987, Mosby.)

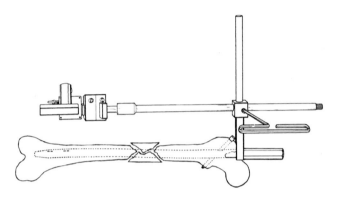

Fig. 11-10. Distal-locking block assembly is attached to the handle of the proximal drill guide. (From Crenshaw AH: *Campbell's operative orthopaedics*, vol 3, ed 7, St Louis, 1987, Mosby.)

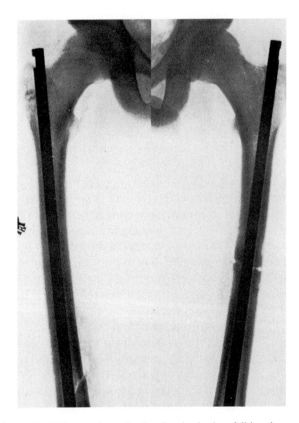

Fig. 11-11. Appearance 2 months after closed reduction of dislocations and medullary nailing of fractures. (From Crenshaw AH: *Campbell's operative orthopaedics*, vol 3, ed 7, St Louis, 1987, Mosby.)

Therapy Guidelines for Rehabilitation

The physical therapy procedures after an open reduction internal fixation (ORIF) procedure for the hip vary depending on several factors, including the health status of the patient before the fracture, the type of ORIF procedure used, and the restrictions ordered by the surgeon. Therefore this chapter provides only general guidelines to assist the therapist and the patient through the rehabilitation process. The physical therapist (PT) must manage the patient's progress carefully and consider the factors listed previously, the patient's ability to heal, and the constraints of the insurance carrier. The rehabilitation process can be described in three phases: the hospital phase, the home care phase, and the outpatient phase. In most cases, depending on lifestyle demands, the patient may only go through one or two of these phases.

Q. During gait training Julie has difficulty maintaining TDWB on the affected lower extremity. She tends to place approximately 20% of her weight onto her affected leg. She attempts to respond to verbal cues but is unsuccessful. A scale was placed under the affected leg so Julie could see and feel how much weight she was transferring onto her leg. Although she improved after using the scale she still could not maintain a safe level of TDWB through the affected leg. What is another way to assist her in maintaining TDWB status?

Phase I: Hospital Phase

TIME: Days 1-7
GOALS: Help patient become independent with transfers and gait (using appropriate assistive devices), discharge from acute care (Table 11-1)

Treatment performed on the day of surgery such as incentive spirometry exercises, management of air compression equipment, and donning thromboembolic disease (TED) hose may be supervised by the PT; however, these tasks are generally assigned to the nursing staff. When a good recovery from surgical trauma is demonstrated, hospital phase physical therapy usually begins on the first day after surgery.

Postoperative day one treatment consists of an evaluation, bed mobility, transfer training, gait training, and a beginning exercise program. The patient's initial goal is to transfer out of bed safely and walk to the bathroom independently using a front-wheeled walker. Some confusion or an emotional reaction to the event that precipitated the surgery may be encountered on the first postoperative day. The patient also may be

groggy or in a great deal of pain, so patience is important. The patient does not have the advantage of a preoperative training session because an ORIF is normally an emergency surgery. However, bed mobility and transfer training may be easier with a patient who has undergone an ORIF than with a patient who has undergone total hip replacement because usually no ROM precautions are necessary.

Patients who received sacral anesthesia often initially show a faster rate of progress than those who received general anesthesia. Coordination with the nursing staff so the patient's pain medications are timed to reach peak effectiveness during therapy sessions can hasten patient progress.

The PT should be informed regarding the patient's WB status and any special ROM restrictions. On postoperative day one the patient attempts to walk to a chair and sit up for approximately an hour before returning to bed. This may be repeated two to three times on the first day. The PT encourages the patient to sit up longer each day as progress is made.

The PT checks the patient's skin daily for pressure sores, especially heel ulcers. Proper positioning in bed precludes the tendency to lie in a frog-legged position with the hips in extreme external rotation and flexion.

Ankle pumps are the first exercises assigned to the patient to prevent blood clots and decrease edema in the legs. The patient performs ten to twenty repetitions every half hour. Quadriceps sets or quadriceps sets with adductor squeezes (Fig. 11-12), gluteal sets, hamstring sets, and hip abduction sets should be performed three times per day with ten repetitions of each to restore proximal hip strength. This program may be expanded to include active assistive and then active hip abduction, adduction, and hip-knee flexion. Repeated encouragement may be necessary. Other exercises to consider are ankle proprioceptive neuromuscular facilitation (PNF) patterns in both diagonal planes to prepare the patient for WB. If needed, lower extremity stretching may be done to avoid contractures and prepare the patient for a normal gait pattern. Stretching of the calves and hamstrings may be done with the help of the therapist or independently by the patient using a towel.

The patient can strengthen the upper extremities using a Theraband or the hospital bed's triangle as a pull-up bar. Pelvic tilts and single knee to chest of the uninvolved extremity can help decrease lumbar spine soreness and stiffness.

The patient's WB status, assigned by the surgeon, can vary depending on the type of procedure performed. A front-wheeled walker is recommended for patients with WB restrictions; however, some patients, especially NWB patients, may feel more stable using a pick-up walker. A platform walker may be necessary if upper extremity injuries are present. More agile pa-

Table 11-1   Hip ORIF

Rehabilitation Phase	Criteria to Progress to this Phase	Anticipated Impairments and Functional Limitations	Intervention	Goal	Rationale

Phase I Postoperative 1-7 days	Postoperative (inpatient)	• Pain
		• Limited bed mobility
		• Limited transfers
		• Limited gait
		• Limited strength of involved lower extremity (LE)
			• Inpatient on pain medication
			• Bed mobility training
			• Transfer training
			• Gait training
			• Isometrics—
			  Quadriceps sets
			  Gluteal sets
			• Assisted active range of motion (A/AROM)—
			  Hip—
			  Flexion, extension, abduction, and adduction
			• Active range of motion (AROM)—
			  Heel slides
			  Ankle pumps
			• Patient education emphasizing safety with all mobility training
				• Independent or stand by assist (SBA) with the following:
				  Bed mobility transfers
				  Gait 200 ft (using a front-wheeled walker [FWW]
				• Independent with home exercise program
				• Caregiver trained to assist with basic skills
				• Discharge to home
					• Emphasize restoration of independence with self care activities (bed mobility, transfers)
					• Ambulate safely to return to home environment with some degree of independence
					• Provide exercises to help patient regain muscular control of involved LE
					• Provide assistance to patient to perform hip range of motion (ROM)
					• Ensure patient and caregiver safety and prevent falls

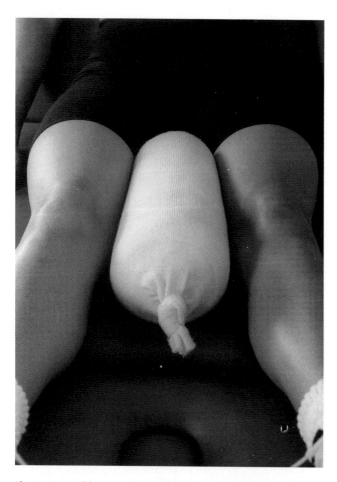

Fig. 11-12. Quadriceps set with the adductor squeezed. The patient sits with the legs stretched out in front. With a pillow between the knees and thighs, the patient squeezes the knees together and tightens the top of the thighs at the same time, holding for a count of 10 seconds.

tients can be issued axillary crutches immediately regardless of WB status.

Patients having difficulty with TDWB, defined as less than 10 lb of pressure through the affected leg,[10] or partial weight bearing (PWB) on the involved extremity may benefit from weight shift training in the parallel bars. A very thick-soled shoe worn on the uninvolved leg helps lift the patient to facilitate TDWB with the involved leg. With PWB status, stepping up on a bathroom scale helps the patient appreciate the appropriate amount of pressure to place on the involved extremity.

Electrical galvanic stimulation can be used to manage edema, and electrical stimulation in the muscle reeducation mode can help facilitate quadriceps (especially vastus medialis oblique) contraction. However, electrical modalities tend to be uncomfortable for most patients in the acute phase, especially those with metal implants. These treatments may be more appropriate at the outpatient stage. The surgeon, as always, should be consulted before the application of these modalities.

Transfer to the skilled nursing facility from acute care is expected on the third day after surgery. Patients are discharged from the hospital when they are medically stable and demonstrate independence with bed mobility, transfers, and ambulation (using an appropriate assistive device). Home caregivers should be trained to assist with these tasks safely before the patient leaves the hospital. Discharge goals are usually attained within 1 or 2 weeks after surgery. Patients may be kept in an extended care wing longer if no home caregiver is available and assistance is still required for basic mobility. The medical facility may present the patient with a written exercise program for home use at the time of discharge. The visiting PT in the home reinforces the skills learned in the hospital.

 $A_{\bullet}$ A very thick-soled shoe worn on the uninvolved foot helps lift the patient and facilitates TDWB status.

Phase II: Home Phase

TIME: Weeks 2-4
GOALS: Improve hip AROM to 90 degrees, educate patient regarding home maintenance program, help patient become independent with transfers and ambulate around the home with appropriate assistive devices, encourage limited community ambulation (Table 11-2)

Home care physical therapy is normally authorized for patients who are homebound and those who would incur undue hardship by leaving home for treatment. Homebound status is a requirement for reimbursement through Medicare and most other insurance. Physical therapy visits occur two to three times per week until the patient is no longer homebound or until goals have been met. This is usually achieved within 2 to 4 weeks of the patient's returning home from the hospital.

The goal of the home care therapist is to ensure the patient's safety at home and enable a return to previous community activities with the use of an appropriate walking device. However, this goal may be unrealistic depending on the patient's overall health status, motivation level, or previous level of function. In such cases the patient is discharged when progress has leveled.

During the initial home care visit the PT evaluates the patient's ROM, strength, bed mobility, transfer ability, safety with ambulation, stair-climbing ability, performance of the home exercise program, endurance, pain level, leg length, and skin and incision status. He or she also investigates equipment needs and the ability of caregivers to attend to the patient. Equipment needs may include a bedside commode, a raised toilet seat (if the patient has not attained 90 degrees of hip

Table 11-2   Hip ORIF

Rehabilitation Phase	Criteria to Progress to this Phase	Anticipated Impairments and Functional Limitations	Intervention	Goal	Rationale

Phase II Postoperative 2–4 weeks	No signs of infection
	No increase in pain
	Usually home health status but may be transitioned to outpatient when appropriate
		• Limited hip ROM
		• Limited LE strength
		• Limited with transfers in and out of car
		• Limited gait
			Continuation of exercises as in Phase I
			• Passive range of motion (PROM)—Stretches as indicated
			  Calf
			  Hamstring
			  Quadriceps
			  Single knee to chest
			• AROM—
			  Standing—
			  Hip flexion, extension, abduction, and adduction
			  Mini-squats
			  Lunges
			  Heel raises
			  Wall slides
			  Sitting—
			  Long arc quadriceps
			  Pelvic tilt
			• Elastic tubing exercises for upper extremities (UEs)
			• Gait/stair training
			• Standing balance training (balance boards) with assistance as needed
			• Car transfers
				• Increase AROM to Hip flexion 90° abduction 20° Knee flexion 90°
				• Independent with home exercises
				• Increase strength in Hip to 60% Knee to 70%
				• Initiate UE strengthening program
				• Gait—
				  Independent with cane at home
				  SBA with cane in community (1000 ft)
				• Improve balance
				• Perform independent transfers
					• Develop flexibility to improve sitting posture and tolerance
					• Improve strength to ensure safety with ambulation and transfers, decreasing dependence on uninvolved LE
					• Restore presurgical UE strength
					• Promote independence with community ambulation
					• Improve balance to prevent falls
					• Encourage return to previous ADLs and community activities

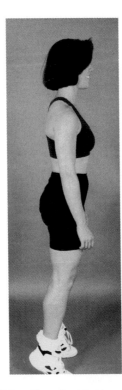

Fig. 11-13. Bilateral tiptoes. The patient stands on the floor with the knees straight and then lifts onto the toes, holds for 5 seconds, and slowly releases downward.

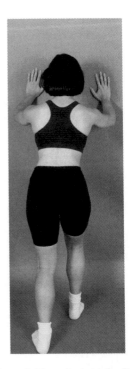

Fig. 11-14. Heel cord stretch. The patient stands with the involved leg and foot back, and the toes turned in slightly. He or she then places the hands against a wall and leans forward until a stretch is felt. The patients keeps the heel down, holds for 15 seconds, and slowly releases.

flexion), a shower chair, grab bars installed in the bathroom, railings installed by stairways, and appropriate assistive devices for the progression of gait. Moving furniture and light cords to ensure a clear pathway may be necessary. The PT reviews the skills learned in the hospital during the home evaluation and questions the patient's understanding of the WB restrictions and ROM precautions prescribed by the physician. Caregivers also should be present during this review.

PTs are now being trained to remove staples because of constraints imposed on nursing visits by insurance carriers. Staples are usually removed at about the fourteenth postoperative day. Proper sanitary technique protocols must be followed. The PT should consult the physician if any irregularity in scar healing is noted.

The patient advances from performing exercises isometrically to performing them actively during this phase. Exercises that require active assistance should soon be performed independently. Bilateral tiptoes (Fig. 11-13) and heel cord stretches (Fig. 11-14) performed while standing can be added, with a walker used for support. Other closed-chain exercises such as modified lunges and wall slides (Fig. 11-15) may be added as appropriate.

Hip flexion, extension, and abduction (performed with legs straight and then with legs bent) performed while standing are beneficial for the involved leg. They may be alternated bilaterally depending on the WB re-

strictions in place. With weight bearing as tolerated (WBAT) status, the patient may attempt balancing exercises on the involved leg. The PT should address chronic deficits in flexibility, strength, and balance that may have precipitated the patient's injury. A balance retraining program may benefit patients with vestibular or neurologic involvement. Vision problems should be referred to the physician.

Hamstring and calf stretching may be done using a towel (Fig. 11-16). The quadriceps also can be stretched using a towel, with the patient lying prone with knees bent. Pelvic tilt, knee to chest, hip rotator stretches, and trunk rotation exercises benefit the low back as well as the hip.

The patient progresses from using a front-wheeled walker or two crutches to a cane during this phase. The ability to ambulate safely without an assistive device is sometimes attainable within the time period authorized. The PT must take special care to correct uneven stride length (leading with the involved extremity and stepping-to with the uninvolved extremity), knee flexion in late stance phase, forward flexion at the waist, and overstriding with crutches.[10] Gait training includes stair climbing. Initially the patient should lead up the stairs with the strong leg and lead down the stairs with the involved leg in a step-to pattern. The patient with WBAT status can practice step-ups onto a book or step with a very narrow rise (Fig. 11-17). An initial isomet-

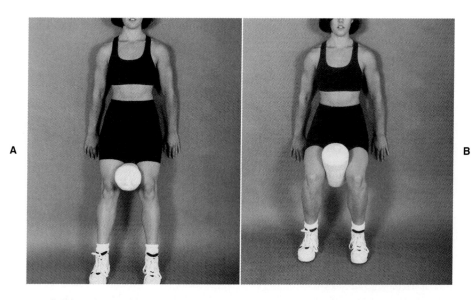

Fig. 11-15. Wall slides using an adductor pillow: **A,** The patient stands with the back against a wall, feet shoulder-width apart with a pillow between the thighs. **B,** He or she then bends the knees to a 45-degree angle, tightens the thighs, and squeezes the pillow. The patient holds for 10 seconds, then extends the knees and slides up the wall.

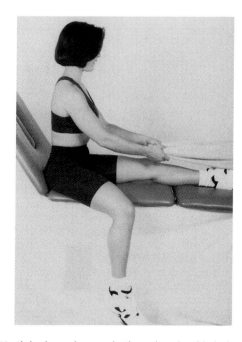

Fig. 11-16. Sitting hamstring stretch. The patient sits with the involved leg straight, and the other leg bent off the edge of a table or bed. He or she then hooks a towel around the foot, keeps the back straight, and leans forward until a stretch is felt. The patient holds this position for 15 seconds and slowly releases.

Fig. 11-17. Step-ups. **A,** The patient slowly steps onto a step with the involved extremity while tightening the muscles of the thigh. **B,** The patient must control the knee while stepping up.

ric contraction can proceed to stepping up isotonically onto progressively taller rises until the patient is able to walk up and down stairs in a normal step-over-step pattern. Training to step up and down from curbs, walk on uneven surfaces, and transfer in and out of a car safely also is provided in the home phase.

Home health physical therapy is usually finished within 2 to 4 weeks. The patient should have 80 to 90 degrees of hip flexion and 20 degrees of hip abduction at this point. The quadriceps and hip abductor strength should be fair to fair plus (3/5 to 3+/5 on the Manual Muscle Test [MMT]), and the patient should be able to perform all exercises actively. The majority of patients who undergo ORIF are elderly and lead fairly sedentary lifestyles. Further rehabilitation is unnecessary for them at this point. Activities such as walking, swimming, and bicycle riding are recommended, when realistic, for long-term exercise programs. Tai Chi has been shown to decrease the risk of falls in the elderly.[7] A few active patients with more rigorous lifestyle requirements may go on to outpatient therapy for further strengthening.

> **Q.** Ruth is 70 years old. She sustained a hip fracture at home when she tripped and fell. She had an ORIF on her left hip 3 months ago. Before her fall she could walk without an assistive device. Presently she walks at home without an assistive device but needs a cane to ambulate around the community. She rarely goes out because she is so fearful of falling. She has maintained a strengthening home exercise program. Ruth feels that her leg remains weak despite all her exercising. Her lower extremity flexibility is generally restricted throughout. The left leg is more restricted than the right. Ruth's balance and coordination also are impaired. Movements other than forward gait appear labored and slow. Left hip strength is generally 4−/5. Should strengthening, stretching, ROM, balance training, or coordination training be emphasized initially during treatment?

Phase III: Outpatient Phase

TIME: Weeks 5-8
GOALS: Encourage patient self-management of exercises, help patient become independent in community ambulation, increase strength of lower extremity (Table 11-3)

Outpatient physical therapy is intended to increase the involved extremity's flexibility to full ROM and increase its strength to at least the good minus level (4−/5 MMT). Gait pattern irregularities are to be normalized. Cardiovascular capacity also may be improved. These treatments should be conducted two to three times per week. The duration of outpatient rehabilitation depends on the patient's ability to make objective progress and on whether the intervention or treatment requires the skill of a physical therapist.

All exercises should be done actively by this time. Exercises previously performed in gravity-eliminated positions such as supine hip abduction (Fig. 11-18) and adduction (Fig. 11-19) are progressed to gravity-resisted positions; ankle weights can be added if appropriate. The closed-chain exercises mentioned previously also are performed in the outpatient clinic.

Mini-squats and wall squats can emphasize a vastus medialis oblique contraction with the addition of an isometric hip adductor squeeze employing a pillow or small ball. Lunges with the involved leg on a small step can progress to stair climbing on larger, more normal-sized steps. Standing balance exercises on the affected leg are appropriate with WBAT status.

Cardiovascular exercise is important during this phase to increase circulation throughout the body and increase endurance for ambulation. An upper body ergometer (UBE) or a stationary bicycle can be introduced at this phase. The patient's tolerance should be built up to a combined 15 to 30 minutes if possible.

The modalities mentioned in the hospital phase may be performed here with the approval of the surgeon. Balance retraining programs may be expanded to include various balance boards. Spine stabilization exercises can include those done in the prone and quadruped positions. Inclusion of the leg press (Fig. 11-20) and other weight training equipment may be appropriate in the clinic phase. At the PT's discretion, a treadmill also may be used to contribute to balance and gait retraining. Placement of the treadmill in front of a mirror can help the patient correct gait pattern irregularities.

By the end of the outpatient phase the patient should have a well-rounded program that can be continued at home or at a fitness center. Bicycling, recreational walking, tai chi, and swimming are excellent long-term options for the patient recovering from hip ORIF.

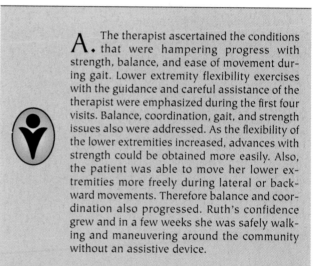

> **A.** The therapist ascertained the conditions that were hampering progress with strength, balance, and ease of movement during gait. Lower extremity flexibility exercises with the guidance and careful assistance of the therapist were emphasized during the first four visits. Balance, coordination, gait, and strength issues also were addressed. As the flexibility of the lower extremities increased, advances with strength could be obtained more easily. Also, the patient was able to move her lower extremities more freely during lateral or backward movements. Therefore balance and coordination also progressed. Ruth's confidence grew and in a few weeks she was safely walking and maneuvering around the community without an assistive device.

Troubleshooting

Complications may arise in the course of rehabilitation. Examples that should be referred to the surgeon include the following:
- Thigh pain with walking that clears with sitting, possibly intermittent claudication
- A positive Trendelenburg sign that does not resolve with treatment, possibly resulting from damage to the gluteal innervation
- Severe rubor and swelling at the surgical site with accompanying fever, possibly indicating a septic infection
- Persistent, severe pain, possibly resulting from an expansion of the fracture or loosening of the fixation devices

Table 11-3　Hip ORIF

Rehabilitation Phase	Criteria to Progress to this Phase	Anticipated Impairments and Functional Limitations	Intervention	Goal	Rationale
Phase III Postoperative 5-8 weeks	Independence with transfers in and out of car • No loss of hip ROM	Limited AROM and strength of involved LE • Limited tolerance to community ambulation • Limited tolerance to cardiovascular exercises • Limited with resuming more advanced activities	Progression of exercises in Phase I and II, adding resistance where appropriate • Modalities as necessary: heat, ice, electrical stimulation • Trunk stabilization exercises • Upper body ergometer • Stationary bicycle • Treadmill • Gait training for uneven surfaces and stairs	• Control pain • Regain full AROM of involved LE • Increase LE strength to 75% • Become independent with community ambulation	• Progress strength and ROM of involved LE • Use modalities to control any residual activity or prepare tissue for stretching • Promote safety with ambulation on all types of surfaces • Regain cardiovascular conditioning • Resume all ADLs and community activities

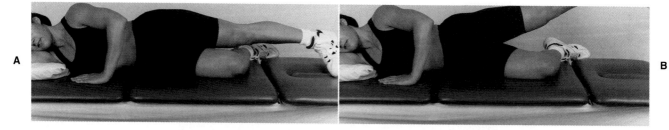

Fig. 11-18. Active hip abduction. **A,** The patient lies on the uninvolved side with the bottom knee bent. **B,** Keeping the top leg straight, he or she lifts upward, holds for 5 seconds, then slowly returns to the starting position.

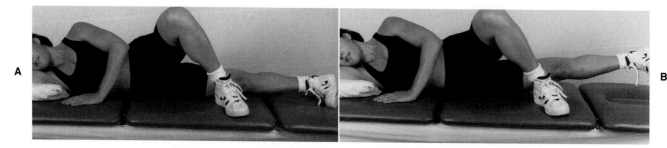

Fig. 11-19. Active hip adduction. **A,** The patient lies on the involved side with the bottom leg straight. **B,** He or she then bends the top knee and places the foot in front of the bottom leg. The patient lifts the bottom leg up approximately 6 to 8 inches and holds for 5 to 10 seconds before slowly returning the leg to the starting position.

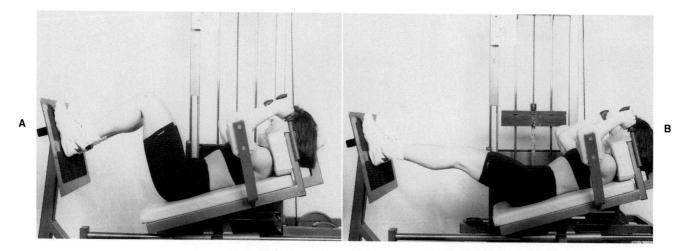

Fig. 11-20. Leg press machine. **A,** The patient should adjust the machine so the knees are bent approximately 90 degrees while the back is flat. **B,** The patient straightens the legs while exhaling without locking the knees, then slowly releases.

Other problems that may arise are the responsibility of the surgeon, but the PT can use palliative measures to assist the patient. Leg length discrepancy is an example. The patient can continue gait training with a temporary shoe insert or with shoes of different heel heights. The surgeon may later prescribe a permanent orthotic. Persistent edema may be treated with medication. Patients should be advised to elevate their legs, rest more often, wear TED hose, pump their ankles, and apply ice to a swollen area. Pain exacerbations are usually treated with medication. Possible side effects of the medication include nausea, constipation, and hypertension. The therapist can assist in pain reduction with modalities, exercise, and positioning.

REFERENCES

1. American Academy of Orthopaedic Surgeons: *Orthopedic knowledge update 3: home study syllabus,* Rosemont, IL, 1990, the Academy.

2. American Academy of Orthopaedic Surgeons: *Orthopedic knowledge update 4: home study syllabus,* Rosemont, IL, 1992, the Academy.

❧ Suggested Home Maintenance for the Postsurgical Patient

Days 1-7 (in hospital)

GOALS FOR THE PERIOD: Increase volitional control of involved lower extremity, improve and maintain ROM
Isometric Exercises
1. Quadriceps sets
2. Gluteal sets
AROM Exercises
3. Heel slides
4. Ankle pumps

Weeks 2-4

GOALS FOR THE PERIOD: Increase lower extremity strength and functional ROM, initiate upper extremity strengthening program
1. Stretching as indicated by evaluation
AROM
2. Standing hip flexion, extension, abduction, and adduction
3. Mini-squats
4. Lunges
5. Wall slides
6. Pelvic tilt
7. Long-arc quadriceps
8. Upper body exercises as indicated

Weeks 5-8

GOALS FOR THE PERIOD: Promote return to previous level of function (as cleared by physician)
1. Continue exercises from weeks 2-4
2. Progress to gym activities as indicated and prepare for discharge to community or home gym (treadmill, stationary bicycle)

3. Bray TJ et al: The displaced femoral neck fracture: internal fixation versus bipolar endoprosthesis. Results of a prospective randomized comparison, *Clin Orthop* 230:127, 1988.

4. Brumback RJ et al: Intramedullary nailing of femoral shaft fractures. Part I: decision making errors with interlocking fixation, *J Bone Joint Surg* 70A:1441, 1988.

5. Brumback RJ et al: Intramedullary nailing of femoral shaft fractures. Part II: fracture healing with static interlocking, *J Bone Joint Surg* 70A:1453, 1988.

6. Brumback RJ et al: Intramedullary nailing of femoral shaft fractures. Part III: long-term effects of static interlocking fixation, *J Bone Joint Surg* 74A:106, 1992.

7. Clark GS, Siebens HC: Geriatric rehabilitation. In DeLisa JA, editor: *Rehabilitation medicine: principles and practice*, ed 3, Philadelphia, 1988, JB Lippincott.

8. Crenshaw AH et al: *Campbell's operative orthopaedics*, ed 9, St Louis, 1998, Mosby.

9. Elmerson S, Zetterberg C, Andersson G: Ten-year survival after fractures of the proximal end of the femur, *Gerontology* 34:186, 1988.

10. Fagerson TL: *The hip handbook*, Newton, MA, 1998, Butterworth-Heinemann.

11. Hoppenfeld S, deBoer P, Thomas HA: *Surgical exposures in orthopedics: the anatomic approach*, Philadelphia, 1984, JB Lippincott.

12. Ions GK, Stevens J: Prediction of survival in patients with femoral neck fractures, *J Bone Joint Surg* 69B:384, 1987.

13. Jensen TT, Juncker Y: Pressure sores common after hip operations, *Acta Orthop Scand* 58:209, 1987.

14. Jette AM et al: Functional recovery after hip fractures, *Arch Phys Med Rehabil* 68:735, 1987.

15. Rehnberg L, Olerud C: The stability of femoral neck fractures and its influence on healing, *J Bone Joint Surg* 71B:173, 1989.

16. Ruff ME, Lubbers LM: Treatment of subtrochanteric fractures with a sliding screw-plate device, *J Trauma* 26:75, 1986.

17. Sexson S, Lehner J: Factors affecting hip fractures mortality, *J Orthop Trauma* 1:298, 1988.

18. White BL, Fisher WD, Laurin CA: Rate of mortality of elderly patients after fracture of the hip in the 1980's, *J Bone Joint Surg* 69A:1335, 1987.

Chapter 12

Anterior Cruciate Ligament Reconstruction

Luga Podesta
Jim Magnusson
Terry Gillette

Anterior cruciate ligament (ACL) injuries occur most often in the relatively young active (athletic) population.[33,88] The extent of the injury and desired level of activity usually dictate when surgical intervention is required. This chapter describes the current surgical considerations, techniques, and rehabilitative guidelines with supportive rationale. The individual clinician must determine the speed and intensity appropriate for each patient.

Surgical Indications and Considerations

Etiology and Epidemiology

The mechanism of ACL injury has been well documented and classically involves a deceleration and pivoting motion.[38] However, factors that predispose an individual to ACL injury include the following: narrow intercondylar notch, tibial rotation, hypermobility and alignment of the foot, and width of the pelvis in the female athlete. Other anatomic relationships have been discussed, but no studies have found a conclusive relationship between ligament failure and the predisposing factors. The incidence of individuals sustaining a ruptured ACL has been reported at 1 in 3000.[38] The individual describes feeling and sometimes hearing a "pop."[76] The person is 1000 times more likely to be participating in a sporting event.[31] Swelling is immediate, which implicates a ligamentous injury because of its associated vascularity. Patients exhibiting an instability of the knee that affects pivot shift, a positive Lachman's test, and positive magnetic resonance imaging (MRI) for ACL rupture should be thoroughly evaluated for surgical considerations. Functionally these individuals have difficulty performing pivoting and deceleration activities related to activities of daily living (ADLs) or sports. The age group more commonly associated with ACL ruptures is between 15 and 25 years old, but this injury also is seen in active individuals up to and into their fifth decade.[9,31,73] Although individuals who have sustained isolated rupture of the ACL may continue to be functional, their level of function is compromised and may require future surgical intervention because of secondary restraint pathology.[50]

Researchers have speculated regarding the age at which reconstruction is not recommended; however, to date no literature has noted any detrimental outcomes based on the age of the patient. In fact, studies have shown no significant difference in outcomes in comparing individuals at the age breaks of 35 and 40 years.[9,73] However, the anticipated functional limitations (modification of activities involving pivoting and deceleration) must be explored and explained to the patient who chooses not to have an ACL-deficient knee reconstructed. Ciccotti et al[20] reported on nonoperative management of patients from 40 to 60 years. They found that 83% of the patients had a satisfactory result with guided rehabilitation. However, they also mentioned that surgery may be an option for individuals wishing to continue sporting and pivoting activities.

Treatment Options

Surgical techniques to replace the deficient ACL have evolved over the past decade and continue to be refined. Advances in arthroscopic surgery now provide surgeons with the ability to perform these reconstructive procedures using a one-incision endoscopic technique. Research continues in the search for the optimal graft, fixation technique, and surgical reconstructive procedure. The biologic grafts most widely used today are the central third patellar tendon or hamstring tendon grafts. Hey-Groves[45] in 1920 and Campbell[17] in 1939 first described the use of the patella tendon as an ACL graft. Since these original surgical descriptions, numerous procedures to repair or reconstruct the ACL have been advocated. Attempts at primary repair of the ACL with and without augmentation[16,66,67] were of limited success.[94] Extraarticular ACL reconstruction also was suggested as a technique to reconstruct the ACL-deficient knee.[34,60] However, long-term results were disappointing.[99] Intraarticular ACL reconstruction using various tissues, including the patellar tendon, iliotibial band, and combinations of hamstring tendons (semitendinosus, semitendinosus-gracilis), has been extensively described in the literature.[2,19,49,52,72]

Graft Selection

The selection of the appropriate graft to replace the ACL is crucial to the ultimate success of the reconstruction. Primary concerns in the selection of an autogenous graft to replace the incompetent ACL include the biomechanical properties of the graft (e.g., initial graft strength and stiffness relative to the normal ACL), ease of graft harvest and fixation, potential for donor-site morbidity, and individual patient concerns. Other factors that ultimately influence graft performance include biologic changes in graft materials over time and their ability to withstand the effects of repetitive loading and stress.[24] Noyes et al[75] studied the biomechanical properties of a number of autograft tissues and showed that an isolated 14 mm wide bone–patella tendon–bone complex (BPB) graft has 168% the strength of an intact ACL. A graft 10 mm wide is about 120% as strong. The study also determined that a single-strand semitendinosus graft displayed only 70% of the normal ACL strength. The data show that BPB grafts have comparable tensile strength but increased stiffness in relation to the normal ACL, whereas single-strand semitendinosus grafts have decreased tensile strength but comparable stiffness. Other researchers have shown that multiple strands of semitendinosus or semitendinosus-gracilis composite grafts are stronger relative to the normal ACL.

The graft of choice varies among surgeons. They currently include BPB autografts and allografts; single-, double-, and quadruple-stranded semitendinosus autografts; and composite grafts using semitendinosus-gracilis autografts.

The enthusiasm surrounding the use of allograft replacement of the ACL has recently declined because of the small but tangible risk of infectious disease transmission. The risk of human immunodeficiency virus (HIV) transmission has been estimated to be 1 in 1.6 million using currently available bone- and tissue-banking techniques.[12] Both gamma radiation and ethylene oxide have been used to sterilize allograft tissue of bacterial and viral contamination. Fielder et al[36] have determined that 3 mrads or more of gamma radiation are required to sterilize HIV. Furthermore, sterilization procedures have been associated with alterations in graft properties and shown to cause a significant average decrease in stiffness (12%) and maximal load (26%)[81] and a marked inflammatory response with ethylene oxide use. Further studies must be conducted regarding post-sterilization ACL allograft performance. Although the use of allografts as ACL replacements can diminish operative time and prevent graft harvest site

morbidity, they are not recommended for routine use in primary ACL deficiency. Currently, either BPB or semitendinosus autografts are the most widely used ACL substitutes to reconstruct the ACL-deficient knee.

Graft Fixation

Adequate fixation of the biologic ACL graft is crucial during the early postoperative period after ACL reconstruction. Fixation devices must transfer forces from the fixation device to the graft and provide stability under repetitive loads and sudden traumatic loads. Various techniques are now available for fixation, including interference screws, staples, sutures through buttons, sutures tied over screw posts, and ligament and plate washers. Kurosaka et al[55] determined the interference screw to be the strongest method of fixation of BPB grafts. Interference screw strength depends on compression of the bone plug,[24] bone quality,[24,55] length of screw thread-bone contact,[24] and direction of ligament forces.[24] Robertson et al[85] studied soft tissue fixation to bone and determined the screw with washer and the barbed staple to be the strongest methods of fixation.

Graft Maturation

Graft maturation has an influence on the patient whose goals include a return to sports, most of which require pivoting and cutting. The healing properties of autografts have been discussed in the literature,[5,6,22,40,59] and although a majority of the studies the authors of this chapter have reviewed describe maturity of the graft at 100% 12 to 16 months postoperatively, return to sports participation in some protocols occurs at 6 months (if functional tests and isokinetics meet criteria).[28,92]

The graft maturation process begins at implantation and progresses over the next 1 to 2 years. Autografts are strongest at the time of implantation. The implanted graft undergoes a process of functional adaptation (ligamentization), with gradual biologic transformation. The tendon graft undergoes four distinct stages of maturation[5,6,40]:

1. Necrosis
2. Revascularization
3. Cellular proliferation
4. Collagen formation, remodeling, and maturation.

Within the first 3 weeks after implantation, cell necrosis of the patella tendon intrinsic graft cells occurs. The graft consists of a collagen network that to this point has relied on a blood supply. As this blood supply is interrupted, the graft undergoes a necrotizing process. Necrosis commences immediately and generally lasts 2 weeks.[22,40,59] Native patella tendon (graft) cells diminish, and replacement cells can be present as early as the first week. Cellular repopulation occurs before revascularization. These cells are thought to arise from both extrinsic sources (synovial cells, mesenchymal stem cells, bone marrow, blood, and the ACL stump) and intrinsic sources (surviving graft cells). Early full range of motion (ROM) is desirable because as new collagen is formed, its formation and strength are dictated by the stresses placed on it.

As the new cells find their way to this frame and add stability to this weak structure, rehabilitation must be careful not to disrupt or stretch them. Necrosis of the graft allows the metamorphosis of the graft from tendon to ligamentous process. Necrosis of the graft is highlighted by the formation of granulation tissue and inflammation. The bone blood supply and synovial fluid nourish the graft by synovial diffusion.[3] Revascularization occurs within the first 6 to 8 weeks after implantation. By this time the graft is revascularized via the fat pads, synovium, and endosteum,[22,40,59] and the inflammatory response should be under control. Further inflammatory problems signify a delayed healing process and potential graft problems; the physician and therapist should be alert for them.[65,101]

Amiel et al[3] in 1986 described ligamentization of the rabbit patella tendon ACL graft. However, the graft never obtained all the cellular features of normal ACL tissue. Although the graft takes on many of the physical properties of the normal ACL, the cellular microgeometry of the remodeling graft does not closely resemble that of a normal ACL. The revascularization process progresses from peripheral to central.

Bone plugs incorporate into their respective bone tunnels over a 12-week period but are felt to near completion by approximately the sixth postoperative week. The comparative strength of the healed tendon-to-bone attachment versus the healed bone-plug attachment is unknown. Tendon-bone healing begins as a fibrovascular interface develops between the bone and tendon. Bony ingrowth occurs into these interfaces, which extend into the outer tendon tissue. A gradual reestablishment of collagen fiber continuity between bone and tendon occurs, and the attachment strength increases as collagen fiber continuity increases. These ACL autografts approximate 30% to 50% of the normal ACL strength 1 to 2 years postoperatively.[40]

Cellular proliferation and collagen formation take place as a continuing process throughout the maturation process. The function of collagen in the ligament is to withstand tension, and certain types of catalysts are present during the healing process. Transforming growth hormone factor β1 has been isolated during the healing of the medial collateral ligament (MCL) in rats. Administration of this growth hormone during the first 2 weeks after injury was found to increase strength,

stiffness, and braking energy of the ligament.[59] Other catalysts of collagen formation (platelet-derived growth factor 1 [basic fibroblast growth factor]) have had equally good results in improving the tensile strength of healing ligaments. Future studies should be performed to validate this intervention.

During the rehabilitation program assessment using the KT-1000 (Medmetric, San Diego, CA) to monitor pain, ROM, and edema should dictate the speed at which the patient may progress through the program.*

Surgical Procedure: Endoscopic BPB ACL Reconstruction

The procedure begins with a complete examination of the knee under anesthesia followed by a thorough diagnostic arthroscopic evaluation. The menisci, joint surfaces, and ligamentous structures are evaluated and additional injuries assessed arthroscopically. The leg is then exsanguinated and a tourniquet inflated with 350 mm of pressure. A medial parapatellar incision is made from the inferior pole of the patella to the tibial tuberosity. The skin is dissected down to the peritenon, and skin flaps are made superiorly, inferiorly, medially, and laterally. The peritenon is incised and the patella tendon is exposed. The width of the patellar tendon is noted, and a 10 mm graft is measured from the midpatellar tendon. Two small incisions 10 mm apart are made in the patellar tendon and then extended superiorly and inferiorly with a hemostat. The patellar and tibial bone plugs are measured to provide graft lengths of 20 to 25 mm of patella and 25 to 30 mm of tibial bone. To facilitate bone graft harvest, the corners of the bone plugs are pre-drilled with a 2-mm drill to decrease stress risers. The perimeters of the bone plugs are then sawed out with a reciprocating saw to a depth of 10 to 11 mm, depending on the size of the patella and tibial tubercle. The graft is then taken to the back table where it is prepared and fashioned to allow passage through the appropriate guides. The graft is completed by placing one #5 Tycron suture in the femoral and three #5 Tycron sutures into the tibial bone plugs to facilitate graft passage through the knee. The graft is preserved in a saline-moistened gauze sponge for later use.

The remnant of the ACL is resected, along with any hypertrophic tissue. Arthroscopically, the intercondylar notch is then prepared with the aid of a burr to prevent graft impingement. A site is chosen for placement of the tibial tunnel. Through the mid-line incision, a small area medial to the tibial tubercle is prepared with subperiosteal elevation. Using a tibial guide and under direct visual-

---

*References 1, 28, 30, 90, 91, 93, 95.

ization, the surgeon drills a guide pin into the knee from the outside in, exiting within the knee at a site chosen anteromedial to the ACL insertion. The tibial tunnel is reamed to the size of the harvested graft. A curette placed over the guide pin during reaming helps protect the articular cartilage and posterior cruciate ligament from damage. The tibial tunnel must be larger than the femoral tunnel to allow passage of the graft into the knee. The tibial tunnel edges are smoothed with a rasp to prevent graft abrasion after implantation. A fenestrated plug is then placed into the tibial tunnel to prevent fluid extravasation yet allow passage of instruments.

The femoral isometric point is determined on the medial aspect of the lateral femoral condyle, usually 3 to 5 mm anterior to the posterior cortex near the superior intercondylar notch margin (over-the-top position); it is marked with a curette or burr. With the knee flexed past 90 degrees, a fenestrated guide pin is inserted into the knee through the tibial tunnel and drilled through the femoral isometric point and out through the skin with the aid of an over-the-top guide. The femoral tunnel is then reamed to the size of the femoral bone plug to a depth of 30 mm.

The sutures from the femoral bone plug are inserted into the femoral pin and pulled out through the skin. The graft is delivered into the knee, through the tibial tunnel, and into the femoral tunnel under direct visualization. A cannulated interference screw is then inserted into the knee over a nidal guide pin and screwed into the femoral tunnel, compressing the femoral bone plug within the tunnel. Graft isometry is evaluated. The tibial bone plug within the tibial tunnel is secured with interference screw fixation. ROM and stability testing are then performed. The graft is evaluated arthroscopically to assess graft excursion and placement within the intercondylar notch.

The tourniquet is released, hemostasis is obtained, and the knee is irrigated. Loose closure of the patellar tendon is performed with the peritenon approximated to close the anterior defect. The subcutaneous tissue is approximated, and a continuous subcuticular skin closure is performed. The wounds are dressed sterilely. A light compressive wrap and continuous ice water cryotherapy system are applied, and the patient is taken to the recovery room with the knee in a knee immobilizer in full extension.

Therapy Guidelines for Rehabilitation

Rehabilitation of the ACL depends on a number of factors. This chapter does not give a precise time frame during which to progress from double-leg squats to single-leg squats; however, the physical therapist should respond as further data emerge and make modifications as indicated. Interpretation of response is usually performed via observation, palpation, and measurement.

Much has been written regarding the rehabilitation of the patient who has undergone ACL reconstructive surgery. A body of literature has addressed the BPB graft because this has been the gold standard. Many protocols have been presented to manage such patients.* This chapter focuses on effective guidelines for autograft rehabilitation because it is currently the most common graft selection. The guidelines in this chapter are tailored for an isolated ACL reconstruction, but it is important to be able to modify these guidelines if any additional pathologies are present such as meniscal repair or additional ligamentous injury. The rationale behind each component of rehabilitation is discussed. The factors in developing a program should be as follows:

1. To comprehend the healing constraints of the ACL graft when making a clinical decision regarding modification or progression of the patient's program
2. To use closed-chain (functional) in addition to open-chain exercises
3. To emphasize early ROM (especially full extension)

Preoperative Management

A 1- to 4-week program of rehabilitation can be used after acute ACL rupture to control edema, improve gait (education), and increase motion and strength.[31,86] The length of the program depends on the degree of swelling and ROM present. During the preoperative examination the physical therapist should assess the patient's gait, lower extremity ROM, patellofemoral (PF) alignment, degree of edema, and weight-bearing capacity. Passive accessory and functional tests also should be performed as appropriate. The therapist may wish to seek out educational sources (continuing education programs) for a thorough understanding of rationales and applied techniques.

Gait evaluation focuses on tolerance of weight bearing on the involved leg, stride length, and step length. Lower extremity alignment should be assessed from the ground up. After surgery the patient's safety regarding gait must be ensured. Ambulation with crutches in varying degrees of weight bearing on the involved leg on level surfaces and stairs is performed to make the patient familiar with one of their first postoperative demands. Evaluation of preoperative knee ROM and PF alignment is helpful in beginning the postoperative planning process. The physical therapist must evaluate both the ankle and the hip (in addition to the knee)

---

*References 28, 30, 31, 39, 40, 43, 51, 63-65, 74, 77, 79, 87-93, 95, 97, 103.

Table 12-1   ACL Reconstruction

Rehabilitation Phase	Criteria to Progress to this Phase	Anticipated Impairments and Functional Limitations	Intervention	Goal	Rationale

Phase Ia Preoperative 1-4 weeks	Preoperative	• Pain
		• Edema
		• Limited ROM
		• Limited weight bearing
		• Gait on crutches with brace (non–weight bearing to weight bearing as tolerated)
		• Poor thigh muscle recruitment
			• Cryotherapy 20-30 minutes
			• Elevation 20-30 minutes
			• Gait training
			• Passive range of motion (PROM)—Stretches as needed
			  Supine knee extension
			  Wall slides
			  Seated knee flexion
			• Isometrics—
			  Quadriceps/hamstring isolation and co-contraction, 10-30 repetitions (can also be done with elevation)
			• Assisted active range of motion (A/AROM)—Stretches as needed
			  Seated knee flexion
			• AROM progressive resistance exercises (PREs)—Ankle pumps, 10 repetitions per minute with elevation (20 minutes)
			  Hip abduction, adduction, flexion (SLR with brace locked at 0°)
			  Heel slides, standing hamstring curls
			• Joint and soft tissue mobilization
				• By the end of 4 weeks
				• Self-manage pain
				• Decrease edema
				• ROM 0°–10° extension
				• 75%–100% weight bearing using brace and crutches as appropriate
				• Fair to good muscle recruitment
				• Active motion 0° to –10° extension, 130° flexion
				• Prevent weakening of lower extremity
				• Independent straight leg raise (SLR) during supine–sit
				• Improve PROM as above
					• Pain control
					• Edema management
					• Gait training for safety and ease with transition postoperatively
					• ROM stretches to prevent complications going into surgery
					• Muscle pump and elevation to assist lymph drainage
					• Graduated exercise to improve neuromuscular coordination
					• Emphasize self-management of ROM program
					• Prepare for transfers (supine–sit)
					• ROM and muscle contraction to assist edema management and improve ROM
					• Decrease pain through input to joint receptors

to identify any ROM limitations and strength deficits. ROM limitations greater than −10 degrees extension have been associated with an increased incidence of arthrofibrosis (which is discussed in the section on complications).[23] Passive accessory testing includes assessing the secondary restraints of the knee, the superior and inferior tibial-fibular articulations, PF complex, and a brief appraisal as described by Maitland of the hip and ankle as appropriate.[61] Mid-patellar girth measurements are effective in comparing edema of the uninvolved with the involved knee and monitoring progress. PF alignment and mobility are important to assess because of their influence on the pace of the rehabilitation process. Preoperative PF crepitus is a factor in determining postoperative complications.[1] Therefore treatment of this dysfunction should be initiated early to avoid setbacks in functional progression. (Refer to Chapter 15 for PF rehabilitation.) Weight-bearing tolerance measurement can be as easy as using a weight scale and having the patient perform weight shifting until pain or instability is noted. Other assessments of weight acceptance on the involved leg can include sit-to-stand simulation (90-degree squat) using an inclined sled (calculating the percentage body weight based on the degree of incline) or shuttle (using resistive bands). Treatment for the preoperative phase is listed in Table 12-1. It is useful to initiate a progressive program to increase ROM, decrease edema and pain, and ultimately improve function.

Edema and pain management. The control of edema and pain is important both preoperatively and postoperatively. The modalities of choice are ice, electrical stimulation, passive motion with progression to active motion, and elevation. After surgery an inflammatory response occurs as a necessary part of the healing process. However, edema management and pain control should be balanced. Swelling in the knee joint and its surrounding soft tissues is a painful side effect. Joint effusion can inhibit muscle function[96] and limit motion. The percentage of patients with persistent hemarthrosis after reconstruction has been reported to be as high as 12%.[65] Therefore it is important to manage edema and pain from the outset. A good healing environment must be provided to allow the graft to mature. Cryotherapy is commonly used to manage edema and pain.[54] However, no studies have shown cryotherapy to be effective in reducing swelling. Nevertheless, cryotherapy can be used to manage and decrease secondary hypoxia, a side effect of swelling.[68] Although the literature has been a forum for debating the effectiveness of cryotherapy,[25] the clinical experiences of the authors of this chapter are similar to those of Cohn et al and Lessard et al,[21,58] who found that patients receiving cryotherapy were more compliant, had less pain, and

took less pain medication. Cryotherapy is effective in pain management. Elevation and intermittent compression are used in conjunction with cold to manage postoperative pain and edema.[28,31,65,79]

Initially a cryotherapy device is used immediately postoperatively and at home; cold packs can be used in the outpatient clinic. The temperatures commonly used are 10° to 20° C.[54] The use of a Cryocuff accomplishes intermittent compression and cooling to maximize efficiency. Ice and exercise are used in an active combination to battle continued edema and pain. Cryotherapy in the form of cold packs or crushed ice can be used for as long as 20 or 30 minutes in conjunction with limb elevation[13,56,69] (above heart level) and exercise (ankle pumps, quadriceps sets, quadriceps/hamstring co-contraction). Elevation and muscle pumping help the lymph system remove tissue debris and inflammatory by-products (free-floating proteins too large to filter through the capillaries).[54] Cryotherapy also has been used effectively in conjunction with early motion (cryokinetics) to shorten rehabilitation time in acute ankle sprains.[10] The use of cold may be effective in the pain-dominant patient, allowing the therapist to progress ROM exercises. Electrical stimulation also is an effective tool used in the management of pain through the intermittent use of transcutaneous electrical nerve stimulation (TENS).[79]

The types of cold packs used affect the efficiency of cooling. Frostbite is a common concern, as is nerve palsy.[33,80] The optimal delivery mechanism is crushed ice in a plastic bag secured in place by an elastic wrap. Care should be taken to avoid compression or ice over the proximal fibular head (because of the risk of affecting the peroneal nerve). If the use of a gel pack is considered, compression wrap should not be used and precautions should be taken to avoid frostbite. A cryotherapy application of 20 to 30 minutes (which includes exercises as noted previously) is reinforced as part of the home exercise program, and the patient is instructed to perform it as often as four times daily, depending on the level of edema and pain. Although little consensus exists on this issue, in the management of edema and pain, cryotherapy is the authors' modality of choice for patients who tolerate cold temperatures.

Initial Postoperative Examination

Subjective information is reviewed with the patient regarding medication needs, edema and pain management program compliance, and other pertinent history (if not obtained preoperatively).[61] Baseline measurements of ROM (knee flexion-extension), girth, and PF mobility are included in the objective examination, along with palpation and observational findings (e.g., gait, transfers).

Many subjective measurements can be obtained using questionnaires. Some of the tests cited in studies are the Gillquist, Lysholm, Noyes, Patient-Specific Functional Scale (PSFS), and Tegner.* Although these tests strive to objectify outcome studies, there is no consensus concerning which test is appropriate to use for all ACL reconstructions. Neeb et al[71] attempted to identify a "package" of tests (subjective, functional, and clinical) and found that the clinician must use a comprehensive package to identify impairment and disability.

ROM measurements are essential to monitor each treatment until full motion and function are restored. Patients seen during the first couple of days after surgery should have close to full extension (0 to −10 degrees) and limited flexion (80 to 100 degrees). Full extension must be given the utmost emphasis early on.† Full ROM is expected anywhere from 3 to 10 weeks after surgery.[28,101] Lack of early progress with motion is a red flag for complications and delay in progression through rehabilitation (see the discussion of complications).

Edema can be observed about the knee, leg, and at times the ankle and foot. Girth measurements are typically taken at the mid-patella and 10 cm proximally and distally. The authors use the mid-patellar measurement to monitor edema. Proximal and distal assessments are continued to monitor progress; they also objectively monitor inhibition.[70,96] Girth measurements have long been taken in an effort to relate to muscle strength. Clinically there seems to be no significant relationship between muscle girth and function or strength. Measurements of PF alignment should be undertaken in the first postoperative visit and continued during rehabilitation to avoid additional surgeries, slow progression of rehabilitation, and early plateau of exercises.

Palpation assessment of the PF articulation helps confirm any static malalignment problems (glides, tilts, patella alta or baja). Physical therapists can further their evaluation skills with continuing education that emphasizes PF assessment and treatment. (See Chapter 15.)

Skin temperature should be assessed on a continuing basis to monitor the inflammatory response phase. The physical therapist should assess the incision wound regularly to monitor healing; healing should be complete by 2 weeks after surgery. When appropriate, scar mobilization can be performed in a multidirectional pattern to prevent adhesions.

ROM, edema, pain, and stability testing ultimately determine the progression of exercises throughout rehabilitation. However, the authors feel that the KT-1000

assessment of the anterior drawer is the hallmark measurement of how rapidly to progress rehabilitation. Increases of 2 mm or more indicate imminent graft failure[65] and require highly conservative treatment that avoids any stress on the graft for a period of 2 weeks, until two KT-1000 readings do not indicate increased laxity. Rehabilitation is then progressed conservatively.

In addition to the use of positioning and modalities, the authors feel that joint mobilization effectively decreases pain.[61] The Continuous Passive Motion (CPM) device can be used to assist in managing postoperative pain (in addition to restoring ROM). Although CPM may produce no long-term benefits,[64,65,83] it appears helpful for patients with preoperative ROM difficulties.[30]

Postoperative Guidelines and Rationales

The general guidelines listed here are for ACL reconstruction using the BPB graft. On initial assessment, physical therapists must set treatment goals with patient input to avoid any potential misunderstandings. They also should provide education about graft maturation and the need to progress the rehabilitation program gradually and systematically. The treating therapist can modify the program based on the patient's response to treatment and the healing time frame of the graft.

The use of *closed-chain* versus *open-chain* exercises should be explored when planning rehabilitation of the lower extremity. Closed-chain rehabilitation makes sense for a variety of reasons. Closed-chain activities are less stressful on the graft, have a functional relationship, and are easy for patients to perform at home. Open-chain exercises place the graft at risk in certain ROMs, appear to be non–activity-specific (except for kicking), and require equipment to progress resistance.

In strengthening the muscles affecting the knee, activation of the quadriceps has the most potential to place increased stress on the graft.[44,82] Grood et al[42] and Palos et al[77] noted increased anterior tibial translation during the last 30 degrees of extension in an open-chain environment. A number of other researchers and clinicians also support the idea of avoiding open-chain terminal knee extension.* Performing closed-chain exercises with the foot in a fixed load–bearing position places less stress on the graft.[44,90,91,105] Closed-chain exercises make the exercise more specific to function, thus enhancing functional skills and transitional movements (e.g., weight shifting, sit-stand) in a safe manner.[102] Although open-chain exercises have a place in rehabilitation, the range of these exercises must be limited until graft maturation is adequate to support the stress. Ranges

---

*References 8, 18, 20, 71, 84, 98.
†References 31, 65, 74, 91, 92, 103.

* References 4, 37, 46, 47, 75, 78, 87, 89, 102.

commonly found in the literature are 90 to 30 degrees, again avoiding the last 30 degrees of extension in an open-chain environment.[32,74]

The most common brace used initially is the immobilizer or locked hinged brace. It is used 24 hours a day and is taken off or unlocked only for bathing and appropriate exercises. As the patient gains muscular (quadriceps/hamstrings) control in a weight-bearing position the brace is unlocked (hinged brace) or discarded (immobilizer). The physical therapist should caution the patient to avoid ambulation on uneven surfaces until adequate dynamic stability is apparent (usually 4 to 6 weeks).

Functional bracing that uses custom or prefabricated (off-the-shelf) braces is controversial. Malone and Friedhoff[62] found the custom-fitted double upright brace to be the most effective, allowing less slippage or migration. Debate continues regarding the necessity and type of brace that is most appropriate. The authors' preference during phases II and III is to use braces sparingly and determine individually whether bracing is indicated for a specific activity.

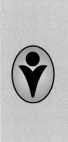

Q. Tracy is a 45-year-old woman. She tore her ACL while skiing. Tracy had surgery 3 weeks ago to reconstruct her ligament. Knee flexion ROM is progressing nicely. Knee extension is limited, with a passive range of motion (PROM) of −10 degrees. Inflammation is decreasing. Tracy has complaints of pain while performing quadriceps sets and straight-leg raises. What treatment techniques may be helpful for gaining knee extension?

Phase I

TIME: Weeks 1 to 4 after surgery
GOALS: Patient education and reinforcement of goals, quadriceps contraction, full knee extension, increase active ROM, and initiate joint mobilization (Table 12-2)

The first postoperative visit takes place between 1 and 7 days after surgery. Measurements are taken as appropriate (the reader should refer to the section on preoperative evaluation). This is the time to re-educate the patient about treatment goals and mechanisms to obtain those goals (including the edema and pain management program) and to initiate mild cardiovascular exercises (stationary bicycling using the uninvolved leg, upper body ergometer [UBE]). Education at this point regarding graft maturation and expectations regarding home exercise follow through is essential and saves time in future sessions.

DeCarlo and Sell[27] retrospectively examined the number of treatments used in two groups of patients who had undergone ACL reconstruction. One group averaged a mere seven treatments (range of 3 to 18) over a 6-month program that emphasized patient education concerning ROM. Patients "followed written instructions prescribed by a physical therapist for increasing muscle strength." Although this underscores the importance of patient education, these authors cautioned that limited visits for therapy should be considered on an individual basis and should reflect sound clinical rationale. The authors of this chapter suggest a range of 12 to 24 visits over a 6-month period. Most of these visits take place during the first 6 weeks and taper off as clinically indicated; the program places greater emphasis on patient self-management. The vast majority of the literature emphasizes early full extension, progressive weight bearing, and early ROM and mobility.[28,74,90-92,103]

After collecting all data, the physical therapist begins treatment. The patient may be brace free during PROM exercises, but the brace must be used when performing squatting activity and locked at 0 degrees (extension) with hip active range of motion (AROM) exercises until muscle contraction is adequate.

Initially electrical stimulation (ES) is used to assist in obtaining quadriceps contraction. This can be done in conjunction with ES to the hamstrings to facilitate co-contraction. Co-contraction helps stabilize the knee and control tibial translation.[11] Isometrics (quadriceps/hamstring sets) are initiated along with AROM (ankle pumps) and cryotherapy in an elevated position (as mentioned in the edema and pain management program). One effective exercise is a quadriceps/hamstring isometric contraction using a closed-chain environment (Fig. 12-1). These are called *spider killers* because the patient performs the isometric exercise while applying pressure to the ground via the heel (pretending that a spider is under the heel). Passive stretches are used to obtain early full knee extension. With prone hangs (Fig. 12-2) and supine passive knee extension (Fig. 12-3) (towel roll propped under the heel), patients should be well on their way to obtaining full extension. Flexion ROM is emphasized to a lesser extent than extension but it is still important. Supine wall slides are included in a home exercise program. The goal by 4 weeks is for the knee to be at 125 degrees of flexion. However, edema, pain, and overall tolerance of the knee to rehabilitation may limit flexion ROM progress.

AROM exercises are performed for the hip and ankle initially to improve strength and endurance. Supine heel slides and standing hamstring curls assist in gaining flexion ROM and strength. The patient should use a brace with exercises that place stress about the knee

Table 12-2   ACL Reconstruction

Rehabilitation Phase	Criteria to Progress to this Phase	Anticipated Impairments and Functional Limitations	Intervention	Goal	Rationale

Phase 1 Postoperative 1–4 weeks	Postoperative	• Postoperative edema
		• Postoperative pain
		• Limited ROM
		• Limited strength
		• Limited weight bearing
		• Limited gait
		• Limited transfers
			• Brace should be worn for all exercises in **bold type**
			• Edema and pain management program
			• PROM–Supine knee extension
			  Prone heel hangs
			  Supine wall slides
			• Isometrics–Quadriceps/ hamstring sets
			  Towel squeeze
			• AROM–Heel slides
			  SLR (brace locked at 0°)
			  Hip: Flexion
			  Extension
			  Abduction
			  Adduction
			  Standing hamstring curls
			• PREs–Supine leg press (0°–90° as indicated)
			  Heel raises
			  Bicycle
			  Step-up exercises (initiate on a 2-inch step)
			• Gait training using crutches: weight bearing as tolerated, weaning as appropriate
			• Weight shifting
			• Joint mobilization as indicated
			  Patella glides
			  Tibia-femoral (posterior) glides
				Achieve the following by the end of week 4:
				• ROM 0°–125°
				• Transfers (supine–sit) without assisting involved leg (SLR independent)
				• Good quality thigh and calf muscle contraction
				• Full weight bearing
				• Walk without crutches or cane (household and limited community distances)
				• Self-manage edema/pain
					• Provide support and proprioceptive feedback
					• Prevent complications
					• Control pain
					• Manage edema
					• Provide PROM to improve joint mobility and decrease pain
					• Initiate home exercise program
					• Teach isometrics to improve muscle recruitment in preparation for functional activities
					• Provide AROM to improve neuromuscular coordination, strength, transfers, and gait
					• Promote self-management of pain
					• Educate that closed-chain exercises placed decreased stress on the graft
					• Provide gait training to progress independent ambulation
					• Increase strength and tolerance to weight bearing
					• Perform joint mobilization to improve ROM and prevent complications

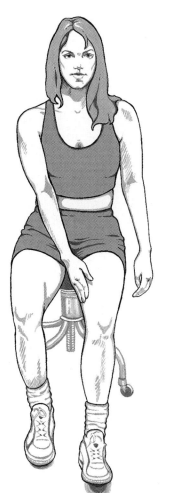

Fig. 12-1. Spider killers. Patient is seated with the involved knee (in this case the left) flexed to a comfortable position (70 to 90 degrees). The patient is instructed to palpate over the vastus medialis oblique while applying pressure down through the heel (ankle dorsiflexed) eliciting a quadriceps/hamstring co-contraction.

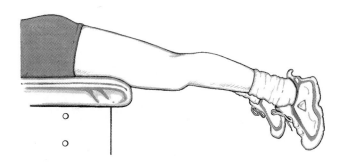

Fig. 12-2. Prone heel hangs. Patient is in the prone position with the involved leg hanging over the edge of the table or bed. Care is taken to avoid pressure on the patella.

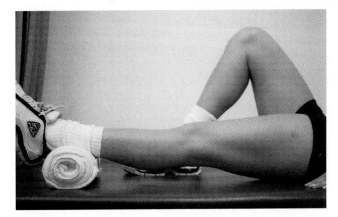

Fig. 12-3. Passive knee extension. Patient is supine or sitting with involved leg straight, into full extension. A towel is placed under the heel, allowing the knee to hang. Care is taken to avoid rotating the hip.

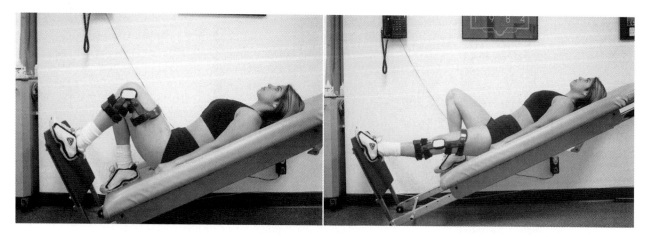

Fig. 12-4. Inclined sled. The use of an inclined sled can be initiated early to recruit volitional muscle contraction in a limited weight-bearing (resistance) environment.

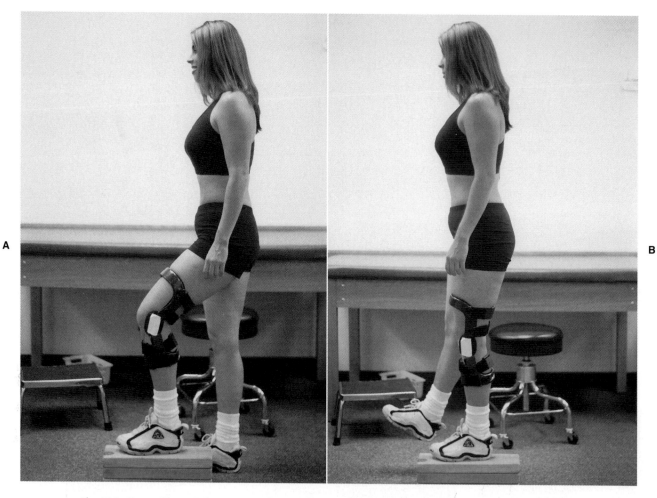

A

B

Fig. 12-5. Step up/down. Patients progress from 2-inch to 6-inch high steps. Care is taken to avoid increased stress on the graft and patella (knee is kept in line with the foot and not allowed to migrate anterior to the toes during the exercise).

to give a sense of security initially. Exercises that require brace support (locked at 0 degrees) initially include the following:

- Proprioceptive neuromuscular facilitation (PNF) patterns of the hip[35]
- Hip flexion, extension, abduction, and adduction
- Inclined sled (Fig. 12-4)
- Leg presses

Step-up activities (Fig. 12-5) are performed (when appropriate) with the brace unlocked and motion limited. An inclined sled or leg press can be used for ankle plantar flexion strengthening and initial bilateral squatting activity within pain-free ranges (usually 20 to 70 degrees, but progressing to 0 to 90 degrees as able). Stationary bicycling is performed with both legs after a ROM of 100 degrees flexion is obtained; it is initiated not for cardiovascular but for neurophysiologic purposes. The brace should be locked during ambulation until adequate quadriceps contraction is available to control the knee during the stance phase. The physical therapist can wean the patient from crutches as tolerance to weight bearing dictates. Exercise repetitions should be carried out to the point of fatigue, or 30 repetitions per set. Resistance may be added as appropriate above the knee for hip exercises and at the ankle for standing hamstring curls. Exercise progression throughout rehabilitation is guided by the Delorme method.[29] Depending on the duration of therapy, the therapist should vary the exercises to keep the treatments from becoming prosaic.[100]

Joint mobilization is initiated in the form of early PF and tibiofemoral (TF) mobilization. To avoid complications, all PF glides are initiated after consideration of incision integrity. The physical therapist instructs patients in self-mobilization techniques as part of the home exercise program. Mobilization of the TF joint also improves extension. Techniques described by Maitland[61] have proven successful in this regard. Posterior gliding of the tibia on the femur also is helpful in gaining flexion ROM.

Phase II

TIME: Weeks 5 to 8 after surgery
GOALS: Increased ROM, increased independence in performing transfers and in gait performance, full weight bearing, good management of pain and edema (Table 12-3)

By the end of the fourth week after surgery the physical therapist should be concerned with lingering ROM deficits, edema, and increases in the intensity of pain because these could signal potential complications (e.g., arthrofibrosis, PF dysfunction, patient noncompliance). At the beginning of the second phase of rehabilitation the patient should have the following:

- No increase in KT-1000 readings
- 0 to 110 degrees ROM (ideally 125 degrees flexion)
- Independence in lifting the involved leg when performing transfers
- Full weight bearing
- Independence with gait (no crutches or cane) in walking household and limited community distances
- Good management of pain and edema

The hallmark of this phase is the progression to an independent functional status for activities of daily living (ADLs). In weeks 5 through 8, joint mobilization is continued on an as-needed basis to maintain extension and improve flexion. By this time patients should continue performing home exercises without much cueing. The brace is worn for the exercises already listed as well as for gait activities. The therapist increases the exercise intensity from AROM to progressive resistance exercises (PREs). Stepping activities are progressed on a height basis (2 to 6 inches) to prepare the patient for community ambulation. Isokinetic exercises are performed in a limited ROM (90-30 degrees), as before. The patient continues gait training, shifting the focus from increasing weight-bearing tolerance to normalizing the gait pattern. The therapist adds balance exercises to work on proprioception. By the end of the eighth week, patients should be walking through figure-eight and box patterns.

A. Anteroposterior mobilization movements into resistance at end range (using grades III and IV) were applied to the tibia while the knee was in extension. PROM for knee extension increased immediately and pain with quadriceps sets was alleviated. It was postulated that the tibia was not articulating with the femur at its normal contact point during knee extension and terminal knee extension movements. After the mobilizations the tibia was better able to contact the femur, thus improving the arthrokinematics of the joint.

Q. Doug is a 45-year-old fireman. He had an ACL reconstruction 9 weeks ago on his left knee. Because of mishaps and personal reasons, physical therapy was not initiated until 5 weeks ago. Presently (9 weeks after surgery) PROM for knee flexion is 110 degrees. The end range is beginning to feel leathery. The quadriceps muscles also are restricted. Swelling and complaints of pain are usually minimal. Strength is gradually progressing. What treatment techniques could promote increased knee flexion?

Table 12-3   ACL Reconstruction

Rehabilitation Phase	Criteria to Progress to this Phase	Anticipated Impairments and Functional Limitations	Intervention	Goal	Rationale
Phase II Postoperative 5-8 weeks	• ROM 0°-110° • No increase in edema • No increase in pain • No increase in laxity as measured by KT-1000	• Limited ROM • Limited strength • Limited gait • Limited transfers • Minimal pain: unable to run, jump, or pivot	• Braces should be worn for all exercises in **bold type** • Continue phase I exercises (patient may have functional brace by 6 weeks, depending on physician) • Exercise intensity progressed from AROM to PREs • **PREs–Step up/down, progress to 6-inch step** • **Isokinetics–Limited range (90°-30°)** • **Walking program inclusive of boxes and figure 8s** • **Balance exercises** • **Patient education** • Continue joint mobilization	Achieve the following by the end of week 8: • ROM 0°-135° • 100% single leg squat 90°-0° • Gait with functional brace 1 mile • Transfer sit-stand (equal weight bearing) • Self-manage pain • Stand for 1 hour	• Wear brace for additional proprioceptive input to the knee and to increase stability • Increase muscle strength to progress functional activities • Use limited range on open-chain exercises to protect graft • Prepare for return to sport or activity • Increase patient self-reliance for exercise and self-management • Improve joint mechanics and normalize arthrokinematics

A. Doug assumed a prone position and the therapist performed gentle contraction/relaxation stretches to the quadriceps. Doug then moved into the supine position with his left knee flexed to its end range. Tibial antero-posterior glides were performed with vigor, followed by PROM for knee flexion with over pressures. Next, Doug rode the stationary bicycle. Massage and cryotherapy were used during treatments to decrease swelling. After two or three of these treatments, Doug's knee flexion increased to 0 to 125 degrees.

Phase III

TIME: Weeks 9 to 16 after surgery
GOALS: Independence in ADLs and readiness for sports participation (Table 12-4)

By the ninth week postoperatively, patients should have close to full ROM; be able to perform a unilateral squat with 100% body weight (0 to 90 degrees); walk up to 1 mile; tolerate standing for up to 1 hour; and demonstrate independence in self-management of exercises. The hallmark of this phase is progression from being a functionally independent person with ADLs to resumption of the previous level of physical activity (running, hiking, sports).

The physical therapist should progress the exercises as in prior phases and continue with PREs in the form of open- and closed-chain exercises. Resistance may be added to gait training exercises in the form of elastic tubing, thus improving multidirectional (forward, backward, side-to-side, diagonally) weight acceptance of the involved leg. The patient may use a variety of equipment to improve strength, balance, proprioception, and cardiovascular conditioning (see Fig. 13-9).

After the patient tolerates prolonged walking on a level surface (45 minutes to 1 hour) without any pain or edema and has been cleared by the physician, the patient can initiate a running program under the direction of the physical therapist. This usually takes place after the third month. This return to activity depends on the patient's status and must be initiated as appropriate to the patient's previous level of function. A trampoline can be used initially to increase tolerance to landing on the involved side with some cushioning. The authors of this chapter suggest a simple progression for the return to running. It is based on activity or sport need and allows a rest day between runs, as follows:

Running Program
Week 1
¼ mile walk then ¼ mile run (50% effort) for 4 repetitions, 3 times a week

Week 2
¼ mile walk then ½ mile run (50% effort) for 2 repetitions, 3 times a week
Week 3
¼ mile walk then 1 mile run (50% effort) then ¼ mile walk for 1 repetition, 3 times a week
Week 4
¼ mile walk then ¼ mile run (50% effort) then ¼ mile walk then ½ mile run (75% effort) then ¼ mile walk for 2 repetitions, 3 times a week
Week 5
¼ mile walk then 1 mile run (75% effort) then ¼ mile walk for 2 repetitions, 3 times a week
Week 6
¼ mile walk then ¼ mile run (75% effort) then ¼ mile walk then ½ mile run (100% effort) then ¼ mile walk for 2 repetitions, 3 times a week
Week 7
¼ mile walk then 1 mile run (100% effort) then ¼ mile walk for 2 repetitions, 3 times a week

The program is modified to fit the individual's needs and abilities. The patient should run on level surfaces, using a school track if possible. Along with the running program, the physical therapist should incorporate conditioning for other parts of the body (e.g., abdominals, upper extremities) as applicable to the sport or activity the patient wishes to resume.

Phase IV

TIME: 4 to 6 months after surgery
GOALS: Return to activity or sport (Table 12-5)

The last phase of rehabilitation focuses on the actual return to the activity or sport. Although the time frame varies with the demands of the activity, Malone and Garrett[63] note that it is possible to return to the sport at 6 months if the patient has successfully completed "controlled physiologic rehabilitation." Thus initiating the training at the 4-month point allows 2 months of functional training and progression. Isokinetic testing is another piece of the puzzle used to determine whether the patient is ready to return to sport.[41] Shelbourne et al[91] described criteria for return as follows:

- Full ROM
- 65% strength
- Completion of prescribed running and agility drills

The factors that most rehabilitation programs use to evaluate readiness for return to sport are KT-1000 stability, isokinetic equivalence, and functional tests.* The most useful of these, without denying the importance of others, is functional testing. By using a complement of functional and isokinetic tests the therapist and physician can determine when return to sport is appropriate.

---

*References 28, 30, 31, 53, 57, 64, 74, 92.

Table 12-4 ACL Reconstruction

Rehabilitation Phase	Criteria to Progress to this Phase	Anticipated Impairments and Functional Limitations	Intervention	Goal	Rationale
Phase III Postoperative 9-16 weeks	• Same as in phase II • No loss in ROM • No increase in edema or pain	• Limited strength • Limited balance and coordination • Unable to run, jump, or pivot	• Brace should be worn for all exercises in **bold type** • Phase I and II exercises as indicated • PREs using closed and open chain (isokinetic) (open chain 90°-30°) • **Trampoline jogging progressing to single leg balance/hop** • Initiate running when cleared by physician (usually by third month) • Sport-/and activity-specific drills as appropriate	Achieve the following by the end of week 16: • Come within 10% of full range flexion • Isokinetic test within 25% of uninvolved knee • Run 1+ miles without pain (patient dependent) • Initiate sport- or activity-specific training, modifying appropriately	• Increase stability of the knee while limiting stress on the graft • Prepare for functional activities such as jumping and hopping • Prepare to return to sports

Table 12-5   ACL Reconstruction

Rehabilitation Phase	Criteria to Progress to this Phase	Anticipated Impairments and Functional Limitations	Intervention	Goal	Rationale
Phase IV Postoperative 17+ weeks	• Same as in phase III	• Limited strength with jumping, hopping, and cutting activities	• Continuation of exercises from phases I-III as indicated • Plyometrics: hopping and jumping activities • Sport-specific activities	• Achieve the following before return to sport or activity: • Isokinetic test within 10% • Functional tests within criteria to return to sport • Return to sport by 8-12 months	Return to sport or activity safely and confidently

The hop and stop,[53] vertical jump, single-leg hop (6 meters for time and distance),[14] triple jump,[14,84] and stair hopple[84] are the most common functional tests referenced in the literature to assess stability and strength after ACL reconstruction. To evaluate readiness to return to previous activities, the authors of this chapter follow an eclectic approach similar to that of Lephart et al,[57] who use a combination of functional tests and self-assessment of ability. Two tests are used regularly:

1. *Single-leg hop (for distance)*—Patient stands on involved leg and performs a long jump type movement. Distance is measured from take-off (toe) to landing (heel). The physical therapist compares the distance with the uninvolved side (three trials each, take best effort of the three).
2. *Single-leg hop (for time)*—The physical therapist measures off 6 meters, and the patient performs single-leg hops over the measured distance. Time is measured with a stopwatch or other device. The physical therapist compares the distance with the uninvolved side (three trials each, take the best effort of the three).

Suggested Home Maintenance for the Postsurgical Patient

An exercise program has been outlined at the various phases. The home maintenance box on page 223 outlines the rehabilitation the patient is to follow. The physical therapist can use it in customizing a patient-specific program. Home exercises are progressed through the four phases of rehabilitation based on the patient's tolerance to activity. Any increase in edema, pain, or laxity should be addressed early and exercises should be modified to eliminate complications.

Troubleshooting

The most frequent problems encountered after ACL surgery are joint stiffness, flexion contractures, patellar irritability, and quadriceps weakness.[101,104] Less frequently, complications include reflex sympathetic dystrophy (<1%), neurovascular injury (<1%), deep venous thrombosis, infection and possible fluid extravasation, and compartment syndromes (especially with endoscopic techniques).

The incidence of stiffness after ACL reconstruction is reduced by using proper surgical technique combined with an aggressive rehabilitation program. Improper graft placement with the tibial tunnel too far anterior or inadequate notchplasty can cause graft impingement, blocking terminal knee extension. Intraoperative inspection of the graft throughout a full ROM should always be conducted to ensure that the graft is not impinging within the intercondylar notch.[48]

One of the most devastating complications after ACL reconstruction is the development of arthrofibrosis. The knee synovium and fat pad become inflamed, leading to a thickened joint capsule. This in turn begins to obliterate the medial and lateral gutters and suprapatellar pouch. The patellar tendon can shorten, produce patella baja, and eventually cause articular damage. Paulos et al[78] have defined three stages in the arthrofibrotic knee:

1. In the early stage, stage 1 (2 to 6 weeks), decreased extension is noted in addition to quadriceps lag, diminished patellar mobility, joint swelling, and failure to progress in rehabilitation.
2. Stage 2, the active stage (6 to 30 weeks), is defined by a marked decrease in ROM, decreased patellar mobility, quadriceps atrophy, skin changes, and osteopenia. These patients walk with a significant limp.

3. The residual stage, stage 3 (beyond 8 months), is defined by a marked decrease in ROM, patellar rigidity, quadriceps atrophy, patella baja, osteopenia, and possibly arthrosis.

The physical therapist should manage arthrofibrosis early to attempt restoration of full mobility. A knee with a significant flexion contracture can cause greater impairment than an ACL-deficient knee. Antiinflammatory agents, aggressive physical therapy, and patellar mobilization are the initial treatments for all stages of arthrofibrosis. Arthroscopic debridement, open debridement, and dynamic splinting are usually required in the later stages.

PF pain commonly occurs after ACL reconstruction, although more frequently after BPB autograft reconstructions than with hamstring autograft reconstructions. Bach et al[7] reported an 18% incidence of mild PF symptoms in a 2- to 4-year follow-up study.

Patellar fractures have been reported in the literature as a late complication of BPB graft harvest. These are believed to be stress fractures that develop because of the decreased vascularity of the patella. Patellar fracture also can occur intraoperatively during graft harvest and has been reported postoperatively. Brownstein and Bronner[15] reported the incidence of patellar fractures at 0.5% and note that it usually occurs as a result of a fall. They put the patella at highest risk for fracture during rehabilitation at 10 to 14 weeks postoperatively. Pain over the tibial tubercle is less frequently encountered but may occur in those with prominent tibial tubercles. If the patient has limited joint motion preoperatively, especially in extension, a continuous passive motion device should be used immediately postoperatively.[30]

During the first postoperative phase, ROM complications, if present, usually occur in extension. If mobilization and home exercises are not effective, the patient should try adding weight to the ankle during the prone hanging exercises. Duration and intensity are determined individually, but the authors of this chapter generally start with 3 to 5 lb for a 5-minute increment and have the patient follow through at home three to five times a day. In addition, the patient can add weights to the knee while performing supine knee extension (towel propped under the heel) and progress in a similar manner.

Strength complications are addressed using electrical stimulation over the muscles in conjunction with exercise. The physical therapist also can initiate biofeedback. Taping of the patella (after the incision has healed) can be useful in addressing PF issues.

Persistent swelling may indicate hemarthrosis, synovitis, reinjury, or infection.[30] If by 4 to 6 weeks the patient has not gained full extension, the cause may be patellar entrapment. Use of patellar mobilization to a greater extent and with more vigor and serial casting may be considered. Arthroscopy is usually considered if full extension is not obtained by the eighth week.[101] If reflex sympathetic dystrophy occurs, it is usually seen by the fifth week postoperatively.

Complications also can occur in phase II. Motion limitations are of primary concern and require aggressive management, as mentioned earlier. Some patients may need to be manipulated or evaluated for surgery during this phase. As the patient progresses with strengthening exercises, the physical therapist should pay careful attention to the PF articulation. This mechanism must be continually evaluated as the resistance of the exercises is progressed.

Pool exercises may be a helpful adjunct in developing strength, ROM, and weight-bearing tolerance. For phases III and IV, pool exercises in the form of deep-water running and activity-specific drills are a good adjunct to land-based rehabilitation. Plyometric exercises have long been used to improve athletic performance; they should be initiated as early as appropriate.

Summary

Clinical management after ACL reconstruction can follow many directions. The most efficient management is one in which the patient is an educated and active participant in rehabilitation. Early restoration of full extension (1 to 4 weeks) is imperative to a successful outcome, as is awareness of potential complications that may limit progress. The number of visits depends on the patient's involvement, functional goals, and complications. Return to sports depends on strength, skill acquisition, and response of the knee to the activity.

❧ Suggested Home Maintenance for the Postsurgical Patient

Phase I—Weeks 1-4

GOALS FOR THE PERIOD: Mobilization and stretching
1. Use heel slides, wall slides (supine with involved foot against the wall, gravity assisted into flexion), prone heel hangs, supine passive knee extension, quadriceps/hamstring co-contraction isometrics, four-way SLR (flexion/extension/adduction/abduction) with brace, standing hamstring curls, and self-patella mobilization.
2. Perform exercises 3 times a day with repetitions and sets determined by strength—usually 2 sets of as many as 30 repetitions.

Phase II—Weeks 5-8

GOALS FOR THE PERIOD: Progressively more difficult exercises based on tolerance to activity
1. Do the same exercises as for weeks 0 to 4.
2. Continue PROM exercises on an as-needed basis.
3. Add seated passive flexion.
4. Add step up/down with appropriate-height object (local phone book versus county phone book) and single limb balance activities.
5. Follow a walking program (as much as 45 minutes of continuous walking on level surfaces daily).
6. Try box and figure-eight exercises.

Phase III—Weeks 9-16

GOALS FOR THE PERIOD: Education for return to sport
1. Prescribe activities designed to allow a return to gym-based exercises.
2. Begin foundational exercises for return to sport.

Phase IV—Week 17 and Beyond

GOALS FOR THE PERIOD: Return to pre-injury level of participation
1. Add one-legged hopping and jumping activities.
2. Perform exercises specific to sport.

REFERENCES

1. Aglietti P et al: Patellofemoral problems after intraarticular anterior cruciate ligament reconstruction, *Clin Orthop Rel Res* 288:195, 1993.
2. Alm A, Lijedahlso SO, Stromberg B: Clinical and experimental experience in reconstruction of the anterior cruciate ligament, *Orthop Clin North Am* 7:181, 1976.
3. Amiel D et al: The phenomenon of 'ligamentization': anterior cruciate ligament reconstruction with autogenous patellar tendon, *J Orthop Res* 4:162, 1986.
4. Arms SW et al: The biomechanics of anterior cruciate ligament rehabilitation and reconstruction, *Am J Sports Med* 12(1):8, 1984.
5. Arnoczky SP: The vascularity of the anterior cruciate ligament and associated structures. Its role in repair and reconstruction. In Jackson DW, Drez D, editors: *The anterior cruciate deficient knee: new concepts in ligament repair*, St Louis, 1987, Mosby.
6. Arnoczky SP, Tarvin GB, Marshall JL: Anterior cruciate ligament replacement using patellar tendon, *Am J Bone Joint Surg* 643:217, 1982.
7. Bach BR, Jr et al: Arthroscopy-assisted anterior cruciate ligament reconstruction using patellar tendon substitution. Two-to-four-year follow-up results, *Am J Sports Med* 22(6):758, 1994.
8. Bach BR et al: Arthroscopically assisted anterior cruciate ligament reconstruction using patellar tendon autograft. Five- to nine-year follow-up evaluation, *Am J Sports Med* 26(1):20, 1998.
9. Barber FA et al: Is an anterior cruciate ligament reconstruction outcome age dependent?, *Arthroscopy* 12(6):720, 1996.
10. Barnes L: Cryotherapy: putting injury on ice, *Phys Sports Med* p. 7130, 1979.
11. Barrata R et al: Muscular coactivation: The role of the antagonist musculature in maintaining knee stability, *Am J Sports Med* 16(2):113, 1988.

12. Bock B, Malinin T, Brown M: Bone transplantation and human immunodeficiency virus: an estimate of the risk of acquired immunodeficiency syndrome (AIDS), *Clin Orthop* 240:129, 1989.

13. Boland AL: Rehabilitation of the injured athlete. In Strauss RH, editor: *Sports medicine and physiology*, Philadelphia, 1979, WB Saunders.

14. Bolga LA, Keskula DR: Reliability of lower extremity functional performance tests, *JOSPT* 26(3):138, 1997.

15. Brownstein B, Bronner S: Patella fractures associated with accelerated ACL rehabilitation in patients with autogenous patella tendon reconstructions, *JOSPT* 26(3):168, 1997.

16. Cabaud ME, Rodkey WG, Feagin JA: Experimental studies of acute anterior cruciate ligament injury and repair, *Am J Sports Med* 7:18, 1979.

17. Campbell WC: Reconstruction of the ligaments of the knee, *Am J Surg* 43:473, 1939.

18. Chatman AB et al: The patient-specific functional scale: measurement properties in patients with knee dysfunction, *Phys Ther* 77(8):820, 1997.

19. Cho KO: Reconstruction of the ACL by semitendinosus, *J Bone Joint Surg* 68B:739, 1986.

20. Ciccotti MG et al: Non-operative treatment of ruptures of the anterior cruciate ligament in middle-aged patients. Results after long term follow-up, *JBJS* 76A(9):1315, 1994.

21. Cohn BT, Draeger RI, Jackson DW: The effects of cold therapy in the postoperative management of pain in patients undergoing anterior cruciate ligament reconstruction, *Am J Sports Med* 17(3):344, 1989.

22. Corsetti JR, Jackson DW: Failure of anterior cruciate ligament reconstruction: the biologic basis, *Clin Orthop Rel Res* 323:42, 1996.

23. Cosgarea AJ, Sebastianelli WJ, DeHaven KE: Prevention of arthrofibrosis after anterior cruciate ligament reconstruction using the central third patellar tendon autograft, *Am J Sports Med* 23(1):87, 1995.

24. Daniel DM: Principles of knee ligament surgery. In Daniel DM, Akeson WH, O'Connor J, editors: *Knee ligaments: structure, function and repair*, New York, 1990, Raven.

25. Daniel DM, Stone ML, Arendt DL: The effect of cold therapy on pain, swelling, and range of motion after anterior cruciate ligament reconstructive surgery, *Arthroscopy* 10(5):530, 1994.

26. Daniel DM et al: Fate of the ACL-injured patient. A prospective outcome study, *Am J Sports Med* 22(5):632, 1994.

27. DeCarlo MS, Sell KE: The effects of the number and frequency of physical therapy treatments on selected outcomes of treatment in patients with anterior cruciate ligament reconstruction, *JOSPT* 26(6):332, 1997.

28. DeCarlo MS et al: Traditional versus accelerated rehabilitation following ACL reconstruction: a one-year follow-up, *JOSPT* 15(6):309, 1992.

29. DeLorme TL, Watkins A: *Progressive resistance exercise*, New York, 1951, Appleton-Century.

30. DeMaio M, Noyes FR, Mangine RE: Principles for aggressive rehabilitation after reconstruction of the anterior cruciate ligament. Sports medicine rehabilitation series, *Orthopedics* 15(3):385, 1992.

31. Dietrichson J, Souryal TO: Physical therapy after arthroscopic surgery, 'preoperative and post operative rehabilitation after anterior cruciate ligament tears', *Orthop Phys Ther Clin North Am* 3(4): , 1994.

32. Doucette SA, Child DD: The effects of open and closed chain exercise and knee joint position on patellar tracking in lateral patellar compression syndrome, *JOSPT* 23(2):104, 1996.

33. Drez D, Faust DC, Evans IP: Cryotherapy and nerve palsy, *Am J Sports Med* 9:256, 1981.

34. Ellison AE: Distal iliotibial-band transfer for anterolateral rotatory instability of the knee, *JBJS* 61:330, 1979.

35. Engle RP, Canner GC: Proprioceptive neuromuscular facilitation (PNF) and modified procedures for anterior cruciate ligament (ACL) instability, *JOSPT* 11(4):230, 1989.

36. Fielder B et al: Effect of gamma irradiation on the human immunodeficiency virus, *JBJS* 76A:1032, 1994.

37. Fitzgerald GK: Open versus closed kinetic chain exercises: issues in rehabilitation after anterior cruciate ligament reconstructive surgery, *Phys Ther* 77(12):1747, 1997.

38. Frank CB, Jackson DW: The science of reconstruction of the anterior cruciate ligament, *JBJS* 79A(10):1556, 1997.

39. Fu FH, Schulte KR: Anterior cruciate ligament surgery 1996 state of the art?, *Clin Orthop Rel Res* 325:19, 1996.

40. Fu FH, Woo SL-Y, Irrgang JJ: Current concepts for rehabilitation following anterior cruciate ligament reconstruction, *JOSPT* 15(6):270, 1992.

41. Grace TG et al: Isokinetic muscle imbalance and knee-joint injuries, *Am J Bone Joint Surg* 66:734, 1984.

42. Grood ES et al: Biomechanics of the knee-extension exercise. Effect of cutting the anterior cruciate ligament, *Am J Bone Joint Surg* 66:725, 1984.

43. Hardin JA et al: The effects of "decelerated" rehabilitation following anterior cruciate ligament reconstruction on a hyperelastic female adolescent: a case study, *JOSPT* 26(1):29, 1997.

44. Henning C, Lych M, Glick J: An in vivo strain gauge study of the elongation of the anterior cruciate ligament, *Am J Sports Med* 13(1):22, 1985.

45. Hey-Groves EW: The crucial ligaments of the knee joint. Their function, rupture, and operative treatment of the same, *Br J Surg* 7:505, 1920.

46. Hirokawa S et al: Anterior-posterior and rotational displacement of the tibia elicited by quadriceps contraction, *Am J Sports Med* 20(3):299, 1992.

47. Howell SM: Anterior tibial translation during a maximum quadriceps contraction: is it clinically significant?, *Am J Sports Med* 18(6):573, 1990.

48. Howell SM, Taylor MA: Failure of reconstruction of the anterior cruciate ligament due to impingement by the intercondylar roof, *J Bone Joint Surg* 75A:1044, 1993.

49. Insall JJ et al: Bone block iliotibial-band transfer for ACL insufficiency, *JBJS* 63:560, 1981.

50. Jacobsen K: Osteoarthritis following insufficiency of the cruciate ligaments in man. A clinical study, *Acta Orthop Scan* 48:520, 1977.

51. Johnson RJ et al: Five to ten year follow-up evaluation after reconstruction of the anterior cruciate ligament, *Clin Orthop* 83:122, 1984.

52. Jones KG: Reconstruction of the anterior cruciate ligament using the central one-third of the patella ligaments, a follow-up report, *JBJS* 63A:1302, 1970.

53. Juris PM et al: A dynamic test of lower extremity function following anterior cruciate ligament reconstruction and rehabilitation, *JOSPT* 26(4):184, 1997.

54. Knight KL: *Cryotherapy in sport injury management*, Champaign, IL, 1995, Human Kinetics.

55. Kurosaka M, Yoshiyas S, Andrish JT: Biomechanical comparison of different surgical techniques of graft fixation in anterior cruciate ligament reconstruction, *Am J Sports Med* 15:225, 1987.

56. Lange GW et al: Electromyographic and kinematic analysis of graded treadmill walking and the implications for knee rehabilitation, *JOSPT* 23(5):294, 1996.

57. Lephart SM et al: Relationship between selected physical characteristics and functional capacity in the anterior cruciate ligament insufficient athlete, *JOSPT* 16(4):174, 1992.

58. Lessard LA et al: The efficacy of cryotherapy following arthroscopic knee surgery, *JOSPT* 26(1):14, 1997.

59. Liu SH et al: Collagen in tendon, ligament, and bone healing: a current review, *Clin Orthop Rel Res* 318:265, 1995.

60. MacIntosh DL, Tregonning RJA: A follow-up and evaluation of the over-the-top repair of acute tears of the anterior cruciate ligament, *J Bone Joint Surg* 59B:511, 1977.

61. Maitland GD: *Peripheral manipulation*, ed 3, London, 1991, Butterworth-Heinemann.

62. Malone T, Friedhoff GC: Knee bracing—the prophylactic knee bracing debate, *Biomechanics* (special report) p. 23, May 1997.

63. Malone TR, Garrett WE, Jr: Commentary and historical perspective of anterior cruciate ligament rehabilitation, *JOSPT* 15(6):265, 1992.

64. Mangine RE, Noyes FR: Rehabilitation of the allograft reconstruction, *JOSPT* 15(6):294, 1992.

65. Mangine RE, Noyes FR, DeMaio M: Minimal protection program: advanced weight bearing and range of motion after ACL reconstruction—weeks 1-5, *Orthopedics* 15(4):504, 1992.

66. Marshall JL, Warren RJ, Wickiewicz TL: The anterior cruciate ligament. A technique of repair and reconstruction, *Clin Orthop* 143:97, 1979.

67. Marshall JL, Warren RJ, Wickiewicz TL: Primary surgical treatment of anterior cruciate ligament lesions, *Am J Sports Med* 10:103, 1982.

68. McLean DA: The use of cold and superficial heat in the treatment of soft tissue injuries, *Br J Sports Med* 23:53, 1989.

69. McMaster WC: A literary review on ice therapy in injuries, *Am J Sports Med* 5:124, 1977.

70. Morrissey MC: Reflex inhibition of thigh muscles in knee injury, *Sports Med* 7:263, 1989.

71. Neeb TB et al: Assessing anterior cruciate ligament injuries: the association and differential value of questionnaires, clinical tests, and functional tests, *JOSPT* 26(6):324, 1997.

72. Nicholas JA, Minkoff J: Iliotibial band transfer through the intercondylar notch for combined anterior instability, *Am J Sports Med* 6:341, 1978.

73. Novak PJ, Bach BR, Jr, Hager CA: Clinical and functional outcome of anterior cruciate ligament reconstruction in the recreational athlete over the age of 35, *Am J Knee Surg* 9(3):111, 1996.

74. Noyes FR, Barber-Westin SD: Revision anterior cruciate ligament surgery: experience from Cincinnati, *Clin Orthop Rel Res* 325:116, 1996.

75. Noyes FR et al: Biomechanical analysis of human ligament grafts used in knee ligament repairs and reconstructions, *J Bone Joint Surg* 66A:344, 1984.

76. Gould JA, Davies GJ: *Orthopedic and sports physical therapy*, vol 2, St Louis, 1985, Mosby.

77. Paulos L et al: Knee rehabilitation after anterior cruciate ligament reconstruction and repair, *Am J Sports Med* 9(3):140, 1981.

78. Paulos LE et al: Infrapatellar contracture syndrome: an unrecognized cause of knee stiffness with patella entrapment and patella infera, *Am J Sports Med* 15:331, 1987.

79. Podesta L et al: Rationale and protocol for postoperative anterior cruciate ligament rehabilitation, *Clin Orthop* 257:262, 1990.

80. Proulx RP: Southern California frostbite, *J Am Coll Emerg Phys* 5:618, 1976.

81. Rasmussen T et al: The effects of 4 mrad of gamma irradiation on the internal mechanical properties of bone-patella tendon-bone grafts, *Arthroscopy* 10:188, 1994.

82. Renstrom P et al: Strain within the anterior cruciate ligament during a hamstring and quadriceps activity, *Am J Sports Med* 14(1):83, 1986.

83. Richmond JC, Gladstone J, MacGillivray J: Continuous passive motion after arthroscopically assisted anterior cruciate ligament reconstruction: comparison of short versus long-term use, *J Arthr Rel Surg* 7(1):39, 1991.

84. Risberg MA, Ekeland A: Assessment of functional tests after anterior cruciate ligament surgery, *JOSPT* 19(4):212, 1994.

85. Robertson DB, Daniel DM, Biden E: Soft tissue fixation to bone, *Am J Sports Med* 14:398, 1983.

86. Rochman S: Accelerating ACL rehab, *Training and Conditioning* 7(2):33, 1997.

87. Rubenstein RA et al: Effect on knee stability if full hyperextension is restored immediately after autogenous bone-patellar tendon-bone anterior cruciate ligament reconstruction, *Am J Sports Med* 23(3):365, 1995.

88. Sandberg R, Balkfors B: Reconstruction of the anterior cruciate ligament: a 5-year follow-up of 89 patients, *Acta Orthop Scand* 59(3):288, 1988.

89. Seto JL et al: Rehabilitation of the knee after anterior cruciate ligament reconstruction, *JOSPT* 11(1):8, 1989.

90. Shelbourne KD, Klootwyk TE, DeCarlo MS: Update on accelerated rehabilitation after anterior cruciate ligament reconstruction, *JOSPT* 15(6):303, 1992.

91. Shelbourne KD et al: Ligament stability two to six years after anterior cruciate ligament reconstruction with autogenous patellar tendon graft and participation in accelerated rehabilitation program, *Am J Sports Med* 23(5):575, 1995.

92. Shelbourne KD, Nitz P: Accelerated rehabilitation after anterior cruciate ligament reconstruction, *JOSPT* 15(6):256, 1992.

93. Shelbourne KD et al: Correlation of remaining patellar tendon width with quadriceps strength after autogenous bone-patellar tendon-bone anterior cruciate ligament reconstruction, *Am J Sports Med* 22(6):774, 1994.

94. Sherman MF et al: The long-term follow up of primary anterior cruciate ligament repair. Defining a rationale for augmentation, *Am J Sports Med* 19:243, 1991.

95. Silverskiold JP et al: Rehabilitation of the anterior cruciate ligament in the athlete, *Sports Med* 6:308, 1988.

96. Spencer JD, Hayes KC, Alexander IJ: Knee joint effusion and quadriceps reflex inhibition in man, *Arch Phys Med Rehabil* 65:171, 1984.

97. Tegner Y: Strength training in the rehabilitation of cruciate ligament tears, *Sports Med* 9(2):129, 1990.

98. Tegner Y, Lysholm J: Rating systems in the evaluation of knee ligament injuries, *Clin Orthop* 198:43, 1985.

99. Teitge RA, Indelicato PA, Kerlan RK: Iliotibial band transfer for anterolateral rotatory instability of the knee: summary of 54 cases, *Am J Sports Med* 8:223, 1980.

100. Tippett SR, Voight ML: *Functional progressions for sport rehabilitation,* Champaign, IL, 1995, Human Kinetics.

101. Tomaro JE: Prevention and treatment of patellar entrapment following intra-articular ACL reconstruction. Athletic training, *JNATA* 26:11, 1991.

102. Tovin BJ, Tovin TS, Tovin M: Surgical and biomechanical considerations in rehabilitation of patients with intra-articular ACL reconstructions, *JOSPT* 15(6):317, 1992.

103. Wilk KE, Andrews JR: Current concepts in the treatment of anterior cruciate ligament disruption, *JOSPT* 15(6):279, 1992.

104. Wilk KE, Andrews JR, Clancy WG: Quadriceps muscular strength after removal of the central third patellar tendon for contralateral anterior cruciate ligament reconstruction surgery: a case study, *JOSPT* 18(6):692, 1993.

105. Yack HJ, Riley LM, Whieldon TR: Anterior tibial translation during progressive loading of the ACL-deficient knee during weight-bearing and nonweight-bearing isometric exercise, *JOSPT* 20(5):247, 1994.

Chapter 13

Arthroscopic Lateral Retinaculum Release

Andrew A. Brooks
Dan Farwell

Surgical Indications

Adaptation resulting from chronic compression in the patellofemoral joint can lead to significant arthrosis in a wide variety of patients, both young and old. Pain, attributed to increased patellofemoral compression, occurs in different aspects of the joint, but the most common site is along the lateral aspect. This patellofemoral pain can originate from mechanical malalignment, the static or dynamic soft tissue stabilizers, or increased load placed across the joint as a result of various activities.[38] Symptoms may include diffuse aches and pains that are exacerbated by stair climbing or prolonged sitting (flexion of the knees). Crepitus and mild effusion are often associated with patellofemoral arthralgia. Although complaints of "giving way" or collapse are more often linked with ligamentous instability, these symptoms also can be associated with patellofemoral pain. Patients may even complain of joint pain and "locking" when they are experiencing poor patella stabilization during flexion of the knee.

In examining the way lateral retinacular release procedures may affect the arthrokinematics of the patellofemoral joint, the focus should be on the relationship between patella tilt compression and associated tightness in the lateral retinaculum. The function of the patella is to increase the lever of the quadriceps muscle, thus increasing its mechanical advantage. For functional and efficient knee motion the patella must be aligned so it can travel in the trochlear groove of the femur. The ability of the patella to track properly depends on the bony configuration of the trochlear groove and the balance of forces of the connective tissue surrounding the joint.

One of the primary factors in the development of poor patella alignment is iliotibial band (ITB) tension. Tensor fascia latae and gluteus maximus fibers combine to form this very thick, fibrous structure that attaches distally into the lateral tibial tubercle (Gerdy's tubercle).[20] The ITB slips into the lateral border of the patella, which interdigitates with the superficial and deep fibers of the lateral retinaculum. This design often leads to excessive compression over the lateral condyle and lateral border of the patella during dynamic activity.

Tilt compression is a clinical radiographic condition of the patellofemoral joint that can lead to retinacular strain (peripatellar effect) and excessive lateral pressure syndrome (ELPS; articular effect).[10] A case can definitely be made for a cause-and-effect relationship between tilt compression and retinacular strain. Chronic patella tilting and associated retinacular shortening cannot only produce significant lateral facet overload but also a resultant deficiency in medial contact pressure. This tilt compression syndrome may present as simple soft tissue pain related to the shortening of the lateral retinacular tissue. If left untreated, histologic studies of painful retinacular biopsies may reveal degenerative fibroneuromas within the lateral retinaculum of patients with chronic patellofemoral malalignment.[13] ELPS results from chronic lateral patella tilt, adaptive lateral retinacular shortening, and resultant chronic imbalance of facet loads. It is prevalent in active, middle-aged adults. In younger patient populations, excessive lateral pressure during growth and development can alter the shape and formation of both the patella and trochlea.[12]

Nonoperative treatment of patella tilt should focus on mobilization of tight quadriceps muscles and the lateral retinaculum. Patellofemoral taping, bracing, and antiinflammatory medications also are quite helpful. Gait deviation and excessive foot pronation should be corrected to eliminate possible secondary influences on patellofemoral malalignment.[38] The use of resistant weight training or isokinetic exercise (in conjunction with patella taping) can be beneficial in building quadriceps muscle strength.[40]

Patellofemoral Taping

McConnell patellofemoral taping has become a useful technique in the conservative (nonsurgical) rehabilitation of patellofemoral pain, but it can be beneficial in assisting patients after surgical lateral release as

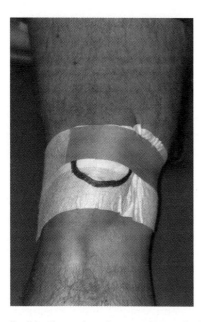

Fig. 13-1. Patella glide. Place a piece of tape on the superior half of the lateral border of the patella and pull the tape medially. Lift the soft tissue over the medial femoral condyle toward the patella to ensure a more secure fixation and less tape slippage.

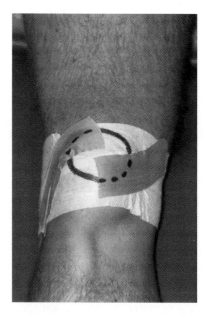

Fig. 13-3. Patella rotation. Place a piece of tape on the inferior-medial quarter of the patella and perform an upward rotation movement of the patella. Place another piece of tape on the superior-lateral half of the patella and perform a downward rotation movement of the patella.

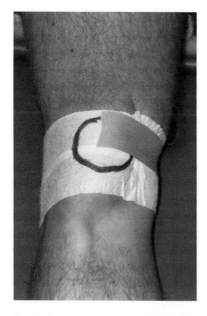

Fig. 13-2. Patella tilt. Place the tape on the medial superior half of the patella. Pull the tape medially to lift the lateral border. Lift the soft tissue over the medial femoral condyle toward the patella to ensure a more secure fixation.

well. This program emphasizes closed-chain exercises to correct patella glide (Fig. 13-1), tilt (Fig. 13-2), and rotation (Fig. 13-3) and allow for pain-free rehabilitation. The patient is evaluated dynamically during a functional activity such as walking, stepping down, or squatting. According to Maitland[25] "the aim of examining movements is to find one or more comparable signs in an appropriate joint or joints." These compa-

rable signs, or reassessment signs, are reevaluated after each patella correction to determine the effectiveness of the treatment. After an assessment of patella orientation, a specifically designed tape is used to correct for each patella orientation. The patellofemoral joint is principally a soft tissue joint, which suggests that it can be adjusted through appropriate mechanical means (i.e., physical therapy). Two primary components (glide and tilt) may be present either statically or dynamically. Patella orientation varies among patients and even from left to right extremities.

Glide component. The amount of glide correction depends on the tightness of the structures and the relative amount of activity in the entire quadriceps musculature. The corrective procedure involves securing the edge of the tape over the lateral border of the patella and pulling or gliding the patella more medially. Although this technique is useful for most patellofemoral pain, it is not often used in the postoperative care of patients recovering from lateral retinacular release (see Fig. 13-1).

Tilt component. Tilt correction is quite often used to stretch the deep retinacular fibers along the lateral borders of the knee. Increased tension in the lateral retinaculum along with a tight ITB (which inserts into the lateral retinaculum) can produce a lateral "dipping," or tilt, of the lateral border of the patella (see Fig. 13-2).

When focusing on patients recovering from lateral retinacular release, the physical therapist should remember that the very tissues these taping techniques address have been surgically released. Although patella orientations have most definitely been altered in patients after surgical release, muscle recruitment patterns and joint loading characteristics that may have contributed to the symptoms are still present. McConnell taping procedures produce improved joint loading and allow the patient to return to a more active, pain-free lifestyle when used in conjunction with closed-chain functional exercises.[37]

Surgical Considerations

Although conservative management remains the cornerstone of treatment for patients with anterior knee pain, some patients will not respond and continue to have pain and functional disability. If conservative (nonsurgical) treatment is unsuccessful in providing the patient with appropriate pain relief and function, surgical intervention should be considered.[31]

In addition to subjective complaints and functional limitations, other indications for surgery include dislocation, subluxation, and failure of previous surgery with or without medial patella position.

Operative procedures that modify patella mechanics are most successful in treating patients with patella articular cartilage lesions. Lateral release procedures should ultimately produce a mechanical benefit to the patient, such as relieving documented tilt.[39]

Surgical Procedure

Review of the literature suggests strict indications for lateral release:[11]
1. Chronic anterior knee pain despite a trial of a nonoperative program for at least 3 months
2. Minimal or no chondrosis (Outerbridge grade 2 or less)
3. A normal Q angle
4. A tight or tender lateral retinaculum with clinically and radiographically documented lateral patella tilt.

Results may be disappointing for lateral release in the presence of the following conditions:
1. Patellofemoral pain syndrome (anterior knee pain)
2. Advanced patellofemoral arthritis
3. A Q angle greater than 20 degrees

Patients with instability may require medial retinacular imbrication or a distal realignment in addition to an isolated lateral release.

The Southern California Orthopedic Institute (SCOI) technique of arthroscopic lateral release is performed in the supine position without the use of a leg holder; the tourniquet is inflated only when necessary. The procedure is performed with the arthroscope in the anteromedial portal. Routine arthroscopic fluid is used. An 18-gauge spinal needle is inserted at the superior pole of the patella and is used as a marker for the proximal extent of the release. The needle must be withdrawn as the electrosurgical electrode approaches it. With experience, the surgeon can omit the needle marker. The electrosurgical lateral release electrode is inserted through the inferior anterolateral portal using a plastic cannula to protect the skin. The procedure is performed with the generator setting at approximately 10 to 12 watts of power. With the patient's knee extended, the surgeon performs the release approximately 1 cm from the patella edge, progressing from distal to proximal using the cutting mode. The deep and superficial retinaculum as well as the lateral patellotibial ligament are released under direct visualization until subcutaneous fat is exposed. The extent of the proximal release is only to the deforming tight structures and should never extend beyond the superior pole of the patella.

An incomplete release is often secondary to inadequate release of the patellotibial ligament. Again, the tourniquet is not inflated during the procedure and vessels are coagulated as they are encountered. An adequate release is confirmed by the ability to evert the patella 60 degrees. After the release the knee is passively moved through a range of motion (ROM) and correction of lateral overhang during knee flexion is confirmed. The arthroscope should be switched back to the accessory superolateral portal for this assessment. Usual postoperative dressings are applied after the arthroscopic procedure— sterile dressings and an absorbent pad held in place by an elastic toe-to-groin support stocking previously measured for the patient.

Postoperative rehabilitation includes muscle strengthening and ROM exercises the day of surgery, including quadriceps sets and straight leg raising. The patient continues to do these exercises at home the night of surgery and is given weight bearing as tolerated status with crutches immediately. Crutches are discontinued when adequate quadriceps muscle control has been obtained and patients can walk safely. The vast majority of patients use their crutches for less than 7 days, although some may need them for 2 to 3 weeks depending on quadriceps control.

The SCOI experience with arthroscopic lateral retinaculum release (ALRR) has been reported previously.[32] The researchers followed 45 knees in 39 patients with a history of recurrent patella subluxation or dislocation for an average of 28 months and noted good to excellent results in 76% of patients. Similar experiences with ALRR have been reported in the literature, with favorable results in 60% to 85% of cases.[1] Arthroscopic treatment compares favorably with open realignment and has a lower complication rate. No postoperative hemarthrosis occurred in the SCOI series; hemarthrosis is the main complication reported in the literature, occurring in 2% to 42% of cases. Small's[35]

Table 13-1   Lateral Retinaculum Release

Rehabilitation Phase	Criteria to Progress to this Phase	Anticipated Impairments and Functional Limitations	Intervention	Goal	Rationale
Phase I Postoperative 1-2 weeks	Postoperative	• Postoperative pain • Postoperative edema • Gait deviations • Limited tolerance to weight-bearing activities • Limited ROM • Limited strength	• Ice • Vasopneumatic compression • Grade II patella mobilization • Neuromuscular stimulation • Patellar taping • Knee active range of motion (AROM)— Ankle pumps • Knee passive range of motion (PROM)— Hamstring and ITB stretches • Isometrics— Quadriceps/hamstring sets Quadriceps sets at 20°-30° • Home exercises (Refer to Suggested Home Maintenance section)	• Decrease pain • Manage edema • Decrease gait deviations • Increase tolerance to weight-bearing activities • ROM 0°-135° • Quality contraction of the quadricep	• Decrease edema and pain • Increase neuromuscular coordination with muscle contraction • Restore joint mechanics • Improve joint mobility and stability • Prevent adhesions • Initiate volitional muscle control and increase strength • Increase patient self-management

review of 194 cases of ALRR performed by 21 arthroscopic surgeons found hemarthrosis associated with 89% of the 4.6% total complication rate. Careful coagulation of vessels without an inflated tourniquet can reduce hemarthrosis. If strict criteria are met and proper surgical techniques employed, a consistent result can be obtained with these patients.

The complexity of the patellofemoral articulation and its associated disorders are evident by the significant body of literature on the subject and the abundant surgical procedures involving the joint. A thorough clinical evaluation, including history and physical and radiographic examination, helps clarify the diagnosis of patellofemoral disorder. Use of the arthroscope for the electrosurgical lateral release is an effective component in the armament of knee surgeons for patients with persistently symptomatic patellofemoral disorders who meet the surgical indications described.

Therapy Guidelines for Rehabilitation

Phase I: Acute Phase

> TIME: Weeks 1-2
> GOALS: Decrease pain, manage edema, increase weight-bearing activities, facilitate quality quadriceps contraction (Table 13-1)

After knee surgery the goal of rehabilitation is to prevent loss of muscle strength, endurance, flexibility, and proprioception. These issues often are difficult to address immediately after lateral release. The procedure is often associated with significant hemarthrosis resulting from sacrifice of the lateral geniculate artery.[2] Therefore the acute phase of treatment should focus on managing edema and decreasing pain. The use of vasopneumatic compression, electrical stimulation (ES), ice, and intermittent elevation of the limb can assist in decreasing the patient's swelling. Other strategies to both decrease joint effusion and begin restoring joint mobility include grade II (mobilizations performed shy of resistance in an effort to decrease pain)[24] patella mobilizations, active calf pumping exercises, and the application of McConnell taping[26] specific to acute lateral release rehabilitation (Fig. 13-4). This procedure places a very mild tilt on the patella, providing a small amount of length to the repair site or lateral retinacular tissue. The tape maintains the new alignment, preventing adhesions that may bind down the released retinaculum during tissue healing. Other taping procedures such as unloading the lateral soft tissue may assist in decreasing pain and discomfort during exercise (Fig. 13-5). This procedure is beneficial in decreasing joint effusion and adds joint stability. It is often used in combination with a patella tilt correction.

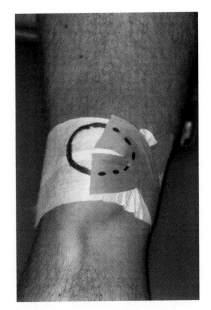

Fig. 13-4. Stabilization taping. After surgery the lateral tissue is often hypersensitive to any type of stretching or pull. The application of a taping correction for both internal and external rotation results in a low-level patella stabilization that the patient finds much easier to tolerate. Taping enables the patient to perform normal knee flexion-extension activity without pain or with less pain. It also decreases effusion.

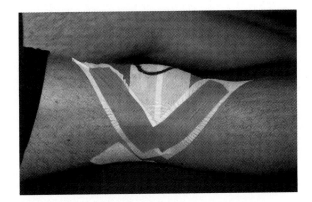

Fig. 13-5. Unloading of lateral soft tissue structures. Taping allows for a decrease in the tension produced over the surgical repair site by inhibiting the effective pull from the ITB and vastus lateralis. Unloading the lateral retinaculum may significantly reduce the patient's symptoms. Tape from the posterior aspect of the lateral joint line down to the tibial tubercle and from the posterior lateral joint line to the distal mid-thigh (approximately 2 to 3 inches above the patella). The tissue inside the tape should be pulled toward the joint line as you pull and secure the tape. The tape should look like a wide V lateral to the knee and should not inhibit active motion.

Q. Rebecca is 24 years old. She had an arthroscopic lateral release done on her right knee 18 days ago. Treatment has focused on decreasing joint effusion, pain, and discomfort. Over the past 2 days her pain has increased, with redness around the knee. What should be done?

Table 13-2   Lateral Retinaculum Release

Rehabilitation Phase	Criteria to Progress to this Phase	Anticipated Impairments and Functional Limitations	Intervention	Goal	Rationale
Phase II Postoperative 3–4 weeks	Incision healed Edema controlled Full weight bearing although full ROM and strength may be deficient	• Pain with squatting and sit-stand • Gait deviations • Limited stability of patellofemoral joint • Limited tolerance (if any) to prolonged walking, standing, running, or jumping	Continuation of interventions from phase I, progressed as indicated • Moist heat and ultrasound (if edema is under control) • Soft tissue mobilization • Neuromuscular stimulation • Closed-chain exercises, lunges, standing wall slides, and step-downs (see Figs. 13-6 through 13-8) • Biofeedback in conjunction with exercises • Patellofemoral taping (refer to weaning protocol) • Home exercises	• Achieve full ROM • Decrease pain • Increase mobility • Increase strength • Sit-stand without pain • Decrease gait deviations • Increase stability of patellofemoral joint • Tape only for skill-specific activity	• Decrease swelling and pain • Increase neuromuscular coordination with muscle contraction • Restore joint mechanics • Functional strengthening using closed-chain exercises • Biofeedback with exercise to improve VMO tonic activity • Improve joint mobility and stability • Increase patient self-management

Phase II: Subacute Phase

TIME: Weeks 3-4
GOALS: Continue to manage edema and pain, improve sit-stand transfer activities, improve strength and stability of the patellofemoral joint, progress functional training to return activity to previous levels (Table 13-2)

As the patient's swelling and pain subside (1 to 2 weeks) the patient moves into a subacute phase. During this phase a more direct and aggressive type of treatment to the knee is implemented. Heat modalities (moist heat, ultrasound) are used to assist in the absorption and removal of waste products within the joint. Their influence on the cardiovascular system produces increased capillary permeability and vasodilation. The vasodilation brings increased oxygen and nutrients to the knee, which assist in the healing and repairing of the surgically altered tissue.[21] Increased blood flow produces increased capillary hydrostatic pressure. Therefore heat modalities can be very beneficial at this stage of rehabilitation, *but only if the patient's effusion is under control.* If the patient's effusion is displacing the patella from the trochlear groove or the patient cannot perform active isometric quadriceps contractions, the joint effusion is significant. Heat applications may be contraindicated until edema is no longer a concern.

Soft tissue mobilization can be beneficial at this stage to increase circulation, decrease swelling, mobilize healing tissue, and decrease hypersensitivity in the knee joint.[12] Deep massage can assist in the reabsorption of fluid within the knee, yet manipulation of soft tissue structures over the lateral aspect of the knee should be avoided to prevent aggravation of the trauma from surgery. Soft tissue mobilization should not be initiated in the area of lateral structures before the tissues have begun to heal (1 to 2 weeks) and pain is significantly diminished on palpation of the entire patellofemoral joint.

ES is used to assist in activation of the quadriceps muscle. Specific benefits include decreasing joint edema, increasing local blood flow to the muscle, promoting increased muscle tone, and controlling postoperative pain.[22,29] Electricity also can be used to retard quadriceps atrophy, which results from immobilization or inhibition of the muscle.[14] When used in combination with active isometric and isotonic exercises, ES retrains transposed muscles and promotes muscle awareness in regaining volitional muscle control postoperatively.[21]

Experiments conducted by scientists in the USSR in the 1970s examined the possibility of producing greater intensity of muscle contraction with electrical current. Some studies have found the use of ES during immobilization produces a significant increase in muscle strength.[26,35] By using ES early in the rehabilitative process, physical therapists can prevent the loss of oxidative capacity, thus shortening postoperative rehabilitation and conditioning time and allowing a more rapid return to functional activities.[6] Although ES can be of great benefit, it should not be used as a replacement for postoperative rehabilitation and strengthening exercise programs.[5]

In summary the use of modalities is beneficial in aiding healing by decreasing acute reactions and altering blood flow, which may provide low-level analgesic effects.[22,29] Understanding the action of these modalities and the way they influence healing is important in predicting their usefulness and appropriateness in the rehabilitation of patients after lateral retinacular release.

Strengthening. Strengthening of the entire lower kinetic chain is the goal in most patients suffering from anterior knee pain. This goal is no different for patients after lateral retinacular release. Although special attention is paid to the quadriceps muscle, particularly the vastus medialis oblique (VMO), it is the balanced contraction in the vasti group as a whole that is the ultimate goal. Richardson[31] examined the activity level of the quadriceps, specifically the VMO, to better understand the activation patterns of the quadriceps during dynamic motion. The quadriceps were monitored with surface electromyography (EMG) through a full arc of motion in both patients suffering from patellofemoral pain and normal patients. The VMO produced a tonic (constant) pattern of activation throughout a full (0 to 135 degrees) arc of motion in pain-free patients; a phasic (intermittent) activity pattern was observed in patients with patellofemoral pain. A consistent activation of the entire quadriceps is the goal in quadriceps strengthening. Quality of motion should be emphasized over relative quantity. Exercise beyond 20 degrees flexion (20 to 135 degrees) increases the surface area of contact and gives better stability within the trochlear groove. Although the development of muscle strength is important, it is not the only goal of rehabilitation. Muscle endurance, flexibility, and the development of correct proprioceptive loading through the entire lower extremity must be addressed as well. These goals can be accomplished in patients recovering from surgical lateral release by protecting the surgical repair through modalities that speed the tissue repair process and protective taping that adds stability and promotes early functional rehabilitation. Early quadriceps activation includes isometric quadriceps sets in varying degrees of flexion produced by a proximal load-bearing shift with increased knee flexion.[33] This allows for early muscle strengthening even while joint effusion may still be causing pain in a closed-chain (joint loaded) position. When effusion and pain have been eliminated for 7 to 14 days, a gradual increase in activity may begin, with

Table 13-3   Lateral Retinaculum Release

Rehabilitation Phase	Criteria to Progress to this Phase	Anticipated Impairments and Functional Limitations	Intervention	Goal	Rationale
Phase III Postoperative 4-6 Weeks	• Pain-free during functional activity (sit-stand, squat 0°-90°) • Limited tolerance to walking, running, and standing	• Limited endurance with prolonged functional activities • Mild instability of patellofemoral joint during skill-specific exercises • Continued reliance on patellofemoral taping	• Closed-chain and stretching exercises as listed in Tables 13-1 and 13-2 • Patella taping • Patella mobilization • Lunges with weights, increased repetitions and speed with exercises • Progressive resistive exercises on leg press • Functional specific activity Isokinetic training • Knee flexion and extension 270°-300°/sec 10 repetitions at each speed = 1 set 2-10 sets • Home exercises	• No gait deviations • Good patella stability without taping • Unlimited community ambulation • Leg press body weight • Pain-free with specific activity • Increase strength and velocity of muscle contraction • Patient can self-manage symptoms	• Functional strengthening • Decrease pain with functional activities • Improve joint mechanics • Improve joint mobility and stability • Improve endurance of VMO • Increase strength • Specificity of training and progression to community-based gym program (if appropriate) • Use isokinetic principles of strength training • Discharge patient

cryotherapy being used after activity. During lower extremity rehabilitation, after the patient can stand or load the joint, the emphasis should be on closed-chain activity because of its relevance to function. The goal is to advance the patient toward functional activities and then slowly introduce a patient-specific exercise program. Specific closed-chain exercises allow for the selection and stimulation of the appropriate muscles at the proper time.[23] These factors, combined with gradual muscle inhibition of the antagonist, produce smooth, coordinated loading of the entire lower extremity.

Although McConnell patellofemoral taping is the modality of choice used by the authors of this chapter to bolster stability at the onset of exercise, a variety of braces may be beneficial in supporting the patellofemoral joint after surgery. Almost any elastic, compressive support around the patellofemoral joint produces an improved ability to exercise. The concept of proprioceptive feedback, together with comfort and affordability, makes postoperative McConnell patellofemoral taping or nonspecific bracing of the knee desirable in patients who do not respond to exercise alone.

A. These are signs of infection. The physical therapist should notify the physician immediately.

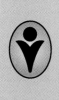

Q. Diane is 33 years old. She has a history of anterior knee pain for 2 years. Before having an arthroscopic lateral retinacular release, she used orthotics because she over-pronated during gait. She had surgery 6 weeks ago. Complaints of pain are minimal to nonexistent if she avoids all aggravating factors. However, she generally has some soreness from activities of daily living around the home and from taking care of two young children. Diane is performing all the exercises mentioned in phase I and most exercises in phase II without pain. However, she has pain during functional double-limb squats with knee flexion exceeding 60 degrees and knee pain with step-downs from a 4-inch step. What may help Diane progress with her exercise program?

Phase III: Advanced Phase

TIME: Weeks 5-6
GOALS: Patient self-manages edema and pain, performs gait without deviations, and has unlimited ambulation (Table 13-3)

By phase III patients should have their pain under control using little if any external support (brace or tape). They may continue to benefit from stretching, patella

mobilization, and taping in addition to ice after exercise. However, this phase is designed to take the patient back to the pre-injury level of function. Exercises are progressed through specificity of training principles. By breaking down the activity into its core components, the physical therapist can assess patellofemoral and lower extremity function for any deviations or barriers to performance.

Closed kinetic chain progression consists of the following:

1. Lunges with 5 lb weights in a long stride position (Fig. 13-6). Patients must activate the quadriceps and hold the contraction from 0 to 30 degrees eccentrically and back to 0 degrees concentrically without stopping, moving slowly, and maintaining proper alignment.
2. Wall slides at various degrees of flexion with 1-minute holds to promote fatigue (Fig. 13-7). The patient should progress from 0 to 45 degrees; if a certain angle in the arc of motion appears weaker, the patient can perform isometric holds at the angle of weakness.
3. Functional single-limb squats from 0 to 30 degrees. Deep flexion squats can be performed by two different methods. In the first, both lower extremities are aligned directly below the hips, and bilateral knee flexion is initiated. The patient should maintain proper patella alignment directly over the midfoot. The second method is a shortened stride position with the involved lower extremity forward. The patient initiates the squat until the knee is flexed 90 degrees and then rises back to full extension.
4. Functional double-limb squats with elastic tubing
5. Sit-to-stand at increased speed and repetition. The patient initiates sit-to-stand activity (and stand-to-sit activity) without upper extremity assistance. This exercise can be adjusted from easier to more difficult by lowering the height of the chair.
6. Step-down exercises with an increase in height of step and speed of movement. Proper alignment is crucial, along with slow, controlled movement. The patient must activate the quadriceps before motion is initiated and hold the contraction until heel contact of the opposite leg (Fig. 13-8).
7. Resistive leg press using progressive resistance exercise (PRE) protocols for weight.[9,42]
8. Standing (four-wall) elastic tubing exercises for hip flexion, extension, abduction, and adduction (the involved knee acts as the stabilizing leg). The lower extremity that anchors the body is the "working" leg. The patient should activate the quadriceps and hold throughout the entire active motion of the opposite leg. This may be performed in terminal extension or 10 to 20 degrees of knee flexion of the involved (stabilizing) leg.

Activity specific exercises (Fig. 13-9) may include the following: stationary cycle, stair climbing machine,

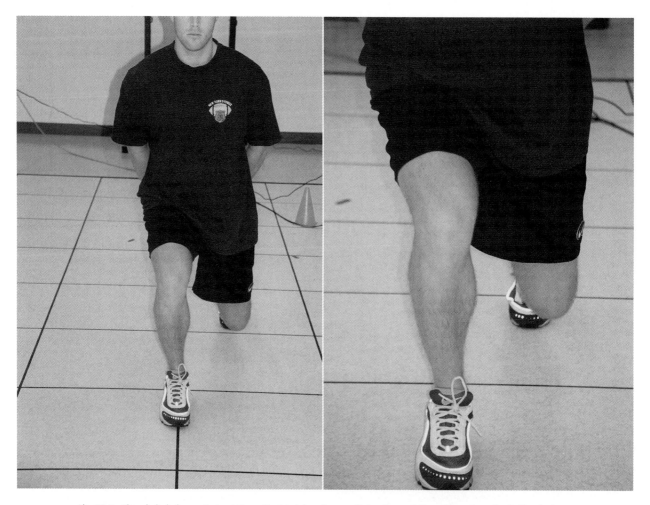

Fig. 13-6. Closed-chain lunge. Instruct the patient to take a "normal" step forward. Have the patient slowly flex the knee to 30 degrees flexion, hold for 3 seconds, and return to 0 degrees extension while maintaining proper postural alignment (anterosuperior iliac spine [ASIS] over mid-patella and second toe). The patient should be able to activate the quadriceps tonically (constantly) during the entire motion.

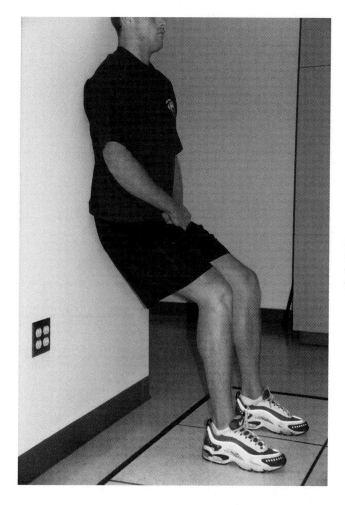

Fig. 13-7. Closed-chain wall slide. This exercise allows the patient to maintain better alignment simply by locking in pelvic tilt. The patient can then move through a particular ROM or the physical therapist can have the patient perform isometric contractions at various ranges of weakness.

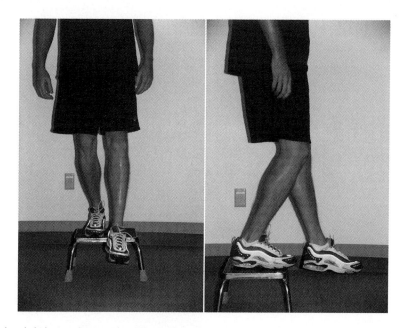

Fig. 13-8. Closed-chain step-down. Patients need to begin on a low-level step (3 to 4 in) and work up to a standard step (8 in). Patients must focus on improved alignment. Because the patient is now performing single-limb support activity, he or she should focus on gluteal muscle activation to better stabilize the femur during dynamic activity.

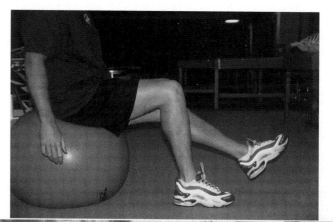

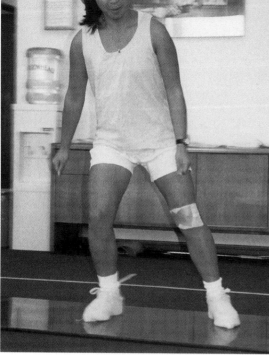

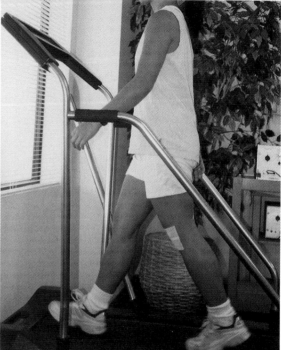

Fig. 13-9. Skill-specific training. After the patient is without pain and has developed a quality contraction that is consistent throughout full knee ROM, a sport- or activity-specific exercise program is needed to aid in the development of an improved loading pattern and promote coordinated balance in patellofemoral mechanics.

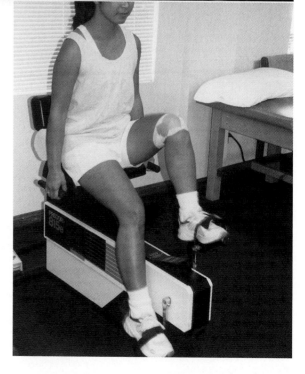

slide board, and treadmill. The authors of this chapter recommend a 6-week progression to pre-surgery activity level. Isokinetic exercise is introduced in this phase at a training velocity spectrum protocol between 270 and 300 degree/sec.[7] The patient performs 10 repetitions at each speed in a ladder progression (50 repetitions equals 1 set). Patient tolerance for exercise determines the number of sets performed (2 to 10 sets).

After patients can perform the exercises with good control of the patellofemoral joint they are weaned from formal physical therapy and encouraged to continue the home exercise program as appropriate.

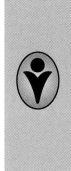

A. Diane was evaluated for patellofemoral symptoms and treated with the McConnell method of taping. She was able to progress with the closed-chain exercises when the appropriate McConnell taping procedure was used. She was able to perform double-limb squats to 80 degrees of knee flexion without pain. She also could perform two sets of 10 repetitions of step-downs on the 4-inch step without pain. Pain with the single-limb squat persisted but lessened. Therefore single-limb squats were not performed until they could be done without pain.

Suggested Home Maintenance for the Postsurgical Patient

An exercise program has been outlined at the various phases. The home maintenance box on pages 240 to 241 outlines rehabilitation ideas the patient may follow. The physical therapist can use it in customizing a patient-specific program.

Troubleshooting

Postural Alignment

A lateral retinacular release procedure produces immediate effects on the patella orientation of the knee, yet the entire lower kinetic chain may still have alignment issues that need to be addressed. When assessing a patient's functional status, the physical therapist should consider equalizing leg lengths, balancing foot posture, restoring normal gait, and regaining appropriate muscle flexibility and strength, which will lead to a restoration of normal posture and balance.[12] By observing static alignment issues, physical therapists can gather valuable information regarding the way the patient will function dynamically. The interaction of poor alignment measures and quadriceps contraction has been examined.[15] This study compared static and dynamic patellofemoral malalignment measures in subjects with anterior knee pain. Quadriceps contraction

altered the malalignment in both type and severity in more than 50% of the cases.

The literature suggests that excessive pronation at the foot is a primary problem because of its association with patellofemoral pain, which inhibits the balance of the entire lower kinetic chain.[38] Increased pronation may lead to increased valgus, compensatory external rotation of the foot and tibia, and a resultant predisposition to lateral patella tracking with dynamic activity.[16] In such cases, orthotic correction may be indicated even after a lateral retinacular release procedure to restore proper loading mechanics through the knee.

Quadriceps Inhibition

Many clinicians tend to use the term *quadriceps inhibition* as though it were synonymous with *quadriceps weakness*, which is not an accurate description. *Reflex quadriceps inhibition* is defined as the inability to perform a quadriceps contraction voluntarily because of direct neurologic suppression.[17,28]

Does true quadriceps inhibition exist? Numerous research articles on the subject describe several mechanisms that could produce a neurogenic influence on voluntary control of the quadriceps.[4,27] The effect of pain on the overall activation of the quadriceps has been examined as a possible cause.[3,41] Effusion also can impair activation of the quadriceps muscle.[8,36] Mechanic receptors within the patellofemoral joint may influence quadriceps function through proprioceptive input.[18,19] Other factors may include training methods, joint position, aging, and even the possible effects of medication.

Any problem resulting in decreased activation of the quadriceps is detrimental to the rehabilitation process. With full activation of the quadriceps femoris muscle, proper strengthening exercises should produce excellent results. However, if voluntary control is absent or compromised, atrophy and weakness may result. If this situation persists, volitional exercise protocols may be ineffective and thus temporarily inappropriate for these patients.

Because of the nature of a lateral retinacular release procedure, pain and especially effusion are quite common after surgery. Therefore any treatment techniques that address pain and swelling will ultimately assist in improved recruitment of the quadriceps femoris muscle.

Patellofemoral Tape Weaning Protocol

Patients using McConnell taping need to learn how to tape themselves. The tape loosens according to the aggressiveness of the patient's activity. The patient should therefore be taught to tighten the tape when necessary.

The patient only needs to wear tape while training the quadriceps to maintain the newly acquired length in the lateral structures. The tape should be removed at night and the skin should be cleaned. This gives the skin a resting period from the pull and friction produced by the tape.

The patient begins closed-chain exercises when pain and effusion are under control. Early home exercises stress "little bits often," meaning multiple VMO sets or quadriceps contractions are performed throughout the day and are linked with a patient's lifestyle. For example, the physical therapist may instruct a patient to perform a quadriceps contraction every time he or she sits down in a chair, palpating the VMO for feedback. When driving a car the patient may perform a quadriceps set at every stop light, taking care to leave the foot firmly on the brake. As the patient begins to recruit a quality quadriceps contraction successfully, goal setting enters into the program and the patient is asked to attempt repetitions of closed-chain exercises (lunges, wall slides, squats, step-downs). The more the patient practices, the faster the skill to activate a quality quadriceps muscle contraction is learned.

The patient is ready to be weaned off the taping protocol and continue the program with specific sports-related activity and training when he or she can do the following:

1. Sustain a quarter squat for 1 minute against the wall without pain
2. Sustain a half squat for 1 minute against the wall without pain
3. Perform 10 step-downs (off an 8-in step) for at least 5 seconds per step with good control and alignment and without pain

If functional activity produces pain and the patient is using patella taping, the physical therapist should first assess the taping procedure to ensure it is correct. The clinician may need to make small adjustments in tension and direction. At the time of discharge from the clinical facility, the patient needs to remember self patella mobilization, proper alignment, and postural issues with closed-chain exercises; the patient should be reminded that exercise should be painless.

❦ Suggested Home Maintenance for the Postsurgical Patient

Weeks 1-2

GOALS FOR THE PERIOD: Decrease pain, manage edema, increase weight-bearing activities, facilitate quality quadriceps contraction
1. Elevate and ice at home two to three times per day (preferably after exercises).
2. Perform ankle pumping and hamstring stretch while elevated on ice (20 to 30 minutes).
3. Perform self patella mobilizations (Fig. 13-10).

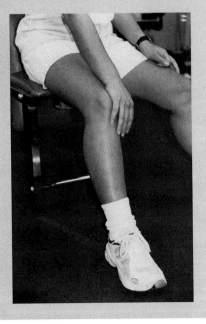

Fig. 13-10. Self mobilization. The patient should be able to perform active self stretching to the lateral retinacular tissues. The patient is instructed to place the heel of the hand over the medial half of the patella and push the medial border of the patella down into the trochlear groove. If the exercise is done properly, the lateral border tilts anteriorly, stretching the lateral retinacular tissue. The knee should be placed in at least 30 degrees of flexion to ensure stability in the trochlear groove and guard against lateral gliding of the patella. The patient progresses into deeper ranges of flexion as pain and lateral tissue tension subside. Each stretch should be held for 5 seconds for two to three repetitions, three to four times a day.

❧ Suggested Home Maintenance for the Postsurgical Patient—cont'd

Weeks 1-2—cont'd

4. Perform active heel slides: one set of 10 repetitions performed three to four times per day.
5. Perform quadriceps sets: two sets of 10 repetitions performed three to four times per day. The physical therapist should always remember that even though general protocols such as this one may prescribe a number of sets and repetitions, if the patient fatigues and cannot continue to recruit a quality quadriceps contraction, the exercise is over. Patients are only to count repetitions with quality quadriceps contractions. Quadriceps sets are performed in the sitting or long-sitting position with the knee positioned at 20 to 30 degrees flexion. The heel stays on the floor. Quadriceps sets also may be performed standing if patient finds it is easier to activate the quadriceps in this position. The key to early strengthening is to find which position gives the patient the most success in recruiting a quality quadriceps contraction.

Weeks 3-4

GOALS FOR THE PERIOD: Continue to manage edema and pain, improve sit-stand transfer activities, improve strength and stability of the patellofemoral joint, progress functional training to return activity to previous levels
1. Perform the same exercises as in weeks 1-2, but increase the number of repetitions. Generally the patient should perform two sets of 10 to 20 repetitions per day (more or less depending on fatigue).
2. Perform closed-chain exercises (see Figs. 13-6 through 13-9) at home depending on quadriceps and lower extremity control.
3. Perform self-taping as deemed appropriate by the therapist. Taping should be tailored to the activity.
4. Continue using ice after exercises.

Weeks 5-6

GOALS FOR THE PERIOD: Patient self-manages edema and pain, performs gait without deviations, and has unlimited ambulation
1. Depending on remaining deficits exercises from weeks 1-4 are continued. The need for taping should be minimal, but if continued taping is required patients should be instructed in self-taping techniques.
2. Patient should gradually return to functional activities, with both patient and therapist monitoring for pain and joint effusion.

REFERENCES

1. Aglietti P et al: Arthroscopic lateral release for patellar pain or instability, *Arthroscopy* 5:176, 1989.
2. Armato DP, Czamecki D: Geniculate artery pseudoaneurysm: a rare complication of orthroscopic surgery, *ATR Am J Roentgenol* 155(3):659, 1990.
3. Arvidsson I et al: Reduction of pain inhibition on voluntary muscle activation by epidural analgesia, *Orthop* 9:1415, 1986.
4. Chaix Y et al: Further evidence for non-monosynoptic group I excitation of motoneurons in the human lower limb, *Exp Brain Res* 115(1):35, 1997.
5. Currier DP, Lehmon J, Lightfoot P: Electrical stimulation in exercise of the quadriceps femoris muscle, *Phys Ther* 59(12):1508, 1979.
6. Currier DP, Petrilli CR, Threlkeld AJ: Effect of graded electrical stimulation on blood flow to healthy muscle, *Phys Ther* 66(6):937, 1986.
7. Davies GJ: *A compendium of isokinetics in clinical usage and rehabilitation techniques,* ed 2, 1984, S&S Publishers.
8. DeAndrade JR, Grant C, Dixon ASJ: Joint distension and reflex muscle inhibition in the knee, *J Bone Joint Surg* 47A:313, 1965.
9. DeLorme TL: Restoration of muscle power by heavy resistance exercise, *J Bone Joint Surg* 27:645, 1945.
10. Ficat P, Hungerford D: *Disorders of the patellofemoral joint,* Baltimore, 1977, Williams and Wilkins.
11. Fu F, Maday M: Arthroscopic lateral release and the patellar compression syndrome, *Orthop Clin North Am* 23:601, 1992.
12. Fulkerson JP: *Disorders of the patellofemoral joint,* ed 3, Baltimore, 1997, Williams and Wilkins.

13. Fulkerson J et al: Histological evidence of retinacular nerve injury associated with patellofemoral malalignment, *Clin Orthop* 197:196, 1985.

14. Gould N et al: Transcutaneous muscle stimulation to retard disuse atrophy after open meniscectomy, *Clin Orthop* 178:190, 1983.

15. Guzzanti V et al: Patellofemoral malalignment in adolescents: computerized tomographic assessment with or without quadriceps contraction, *Am J Sports Med* 22(1):55, 1994.

16. Heckman TP: Conservative vs. postsurgical patellar rehabilitation. In Margine R, editor: *Physical therapy of the knee*, New York, 1988, Churchill Livingstone.

17. Hensyl WR: *Steadman's pocket medical dictionary,* Baltimore, 1987, Williams and Wilkins.

18. Hurley MV et al: Rehabilitation of the quadriceps inhibited due to isolated rupture of the anterior cruciate ligament, *J Ortho Rheum* 5:145, 1992.

19. Johansson J: Role of knee ligaments in proprioception and regulation of muscle stiffness, *J Electromyogr* 1:158, 1991.

20. Krivickes LS: Anatomical factors associated with overuse sports injuries, *Sports Med* 24(2):132, 1997.

21. Kues JM, Mayhew TP: Concentric and eccentric force-velocity relationships during electrically induced submaximal contractions, *Physiother Res Int* 1(3):195, 1996.

22. Lehmann JF et al: Effect of therapeutic temperatures on tendon extensibility, *Arth Phys Med Rehabil* 51:481, 1970.

23. Lui HI, Corrier DP, Threlkeld AJ: Circulatory response of digital arteries associated with electrical stimulation of calf muscles in healthy subjects, *Phys Ther* 67(3):340, 1987.

24. Lutz GE et al: Rehabilitative techniques for athletes after reconstruction of the anterior cruciate ligament, *Mayo Clin Proc* 65(10):1322, 1990.

25. Maitland GD: *Peripheral manipulation,* ed 5, Newton, MA, 1986, Butterworth-Heinemann.

26. McConnell Patellofemoral Program Course Notes, 1997.

27. McMiken DF, Todd-Smith M, Thompson C: Strengthening of human quadriceps muscles by cutaneous electrical stimulation, *Scand J Rehab Med* 15(1):25, 1983.

28. Meunier S, Pierrot-Deseilligny E, Simonetta-Moreau M: Pattern of heteronymous recurrent inhibition in the human lower limb, *Exp Brain Res* 102(1):149, 1994.

29. Morrissey MC: Reflex inhibition of thigh muscles in knee injury. Cases and treatment, *Sports Med* 7:263, 1989.

30. Randall, Iming, Hines: Effect of electronic stimulation flow and temperature of skeletal muscle, *Am J Phys Med* 1953.

31. Richardson C: *The role of the knee musculature in high speed oscillative movements of the knee,* MTAA 4th Biennial Conference Proceedings, Brisbane, Australia, 1985, p 59.

32. Shelton GL: Conservative management of patellofemoral dysfunction, *Prim Care* 19(2):331, 1992.

33. Sherman OH et al: Patellar instability: treatment by arthroscopic electrosurgical lateral release, *Arthroscopy* 3:152, 1987.

34. Singerman R, Berilla J, Davy DT: Direct in vitro determination of the patellofemoral contact force for normal knees, *J Biomech Eng* 117:8, 1995.

35. Small NC: An analysis of complications in lateral retinacular release procedures, *Arthroscopy* 5:282, 1989.

36. Soo CL, Currier DP, Threlkeld AJ: Augmenting voluntary torque of healthy muscle by optimization of electrical stimulation, *Phys Ther* 68(3):333, 1988.

37. Spencer JDC, Hayes KC, Alexander IJ: Knee joint effusion and quadriceps reflex inhibition in man, *Arch Phys Med Rehab* 65:171, 1984.

38. Steine HA et al: A comparison of closed kinetic chain and isokinetic joint isolation exercise in patients with patellofemoral dysfunction, *J Orthop Sports Phys Ther* 24(3):136, 1996.

39. Tiberio D: The effect of excessive subtalar joint pronation on patellofemoral mechanics: a theoretical model, *J Orthop Sports Phys Ther* 9:160, 1987.

40. Vuorinen OP et al: Chondromalacia patellae: results of operative treatment, *Arch Arthoscop Trauma Surg* 104(3):175, 1985.

41. Werner S, Knutsson E, Eriksson E: Effect of taping the patella and concentric and eccentric torque and EMG of knee extensor and flexor muscles in patients with patellofemoral pain syndrome, *Knee Surg Sports Traumatol Arthrosc* 1(3-4):169, 1993.

42. Wild JJ, Franklin TD, Woods GW: Patellar pain and quadriceps rehabilitation: an EMG study, *Am J Sports Med* 10:12, 1982.

43. Zinovieff AN: Heavy resistance exercises: the Oxford techniques, *Br J Phys Med* 14:29, 1951.

Chapter 14

Meniscectomy and Meniscal Repair ————

Andrew A. Brooks
Terry Gillette

Although meniscal repair was introduced more than 100 years ago,[1] only within the past 10 to 20 years has the meniscus successfully outlived its characterization as a "functionless remains of leg muscle."[25] Only a few years ago it was standard practice to excise the meniscus with impunity because of the perception that it played little role in the function of the knee. Fairbanks[10] called attention to the frequency of degenerative changes after removal of the meniscus and stimulated a new era of research into the anatomy and function of this poorly understood structure. Researchers eagerly investigated the role of the meniscus in load transmission and joint nutrition, and soon the pendulum of orthopedic popular opinion swung in the direction of determining new ways to preserve the injured meniscus.

With the advent of arthroscopic surgery, partial meniscectomy rapidly supplanted total meniscectomy, and research continued to determine the healing capacity of the torn meniscus. From these efforts, meniscal repair has evolved as a successful technique. Ultimately, recognition of the intact meniscus as a crucial factor in normal knee function has led to widespread acceptance of preservation of torn menisci through partial meniscectomy or repair.

Surgical Indications and Considerations

Four techniques for repair currently exist:
1. Open meniscal repair
2. Arthroscopic inside-out repair
3. Arthroscopic outside-in repair
4. All-inside arthroscopic repair

Each of these techniques has advantages and disadvantages; application of individual techniques is largely a matter of individual preference.

When assessing the suitability of a meniscal tear for repair the surgeon must consider several factors: patient age; chronicity of the injury; type, location, and length of the tears (the blood supply of the meniscus exists primarily at the peripheral 10% to 25%); and associated ligamentous injuries.[2] The perfect candidate for a meniscal repair is a young individual with an acute longitudinal peripheral tear of the meniscus that is 1 to 2 cm long, to be repaired in conjunction with an anterior cruciate ligament (ACL) reconstruction. Outside of these parameters, little consensus exists on the relative indications for meniscal repair.

The arthroscopic surgeon should be prepared to perform meniscal repair at the time of any knee arthroscopy. The identification of reparable menisci is usually not possible preoperatively, but often magnetic resonance imaging (MRI) can help demonstrate the location of tears.

Surgical Procedure

Open Meniscal Repair

Open meniscal repair is the oldest technique of meniscal repair and has been popularized by Dr. Ken DeHaven.[6] It has a good record of success, even at 1-year follow-up.[7] Open meniscal repairs are best suited for extremely peripheral tears. DeHaven still advocates routine arthroscopic evaluation before considering open repair. The arthroscope is removed from the joint and the knee is prepared. After exposing the capsule through a longitudinal incision, the surgeon prepares the meniscal rim and capsular attachment and places vertically oriented sutures at 3- to 4-mm intervals. The incision is closed in a layered fashion.

Inside-Out Meniscal Repair

The inside-out meniscal repair technique was popularized by Henning[11] in the early 1980s and is the most popular technique for meniscus repair. It is done by using long, thin cannulas to allow placement of vertical or horizontal sutures. After identifying the tear arthroscopically, the surgeon prepares the tear by using a meniscal rasp to create a better biologic environment for healing. A small posterior incision is carried down to the capsule, and sutures are placed arthroscopically using specially designed long Keith needles to pass the suture. The assistant protects the popliteal structures with a retractor while grasping the suture needles. After placing all sutures the surgeon ties them over the capsule.

Outside-In Meniscal Repair

The outside-in meniscal repair technique allows suture placement using an 18-gauge spinal needle placed across the tear from outside the joint to inside. Absorbable polydioxanone suture[12] is passed through the needle into the joint; it is secured with a mulberry knot tied to the end of the sutures. These sutures are tied to adjacent sutures at the end of the procedure over the joint capsule; separate small incisions are made for each pair of sutures.

All-Inside Meniscal Repair

All-inside meniscal repair allows the meniscus to be repaired without any additional incisions outside the knee. This is truly an all-arthroscopic technique. It is popular because it avoids additional incisions and therefore diminishes neurovascular risk.

All-inside meniscal repair can be accomplished with either suture or biodegradable "darts."[20] The suture technique is accomplished using a specially designed cannulated suture hook to pass suture through both sides of the tear. The sutures are then tied arthroscopically using a knot pusher.

The biodegradable darts are passed across the tear using specially designed cannulas. After preparing the torn meniscal surface, the surgeon reduces the tear and holds it in place with a cannula. A thin cutting instrument is used to make a pathway across the meniscal tear, and the biodegradable dart is passed through the same cannula, fixing the tear. The darts generally completely resorb by 8 to 12 weeks.

Therapy Guidelines for Rehabilitation

Limited research is available regarding physical therapy protocols after meniscus repair and long-term outcomes. Clinic protocols vary with the degree of weight bearing, duration of immobilization, control of range of motion (ROM), and return to sports or work. Recent studies have shown the success rates after accelerated rehabilitation programs to be similar to those in conservative rehabilitation programs. These studies found no statistically significant difference in success and repair failure rates between groups using conservative or accelerated programs. The hallmarks of accelerated programs are early full weight-bearing tolerance, unrestricted ROM, and return to pivoting sports.[3,23,24]

An understanding of the clinical implications of knee and meniscus biomechanics helps guide the therapist through the rehabilitation process. Communication among all rehabilitation team members—the physician, therapist, patient, family, and coach—is crucial to a successful rehabilitation outcome. The rehabilitation program must be acceptable to the patient, with goals designed to meet the patient's needs.

Several crucial factors must be considered before initiating a rehabilitation program. These factors influence the speed and aggressiveness of the rehabilitation program. The size of the tear, repair stabilization technique, suture material, number of sutures, and location of the meniscal repair influence initial postoperative weight-bearing tolerance, ROM, and exercise restrictions. Other factors to consider before initiating a rehabilitation program include degenerative pathology in the weight-bearing articulations or patellofemoral joint, previous patella dysfunction, and concomitant injuries and possible joint laxity (i.e., ACL deficiency or reconstruction, medial collateral ligament injury). These injuries do not necessarily indicate a potentially unsatisfactory result. The rehabilitation protocol may require modifications to accommodate the effects of these pathologies. Barber and Click[3] evaluated the results of 65 meniscal repairs in patients who underwent an accelerated rehabilitation program. Successful meniscal healing occurred in 92% of patients with a concomitant ACL reconstruction, compared with 67% of patients with ACL-deficient knees and 67% of patients with meniscal pathology alone.

The meniscal repair rehabilitation protocol must be individually tailored to the patient's needs. The rehabilitation process can be broken down into three phases: initial, intermediate, and advanced. These phases may overlap and should be based on objective and functional findings rather than time.

The early phase of the rehabilitation program should emphasize decreasing postoperative inflammatory reaction, restoring controlled ROM, and encouraging early weight bearing as tolerated. Exercise intensity is increased in the later phases of rehabilitation. Closed kinetic chain exercises are progressed through a variety of positions, from simple linear movements to complex multidirectional motions. The final phase of treatment is directed toward return to normal activity (sport or work).

The length of rehabilitation varies among patients. Treatments may be equally distributed among each of the phases of rehabilitation if the number of patient visits must be managed. Fewer treatments are required in the initial phases of rehabilitation if swelling and pain are adequately controlled and ROM is progressing without complications.

Preoperative Care

Ideally the patient should be seen at a preoperative visit, which includes a brief clinical evaluation to record baseline physical data and identify potential latent biomechanical deficits. The evaluation format encompasses a subjective history as outlined in Maitland, and objective data are gathered primarily to record baseline measurements.[16] The lower extremity is evaluated as a functional unit. Strength and ROM are recorded for the hip, knee, ankle, and foot. Foot mechanics also are evaluated and addressed as indicated. Reassessment continues postoperatively with each progression of weight bearing. Girth measurements also are taken about the knee. The remainder of the preoperative visit should include instruction in proper use of crutches, education regarding ROM (heel slides with a 30-second hold for 10 repetitions), instruction in antiembolic exercises (ankle pumps with a 30-second hold for 10 repetitions), and prescription of lower extremity strengthening exercises in the form of isometrics (quadriceps sets, hamstring sets, and co-contraction of quadriceps and hamstrings; all three exercises should be held for 10 seconds for 10 to 20 repetitions) and active range of motion (AROM) of the hip (working the adductors, abductors, and external rotators for 10 to 20 repetitions). Cryotherapy and elevation (for 15 to 30 minutes) and compression wrapping should be reviewed for postoperative pain and swelling management. Depending on individual clinic and physician preference, the patient may be instructed in the use of electrical stimulation. The patient should be instructed in activity of daily living needs (bathing, dressing) as appropriate. Any preoperative instruction pertaining to exercise and weight-bearing status must be cleared by the physician postoperatively based on the extent and nature of the surgical repair performed. Home exercises are to be performed three times a day until return for the initial postoperative physical therapy evaluation.

Q. Stephen is an active 42-year-old man. He wants to return to skiing as soon as possible. Stephen had a lateral meniscal repair for the posterior horn $2\frac{1}{2}$ weeks ago. The therapist is having Stephen perform co-contraction isometrics of the quadriceps and hamstrings. Stephen wants to know why he cannot start using weights on the seated knee flexion machine (isotonics) for resisted hamstring strengthening. What should the therapist tell him?

Phase I: Initial Phase

TIME: Weeks 1-4
GOALS: Manage pain and swelling, increase ROM and strength, increase weight-bearing activities (Table 14-1)

The patient is typically seen for physical therapy 4 to 7 days after surgery. He or she may complain of mild to moderate pain, swelling, and decreased weight-bearing tolerance. The patient may or may not be using pain medication. Objectively, the patient is non–weight bearing or partial weight bearing to tolerance with crutches for a period of 2 to 6 weeks. Minimal to moderate effusion may be evident. Based on physician preference the patient may have a postoperative protective brace.

Meniscal repairs in the "red zone" (meniscus area that has a blood supply) and larger peripheral repairs may be braced 0 to 90 degrees for up to 14 days. "White zone" (meniscus area that lacks a blood supply) repairs may be braced at 20 to 70 degrees. Extension is increased to 0 degrees and flexion is increased to 90 degrees after 7 to 10 days. ROM is typically limited within constraints of bracing. Strength of the quadriceps and hamstring may be limited.

On the first visit a comprehensive evaluation is performed, with the physical therapist collecting the new objective data and reviewing and updating the previous subjective data.[16] Subjective data that need to be reviewed postoperatively include medication usage, sleep pattern, pain levels at rest and during activity, and aggravating and easing factors. In addition the therapist should review the postoperative report that describes the extent and nature of the repair. Goals and rehabilitation expectations are established and reviewed with the patient during the initial visit.

The new and updated objective and clinical data should include visual examination, gait assessment, ROM measurement, strength assessment, palpation, and girth measurement (as described in the section on the preoperative initial visit). Visual observation should focus on areas of atrophy, in particular the vastus medialis oblique (VMO); healing status of incision sites; and swelling about the knee joint and distal lower extremity. Depending on the patient's weight-bearing status or tolerance, gait assessment is either brief or detailed. The primary focus of the brief assessment is safety, correct mechanics, and weight bearing in patients with restricted tolerance. If the patient does not have weight-bearing restrictions and has good gait tolerance, a more detailed assessment of gait can be made. Gait assessment should focus on proper mechanics and weight-bearing tolerance. The patient's ability to ambulate with normal mechanics throughout each phase of gait should be assessed. Remedial corrective actions are required to decrease potentially harmful loading onto healing structures. Typically patients require cueing to avoid hip external rotation during the stance phase because this puts abnormal stresses through the knee, ankle, and foot. Crutches should be used throughout the initial phase of treatment until adequate strength, ROM, and normal gait mechanics are achieved. Static and dynamic foot function, as related to normal gait mechanics, continue to be assessed during this phase of rehabilitation. Dysfunctions must be addressed to decrease abnormal tensile or compressive force affecting healing of the meniscus repair.

Typically, on initial evaluation the patient exhibits a loss of extension of 5 to 10 degrees; flexion ROM is 70 to 90 degrees. The patient exhibits a guarded end feel with motion improving with repetition. Flexibility of the hip musculature, hamstring, and gastrocnemius-soleus complex should be assessed. Appropriate remedial flex-

Table 14-1　Meniscus Repair

Rehabilitation Phase	Criteria to Progress to this Phase	Anticipated Impairments and Functional Limitations	Intervention	Goal	Rationale
Phase I Postoperative 1-4 weeks	Postoperative	• Mild to moderate pain • Non-weight bearing to partial weight bearing to tolerance • Decreased strength • Minimal to moderate effusion • Decreased ROM	• Cryotherapy, heat and ice contrast, electrical stimulation • Passive range of motion (PROM)— 　Hamstring stretches 　Gastrocnemius-soleus stretches • Wall slides or passive heel slides (Fig. 14-1) • Isometrics—Co-contraction quadriceps and hamstring (depending on the repair site) 　Quadriceps sets 　Hip adductor sets 　Hamstring sets 　Resistive exercises • "4 quad" program, weight added distally as tolerated • Elastic tubing exercises • Gait training • Low-resistance, moderate-speed stationary cycling • Aquatic therapy 　Closed kinetic chain activities (initiate near end of phase) • Leg press machine • Partial squats • Heel raises • Standing terminal knee extension with tubing	• Manage pain and swelling • Knee ROM 0°-120° • Increased muscle strength and endurance • Normalization of gait within healing and weight-bearing limitations	• Decrease pain and minimize swelling • Prevent ROM complications • Assist in restoration of joint mechanics • Facilitate return of neuromuscular control • Minimize disuse atrophy • Strengthen knee musculature while protecting the repair site • Increase muscle endurance • Use properties of water during exercise performance • Functional strengthening

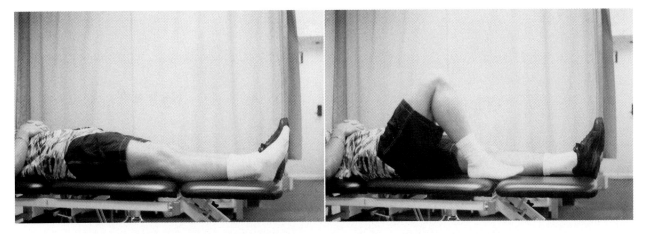

Fig. 14-1. Heel slides. While lying supine the patient slides the involved heel toward the buttock, maintaining the knee in a straight plane and avoiding any hip or tibial rotation.

ibility exercises can be implemented as tolerated in this phase, with the patient avoiding forced knee flexion and rotation about the knee joint. Patients should perform slow static stretches, avoiding ballistic movements, to maintain control of the lower limb and minimize the chance of affecting the healing meniscus repair.[9,13]

The patellofemoral joint should be assessed, especially if the patient reports previous or present patella symptoms. Patella tracking and glides are part of this assessment. Joint mobilization or patellofemoral taping may be helpful in mitigating these symptoms[18] (see Figs. 13-1 through 13-3 and 13-10). All major muscle groups in the lower extremity should be assessed bilaterally. In addition, visible observation and palpation of the VMO during a muscle contraction of the quadriceps indicates VMO function and potential patellofemoral complications. The remaining lower extremity musculature should be assessed, with the therapist identifying any potential weakness that may alter normal closed kinetic biomechanics and therefore increase tensile or compressive forces across the meniscus repair site.

No standard method has been established for assessing girth about the knee joint. Consistency among the team members providing patient care is important when reassessing the patient's condition. Atrophy as measured by girth measurements is not diagnostic of weakness or atrophy in a specific muscle group. Circumference measurement assesses girth of all muscle and joint structures underlying the measurement area. Typical measurement sites for a bilateral comparison include the mid-patella, 5 and 10 centimeters above the knee joint and 5 and 10 centimeters below the knee joint.

Treatment is initiated after the clinical evaluation is completed (see Table 14-1). Initial phase treatment goals are to decrease pain and manage swelling, restore ROM, increase muscle strength and endurance, and normalize gait within healing and weight-bearing limitations.

Modalities such as heat and ice contrast, electrical stimulation, and cryotherapy can be used to decrease pain and swelling.[5,15,27] Instructions in home use of cryotherapy, compression wrapping, and elevation as discussed in the section on preoperative management is initiated for postoperative pain and swelling. The importance of home cryotherapy cannot be overemphasized. Lessard et al's[15] study of cryotherapy use after meniscectomy found statistically significant differences between groups with and without postoperative cryotherapy. Patients reported decreased pain ratings per the McGill pain questionnaire, decreased medication consumption, improved exercise compliance, and improved weight-bearing status.

Restoration of ROM is important. The time parameter to achieve full ROM is longer than it is in partial arthroscopic meniscectomies. Although early restoration of ROM is important to normalize joint function, the healing process of the meniscus repair dictates caution, especially with full circumferential peripheral repairs. Any exercises used to increase ROM should not be forced because of the risk of stressing healing repair sites. Wall slides or passive heel slides (Fig. 14-1) may be used to increase knee flexion. ROM exercises are to be performed within pain tolerance, held at least 30 seconds, and repeated as tolerated (generally 5 to 10 times). As part of the home exercise program, ROM activity can be repeated two to three times per day.

Hamstring and gastrocnemius-soleus flexibility exercises can be initiated to the patient's tolerance. Stretches should be held at least 30 seconds and repeated 5 to 10 times, three times a day. Stretches should be sustained and passive in nature, allowing the patient or therapist to control knee joint motions, avoiding potential complications from ballistic-type stretching.[28] The hamstring group can be stretched passively using a long-sit position (with legs straight out in front of the body). A towel can be used to assist with pas-

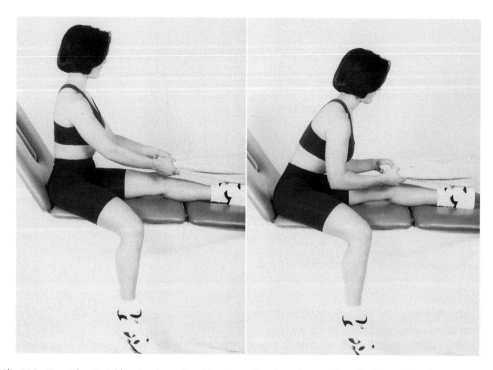

Fig. 14-2. Hamstring stretching. In a long-sit position the patient leans forward from the hip, avoiding lumbar flexion.

sive ankle dorsiflexion to intensify the stretch. The physical therapist should instruct the patient to maintain a "neutral spine" while performing the stretch (Fig. 14-2). The gastrocnemius-soleus can be stretched using a towel or strap in the early phases of rehabilitation. Progression to stretching of the hip musculature and quadriceps can be performed as the patient's increase in knee ROM dictates. The knee needs to be kept in a relative neutral position to avoid any rotational or compressive forces on the repaired meniscus site. Standing gastrocnemius-soleus stretching can be initiated as weight-bearing tolerance increases. The foot is kept in a neutral position to avoid any tibia rotation caused by supination or pronation, which may increase knee joint compression and tensile forces across the repaired meniscal site.

Initial strengthening is performed as tolerated in open-chain positions. Closed kinetic strengthening (as discussed in Chapter 12 and shown in Figs. 12-1 and 12-4) can be initiated depending on the weight-bearing status and tolerance of the patient. All strengthening exercises should be closely monitored for potential adverse reactions and increased pain or swelling.

Strengthening exercises for all lower extremity musculature are initiated with an emphasis on restoration of quadriceps muscle function to minimize potential patellofemoral dysfunction. Isometric exercises should be held for 10 seconds and performed for 10 to 20 repetitions. Quadriceps sets can be performed within the patient's tolerance. A small towel may be required under the posterior aspect of the knee if the patient lacks

full extension or if muscle setting in full extension is painful to the knee joint area. The patient is instructed to extend at the hip while tightening the quadriceps muscle, straightening the knee as tolerated. This exercise also may help restore knee extension. The towel should be removed as knee extension increases or becomes less painful. Adductor isometric contractions can be performed isolated or in conjunction with quadriceps sets (see Fig. 11-12). The role of the VMO in patella dysfunction is debatable.[22] Adductor contractions theoretically may facilitate VMO contraction based on the anatomic origin of the horizontal fibers of the VMO to the intermuscular septum of the hip adductor group and the distal adductor tendon insertion into the suprapatellar tendon.[4]

Hamstring isometrics can be performed; they should initially be performed at a submaximal level, with vigor increased based on patient tolerance and response. Caution should be exhibited when performing hamstring exercises early in rehabilitation, especially with larger peripheral rim or posterior horn meniscus repairs. Active knee flexion pulls the medial and lateral meniscus posterior. Because the lateral meniscus is more loosely attached it can migrate posteriorly as much as 1 cm as a result of pull from the popliteus muscle. The medial meniscus may move a few millimeters via the posterior attachment to the joint capsule and influence from the nearby semimembranosus attachment.[2] Co-contraction isometrics of the quadriceps and hamstrings may be used in the first 2 to 4 weeks in patients with the aforementioned repairs to allow adequate meniscal healing.[17]

An open-chain straight leg raise (SLR) "4 quad" program (four quadrant: hip flexion, abduction, adduction, and extension) can be initiated with the knee fully extended if the patient has adequate lower extremity and quadriceps control. Short arc quadriceps exercises can be added if the patient tolerates end-range extension movement. Resistance should be added carefully, with the therapist remaining mindful of the role of the quadriceps in pulling the meniscus anteriorly by way of the meniscopatellar ligament as well as the anterior posterior compressive force exerted by the femoral condyle during knee extension.[21] The 4 quad program is a series of SLR exercises held for 10 seconds and 10 to 20 repetitions:

1. Supine SLR
2. Side-lying hip abduction (see Fig. 11-18)
3. Side-lying hip adduction (see Fig. 11-19)
4. Prone hip extension.

Progression of this program is based on patient signs and symptoms. Resistance can be added distally as tolerated. The DeLorme strength progression protocol can be used, with gradual increases in resistance based on patient signs and symptoms.

Weight-bearing status and patient tolerance may limit the ability to strengthen the distal musculature. Strengthening of the ankle can be aided by exercises using elastic tubing; the patient should perform three sets of 10 to 20 repetitions. Ankle movements of dorsiflexion, plantar flexion, inversion and eversion, and hip proprioceptive neuromuscular facilitation (PNF) patterns (with the knee extended) can be performed to the patient's tolerance. As with other healing collagen structures, controlled tensile and compressive loading may assist in scar conformation, revascularization, and improvement in the tensile properties of the meniscal repair through the maturation process.[14] Gradual progression and reassessment of activity is crucial.

When initiating any of the closed kinetic chain exercises, the patient must keep the knee and lower extremity in a neutral position. In normal gait the compressive forces on the knee joint may be two to three times normal body weight. The meniscus assumes 40% to 60% of the weight-bearing load. Variations in knee joint angulation or rotation can increase the force across the meniscus 25% to 50%.[21] Variations in foot mechanics that cause rotation or angulation of the knee into varus or valgus can have potentially significant effects on meniscal compressive and tensile forces that may affect the repair site.

Partial–weight-bearing, closed kinetic chain activities using leg press (see Fig. 11-20) or inclined squat machines (double leg progressed to single leg [see Fig. 12-4]), partial squats, and heel raises (see Fig. 11-13) can be initiated later in the initial phase. Standing terminal knee extension with tubing can be added to increase quadriceps strength and control with full weight bearing.

Aquatic therapy is an additional treatment option during the initial phase, especially if the patient has limited weight bearing and cannot tolerate traditional therapy because of pain.[26] ROM, lower extremity strengthening, progressive weight bearing, and cardiovascular training can be initiated in the pool.

Low-resistance, moderate-speed stationary cycling can be initiated when knee flexion ROM is around 110 degrees. Toe clips may be optional if hamstring activity is to be minimized because of the location of the repair. Progression is determined by the patient's tolerance to stationary cycling. The goal of initial phase cycling is to increase muscle endurance.

Complications in the initial phase of treatment include persistent pain and swelling, arthrofibrosis, adhesions at the porthole sites, patella tendonitis, and patellofemoral pain. Activity modification, use of modalities, heat and cold contrast, cryotherapy, and electrical stimulation may be helpful in decreasing pain and swelling. Adhesion of the porthole sites within the distal fat pads may cause painful limitation of knee flexion and active knee extension. Ultrasound or phonophoresis, along with soft tissue mobilization of incision sites, may be helpful in mitigating distal patella symptoms. Assessment of patellofemoral mechanics (active and passive) is an ongoing process. Patellofemoral taping should be used to control pain and dysfunction.[19]

ROM gradually increases during the initial phase of treatment, approaching full ROM by the end of this phase. Passive and dynamic splints may be helpful in gaining ROM if the joint does not respond to conservative treatment. Initiation of vigorous stretching or knee joint mobilization should be discussed with the patient and physician. The therapist should be aware of knee joint symptoms, pain, and swelling as attempts to increase ROM (especially knee flexion) continue.

In addition, the therapist should be cognizant of and recognize meniscus lesion signs and symptoms. These include persistent joint effusion, joint line pain, and locking or giving way of the knee (as opposed to buckling or weakness from decreased lower extremity or quadriceps strength).

If activity modification and use of modalities does not improve the patient's symptoms and objective findings or if the patient exhibits classic signs of a meniscus tear, referral to the physician is indicated.

A. Active knee flexion pulls the medial and lateral meniscus posterior. The lateral meniscus migrates 1 cm posterior because the popliteus muscle pulls it during knee flexion. This activity places increased stress on the repaired and healing tissues.

Table 14-2 Meniscus Repair

Rehabilitation Phase	Criteria to Progress to this Phase	Anticipated Impairments and Functional Limitations	Intervention	Goal	Rationale
Phase II Postoperative 5–11 weeks	Minimal pain and swelling 4 to 6 weeks to allow sufficient healing Full weight bearing, normal gait mechanics Good control of the lower extremity musculature	• Decreased strength • Minimal effusion • Decreased ROM (flexion)	• Continue exercises as outlined in Table 14-1 Resistive exercise • Isotonics—Hamstrings • Isokinetics—A sub-maximal multi-spectrum isokinetic program • Closed-chain exercise Heel raises Lateral step-up Forward step up/down Wall squats, knee flexion at 45°–60° Mini-squats Partial lunges Progression in knee flexion ROM • Balance activities, balance board, trampoline • Elastic tubing activity, "T kicks" (see Fig. 14-3) • Stationary cycling, modifying the workload parameters of speed, resistance, and duration • Stair-stepping machine, cross-country ski machine, or treadmill	• Full ROM • 90%–100% lower extremity strength • Normal gait and standing tolerance • Progression to functional activities • Prepare patient for discharge	• Restore knee and lower extremity function • Increase muscle strength • Use specificity of training principles to return the patient to previous level of functional activity • Enhance response of joint proprioceptors and neuromuscular coordination • Emphasize stability/strengthening of involved leg • Improve cardiovascular fitness

Q. Silvia is 40 years old. Before tearing her meniscus she had two episodes of anterior knee pain over the past 3 years. Silvia had a medial meniscal repair 5 weeks ago. She has been progressing nicely with exercises, and the exercises have been advanced. After treatment she reports pain in the anterior inferior patella region with most of the exercises. Silvia is concerned because she almost slipped and fell after her last physical therapy visit. She denies any episode of her knee locking or becoming stuck. What might be the source of her pain?

Phase II: Intermediate Phase

TIME: Weeks 5-11
GOALS: Gain full ROM and 90% to 100% strength, progress functional activities, progress to gym program (Table 14-2)

Objective findings rather than time ranges give an indication of progression into the intermediate phase of rehabilitation. In general this phase occurs around 4 to 6 weeks, in part based on improved patient signs and symptoms but also because enough time has elapsed to allow sufficient healing of the meniscal repair. This phase lasts until the patient is ready to enter a return to sport program (usually by the twelfth week). Pain and swelling should be minimal and easily controlled before initiation of this phase. ROM should be full. However, the patient may have a slight restriction of knee flexion, with discomfort at end ROM. Full weight bearing should be tolerated without pain or swelling. The patient should exhibit normal gait mechanics. Good control of the lower extremity musculature should be evident before activity is progressed. The goals of the intermediate phase are to normalize strength, ROM, gait, and endurance and progress the patient into functional activities. Muscle flexibility exercises are continued as needed during this phase. Quadriceps and iliopsoas stretching to improve knee flexion and hip extension can be initiated. Strength exercises are continued and advanced as tolerated. Hamstring strengthening (with isotonic exercise) can be advanced during this phase. Progression is based on DeLorme's principles.[8] Resistance can be applied to the hamstring group gradually based on patient tolerance.

Closed-chain activity can be advanced during this phase of rehabilitation. Progression of activity should be from simple linear movements to complex multidirectional movements. Patients are instructed to perform three sets of 10 to 30 repetitions as indicated. The patient must demonstrate adequate control of lower extremity mechanics and not have adverse reactions (pain and swelling) from the simple linear movements before progressing to complex multidirectional movements. Variables of time, repetitions, ROM, and resistance are used in functionally progressing the rehabilitation program. Full–weight-bearing heel raises, lateral step-ups, wall squats, mini-squats with tubing, and partial lunges can be performed. ROM should be limited initially, with most activity being from 0 to 90 degrees. Constant reassessment should occur and patient tolerance to the particular activity must be demonstrated before any exercise progression.

Balance and coordination exercises can be added to the rehabilitation program during the intermediate phase. Initial training is done bilaterally and progressed as tolerated to unilateral activities. Balance boards, trampoline, and elastic cords can be used. Single-limb balance and control can be performed with exercise tubing "T kicks" (Fig. 14-3). The uninvolved extremity has a cord attached distally; the involved extremity remains stationary with the knee in about 10 degrees of flexion. The patient moves the uninvolved extremity into flexion, extension, abduction, adduction, and diagonal planes. Initially the patient performs 10 to 15 repetitions for two sets in each plane of movement. The patient may require support for balance. The exercise can be progressed by altering the tubing resistance, increasing the repetition or time (up to 30 seconds in each plane), and altering the speed of movement.

Cycling can be continued, with the patient modifying the workload parameters of speed, resistance, and duration based on response to the activity. Additional cardiovascular activity (e.g., stair-stepping machine, cross-country ski machine, treadmill) can be added based on patient response and tolerance.

A gradual walking to running program can be established toward the end of this phase based on weight-bearing tolerance and adequate closed-chain control and lower extremity strength. Refer to p. 219 for a detailed progressive running program. Assessment of foot function with appropriate modifications may be helpful in minimizing abnormal joint and meniscus stress before initiating a running program. The running program can start with jogging in place on a trampoline and be progressed to treadmill running. Continued progression is based on patient tolerance and absence of pain and swelling.

Isokinetics strength and endurance training can be initiated during this phase. Tolerance to resisted quadriceps and hamstring strengthening must be demonstrated before an isokinetic program is initiated. A submaximal multi-spectrum program with a lower velocity speed of 180 degrees/second (three sets of 15 to 20 seconds) and higher velocity speed of 300 degrees/second (three sets up to 30 seconds) can be initiated. Progression is based on patient tolerance and adequate response to training.

Table 14-3 Meniscus Repair

Rehabilitation Phase	Criteria to Progress to this Phase	Anticipated Impairments and Functional Limitations	Intervention	Goal	Rationale
Phase III Postoperative 12-18 weeks	Tolerance to intermediate phase treatment Full ROM MMT normal Good closed-chain control in linear and multidirectional activity Treadmill 10 to 15 minutes at a pace of 7 to 8 miles per hour without adverse signs and symptoms Isokinetic strength 70% of the uninvolved extremity	• Isokinetic strength and endurance deficit • Decreased ability to perform full squat or lunge • Fair balance and control with higher-level activity	Progression and continuation of exercises as listed in Tables 14-1 and 14-2 • Depending on previous activity level and functional requirements, agility, sprinting, and track running • Isokinetics—Strength and endurance training	• Establish an ongoing training program • Return to pre-injury activity or sport • Appropriate performance functional and isokinetic tests as indicated for return to sport or activity	• Continued progression of endurance and strength training • Safe return to functional activity

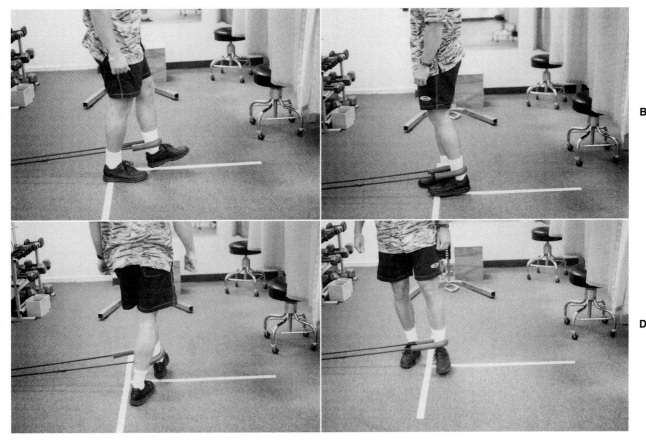

Fig. 14-3. T kicks. This exercise is performed in a standing position, with elastic tubing around the ankle of the uninvolved lower extremity (foot off ground). The uninvolved lower extremity moves into flexion (**A**), extension (**B**), adduction (**C**), and abduction (**D**). The emphasis is on maintaining proper lower extremity alignment and avoiding tibial rotation.

A. Silvia's history, along with the pain distribution pattern, indicate a patellofemoral joint problem that may have become irritated. Meniscal pain often produces complaints of pain near the joint line. Of course, a detailed assessment should be made and the physician notified. In this case the patellofemoral joint was the source of the anterior inferior knee pain. Therefore the patient should be treated for both the patellofemoral symptoms and the meniscal repair. Necessary restrictions should be maintained for each condition. After the patellofemoral symptoms have been significantly reduced or eliminated, the exercise program for the meniscal repair can again be the focus, with consideration of the patellofemoral joint.

Phase III: Advanced Phase

TIME: Weeks 12-18
GOALS: Return to sport or pre-injury activities, establish an ongoing training program (Table 14-3)

Progression to the advanced phase of rehabilitation is based on tolerance to intermediate phase treatment. Typically this phase is initiated around 12 to 18 weeks. ROM should be complete without pain. Caution should be exhibited with full squat or lunge activity. These activities should be avoided early in the advanced phase and gradually introduced with progressive loading toward the end of the phase. Normal strength in all major muscle groups should be exhibited. The patient should exhibit good closed-chain control in linear and multidirectional activity. The goals of this phase are to establish a training program and return to sports or pre-injury activity levels. Progression of strength and endurance training continues. Depending on previous activity level and functional requirements, agility, sprinting, and track running can be initiated. An indicator of patient progress in these activities is the ability to jog on a treadmill 10 to 15 minutes at a pace of 7 to 8 miles per hour without adverse signs and symptoms. As with other knee disorders, adequate isokinetic strength (70% of the uninvolved extremity) can be used as an indication for progression to a running and agility program. A deficit of 10% or less is a reliable indicator of return to sport or activity participation.[24] However, other functional tests (as mentioned in Chapter 12) need to be assessed to ensure safe return.

Suggested Home Maintenance for the Postsurgical Patient

An exercise program has been outlined at the various phases. The home maintenance box on pages 254 to 255 outlines rehabilitation suggestions the patient may follow. The physical therapist can use it in customizing a patient-specific program.

Conclusion

Meniscal repair is an effective technique for preserving certain torn menisci. Although long-term results are still unknown, the meniscus should be preserved whenever possible to avoid the late sequelae of meniscectomy. Numerous techniques are available to achieve this goal and are primarily a matter of surgeon preference. A rehabilitation program must be individually tailored based on scientific evidence, clinical signs and symptoms, and patient needs.

Suggested Home Maintenance for the Postsurgical Patient

Weeks 1-2

GOALS FOR THE PERIOD: Manage pain and swelling, increase ROM and strength, increase weight-bearing activities

1. Heel slides—10 repetitions to be held 30 seconds. Pressure within patient's tolerance.
2. Ankle pumps—20 to 30 repetitions.
3. Isometric muscle contractions—quadriceps, hamstring (if appropriate), adductor, and gluteal isometric contractions—10 to 20 repetitions to be held 10 seconds.
4. Cryotherapy with elevation to be performed as needed throughout the day for 10 to 15 minutes.
5. Additional compression garment or wrapping may be helpful.

Weeks 3-4

GOALS FOR THE PERIOD: Manage pain and swelling, increase ROM and strength, increase weight-bearing activities

1. Supine wall slides or passive heel slides, 10 repetitions to be held 30 seconds. Pressure within patient's tolerance.
2. Co-contraction isometrics of the quadriceps and hamstrings, 10 to 20 repetitions to be held 10 seconds (depending on the repair site).
3. Isometric quadriceps, adductor, and hamstring contractions, 10 to 20 repetitions to be held 10 seconds.
4. Flexibility exercises for the hamstring and gastrocnemius-soleus. Stretches should be held at least 30 seconds and repeated 5 to 10 times.
5. 4-quad program, two to three sets of 10 repetitions, weight added distally as tolerated.
6. Elastic tubing exercises (dorsiflexion, plantar flexion, inversion and eversion, and hip PNF patterns) two to three sets of 10 repetitions.
7. Low-resistance, moderate-speed stationary cycling.
8. Home aquatic therapy (performing AROM exercises of the hip, knee, and ankle in chest-high water).
9. Continued cryotherapy with elevation to be performed as needed throughout the day for 10 to 15 minutes.

Weeks 5-11

GOALS FOR THE PERIOD: Gain full ROM and 90% to 100% strength, progress functional activities, progress to gym program

1. Continued open-chain exercise program, 4-quads, short arc quadriceps (SAQs), and PNF patterns with tubing.

Suggested Home Maintenance for the Postsurgical Patient—cont'd

Weeks 5-11—cont'd

2. Hamstring, gastrocnemius-soleus, quadriceps, and iliopsoas stretching, 5 to 10 repetitions to be held at least 30 seconds.
3. Heel raises, two to three sets of 10 repetitions. Lateral step-ups and forward step up and down (using 2-inch height progressions), two to three sets of 10 repetitions. Wall squats, knee flexion at 45 degrees advanced to 60 degrees, two sets of 10 repetitions to be held 10 seconds. Mini-squats, partial lunges, and progression in knee flexion ROM (add tubing or weight to progress resistance as tolerated), two to three sets of 10 repetitions to be held 5 to 10 seconds.
4. Balance activities (bilateral progressed as tolerated to unilateral)—balance board, trampoline (side-to-side and forward-to-back steps)—2 sets of 1 minute each.
5. Exercise cords activity, T kicks, two to three sets of 10 repetitions.
6. Stationary cycling, modifying the workload parameters of speed, resistance, and duration based on the response to the activity.
7. Stair-stepping machine, cross-country ski machine, or treadmill, with workload progression based on patient response and tolerance.

Weeks 12-18

GOALS FOR THE PERIOD: Return to sport or pre-injury activities, establish an ongoing training program
1. Progression of strength and endurance training.
2. Functional or sport-specific drills.
3. Agility, sprinting, and track running.

REFERENCES

1. Annandale T: An operation for displaced semilunar cartilage, Dr Med J 1:779, 1885.
2. Arnoczky SP, Warren RF: Microvasculature of the human meniscus, Am J Sports Med 10:90, 1982.
3. Barber FA, Click SD: Meniscus repair rehabilitation with concurrent anterior cruciate reconstruction, Arthroscopy 13:433, 1997.
4. Bose K, Kanagasuntheram R, Osman MBH: Vastus medialis oblique: an anatomic and physiologic study, Orthopedics 3:880, 1980.
5. Cohn BT, Draeger RI, Jackson DW: The effects of cold therapy on postoperative management of pain in patents undergoing anterior cruciate ligament reconstruction, Am J Sports Med 17(3):344, 1989.
6. DeHaven KE: Peripheral meniscal repair: an alternative to meniscectomy, J Bone Joint Surg BR63:463, 1981.
7. DeHaven KE, Stone RC: Meniscal repair. In Sahiaree H, editor: O'Connor's textbook of arthroscopic surgery, Philadelphia, 1992, JB Lippincott.
8. DeLorme TL, Watkins A: Progressive resistance exercise, New York, 1951, Appleton-Century.
9. DeVries HA: Evaluation of static stretching, procedures for improvement of flexibility, Res Q 3:222, 1962.
10. Fairbanks TJ: Knee joint changes after meniscectomy, J Bone Joint Surg 30B:664, 1948.
11. Henning CE: Arthroscopic repair of meniscus tears, Orthopedics 6:1130, 1983.
12. Johnson LL: Diagnostic and surgical arthroscopy. The knee and other joints, ed 2, St Louis, 1981, Mosby.
13. Kottke FJ, Pavley DJ, Ptakda DA: The rationale for prolonged stretching for corrections of shortening of connective tissue, Arch Phys Med Rehab 47:345, 1966.
14. Kvist M, Jarvinen M: Clinical, histological and biomechanical features in repair of muscle and tendon injuries, Int J Sports Med 3:12, 1982.
15. Lessard LA et al: The efficacy of cryotherapy following arthroscopic knee surgery, J Orthop Sports Phys Ther 26(1):14, 1997.
16. Maitland GD: Peripheral manipulation, ed 3, London, 1991, Butterworth-Heinemann.
17. Mangine R, Heckman T: The knee. In Saunders B, editor: Sports physical therapy, Norwalk, Conn, 1990, Appleton & Lange.
18. McConnell J: The management of chondromalacia patellae: a long term solution, Aust J Physiother 32(4):215, 1986.
19. McConnell J, Fulkerson J: The knee: patellofemoral and soft tissue injuries. In Zachazewski JE, Magee DJ, Quillen WS, editors: Athletic injuries and rehabilitation, Philadelphia, 1996, WB Saunders.

20. Morgan CD: The all "inside" meniscus repair: technical note, *Arthroscopy* 7:120, 1991.
21. Norkin CC, Levangie PK: *Joint structure and function: a comprehensive analysis*, Philadelphia, 1992, FA Davis.
22. Powers CM: Rehabilitation of patellofemoral joint disorders: a critical review, *J Orthop Sports Phys Ther* 28(5):345, 1998.
23. Rubman MH, Noyes FR, Barber-Westin SD: Technical considerations in the management of complex meniscus tears, *Clin Sports Med* 15:511, 1996.
24. Shelbourne KD et al: Rehabilitation after meniscal repair, *Clin Sports Med* 15:595, 1996.
25. Suton JB: *Ligaments: their nature and morphology*, London, 1897, MK Lewis.
26. Tovin BJ et al: Comparison of the effects of exercise in water and on land on the rehabilitation of patients with intraarticular anterior cruciate ligament reconstruction, *Phys Ther* 74(8):710, 1994.
27. Whitelaw GP et al: The use of the Cryo/Cuff versus ice and elastic wrap in the postoperative care of knee arthroscopy patients, *Am J Knee Surg* 8(1):28, 1995.
28. Zachazewski JE: Flexibility for sports. In Saunders B, editor: *Sports physical therapy*, Norwalk, Conn, 1990, Appleton & Lange.

Chapter 15

Patella Open Reduction and Internal Fixation

Craig Zeman
Dan Farwell

Patella fractures can occur in a wide variety of individuals. Both genders have similar fracture rates. Age-related incidence of patella fractures tends to be shifted to a mature population. Patella fractures are usually caused by direct trauma or a blow to the patella.[4,23,25,35] Depending on the force of the injury the fracture can be nondisplaced or highly comminuted with significant injury to the extensor mechanism complex. Active extension of the knee is usually preserved with a nondisplaced fracture. However, in a displaced fracture the extensor mechanism is disrupted to the extent that active extension is not possible. Displaced fractures require open reduction and internal fixation (ORIF) to maximize active extension of the knee and decrease the incidence of posttraumatic arthritis.

Surgical Indications and Considerations

Physicians use two main criteria to determine whether surgery is indicated:
1. Fracture displacement of more than 3 or 4 mm
2. Loss of ability to extend the knee actively

Different surgical treatments are based on the type or severity of the fracture. Currently, tension band wiring is the most accepted treatment for displaced patella fractures.[6,15,19] Weber[36] noted stability and early range of motion (ROM) is to be performed, there must be a stable repair of the fracture site to avoid displacement of the repair. He noted increased stability by repairing cadaveric patella fractures with a technique in which the wire is anchored directly in bone. He also noted that the retinaculum should be repaired because it added to stability. Bostman[5] examined several different approaches and techniques to repair patella fractures and discovered the tension band wiring procedure to be far superior to other methods.

Smith and associates[31] performed a retrospective review of postoperative complications after ORIF of patella fractures. They followed 51 patients treated with the tension band fixation technique until complete healing had occurred at a minimum of 4 months. The authors' objective was to focus on acute, short-term complica-

tions after ORIF of patella fracture. Although the study did not specifically assess clinical parameters such as pain or strength, it did point out two important factors to consider during rehabilitation. Approximately 22% of the patella fractures treated with modified tension band wiring and early ROM displaced significantly during the early postoperative period. *Failure of fixation was related to unprotected ambulation and noncompliance. Patient noncompliance in restricting early ROM and weight bearing can cause failure of even technically correct tension band wire fixation.*[5,11,24,25,28]

Joint congruity must be restored to decrease the development of arthritis, and the extensor mechanism must be restored to regain full extension. Most patients with displaced fractures are candidates for ORIF. If the patient was ambulatory before the injury and can medically tolerate surgery, surgery should be performed regardless of age. Situations in which nonambulatory patients with patella fractures lack lower extremity function and sensation (neurologic impairment) can be managed conservatively.

Patients with simple two-part fractures have a better chance of a successful outcome than those with highly comminuted fractures. The variability of outcomes relates to the degree of fixation and the ability of the fracture site(s) to consolidate. In some cases of irreducible comminution the fragments may have to be removed, resulting in a partial or total patellectomy.* Patellectomy procedures have a lower success rate than stable internal fixation procedures.[9,12,30,32]

Surgical Procedure

Most methods of ORIF incorporate tension band wiring techniques.[11,22,24,36] The tension band wire is placed around the proximal and distal pole of the patella through the quadriceps and patella tendons. This wire compresses the fracture site. Rotational control is maintained by one to two screws or Kirschner (k) wires

---

*References 1, 2, 8, 11, 14, 16, 26, 33, 34, 35, 37.

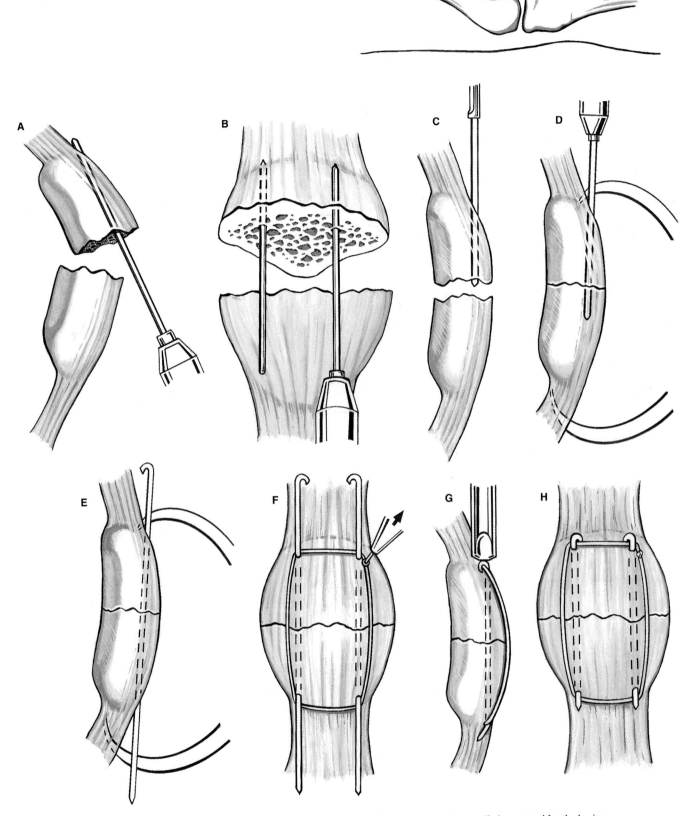

Fig. 15-1. The incision line from which repair of the fracture is initiated.

Fig. 15-2. The ORIF procedure for transverse fracture of the patella. **A** through **C**, The patella is prepared for the k-wires by drilling congruent holes through both pieces of the fracture. **D** and **E**, Bone forceps are used to approximate the fracture while wires are placed through the drill holes. **F** through **H**, The surgeon finishes the process of tension band wiring, creating stable postoperative fixation.

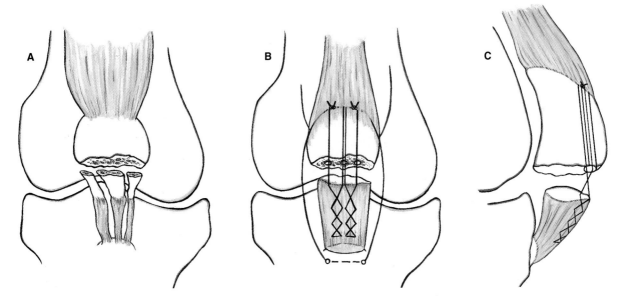

Fig. 15-3. The process of partial patellectomy. **A,** Comminuted fracture involving the inferior pole of the patella. Front view **(B)** and side view **(C)** after débridement of inferior fragments; sutures are woven into the tendon.

placed across the fracture site from the proximal to the distal pole. The tension band wire is passed under the k-wires or screws to add compressive and rotational stability to the fixation. Another method is to use cannulated screws through which the tension band wire may be passed.

The integrity of the skin over the patella must be evaluated before surgery because of its potential to produce postoperative complications. This area should be continually assessed by the therapist for infection and poor healing because vascular supply may have been disrupted during the trauma that caused the patella fracture.

Surgery is performed under either general or regional anesthesia. The patient is positioned supine and a tourniquet is applied to the thigh. The surgeon evaluates knee ROM to determine the stable postoperative ROM. The leg is then prepared and draped in a sterile fashion. If the skin allows, a longitudinal midline incision is made over the patella. This incision (Fig. 15-1) is carried down to the peritenon, and full-thickness flaps are developed both medially and laterally to expose the entire patella and extensor mechanism. The peritenon is then incised to expose the fracture and the tendons. The fracture hematoma is débrided from the fracture site, and the raw cancellous bone is delineated to aid in fracture reduction. Two k-wires are then run from the fracture site of the proximal fragment and out the proximal pole of the patella (Fig. 15-2, A through C). The proximal and distal fragments of the patella are brought together to reduce the fracture. The fracture is then held together with bone-holding forceps while the knee is in extension (Fig. 15-2, D). The k-wires are passed back through the middle of the patella and out the distal pole. The bone-holding forceps are then re-

moved (Fig. 15-2, E). Next the tension band wire is placed around the patella and k-wires. It should be positioned as close to the bone and k-wires as possible to minimize complications after ROM is initiated postoperatively (Fig. 15-2, F).

To place the tension wire as close to the bone and k-wire as possible, the surgeon usually passes a hollow needle under the k-wire and over the bone to guide the tension band wire. The tension band wire is then passed through the needle and brought around the patella. The two ends of the tension band wire are then twisted together with pliers to add tension to the system. The surgeon must be careful not to add too much tension to the wire because this may cause the wire to break early in the rehabilitation process (Fig. 15-2, G and H).

The surgeon then repairs the extensor mechanism. The medial and lateral retinacula are commonly torn in line with the fracture. These tears are simply repaired using nonabsorbable sutures. After this last repair the surgeon checks the ROM to ensure that the patient can easily obtain full extension and at least 90 degrees of flexion. The surgical site is then closed: first the peritenon, then the subcutaneous tissue, and finally the skin. The wound is dressed with a bulky dressing and placed in an immobilizer. A postoperative water cooling system or ice pack may be used to assist with pain control immediately.

A partial patellectomy may be performed in patients with comminuted displaced fractures who have at least 50% of the patella remaining.[33] The inferior pole of the patella usually suffers the most trauma, resulting in its removal (Fig. 15-3, A). The surgeon débrides the bone fragments from the tendon end and then weaves two large 5-0 nonabsorbable sutures into the tendon. He or she then drills two holes longitudinally into the remaining piece of the patella. The sutures in the tendon are brought through the holes in the patella and tied over the bone bridge formed by the two holes (Fig. 15-3, *B* and *C*).

Most patients require a second operation to remove the hardware placed in the patella.[17] The wires and sutures can become prominent and bother the patient during rehabilitation, slowing progress in gaining ROM.

The fixation of simple fractures is usually the most stable immediately after surgery. If the tension band wire is not placed right next to the screw, the wire can cut through the tendon until it butts up against the screw, decreasing the compressive effect of the wire and possibly allowing the fracture to displace. Stable fixation of a simple fracture is usually strong enough to allow early passive range of motion (PROM). The amount of ROM is dictated by the surgical procedure and pain tolerance. Time frames to initiate physical therapy vary depending on the degree of comminution. The repair is most vulnerable between 4 to 6 weeks when the bone and tendon have not completely healed and the pins and wires have loosened. After 8 weeks the repair should be stable enough to allow aggressive therapy with the goal of regaining full ROM.[7] The exception to this time frame is the patient who has a comminuted fracture with unstable fixation. This type of situation may require 12 weeks before the initiation of therapy. Most patients return to pre-injury activities (sports) by 6 months after surgery.

Therapy Guidelines for Rehabilitation

The treatment of patients who have undergone ORIF for patella fractures requires a cooperative approach from the orthopedist and the physical therapist. This concept is most evident when considering the challenge in treating patients after surgery. The goal of treatment is to provide a structurally stable patellofemoral joint and allow for full functional recovery of the involved lower extremity. Factors that influence the choice of treatment include the following:

1. The overall health of the patient and the way it may influence wound and fracture healing
2. The location and configuration of the fracture
3. Immobilization after surgery (osteopenia of the entire lower extremity, muscle atrophy, and possible contracture of the knee joint) versus ORIF (which allows for early ROM and patella mobilization)
4. Patient compliance with prescribed treatment plan (home program)

Although rehabilitation after a patella fracture treated with ORIF is crucial, a wide range of protocols may be used depending on the factors listed previously, the physician's chosen fixation technique, and the patient's goals (which differ among athletes, sedentary adults,

and children). The information the physical therapist collects from both the physician and the patient aids in determining the design and time parameters of the rehabilitation program.

The remainder of this chapter deals only with the simple transverse fracture. However, the clinician is reminded to respect the previously discussed four factors influencing treatment when planning rehabilitation for all patella fractures.

Phase I

TIME: Weeks 1-4
GOALS: Control pain, manage edema, gain 0 to 90 degrees of PROM, improve quadriceps and hamstring contraction (Table 15-1)

The acute phase of rehabilitation (the first 4 weeks) after ORIF of the patella is the time when re-injury is most likely. Attention to detail and communication with the treating physician are crucial during this period.

Controversy exists over when to initiate ROM. Hung[15] initiates knee motion 1 week after surgery, whereas Lotke[20] often immobilizes patients for as long as 3 weeks before beginning any type of motion. Bostman[5,6] not only immobilizes his patients an average of 38 days, but also states that he sees no correlation between the initial time of immobilization and the final outcome. Biomechanical studies that have demonstrated the appropriateness of tension band wiring and early ROM have generally used a simple transverse fracture pattern as the model.[3] Complications such as poor bone quality and comminuted patella fractures may prevent the desired fixation and thus preclude any early joint ROM.

The physical therapist performs an evaluation on the first postoperative visit, respecting the surgical procedure and any restrictions noted by the surgeon. Observation of the surgical site is documented and continually assessed to prevent wound complications. If the surgical site shows any signs of infection the physical therapist should notify the surgeon immediately. Crutches are used postoperatively, and weight bearing is as tolerated with the immobilizer in place. Patients may eventually progress to independent ambulation (with the immobilizer still in place) after they tolerate full weight bearing and are cleared by the physician (usually between 3 to 6 weeks). Smith et al[31] reported four complete failures after ORIF with tension band wiring. No inadequacies were detected during the initial procedures, and all four failures resulted from falls while walking unprotected in the early postoperative period.

ROM measurements of the knee are taken passively, with the physical therapist again observing any restrictions. Quality of muscle contraction in the extensor mechanism is noted and active knee flexion is assessed. Girth measurements may be taken to assess

Table 15-1   Patella ORIF

Rehabilitation Phase	Criteria to Progress to this Phase	Anticipated Impairments and Functional Limitations	Intervention	Goal	Rationale

Phase I Postoperative 1-4 weeks	Postoperative and cleared by physician to initiate therapy
	
	There may be specific precautions depending on the stability of fixation (communicate with physician)
		• Edema
		• Pain
		• Limited ROM
		• Limited strength
		• Limited transfers
		• Limited gait
			• Cryotherapy
			• ES for muscle stimulation
			• PROM—Knee extension Knee flexion supine wall slides
			• Isometrics—Quadriceps/hamstring sets Quadriceps sets at 20°-30°
			• AROM—Standing hamstring curls Supine heel slides
			• Gait training using crutches and weight bearing as tolerated in immobilizer
			• Weight shifting
			• Joint mobilization to the patella (resistance-free)
				• Control pain
				• Manage edema
				• Improve muscle contraction
				• PROM
				  Knee
				  Extension 0°
				  Flexion 90°
				• Initiate volitional muscle contraction
				• Improve tolerance to flexion ROM
				• Avoid excessive stress on the extensor mechanism during ambulation
				• Decrease pain
					• Initiate self-management of pain
					• Use ES to improve muscle contraction
					• Restore joint ROM as indicated by physician
					• Prepare for independence with transfers (straight leg raise [SLR] independent)
					• Begin to prepare extensor mechanism to accept load
					• Restore independence with ambulation
					• Improve stability of involved lower extremity
					• Control pain through resistance-free mobilization to the patella

atrophy of the thigh and calf; however, this has little overall benefit compared with functional assessment.

Early ROM is the goal in any operative treatment of patella fractures, yet the definition of *early ROM* varies depending on who performs the procedure.[5,6,15,20] Although the acute phase of rehabilitation tends to focus on knee joint range, gait deviations can produce problems later in rehabilitation if they are not addressed early. Patients often are treated in some type of immobilizer. A hinged brace can be used to allow for motion while stabilizing the fracture.

Initial treatments focus on restoring ROM (0 to 90 degrees), improving quadriceps and hamstring muscle control, progressing gait (weight-bearing tolerance), managing edema, and controlling pain. A program of elevation and ice (20 to 30 minutes three times a day) is used as necessary to manage edema and control pain. Electrical stimulation (ES) for pain control is avoided because of the proximity of the screw and wires. However, ES can be used to assist in quadriceps contraction when appropriate. Gentle mobilization (grades I and II shy of resistance) of the patella also is employed to control pain.

Initial exercises of the knee involve PROM, active range of motion (AROM), and isometrics. Passive stretches are performed to restore flexion and extension. The vigor of the stretch should be in concert with the guidelines established by the surgeon. In general patients are expected to reach 90 degrees of flexion and full extension by 4 weeks. Supine wall slides can be easily performed in the clinic or at home. (Refer to the section on Suggested Home Maintenance for the Postsurgical Patient.) Regaining full extension is usually not a problem. However, limitations of extension can be treated quite successfully (see Figs. 12-2 and 12-3).

Active exercises primarily focus on using the hamstrings to flex the knee. Heel slides and standing hamstring curls are initiated to aid in increasing muscle control and progressing ROM.

Isometric exercises involve quadriceps and hamstring co-contraction and isolated quadriceps contractions at 20 to 30 degrees flexion. Quality is observed and ES is helpful in recruitment.

Gait training focuses on increasing the acceptance of weight on the involved leg. Weight shifting can be given as part of the home program. After the incision is healed and the surgeon allows it, aquatherapy can be initiated with an emphasis on proper weight shifting and gait mechanics.

Phase II

TIME: Weeks 5-8
GOALS: Self-manage pain, increase strength, increase ROM to 90%, initiate quadriceps AROM (6 to 8 weeks), have minimal gait deviations on level surfaces (Table 15-2)

The subacute or mid-phase of rehabilitation (from weeks 5 to 8) is the transition from limited functional activity to aggressive functional activity. The actual exercise protocol is similar to any other type of patellofemoral rehabilitation. The only real difference with ORIF patella fracture is that a true fixation of the fracture has been obtained. Motion at the fracture site tends to activate secondary callus formation, especially with tension band wiring of a patella fracture. The danger in moving a non-fixated fracture (a fracture with no established callus formation) is that a nonunion may develop. A nonunion of bone is caused by excessive motion directly at the fracture site, which keeps the callus from forming sufficiently. This underlines the importance of maintaining immobility in some patella fractures during the rehabilitative process.[18]

Another factor to consider is that patella fractures involve joint surfaces. Incongruency of the articular surfaces can lead to articular cartilage degeneration and possible early arthritis if not treated. Incongruity of the patellofemoral joint may alter the joint mechanics, producing areas of non-contact or excessive pressure over the patella.[29] Issues of patellofemoral contact area and joint reaction force must be evaluated during this phase of rehabilitation. The use of patellofemoral taping (see Figs. 13-1 through 13-3) can be useful in limiting imbalances over the fractured surface of the patella. By this phase the patient is demonstrating increased competency in ambulating with the brace and decreased reliance (if any) on the crutches. Exercises are progressed as in phase I and the patient is instructed to perform two sets per day, repetitions to fatigue. Closed-chain exercises are initiated on a progressive basis based on patient healing and quadriceps and lower extremity control (see Figs. 12-1, 12-4, and 14-3).

Modalities at this stage are primarily ice for pain control. ES of the quadriceps is continued as indicated to progress muscle recruitment. Moist heat can be used to prepare the knee for stretching after edema is controlled.

PROM stretches are progressed as indicated to obtain full flexion. Vigor of grades of mobilization are increased into resistance as indicated.

AROM for the quadriceps is initiated between 6 to 8 weeks (or when the fracture is deemed stable enough

Q. Jessica is 40 years old. She fractured her patella when she fell off a footstool and onto her knees. She had a patella ORIF surgery 9 weeks ago. Her knee flexion ROM is limited and peri-patella pain is a factor when performing ROM stretches. ROM exercises for knee flexion have been emphasized during the past few treatments along with modalities for pain control. Little progress has been noted. What treatment techniques may be the most helpful?

Table 15-2   Patella ORIF

Rehabilitation Phase	Criteria to Progress to this Phase	Anticipated Impairments and Functional Limitations	Intervention	Goal	Rationale
Phase II Postoperative 5-8 weeks	No signs of infection No significant increase in pain No loss of ROM	• Pain • Limited ROM • Limited strength • Limited gait	• Continuation and progression of interventions from phase I • Patellofemoral taping • Gait training; discontinue crutches when indicated • Lower extremity exercises • Assisted AROM— Stationary Bike used as a ROM assist for flexion • AROM—Knee extension (when cleared by physician, usually between 6-8 weeks)	• Self-manage pain • Decrease gait deviations • Increase lower extremity strength • PROM of knee to 90% • Independent with home exercises	• Prepare patient for discharge • Assist patellofemoral mechanics • Promote return to unassisted gait in the community • Restore lower extremity stability and strength • Obtain close to if not full strength • Promote restoration of normal joint mechanics • Initiate extensor mechanism strengthening and improve tolerance to patellofemoral compression with tracking

to tolerate it). The stationary bike can be used as a ROM assistive device and progressed for strengthening and cardiovascular purposes after flexion allows full revolution without hip hiking.

The rehabilitation at this point begins to mimic that prescribed for the patient recovering from lateral release in terms of exercises and progressions. Taping can be initiated in this phase as deemed appropriate by the therapist.

A. The physical therapist should assess the patella for limited mobility. If mobility is limited, which is likely, patella mobilizations using grades into resistance (grades III and IV) can be helpful. The therapist should receive clearance by the physician before initiating mobilization into resistance. Increasing inferior patella movement if it is limited may particularly help knee flexion ROM. Issues of patellofemoral contact area and reaction forces also must be evaluated. Patellofemoral taping can be useful in limiting imbalances over the fractured surfaces of the patella. Complaints of pain with flexion may decrease, particularly with closed-chain exercises.

Q. Jessica's knee ROM is now full 12 weeks after surgery. She performs a series of exercises for leg strengthening. She begins by stretching her hamstrings and gastrocnemius-soleus muscles. She then performs the following:

- Standing mini-squats against the wall (see Fig. 11-15)
- Leg presses using 100 lb and keeping knee flexion less than 60 degrees (see Fig. 11-20)
- Lunges with 5-lb weights in a long-stride position (see Fig. 13-6)
- Wall slides between 0 and 45 degrees with a 1-minute hold (see Fig. 13-7)
- Sit-stand (see Fig. 16-15)
- Standing (four-wall) elastic tubing hip flexion, abduction, and adduction on the uninvolved side (see Fig. 14-3, *A* through *D*)
- Step-downs on an 8-inch step, holding contraction until the heel of the opposite leg makes contact (see Fig. 13-8)

Although she had minimal discomfort during the exercise regimen, she had increased complaints of pain for 2 days after the exercises. Which of these exercises is most likely to be an aggravating factor?

Phase III

TIME: Weeks 9-12
GOALS: Return to full function, develop endurance and coordination of the lower extremity, continue to address limitations with steps and running (with physician clearance) (Table 15-3)

The advanced stage of rehabilitation (from weeks 9 to 12) focuses on functional, skill-specific activity. Most of the effort and work is spent on building back the patient's quadriceps, hamstring, and gastrocnemius-soleus muscle strength.

Depending on remaining deficits, exercises from the previous two phases are continued. The therapist should keep in mind that the time frame will vary depending on many factors, including type of fracture, fixation, and the patient's response to rehabilitation. Furthermore, isokinetics should be avoided until they have been approved by the physician. The need for taping should be minimal, but if continued taping is needed patients are instructed in self-taping techniques. Monitoring for pain and joint effusion gives the therapist feedback on the way to progress activities aggressively. Long-term strengthening of the muscles surrounding the patellofemoral joint with the development of endurance and coordination over time are the goals of this phase.

By this stage patients should be close to discharge because they are fairly functional with sitting, standing, and walking tolerances. Limitations with stairs and squatting activities continue to be present. Prolonged standing and walking should be continually improving with the focus on a progressive increase in activities. Running and jumping should be initiated on an individual basis as determined by the surgeon (potentially after removal of hardware).

A. The 8-inch step-downs are the most aggressive exercises because they produce the highest patellofemoral compression forces. The knee is most likely flexed beyond 50 degrees while performing an eccentric contraction during full weight bearing on the affected extremity.

Suggested Home Maintenance for the Postsurgical Patient

An exercise program has been outlined at the various phases. The home maintenance box on page 266 outlines rehabilitation guidelines the patient may follow. The physical therapist can use it in customizing a patient-specific program.

Table 15-3 Patella ORIF

Rehabilitation Phase	Criteria to Progress to this Phase	Anticipated Impairments and Functional Limitations	Intervention	Goal	Rationale
Phase III Postoperative 9-12 weeks	• Pain free at rest • ROM 0°-90° • Good quadriceps control during gait • Minimal gait deviations	• Limited endurance with prolonged functional activities • Mild pain of patellofemoral joint during skill-specific exercises • Limited tolerance to stairs and single-limb squat and balance	• Closed-chain and stretching exercises as listed in Tables 15-1 and 15-2 • Patella taping • Patella mobilization • Lunges with weights, increased repetitions and speed with exercises • Progressive resistive exercises on leg press • Function-specific activity: bicycle, stair-climber, slideboard, treadmill, isokinetic training (when cleared by physician) • Home exercises (refer to Suggested Home Maintenance section)	• Unlimited community ambulation • No gait deviations • Good sitting and standing tolerances • Good patella stability without taping • Patient self-management of symptoms	• Decrease pain with functional activities • Improve joint mechanics • Improve joint mobility and stability • Provide functional strengthening • Improve endurance of VMO • Increase reliance on patient self-management

Troubleshooting

Issues that prevent a successful outcome are unstable fixation, incongruous reduction, poor patient compliance, and delays in early PROM exercises. Patients with poor pain tolerance do not regain strength and ROM as easily and may be left with residual deficits. Maximal function after patella fracture has been noted to take as long as 1 year.[10] Residual problems of anterior knee pain and stiffness are common complications.*

*References 2, 12, 13, 26, 32, 38.

An estimated 70% to 80% of patients recovering from patella ORIF have good to excellent results, although 20% to 30% have fair to poor results.[25] Residual loss of extensor strength has been recorded in the 20% to 49% range.

Prolonged immobilization is detrimental to the final result regardless of the treatment.[25] Although it produces a risk of wound infection, the benefits of ROM outweigh the risk of wound complications. However, this situation is especially tenuous in patients who suffer open patella fractures because they are at a higher risk for infection.

Suggested Home Maintenance for the Postsurgical Patient

Weeks 1-4

GOALS FOR THE PERIOD: Control pain, manage edema, gain 0 to 90 degrees of PROM, improve quadriceps and hamstring contraction
1. Elevate and ice at home two to three times per day (preferably after exercises).
2. Perform ankle pumping and hamstring stretches with the extremity elevated and on ice (20-30 minutes).
3. Perform supine wall slides (when appropriate)—one set of five repetitions three to four times a day.
4. Perform active heel slides—one set of 10 repetitions performed three to four times per day.
5. Perform quadriceps sets (on clearance from the physician)—two sets of 10 repetitions performed three to four times per day. Even though general guidelines such as this may prescribe a number of sets and repetitions, if the patient fatigues and cannot continue to recruit a quality quadriceps contraction, the exercise is over. Patients are only to count repetitions with quality quadriceps contractions. The heel should stay on the floor. Quadriceps sets also may be performed standing if the patient finds it easier to activate the quadriceps in this position. The key to early strengthening is to find which position the patient is most successful in recruiting a quality quadriceps contraction.

Weeks 5-8

GOALS FOR THE PERIOD: Self-manage pain, increase strength, increase ROM to 90%, initiate quadriceps AROM (6 to 8 weeks), have minimal gait deviations on level surfaces
1. Perform the same exercises as in weeks 1-4, increasing the number of repetitions. Exercises should generally be performed in two sets of 10 to 20 repetitions per day (based on fatigue).
2. Initiate closed-chain exercises based on patient tolerance to resistance. Spider killers (see Fig. 12-1) are initiated in pain-free ranges. In addition, simulated leg press exercises with elastic tubing can be performed. Patients begin with two sets of 10 repetitions and progress based on tolerance.
3. Perform self-taping as deemed appropriate by therapist.
4. Continue use of ice after exercises.

Weeks 9-12

GOALS FOR THE PERIOD: Return to full function, develop endurance and coordination of the lower extremity, continue to address limitations with steps and running (with physician clearance)
1. Depending on remaining deficits, continue exercises from the previous 8 weeks. The need for taping should be minimal, but if continued taping is required patients are instructed in self-taping techniques.
2. Progress closed-chain exercises to include stepping exercises at home using threshold of doorway for balance.
3. Gradually return to functional activities while monitoring for pain and joint effusion.

REFERENCES

1. Anderson LD: . In Crenshaw AH, editor: *Campbell's operative orthopaedics,* ed 5, St Louis, 1971, Mosby.

2. Andrews JR, Hughston JC: Treatment of patellar fractures by partial patellectomy, *South Med J* 70:809, 1977.

3. Benjamin J et al: Biomechanical evaluation of various forms of fixation of transverse patella fractures, *J Orthop Trauma* 1:219, 1987.

4. Bohler L: *Die Technik der Knochenbruchandlung,* ed 13, 1957, Wein Wilhelm Maudrich Verlag.

5. Bostman O et al: Comminuted displaced fractures of the patella, *Injury* 13:196, 1981.

6. Bostman O et al: Fractures of the patella treated by operation, *Arth Orthop Trauma Surg* 102:78, 1983.

7. Bray TJ, Marder RA: Patellar fractures. In Chapman MD, Madison M, editors: *Operative orthopaedics,* ed 2, Philadelphia, 1993, JB Lippincott.

8. Brooke R: The treatment of fractured patella by excision: a study of morphology and function, *Br J Surg* 24:733, 1937.

9. Burton VW: Results of excision of the patella, *Surg Gynecol Obstet* 135:753, 1972.

10. Crenshaw AH, Wilson FD: The surgical treatment of fractures of the patella, *South Med J* 47:716, 1954.

11. DePalma AF: *The management of fractures and dislocations,* Philadelphia, 1959, WB Saunders.

12. Duthie HL, Hutchinson JR: The results of partial and total excision of the patella, *J Bone Joint Surg* 40B:75, 1958.

13. Einola S, Aho AJ, Kallio P: Patellectomy after fracture. Long-term follow-up results with special reference to functional disability, *Acta Orthop Scand* 47:441, 1976.

14. Heineck AP: The modern operative treatment of fracture of the patella: I. Based on the study of other pathological states of bone. II. An analytical review of over 1,100 cases treated during the last ten years, by open operative method, *Surg Gynecol Obstet* 9:177, 1909.

15. Hung LK et al: Fractured patella: operative treatment using tension band principle, *Injury* 16:343, 1985.

16. Jakobsen J, Christensen KS, Rassmussen OS: Patellectomy—a 20-year follow-up, *Acta Orthop Scand* 56:430, 1985.

17. Johnson EE: Fractures of the patella. In Rockwood CA, Green DP, Bucholz RW, editors: *Fractures in adults,* ed 3, Philadelphia, 1991, JB Lippincott.

18. Klassen JK, Trousdale RT: Treatment of delayed and nonunion of the patella, *J Orthop Trauma* 11(3):188, 1997.

19. Lexack B, Flannagan JP, Hobbs S: Results of surgical treatment of patellar fractures, *J Bone Joint Surg* BR67:416, 1985.

20. Lotke PA, Ecker ML: Transverse fractures of the patella, *Clin Orthop* 158:1880, 1981.

21. MacAusland WR: Total excision of the patella for fracture: report of fourteen cases, *Am J Surg* 72:510, 1946.

22. Magnusen PB: *Fractures,* ed 2, Philadelphia, 1936, JB Lippincott.

23. McMaster PE: Fractures of the patella, *Clin Orthop* 4:24, 1954.

24. Muller ME, Allgower M, Willinegger H: *Manual of internal fixation: technique recommended by the AO group,* New York, 1979, Springer-Verlag.

25. Nummi J: Fracture of the patella: a clinical study of 707 patellar fractures, *Ann Chir Gynaecol Fenn* 60(suppl):179, 1971.

26. Peeples RE, Margo MK: Function after patellectomy, *Clin Orthop* 132:180, 1978.

27. Mehta A: *Physical medicine and rehabilitation: state of the art reviews,* vol 9, no 1, Philadelphia, 1995, Hanley & Belfus.

28. Rorabeck CH, Bobechko WP: Acute dislocation of the patella with osteochondral fracture: a review of eighteen cases, *J Bone Joint Surg* 58A:237, 1976.

29. Sanders R: Patella fractures and extensor mechanism injuries. In Bronner BD et al, editors: *Skeletal trauma,* Philadelphia, 1992, WB Saunders.

30. Sanderson MC: The fractured patella: a long-term follow-up study, *Aust NZ J Surg* 45:49, 1974.

31. Smith ST et al: Early complications in the operative treatment of patella fractures, *J Orthop Trauma* 11(3):183, 1997.

32. Sutton FS et al: The effect of patellectomy on knee function, *J Bone Joint Surg* 58A:537, 1976.

33. Thompson JEM: Comminuted fractures of the patella: treatment of cases presenting with one large fragment and several small fragments, *J Bone Joint Surg* 58A:537, 1976.

34. Watson-Jones R: Excision of the patella (letter), *Br Med J* 2:195, 1945.

35. Watson-Jones R: *Fractures and other bone and joint injuries,* Edinburgh, 1939, E & S Livingstone.

36. Weber MJ et al: Efficacy of various forms of fixation of transverse fractures of the patella, *J Bone Joint Surg* AM62:215, 1980.

37. West FE: End results of patellectomy, *J Bone Joint Surg* 62A:1089, 1962.

38. Wilkinson J: Fracture of the patella treated by total excision: a long-term follow-up, *J Bone Joint Surg* 59B:352, 1977.

Chapter 16

Total Knee Replacement

Geoffrey Vaupel
Nora Cacanindin
Julie Wong

The widespread incidence of osteoarthritis of the knee and its severe affect on disability is well documented.[80] When conservative management fails to restore mobility or decrease pain, surgical intervention is often the treatment of choice. According to the National Center for Health Statistics (on the AAOS web site), 259,000 total knee replacements (TKRs) were performed in 1997. Many were for people aged 65 and older.[81] As the population of "baby boomers" ages, this number will likely grow accordingly. Understanding the various surgical procedures and designing appropriate programs for rehabilitation are essential to ensure successful and cost-effective outcomes in anticipation of this growth.

Surgical Indications and Considerations

The most common indication for a total knee arthroplasty is disabling arthritic knee pain that is refractory to conservative measures (e.g., nonsteroidal antiinflammatory medications, physical therapy, cortisone injections) in elderly patients, ideally over 65 years. Disability and age considerations must be individualized. Contraindications reflecting a greater than normal complication rate include severe peripheral vascular disease, history of infection, and morbid obesity.

Surgical Procedure

Preoperative Evaluation

Preoperative evaluation always includes a thorough history and physical examination, determination of the type of arthritis, other joint involvement and status, walking distance, current and expected activity level, and sports involvement. Other significant concerns include history of deep venous thrombosis or pulmonary embolus and previous surgery such as joint replacement, corrective osteotomy, and internal fixation of a hip, femur, or tibial fracture. Close attention is paid to joint alignment (varus or valgus), stability, range of motion (ROM—especially the presence or absence of flexion contracture), muscle tone, and leg lengths.

Preoperative x-ray films are crucial. Ideally they should include bilateral and single-leg-stance weight-bearing films from hip to ankle on one cassette. This combination demonstrates any femoral or tibial deformity and aids in determining overall lower extremity alignment. The angle between the mechanical and anatomic axis is measured on the femur to ensure that the distal femoral osteotomy will be perpendicular to the mechanical axis and parallel to the proximal tibial osteotomy (Fig. 16-1). Routine roentgenograms should include posteroanterior (PA) standing films of both knees in 45 degrees of flexion and 10 degrees caudad tile (Rosenberg's view) lateral and infrapatellar views.

Procedure

Numerous choices are available for TKR:
1. Cemented, uncemented or hybrid
2. Metal-backed tibia or all-polyethylene tibia
3. Metal-backed patella or all-polyethylene patella
4. Patella resurfacing or patella retaining
5. Posterior stabilization or cruciate retaining
6. Flat-on-flat, round-on-round, or mobile-bearing surfaces

The technique described here is the primary TKR using the cemented implant, metal-backed tibia, all-polyethylene patella with posterior stabilization and round-on-round surfaces (Fig. 16-2). Currently this combination is the most commonly used with the best long-term results published to date.[10,17,64,65,74]

Technique

An anti-thrombotic stocking or pump is placed on the uninvolved leg in the preoperative holding area. The patient is questioned by the surgeon as to which knee is to be replaced as a final check to avoid the indefensible mistake of operating on the wrong knee. Some surgeons have been known to write "Wrong knee!" in permanent marker on the uninvolved knee. An intravenous antibiotic, usually first-generation cephalosporin, is given at least a half hour before the skin incision. The patient is placed supine on the operating

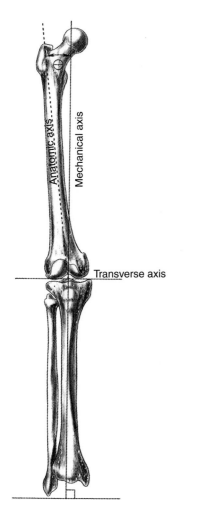

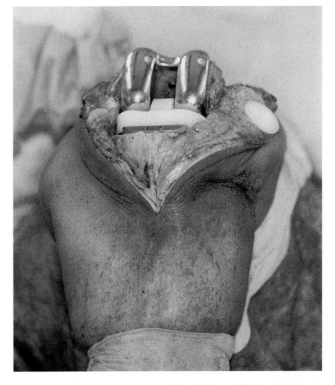

Fig. 16-2. Final result of the author's choice for total knee arthroplasty.

Fig. 16-1. The anatomic axis parallels the femoral shaft, whereas the mechanical axis is a straight line from the center of the femoral head to the center of the knee and the center of the ankle. (Courtesy Zimmer, Inc., Warsaw, Indiana.)

room table with a tourniquet about the proximal thigh. A general endotracheal or regional anesthetic is required. A sandbag is taped to the operating room table, or a commercial leg-holding device is used to help stabilize the leg during the procedure. The entire lower extremity is sterilely prepared and draped. The lower extremity is exsanguinated with an Esmarch bandage, and a tourniquet is inflated to an appropriate pressure.

Exposure. A longitudinal midline skin incision is made extending from proximal to the patella to just distal to the tibial tuberosity. Full-thickness skin flaps, including the deep fascia, are developed medially and laterally (Fig. 16-3). Medial arthrotomy is made extending from the quadriceps tendon and ending medial to the tibial tuberosity. The patella is everted laterally. After flexing the knee to 90 degrees, the surgeon trims osteophytes from about the femoral condyles, intercondylar notch, and tibial plateaus. The cruciate ligaments are excised.

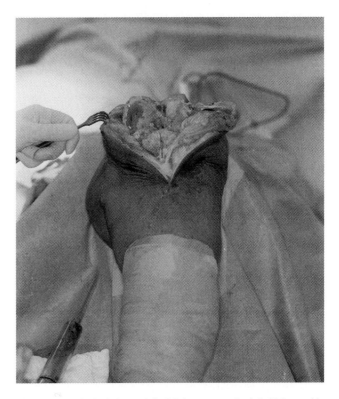

Fig. 16-3. Surgical exposure of the left knee. Note the full-thickness skin flaps, medial arthrotomy, and eversion of the patella. This varus knee demonstrates severe wear of the medial femoral condyle.

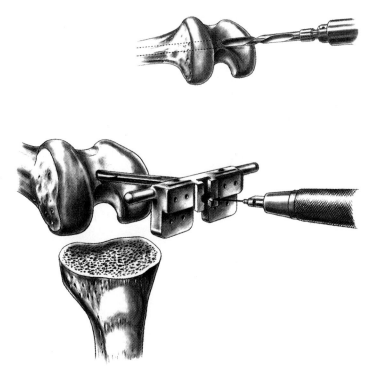

Fig. 16-4. The intramedullary femoral guide ensures placement parallel to the anatomic axis. (Courtesy Zimmer, Inc., Warsaw, Indiana.)

Ligament balancing. Ligamentous balance is then addressed by inserting spreaders in the medial and lateral femoral tibial joints, both in flexion and extension. Equal spacing is then attained by excision of osteophytes and soft tissue releases. The four most common deformities encountered are varus, valgus, flexion, and recurvatum.

VARUS DEFORMITY. Osteophytes protruding off the medial tibia are removed and the medial capsule is incised. If necessary, the medial collateral ligament is subperiosteally stripped off the tibia.

VALGUS DEFORMITY. A lateral retinacular release is commonly required. The iliotibial band may require Z-lengthening. The popliteus tendon, lateral collateral ligament, and posterolateral capsule may be released off the femur. The biceps femoris tendon rarely requires a Z-lengthening. *Peroneal nerve neuropraxia may occur, especially with flexion contracture in association with valgus deformity.*

FLEXION DEFORMITY. A minor contracture is usually addressed by excising posterior femoral osteophytes and releasing posterior capsular adhesions. Further correction requires excision of more bone from the distal femur and possible posterior capsular release.

GENU RECURVATUM. Creation of a slight flexion contracture is done by implanting the components more tightly than usual.

Osseous preparation. The proximal tibia is osteotomized with a power sagittal saw perpendicular to its long axis approximately 5 mm distal to its articular surface and angled posteriorly approximately 3 degrees. Either in-

tramedullary or extramedullary cutting guides are used. Small tibial defects are addressed with cement. Larger defects require either bone grafting or specialized wedge components. Attention is then drawn to the femur. An intramedullary femoral guide is placed through a drill hole in the center of the trochlea (Fig. 16-4). The intramedullary rod must parallel the femoral shaft in both the anteroposterior (AP) and lateral planes, ensuring placement parallel to the anatomic axis of the femur. Cutting guides are attached to the intramedullary guide to allow precise osteotomies of the anterior and distal femur. The distal femoral osteotomy is usually made 6 degrees to the anatomic axis to produce distal femoral alignment perpendicular to the mechanical axis (Fig. 16-5).

An AP measuring guide is used to determine the appropriate site for the femoral component. An AP cutting guide is placed to remove the anterior and posterior femoral condyles. This affords excellent visibility and access to remove any remaining meniscus, cruciate ligament, and osteophytes (Fig. 16-6).

The flexion and extension gaps are measured with standardized blocks. Ideally, the same gap has been produced between the distal femur and tibia in extension and posterior femur and tibia in flexion. This ensures proper soft tissue tension and ligamentous balance. If full extension is not attained, further bone is removed from the distal femur. A guide is then used to chamfer the anterior and posterior femoral condyles and remove the intercondylar notch (Fig. 16-7).

The surgeon then returns his or her attention to the tibia, using sizing guides to determine the proper sized tibial component. After orienting the guide in the AP and

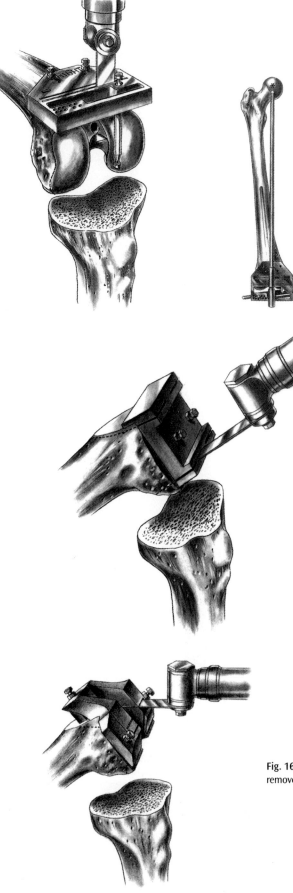

Fig. 16-5. The distal femoral guide attaches to the intramedullary guide with a proper amount of valgus (usually 6 degrees) to ensure the osteotomy is made perpendicular to the mechanical axis.   (Courtesy Zimmer, Inc., Warsaw, Indiana.)

Fig. 16-6. Anterior and posterior femoral osteotomies.   (Courtesy Zimmer, Inc., Warsaw, Indiana.)

Fig. 16-7. Single guide used to perform anterior and posterior chamfers and remove the intercondylar notch.   (Courtesy Zimmer, Inc., Warsaw, Indiana.)

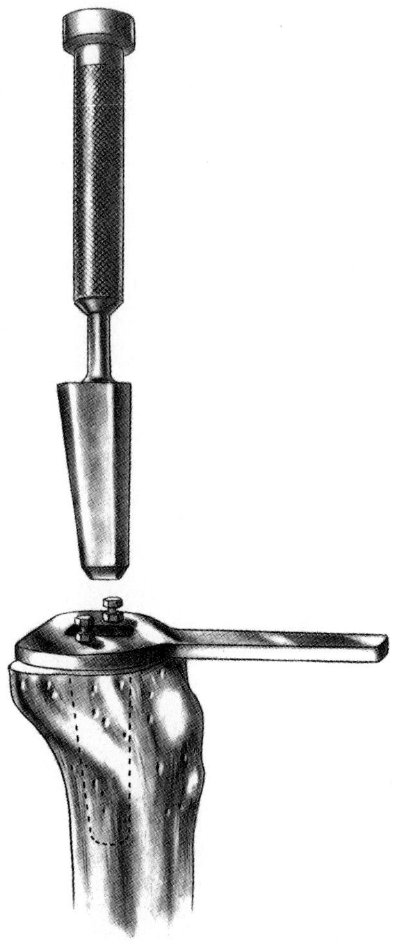

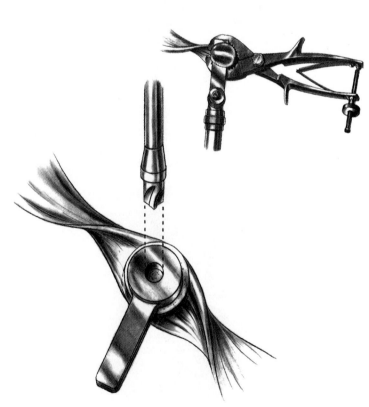

Fig. 16-8. A tibial template is rotationally aligned and sized appropriately to allow proper placement of the tibial stem punch. (Courtesy Zimmer, Inc., Warsaw, Indiana.)

Fig. 16-9. A patella template ensures the proper size and placement of the patella component. (Courtesy Zimmer, Inc., Warsaw, Indiana.)

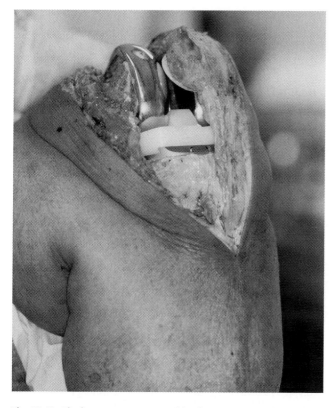

Fig. 16-10. Final component cemented in place. Note central tracking of patella without finger pressure.

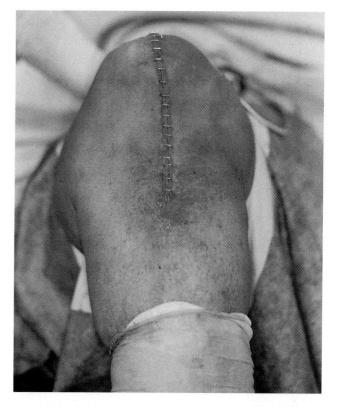

Fig. 16-11. The wound is closed in layers with nonabsorbable sutures in arthrotomy incisions, running absorbable sutures in subcutaneous layer incorporating Scarpa's fascia, and staples in the skin. Suction drainage exits supralaterally to avoid quadriceps mechanism.

medial and lateral planes, the surgeon ensures proper rotation with the use of an alignment rod extending to the middle of the ankle joint. A bone punch is then used to compress the soft cancellous bone in the tibial metaphysis to accommodate the keel on the tibial component (Fig. 16-8). Trial tibial and femoral components are placed to ensure proper sizing, soft tissue tensioning, ligamentous balance, and ROM.

The surgeon measures patella thickness with a caliper. The articular surface is removed with a power saw. A template is used to drill a hole in the center of the proposed patella component position (Fig. 16-9). The component is placed medial on the patella to assist in patella tracking. The thickness is again checked with the caliper, and if thicker than before, more patella is removed to restore normal patella thickness.

Patella tracking is now observed without finger pressure (Fig. 16-10). If the patella tracks laterally, a lateral retinacular release is performed. Efforts are made to preserve the superior lateral geniculate artery, thereby preserving the blood supply to the patella.

All trial components are removed, the tourniquet is deflated, and bleeding is controlled. The tourniquet is reinflated, all bony surfaces are cleansed with pulse lavage, and bone cement is mixed. All components may

be cemented at one time, or a second batch of cement may be prepared to allow sequential implantation of the components. All excess cement is trimmed while soft. After the cement has hardened, the tibial spacer may be exchanged to allow final adjustments with regard to ROM and stability.

The wound is irrigated thoroughly and closed over a suction drain. An anti-thrombotic stocking is applied over a sterile dressing and the patient is transferred to the recovery room (Fig. 16-11).

Therapy Guidelines for Rehabilitation

Successful postoperative management of the patient ideally begins preoperatively with the assembly of a multidisciplinary team consisting of the orthopedic surgeon, nursing staff, physical therapist, occupational therapist, and social service worker, each committed to a common goal of providing the best possible care to get the maximal result. The patient should be educated and familiarized with the surgical procedure and the phases and goals of the rehabilitation process. This identifies any special problems or needs the patient may incur to be anticipated and reinforces the active role of the patient in postoperative care. Good preop-

Table 16-1   Total Knee Replacement

Rehabilitation Phase	Criteria to Progress to this Phase	Anticipated Impairments and Functional Limitations	Intervention	Goal	Rationale

Phase I Inpatient acute care Days 1-5	Postoperative and cleared by physician to initiate therapy	• Edema
		• Pain
		• Limited ROM
		• Limited strength
		• Limited bed mobility and transfers
		• Limited gait
			• CPM set-up and patient education beginning with 0°–40° and progressing 5°–10° as tolerated 5-20 hours a day
			• Inspect for wound drainage, erythema, and excessive pain
			• Breathing exercises
			• Patient education to control edema (elevation and ankle pumps) and positioning to prevent knee flexion contracture
			• PROM—Knee extension
			  Knee flexion
			  Supine wall slides
			• Isometrics—Quadriceps, hamstring, and gluteal sets 10 repetitions three times a day
			• AROM—Ankle dorsiflexion, plantar flexion, and circumduction
			  Supine heel slides
			• Transfer and bed mobility training
			• Gait training with weight bearing as tolerated or as physician orders (using walker or crutches) in immobilizer until adequate quadriceps control is attained
			After second day, progress to:
			• Initiate A/AROM exercises twice a day
			• AROM—Heel slides (supine and seated), TKEs, SLRs
				• Control pain
				• Manage edema
				• Prevent and observe for postoperative complications (DVT, PE, infection)
				• PROM Knee Extension 0° Flexion 90°
				• Improve muscle contraction
				• Initiate volitional muscle contraction
				• Promote independence with bed mobility, transfers
				• Restore independence with ADLs
				• Independent with gait for 100 feet on level surfaces using appropriate assistive device
				• Progress self-management of ROM exercises
				• Decrease pain and edema
					• Restore ROM of knee
					• Improve wound healing, reduce adhesion formation, prevent complications
					• Wound and surgical site protection is important as patient begins to perform exercise and ambulation (Note: infection and DVT are major postoperative complications of TKR)
					• Use gravity feed and muscle pump to minimize edema and prevent DVT
					• Reduce reflex inhibition of quadriceps resulting from edema and pain
					• Prepare for independence with transfers (single-leg raise [SLR] independent)
					• Begin to prepare extensor mechanism to accept load
					• Restore independence with ambulation
					• Improve stability of involved lower extremity
					• Prevent disuse atrophy and reflex inhibition
					• Prepare for home disposition, facilitate independence

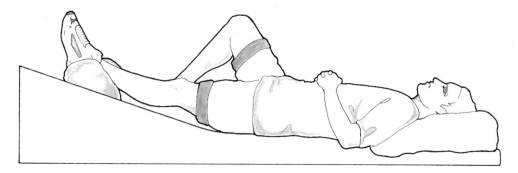

Fig. 16-12. With the leg straight, position a pillow under the ankle to increase end-range extension and venous drainage and decrease compression of the posterior tibial vein.

erative care and communication between the team and the patient can guarantee a smooth transition through the postoperative process.

Phase I: Inpatient Acute Care

TIME: Days 1-5
GOALS: Prevent complications, reduce pain and swelling, promote ROM, restore safety and independence (Table 16-1)

The goals for the initial stage of rehabilitation are standard for postoperative care. The primary goal is to prevent any possible complications. Medical considerations include the following:
1. The prevention of deep venous thrombosis (DVT)
2. The prevention of postoperative infection
3. The prevention of pulmonary embolus (PE)
4. The reduction of pain and swelling
Functional goals include the following:
1. The promotion of ROM
2. Encouragement of independence with bed mobility, transfers, and gait
3. The restoration of safety and independence in activities of daily living (ADLs)
The treatment plan is formulated with these specific goals in mind.

Medical considerations. Intravenous antibiotics are continued for 24 hours. DVT prophylaxis is initiated. This may consist of anti-thrombotic pumps, warfarin (Coumadin) or low–molecular-weight heparin, or any combination of these modalities.

Monitoring the surgical incision for drainage, erythema, excessive pain, and swelling continues throughout the patient's stay in the hospital. The physical therapist must be aware of the signs and symptoms of wound infection, DVT, and pulmonary embolus. Specific signs, symptoms, and tests are discussed in the Troubleshooting section of this chapter. Any symptom must be brought to the immediate attention of the nursing staff and surgeon.

Functional considerations. Because restoration of functional ROM is essential in the successful result of TKR, continuous passive motion (CPM) has been used and shown to be beneficial in regaining mobility. It may be initiated in the recovery room.

In one study patients receiving CPM were able to achieve 90 degrees of flexion in 9.1 days versus their counterparts who did not receive CPM and required 13.8 days to reach the same goal.[8,79] Unfortunately, however, CPM is ineffective in the enhancement of knee extension.[8,34]

Many surgeons choose to begin immediate postoperative CPM.[57,82] Because of wound healing concerns, others choose to begin on the second day after surgery.[54] The beneficial effects of CPM include improved wound healing,[69] accelerated clearance of hemarthrosis,[59] reduced muscle atrophy,[3,16] reduced adhesion formation,[13,14,26,60] reduction in the incidence of DVT,[53] decreased hospital stay,[30] and decreased need for medication.[6,12] Certainly, most surgeons agree that CPM is useful in reducing the frequency of complications after TKR.[31,54,82]

The protocol of CPM application varies in the literature. In general, the initial settings range from 0 to 25 to 40 degrees of flexion. The range is either increased 5 to 10 degrees per day or to patient tolerance. Use of CPM can be from 4 to 20 hours per day. Its use is discontinued at the end of the acute hospital stay or when maximal knee flexion of the CPM machine is attained.

Another modality that has proven to be useful in improving ROM and quadriceps strength is neuromuscular electrical stimulation (NMES). In conjunction with CPM the application of NMES was shown to reduce extensor lag and the length of stay in the acute care setting.[31]

Exercises should be initiated on the second or third postoperative day.[21,57] Breathing exercises can be taught to promote full excursion of the ribcage. Ankle ROM exercises and instruction in proper elevation and positioning of the lower extremity are encouraged (Fig. 16-12). These exercises engage the muscle pump and passive gravity feed to decrease distal edema and avoid DVT.

Strengthening exercises such as isometric gluteal sets, hamstring sets, and quadriceps sets are begun to prevent disuse atrophy and reflex inhibition in the lower extremity. Patients are encouraged to do these exercises independently, thereby increasing their active participation. They should initially be performed in sets of 10 repetitions every hour and progressed to 20 repetitions three times daily.[21]

Advancement of this functional exercise program occurs throughout the first week of rehabilitation. Active assisted range of motion (A/AROM) exercises such as seated heel slides or therapist-assisted knee flexion and passive knee extension are performed to improve mobility. Straight leg raises (SLRs) and terminal knee extensions (TKEs) further strengthen the quadriceps muscles, thus improving the dynamic stabilizers of the knee.[21,73]

The patient also is instructed in ADLs such as dressing, bathing, transfers, reaching, and picking up items. These should be reviewed and performed until the patient can demonstrate safety and independence. Any special precautions or assistive devices are assessed and issued.

Progressive gait training begins with a walker on the second or third postoperative day,[21] proceeding throughout the acute care hospitalization. Ensuring safety and balance and enabling patient independence are the primary goals of this treatment. Negotiating level surfaces, ramps, curbs, and stairs and performing other activities relevant to the patient are practiced.

Current managed care clinical pathways recommend that the average length of stay in the acute hospital setting should be approximately 5 to 7 days,[21,56] with physical therapy sessions received twice a day. The patient is discharged from the hospital when medically stable. Specifically, from a rehabilitation standpoint the patient should be able to demonstrate 80 to 90 degrees of active range of motion (AROM) or A/AROM,[21] transfer supine to sit and sit to stand, ambulate 15 to 100 feet, and ascend and descend three steps[71] or as the home situation dictates.[21] If the patient is unable to do these tasks or has medical postoperative complications, the patient may be sent to an extended care unit (ECU) or skilled nursing facility (SNF) for further care and rehabilitation.

Q. Marc is 69 years old. He had a left TKR 8 days ago. He is now semi-reclined in his hospital bed. When the therapist helps him out of bed during transfer, Marc complains of feeling lightheaded. He usually requires a few moments for his head to clear, but today he needs a little more time to adjust. Gait training is initiated and suddenly Marc has difficulty breathing. What do these symptoms indicate?

Phase IIa: Extended Care Inpatient or Skilled Nursing Facility

TIME: Days 6-14
GOALS: Prevent complications, reduce pain and swelling, promote ROM, restore safety and independence (Table 16-2)

The goals of this short-term rehabilitation phase are the same as those used in the acute hospital. Treatment efforts continue, with physical therapy scheduled twice a day for approximately 3 to 7 days or until the goals are met. Sometimes family members or caregivers must be trained in assisting the patient during gait and transfers. Social services are often necessary to assist in planning home care needs or placement in long-term care facilities.

Phase IIb: Outpatient Home Health

TIME: Weeks 1-3
GOALS: Become safe in home environment with transfers, gait, and most ADLs (see Table 16-2)

After the patient has been discharged home, physical therapy treatments are reduced to three times weekly. During this phase of rehabilitation the goals are expanded to facilitate functional ROM and ensure safe and independent ADLs, transfers, and gait in the community. The home therapist should assess the home for safety and make changes as appropriate. Recommendations may include but are not limited to the installation of nonskid rugs and safety rails and the elimination of potential obstacles around the house.

The home exercise program initiated in the inpatient setting is reviewed and refined. The patient should be able to perform the ROM and isometric strengthening exercises given in the acute care setting. If extension mobility is lacking, more aggressive knee extension exercises are prescribed (Fig. 16-13). If knee flexion is limited, more progressive active and active assisted exercises are given (Fig. 16-14). Functional strengthening exercises are progressed in both the open- and closed-chain positions. Examples of closed-chain exercises are bilateral heel raises, sit-to-stand exercises (Fig. 16-15), quarter squats, and progressive steps up and down (Fig. 16-16). Closed-chain exercises have been shown to be highly effective in recruiting the vastus medialis oblique (VMO) and vastus lateralis (VL) compared with open-chain isometric exercises.[15,28,33,76]

Specific transfers in the home and car are practiced. Progression in gait includes advancing the patient to crutches or cane as balance dictates. Ambulation on uneven surfaces, ramps, and outdoor surfaces also is reviewed. Home physical therapy is discontinued when the patient is not considered homebound.

Table 16-2 Total Knee Replacement

Rehabilitation Phase	Criteria to Progress to this Phase	Anticipated Impairments and Functional Limitations	Intervention	Goal	Rationale
Phase IIa Extended care inpatient or skilled nursing Days 6-14	• No signs of infection • No significant increase in pain • No loss of ROM • Discharge from acute care • Progressive stiffness, wound drainage, other complications that may preclude home discharge • If patient is unsafe for home disposition, transfer to extended care unit (ECU) • Discharged to home	• Edema and pain • Limited ROM • Limited strength • Limited gait tolerance	• Continuation and progression of interventions from Phase I • Transfer training (car, sit-stand) • Gait training using appropriate assistive device • Aggressive knee extension and flexion exercises PROM—Flexion, prone and in standing A/AROM—Flexion, seated, on step, stationary bicycle • AROM—SLR • Heel raises • Leg curls • Step-ups and step-downs • Quarter squats • Joint mobilization • Soft tissue and myofascial release (respecting incision) • Careful ongoing monitoring of edema, pain, and erythema	• Self-manage pain • Independence with transfers • Gait independent in limited community distances (300-500 feet) • Knee PROM 0°-110° • Advance independence with home exercises • Improve functional lower extremity strength	• CPM may be discontinued if ROM is improving • Prepare for discharge from ECU or home health—transition to outpatient • Promote return to unassisted gait in the community • Obtain close to if not full ROM • Restore LE stability and strength • Prevent disuse atrophy • Treat hip weakness resulting from altered weight bearing and compensatory postural strategies • Facilitate ROM (110° necessary for stair climbing) *Note: Postoperative stiffness is a major complication of TKR. Manipulation criteria vary among surgeons (see text).
Phase IIb Home health Weeks 1-3 Depending on need for ECU	Limited ROM Limited strength • Difficulty with gait on uneven surfaces and stairs • Unable to attend outpatient rehabilitation center (homebound)		• Home health intervention usually 2-3 weeks postoperative • Assess home safety and make changes as appropriate • Car transfers and gait training on uneven surfaces • Continuation of exercises as listed previously to increase knee flexion and extension ROM and strength • Progressive weight bearing per physician orders	• Safe and independent in home setting • Independent ambulation using appropriate assistive device • Independent in limited community ambulation • ROM 0°-110°	• Prevent complications (falling) • Return to independent living • Prepare for discharge to outpatient rehabilitation facility • Strengthen lower kinetic chain • Prevent disuse atrophy • 110° necessary for stair climbing and bicycle • Avoid postoperative contracture and need for manipulation

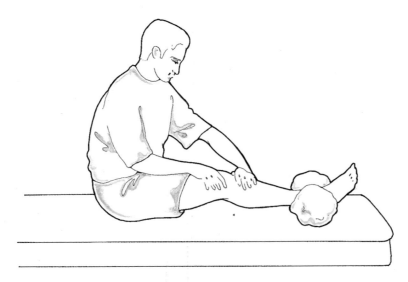

Fig. 16-13. TKE with passive overpressure. With the knee straight, position a pillow under the ankle. Apply manual overpressure above and below the patellofemoral joint to increase TKE passively.

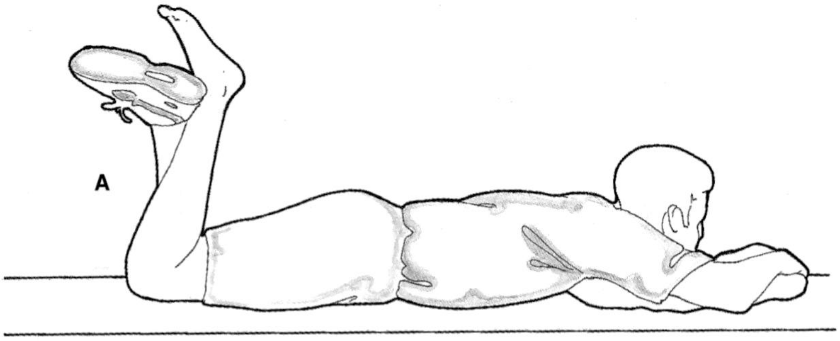

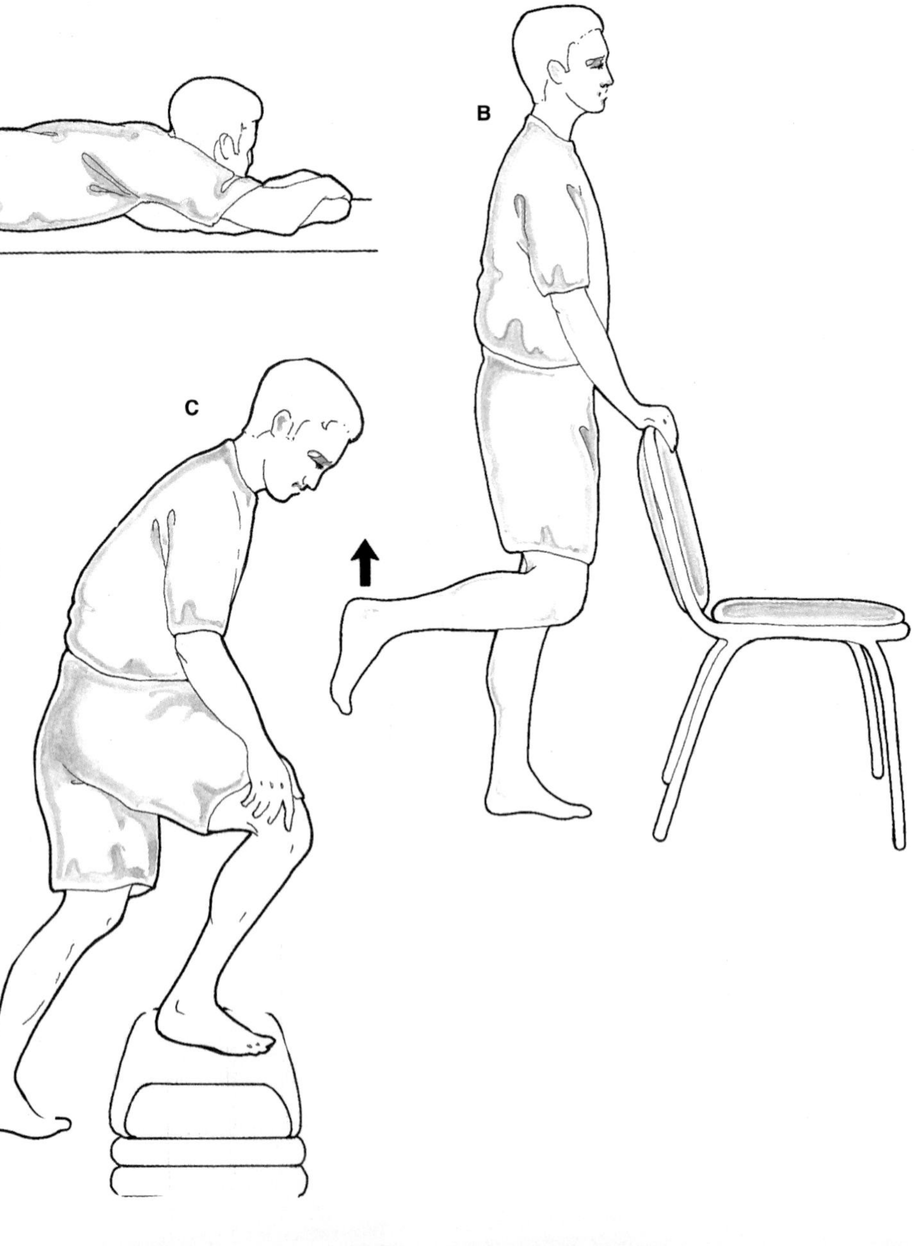

Fig. 16-14. A, Prone knee flexion. In a prone position the patient bends the operated knee as far as possible while using the uninvolved knee to apply passive overpressure to increase knee flexion. **B,** Standing open-chain knee flexion. In a standing position with upper extremity support, the patient actively bends the involved knee, bringing the heel to the buttocks while maintaining upright posture. **C,** Standing closed-chain knee flexion. In a standing position the patient places the foot of the involved leg flat on a step. He or she then places the hands above the knee and slowly leans forward on the involved leg and guides the knee into more flexion.

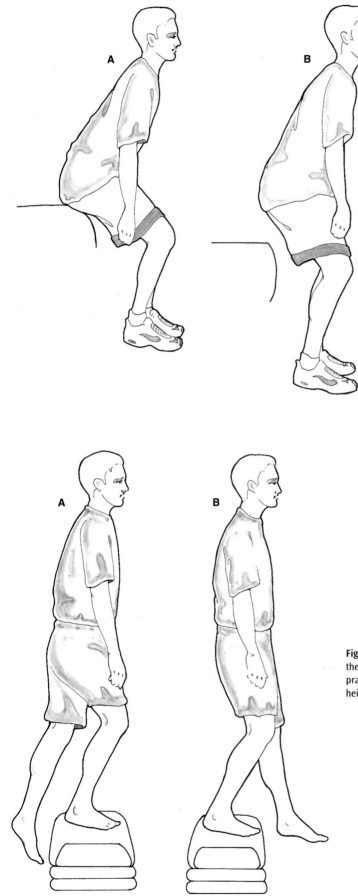

Fig. 16-15. Sit-to-stand exercise. **A,** Start position. **B,** End position. Without using the upper extremities for support, the patient practices controlled and balanced sit-to-stand transfers from various heights.

Fig. 16-16. **A,** Step-up progression. Patient practices controlled steps up with the involved leg from progressive heights. **B,** Step-down progression. Patient practices controlled steps down with the uninvolved leg from progressive heights.

Table 16-3 Total Knee Replacement

Rehabilitation Phase	Criteria to Progress to this Phase	Anticipated Impairments and Functional Limitations	Intervention	Goal	Rationale
Phase III Outpatient care Weeks 3-8 *Frequency and duration per physician's orders—usually three times a week for 1 month, then as appropriate	• No longer homebound • Safe and independent with ambulation using assistive device • Safe and independent with car transfers *Patients may access outpatient care if caregiver or family member is assisting with transfers and gait	• Limited ROM • Limited community ambulation using assistive device • Limited lower extremity strength	• Initiate aquatic therapy if available with concurrent land-based treatment • Continuation of ROM stretches and soft tissue procedures • Progression of (repetitions or weight) intensity with previous exercises • Squats, leg press, and bridging • Bicycle, walking, and/or swimming for cardiovascular conditioning 20 minutes three to five times a week (as indicated per general health issues) • Hip external rotator strengthening • Balance and proprioception exercises (BAPs, foam roller) • Return to previous activities as appropriate (see text)	• Normalize gait pattern and reduce reliance on assistive devices • Increase ROM to 110°-125° or as indicated by comparison with uninvolved knee • Single-leg half-squat to 65% body weight • Full weight bearing with single-limb stance • Improve balance, strength, endurance, and proprioception of lower extremity	• Reduce stress on the compensatory muscles and joints to prevent chronic imbalance issues • Aquatic (buoyant) environment allows for increased ease of mobility • 110°-125° flexion to use bicycle and stairs. The better the flexion, the less "hip hiking" and other compensatory movements • Decrease stress on the uninvolved leg with sit-stand transfers • Increase VMO/VL in closed-chain exercises • Provide aerobic conditioning for weight control • Address hip weakness caused by altered weight bearing and compensatory postural strategies • Improve tolerance to community ambulation and prevent falls • Resume previous activities to restore quality of life

A. Rapid heart rate, hypotension, and dyspnea are signs of a possible pulmonary embolus, a potentially fatal complication. Cardiovascular signs may include tachycardia, distended jugular veins, hypotension, and chest pain. Pulmonary symptoms include tachypnea, rales, wheezing, and pleural effusion. Sudden dyspnea is the most common symptom.

Q. Gemma is 55 years old. She had severe degenerative joint disease (DJD) in her right knee and underwent a TKR 8 weeks ago. She says the pain around the knee has considerably decreased. However, she complains of pain around the area of the fibular neck. The area also is sensitive to palpation. Gemma has intermittent pain radiating down the lateral surface of the lower leg. What is the probable cause of these symptoms?

Phase III: Outpatient Care

TIME: Weeks 3-8
GOALS: Normalize gait, reduce reliance on assistive devices, increase ROM, improve weight bearing, balance, strength, endurance, and proprioception (Table 16-3)

This phase of rehabilitation may begin in the second postoperative week for highly advanced and active patients or the third or fourth week for those proceeding slowly. The length of this stage also depends on factors such as the patient's goals and abilities, and more recently on restrictions on reimbursement for medical services.

Common difficulties encountered with TKR include patella instability and lack of motion. Results are considered successful if ROM is 0 to 110 degrees. Full extension is necessary to normalize the gait cycle[11,37,58] and facilitate quadriceps strength.[46] Normal stair climbing, sitting on a regular toilet seat, and riding a stationary bicycle require 110 degrees of flexion.[1] If this is not achieved, a manipulation under anesthesia may be warranted. General indications for manipulation include the following[52]:

1. Less than 70 degrees of flexion 2 weeks after surgery
2. Less than 90 degrees of flexion 1 month after surgery
3. A progressive loss of flexion
4. Less than 70 degrees total motion 3 months after surgery

Both closed and open manipulation procedures carry risks of fracture and an overall worse outcome than those not requiring manipulation.[52]

Muscle strength and flexibility imbalances of the hip, knee, ankle, and foot can occur after knee injury or surgery.[19,20,36,44,46] Reflex inhibition, faulty joint mechanics, altered gait, presurgical disuse atrophy, immobilization, and nerve injury have been shown to cause altered function of the muscles in the lower kinetic chain.[5,61,66,68] Therefore the physical therapist must fully assess the entire lower extremity for any loss of ROM or muscle strength and then develop a comprehensive treatment program to address the findings. Further rationales and specific details are discussed in the Troubleshooting section of this chapter.

A successful plan must include aerobic conditioning for weight reduction.[80] Because obesity is often associated with osteoarthritis, a patient who has undergone a TKR is likely already overweight. Increased forces such as those found in obesity can be the cause of wear to the weight-bearing surfaces.[70] One study found that subjects were actually 12 to 13 kg heavier and had a 4% to 6% higher percentage of body fat 1 year after TKR.[80] Non-impact activities such as stationary bicycling, distance walking, and swimming are suggested for cardiovascular conditioning.[70]

Aquatic therapy programs have proven to be effective in rehabilitation of total joint replacements.[9,23,77] The buoyant and warm environment can provide pain relief, increased circulation, and decreased weight bearing for the patient. Many patients can immediately start to work on ROM, strengthening, and normalizing gait without the assistance of a walker. The patient can be challenged by progressing from shoulder-deep water (approximately 25% weight bearing) to waist-deep water (50% weight bearing).

Changes in equilibrium after lower extremity injuries have been cited in the medical literature.[27,29,78] Balance activities and single leg exercises should be incorporated to offset any compensatory postural changes that have occurred as a result of decreased weight bearing, altered gait, and pain. The use of rocker boards, foam rollers, and biomechanical ankle platform system (BAPS) can be helpful to improve the patient's proprioception, balance, and postural control strategies.

The patient's primary concern in setting long-term rehabilitation goals should be to maintain a pain-free functional activity level for as long as possible. Certain activity restrictions are warranted after TKR. Generally, recreational activities and sports that involve a large amount of repetitive compression or impact loading are not encouraged because of the possibility of loosening or osteolysis of the joint implant.[2,38,45] Joint forces at the tibiofemoral interface are 1.5 to 4 times body weight when walking,[49] 1.2 times body weight when cycling, and 2 to 8 times body weight when running.[22] Patellofemoral joint forces show comparable increases—0.5 times body weight when walking[24] and 3 to 4 times body weight when running.[63] Failures of

TKRs may occur as a result of loosening of the implant. Therefore patients with joint replacements are encouraged to participate in activities that maintain cardiovascular fitness while subjecting the implant to reduced impact loading stress.

In the gym the use of a treadmill (walking only), ski machine, stair-climbing machine, or stationary bicycle are all acceptable. Outdoor sports that are acceptable include golfing, hiking, cycling, cross-country skiing, swimming, fishing, hunting, scuba diving, sailing, and occasional light doubles tennis.[70] Baseball, basketball, rock climbing, downhill skiing, football, martial arts, parachuting, racquetball, running, soccer, sprinting, and volleyball are strongly discouraged.

Suggested Home Maintenance for the Postsurgical Patient

An exercise program has been outlined at the various phases. The home maintenance box on page 285 outlines rehabilitation suggestions the patient may follow. The physical therapist can use it in customizing a patient-specific program.

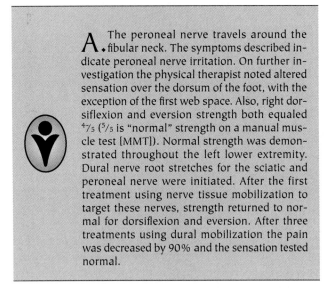

A. The peroneal nerve travels around the fibular neck. The symptoms described indicate peroneal nerve irritation. On further investigation the physical therapist noted altered sensation over the dorsum of the foot, with the exception of the first web space. Also, right dorsiflexion and eversion strength both equaled $^4/_5$ ($^5/_5$ is "normal" strength on a manual muscle test [MMT]). Normal strength was demonstrated throughout the left lower extremity. Dural nerve root stretches for the sciatic and peroneal nerve were initiated. After the first treatment using nerve tissue mobilization to target these nerves, strength returned to normal for dorsiflexion and eversion. After three treatments using dural mobilization the pain was decreased by 90% and the sensation tested normal.

Troubleshooting

Although the treatment guidelines given here provide a framework for postoperative rehabilitation of TKR, they should not be used as strict protocols. In fact, modifications are expected because each patient has individual needs, abilities, and goals. Continual reassessment of the patient's status and subsequent alterations in the treatment plan are necessary to achieve optimal results. The therapist must have the necessary abilities and skills to anticipate any potential complications and implement

appropriate changes in the treatment plan. The following section describes additional procedures and modalities that can be used to refine the therapy further.

Medical Complications

During the initial stage of postoperative care the most serious complications are wound infection, PE, and DVT. As previously noted, the therapist must know all symptoms and signs that may indicate any of the aforementioned medical problems. Any of these complications can severely deter rehabilitation progress in terms of time frame and overall prognosis.

Wound infection. Clinical findings of a potential wound infection include patient complaints of feeling cold, shivering, breaking out in goose bumps, feeling cold in the extremities, and exhibiting minimal diaphoresis. Other symptoms include warmth and erythema about the surgical site and an increase in body temperature up to 104 degrees Fahrenheit.[48] Wound dressings should be checked and changed daily until the staples are removed.[1] Although uncommon, infection remains a serious problem, usually requiring removal of all components, thorough surgical debridement, and long-term intravenous antibiotics. Reimplantation may be possible 3 to 6 months later if the infection has been completely eradicated.

Pulmonary embolus. Equally serious is PE, a potentially fatal, but rare, complication. Cardiovascular signs include tachycardia, distended cervical veins, hypotension, and chest pain. Pulmonary symptoms include tachypnea, rales, wheezing, and pleural effusion.[48] Sudden dyspnea is the most frequent symptom. Pleuritic pain is also common in patients with severe embolization. If any of these signs or symptoms occur, the physical therapist should immediately notify the nursing staff and physician.

Deep venous thrombosis. Significant signs and symptoms of DVT include complaints of pain and swelling in the involved extremity, calf tenderness, and a positive Homan's sign. Specifically, the patient may report a dull ache, tight feeling, or frank pain in the calf or entire leg. The signs and symptoms include slight swelling in the involved calf; distention of the superficial venous collaterals; tenderness, induration, or spasm of the calf muscles, with or without pain, produced by dorsiflexion of the foot (Homans' sign); warmth of the affected leg when both legs are exposed to room temperature; and a slight fever or tachycardia.[48] The risk of DVT may be reduced by using 20 to 30 mm Hg compression thromboembolic disease (TED) hose whenever the patient is out of bed.

Persistent joint effusion. Patients sometimes complain of postoperative stiffness, pain, and swelling. The patient should be reassured that this usually resolves within the first few weeks after surgery. Persistent joint effusion can forestall the rehabilitation process. Manual massage is an effective modality that can enhance muscle recovery and reduce soreness after intense physical activity.[7,50] Increasing blood flow may increase oxygen delivery to the injured tissue, enhance healing, and restore homeostasis.[39] If edema, swelling, and inflammation are significant factors in muscle soreness sensation,[72,75] massage may be able to reduce soreness in the involved muscles. Persistent effusion may be aspirated, not only to relieve pressure and stiffness, but also to rule out an indolent infection.

Functional Complications

Peroneal nerve neuropraxia. Peroneal nerve neuropraxia for flexion contractures can be associated with valgus deformity. The common peroneal nerve and its branches can be entrapped at the fibular neck. Clinical findings of nerve entrapment are local tenderness around the fibular neck with pain, diminished sensation, or paresthesia radiating over the lateral surface of the lower leg and the dorsum of the foot.[47,62] Nerve conduction velocity testing and electromyographic studies will be positive for neuropathic dysfunction in the motor distribution of the common peroneal nerve distal to the entrapment site at the fibular neck. Clinically, the patient displays an inability to walk or stand on the heel because of the weakness of the ankle dorsiflexors. Additionally, instability when attempting toe walking results from the muscle imbalance and associated sensory abnormalities at the ankle joint. The muscles affected are those in the anterior and lateral compartments of the leg.

When the superficial peroneal nerve is compressed, a decrease in sensation is noted over the dorsum of the foot, with the exception of the first web space. The involvement of the deep peroneal nerve produces a diminution of sensation in the first web space of the foot and affects the muscles of the anterior compartment, including the extensor hallucis brevis and the extensor digitorum brevis.

Complete common peroneal nerve palsy results in a severely affected gait pattern. Without an ankle-foot orthosis, the patient suffers from a foot drop with associated steppage gait in profoundly affected cases or foot slapping in milder ones. The ankle is unstable and vulnerable to ankle inversion sprains. The functional result of a partial peroneal nerve palsy depends on which nerve components are the most affected. Loss of the peroneal muscles in the lateral compartment results in a chronically inverted foot, with weight bearing occurring more laterally than normal and invariably affecting the position and stability of the foot and ankle throughout the stance phase of the gait cycle. Loss of the anterior compartment muscles, especially the tibialis anterior, affects the entire gait cycle. The loss of the dorsal intrinsic muscles of the foot has a relatively minor effect on basic weight bearing functions.

Physical therapy interventions for nerve entrapment include examination of the joint mechanics of the proximal and distal tibiofibular joints and determination of the specific muscle weakness and sensory loss. Manual techniques include joint mobilization as appropriate, facilitation of the recruitment of the affected muscles, and dural nerve root stretches for the sciatic and peroneal nerves.

Muscle imbalance. A detailed evaluation of the entire lower kinetic chain is necessary for the successful treatment of patients with TKR. Altered gait, faulty mechanics, and muscle imbalances have more than likely existed before the TKR. These factors contribute greatly to the eventual surgical outcome.

Most of the present understanding regarding muscle imbalances and neuromotor retraining comes from the work of Janda,[42,43] Lewit,[51] and Sahrmann.[68] Muscle imbalance is a multifactorial problem and can be highly complex. In simplistic terms, the result of muscle imbalance is that the tight muscles become tighter, weak muscles become weaker, and motor control becomes asymmetric.[32]

According to Janda, muscle balance is continually adapting the body's posture to gravity. When an injury occurs, faulty posture and weight bearing alter the body's center of gravity, which initiates mechanical responses requiring muscle adaptation. Change in the mechanical behavior of a joint causes neuroreflexive alteration of muscle function through aberrant afferent mechanoreceptor stimulation of articular reflexes.[4]

Postural-tonic muscles respond to dysfunction with facilitation, hypertonicity, and shortening. Dynamic-phasic muscles respond with inhibition, hypotonicity, and weakness. In the lower quadrant, Janda identified a common pattern of muscle imbalance. Hyperactive muscles include the iliopsoas, rectus femoris, tensor fascia latae, quadratus lumborum, the thigh adductors, piriformis, hamstrings, and the lumbar erector spinae musculature. Muscles that display inhibition or reflexive weakness include the gluteus maximus, medius, and minimus; rectus abdominis; and external and internal obliques. Sahrmann,[68] Dorman,[18] and Bullock[5] similarly identified weakness in the entire lower extremity in the presence of knee dysfunction.

Quadriceps weakness, especially in the early stages of TKR rehabilitation, must be addressed. A knee immobilizer may be needed for ambulation in the hospi-

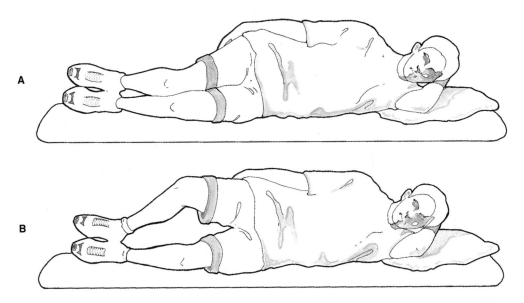

Fig. 16-17. Hip lateral rotation. **A,** Start position. The patient lies on the uninvolved side with the shoulders and hips perpendicular to the table and the knees flexed to 45 degrees. **B,** End position. The patient then lifts the top knee toward the ceiling, keeping the feet in contact. The patient should emphasize movement from the hip and not allow the pelvis to roll backward.

tal setting if quadriceps strength is not great enough to stabilize the knee. Biofeedback or NMES can be beneficial in "jump-starting" the recruitment of the quadriceps. In cases of patella instability, quadriceps strength should be restored as soon as possible. Soft tissue work, friction massage, and assisted stretches to the iliotibial band (ITB) may be beneficial.

Faulty joint mechanics at the hip, knee, and ankle affect the overall surgical result. A study by Dorman[18] found that inhibition or facilitation of the gluteus medius is influenced by the position of the sacroiliac joint. An anterior rotation (an apparent long leg) manifested a significantly weaker muscle than one in posterior rotation (an apparent short leg). Exercises that address gluteus medius weakness include hip abduction and lateral hip rotation (Fig. 16-17).

Altered ankle movements and instability disturb the overall sense of balance and influence gait safety accordingly. Joint mobilization techniques to correct associated dysfunctions in the joints of the lower extremity can be helpful. A stiff knee can be helped with contraction and relaxation techniques to the muscles that may be guarding or fatigued.[9]

Outcomes

TKR is a method to improve quality of life. This is accomplished primarily through pain relief, resulting in increased functional mobility. Results are generally reported according to the Hospital for Special Surgery[40] or the Knee Society[41] rating systems.

Despite extensive rehabilitation efforts, various studies have shown outcomes of diminished functional capacity. Self-report measures of perceived abilities indicate that at 1 year after TKR, most individuals have regained 80% of their normal function. However stiffness and pain still remained a problem.[25] Walsh et al[80] showed that at 1 year after TKR little pain was noted during activities of walking, stair climbing, and concentric muscle strength testing. But slower walking speeds for both males and females were reported (62% and 25% decrease at normal pace and 31% and 6% decrease at fast pace, respectively). Clinical relevance lies in the fact that 17% of these individuals were not able to cross safely at a typical city intersection. Other recent studies have shown slower sit-to-stand and go tests,[35] quadriceps weakness,[55,67] and smaller girth circumferences[67] for individuals more than 1 year after surgery.

With these studies in mind, the development and implementation of a well-thought, comprehensive treatment plan is paramount. Addressing the entire lower quadrant with an appropriate exercise program enhances the course of rehabilitation and ensures a more successful outcome.

Suggested Home Maintenance for the Postsurgical Patient

Days 1-5

GOALS FOR THE PERIOD: Control pain, manage edema, prevent postoperative infection, provide PROM to the knee, improve muscle contraction, promote independence with bed mobility and transfers, restore independence in ADLs

1. Isometric quadriceps sets
2. Isometric gluteal sets
3. Isometric hamstring sets
4. Ankle dorsiflexion, plantar flexion, and circumduction
5. Proper positioning for edema reduction
6. Patient education for purpose and use of CPM
7. Breathing exercises

Days 6-14

8. Straight leg raising
9. Terminal knee extension with overpressure
10. Knee flexion—heel slides (supine)
11. Knee flexion—heel slides (seated)

Weeks 3-8

GOALS FOR THE PERIOD: Normalize gait, reduce reliance on assistive devices, increase ROM, improve weight bearing, balance, strength, endurance, and proprioception

1. Knee flexion—passive
   a. Prone position
   b. Standing open-chain
   c. Standing closed-chain
2. Hip exercises
   a. Straight-leg raises
   b. Abduction in side-lying
   c. Prone extension
   d. Adduction in side-lying
3. Bilateral heel raises
4. Sit-to-stand exercises
5. Bilateral quarter to half squats
6. Step progression
   a. Step up
   b. Step down
7. Leg curls
   a. Prone
   b. Standing
8. Hip lateral rotation exercise
9. Contralateral standing lower extremity hip exercises
10. Bridging
11. Stationary bicycling
12. Walking program
13. Balance activities
    a. Bilateral to single-leg
    b. Level surfaces to uneven surfaces

REFERENCES

1. Aliga NA: New venues for joint replacement rehab, *Adv Dir Rehab* 17(4):43, 1998.

2. Amstutz HC et al: Mechanism and clinical significance of wear debris-induced osteolysis, *Clin Orthop* 276:7, 1992.

3. Anderson MA: Continuous passive motion. In Iglarsh ZA, Richardson JK, Timm KE, editors: *Orthopaedic physical therapy clinics of North America*, vol 1, Philadelphia, 1992, WB Saunders.

4. Bookout MR, Geraci M, Greenman PE: *Exercise prescription as an adjunct to manual medicine*, course notes, Tucson, AZ, Mar 1997.

5. Bullock-Saxton JE, Janda V, Bullock MI: Reflex activation of gluteal muscles in walking, *Spine* 18(6):704, 1993.

6. Burks R, Daniel D, Losse G: The effect of continuous passive motion on anterior cruciate ligament reconstruction stability, *Am J Sports Med* 12:323, 1984.

7. Cafarelli E, Flint F: The role of massage in preparation for and recovery from exercise, *Sports Med* 14:1, 1992.

8. Chiarello CM, Gunderson L, O'Halloran T: The effect of continuous passive motion duration and increment on range of motion in total knee arthroplasty patients, *J Orthop Sports Phys Ther* 25(2):119, 1997.

9. Cocchi R: No pain with gain - aquatic total knee replacement therapy, *Adv Phys Ther* 8(3):7, 1997.

10. Colizza WA, Insall JN, Scuderi GR: The posterior stabilized total knee prosthesis. Assessment of polyethylene damage and osteolysis after a 10 year minimum follow up, *J Bone Joint Surg* 77A:1713, 1995.

11. Corcoran PJ, Peszczynski M: Gait and gait retraining. In Basmajian JV, editor: *Therapeutic exercise*, ed 2, Baltimore, 1978, Williams & Wilkins.

12. Coutts RD et al: The effect of continuous passive motion on total knee rehabilitation (abstract), *Orthop Trans* 7:535, 1983.

13. Coutts RD, Toth C, Kaita JH: The role of continuous passive motion in the rehabilitations of the total knee patient. In Hungerford DS, Krackow DA, Kenna RV, editors: *Total knee arthroplasty: a comprehensive approach*, Baltimore, 1984, Williams & Wilkins.

14. Coutts RD: Continuous passive motion in the rehabilitation of the total knee patient, its role and effect, *Orthop Rev* 15(3):126, 1986.

15. Cuddeford T, Williams AK, Medeiros JM: Electromyographic activity of the vastus medialis oblique and vastus lateralis muscles during selected exercises, *J Man Manip Ther* 4(1):10, 1996.

16. Dhert WJA et al: Effects of immobilization and continuous passive motion of postoperative muscle atrophy in mature rabbits, *Can J Surg* 31:185, 1988.

17. Diduch DR et al: Total knee replacement in young active patients. Long term follow up and functional outcome, *J Bone Joint Surg* 79A(4):575, 1997.

18. Dorman TA et al: Muscles and pelvic clutch, *J Man Manip Ther* 3(3):85, 1995.

19. Elmqvist L et al: Does a torn anterior cruciate ligament lead to change in the central nervous system drive of the knee extensors?, *Eur J Appl Physiol* 58:203, 1988.

20. Elmqvist L et al: Knee extensor muscle function before and after reconstruction of the anterior cruciate ligament tear, *Scand J Rehab Med* 21:131, 1989.

21. Enloe LJ et al: Total hip and knee replacement treatment programs: a report using consensus, *J Orthop Sports Phys Ther* 23(1):3, 1996.

22. Ericson MO, Nisell R: Tibiofemoral joint forces during ergometer cycling, *Am J Sports Med* 14(4):285, 1986.

23. Farina EJ: Aquatic vs. conventional land exercises for the rehabilitation of total knee replacement patients (abstract), *VII World FINA Med & Sci Aspects of Aquatic Sports*.

24. Ficat RD, Hungerford DS: *Disorders of the patellofemoral joint*, Baltimore, 1977, Williams & Wilkins.

25. Finch E et al: Functional ability perceived by individuals following total knee arthroplasty compared to age-matched individuals without knee disability, *J Orthop Sports Phys Ther* 27(4):255, 1998.

26. Frank C et al: Physiology and therapeutic value of passive joint motion, *Clin Orthop* 185:113, 1984.

27. Friden T et al: Disability in anterior cruciate ligament insufficiency - an analysis of 19 untreated patients, *J Orthop Res* 6:833, 1988.

28. Friedhoff G, Davies G, Malone T: Chain links, *Biomechanics* 5(3):59, 1998.

29. Gauffin H et al: Function testing in patients with old rupture of the anterior cruciate ligament, *Int J Sports Med* 11:73, 1990.

30. Gosc JC: Continuous passive motion in the postoperative treatment of patients with total knee replacement: a retrospective study, *Phys Ther* 67(1):39, 1987.

31. Goth RS et al: Electrical stimulation effect on extensor lag and length of hospital stay after total knee arthroplasty, *Arch Phys Med Rehab* 75(9):957, 1994.

32. Greenman PE: *Principles of manual medicine*, ed 2, Baltimore, 1996, Williams & Wilkins.

33. Gryzlo SM et al: Electromyographic analysis of knee rehabilitation exercises, *J Orthop Sports Phys Ther* 20(1):36, 1994.

34. Hansen CH et al: *Meta-analysis of continuous passive motion use in total knee arthroplasty*, research presentation, APTA Scientific Meeting, Orlando, 1998.

35. Hasson S et al: *An evaluation of mobility and self report on individuals with total knee arthroplasty*, research presentation, APTA Scientific Meeting, Orlando, June 1998.

36. Herlant M et al: The effect of anterior cruciate ligament surgery on the ankle plantar flexors, *Isokin Ex Sci* 2(3):140, 1992.

37. Hertling D, Kessler RM: *Management of common musculoskeletal disorders*, ed 2, Philadelphia, 1990, JB Lippincott.

38. Howie DW et al: The response to particulate debris, *Orthop Clin North Am* 24(4):571, 1993.

39. Hunt ME: Physiotherapy in sports medicine. In Torg JS, Welsh RP, Shephard RJ, editors: *Current therapy in sports medicine*, Toronto, 1990, Decker.

40. Insall JN et al: A comparison of four models of total knee-replacement prosthesis, *J Bone Joint Surg* 58A:754, 1976.

41. Insall JN et al: Rational of the knee society clinical rating system, *Clin Orthop* 248:13, 1989.

42. Janda V: *Muscles as a pathogenic factor in low back pain in the treatment of patients,* proceedings of the IFOMT 4th Conference, 1980, Christchurch, NZ.

43. Janda V: Muscles, central nervous motor regulation and back problems. In Korr I, editor: *The neurobiologic mechanisms in manipulative therapy,* New York, 1977, Plenum Press.

44. Jaramillo J, Worrell TW, Ingersoll CD: Hip isometric strength following knee surgery, *J Orthop Sports Phys Ther* 20(3):160, 1994.

45. Jasty M, Smith E: Wear particles of total joint replacements and their role in periprosthetic osteolysis, *Curr Opin Rheumatol* 4(2):204, 1992.

46. Kisner C, Colby LA: *Therapeutic exercise foundations and techniques,* ed 2, Philadelphia, 1990, FA Davis.

47. Kopell HP, Thompson WAL: Peripheral entrapment neuropathies of the lower extremity, *N Engl J Med* 262(2):56, 1960.

48. Krupp MA, Chatton MJ: *Current medical diagnosis and treatment,* Los Altos, CA, 1979, Lange Medical.

49. Kuster MS et al: Joint load considerations in total knee replacement, *J Bone Joint Surg* 79B(1):109, 1997.

50. Lehn C, Prentice WE: Massage. In Prentice WE, editor: *Therapeutic modalities in sports medicine,* St Louis, 1995, Mosby.

51. Lewit K: *Manipulative therapy in rehabilitation of the motor system,* London, 1975, Butterworth.

52. Lux PS, Hoernschemeyer DG, Whiteside LA: *Manipulation and cortisone injection following total knee replacement (abstract),* 64th Annual Meeting of the American Academy of Orthopedic Surgeons, San Francisco, Feb 1997.

53. Lynch JA et al: Mechanical measures in the prophylaxis of postoperative thromboembolism in total knee arthroplasty, *Clin Orthop* 260:24, 1990.

54. Maloney WJ et al: The influence of continuous passive motion on outcome in total knee arthroplasty, *Clin Orthop* 256:162, 1990.

55. Marks R: The effects of 16 months of angle-specific isometric strengthening exercises in midrange on torque of the knee extensor muscles in osteoarthritis of the knee: a case study, *J Orthop Sports Phys Ther* 20(2):103, 1994.

56. Mukand J et al: Critical pathways for TKR - protocol saves time and money, *Adv Dir Rehab* 6(8):31, 1997.

57. Munin MC et al: Early in-patient rehabilitation after elective hip and knee arthroplasty, *JAMA* 279(11):880, 1998.

58. Murray MP: Gait as a total pattern of movement, *Am J Phys Med* 46(1):290, 1967.

59. O'Driscoll SW, Kumar A, Salter RB: The effects of continuous passive motion in the clearance of hemarthrosis from synovial joint: an experimental investigation in the rabbit, *Clin Orthop* 176:305, 1983.

60. Parisien JS: The role of arthroscopy in the treatment of postoperative fibroarthrosis of the knee joint, *Clin Orthop* 229:185, 1988.

61. Patla-Paris C: Kinetic chain: dysfunctional and compensatory effects within the lower extremity (manual), *Orthop Phys Ther Home Study Course* 91(1):1, 1992.

62. Piegorsch K: Peripheral nerve entrapment syndromes of the lower extremity (manual), *Orthop Phys Ther Home Study Course* 91(1):1, 1991.

63. Pitman MI, Frankel VH: Biomechanics of the knee in athletes. In Nicholas JA, Hershman EB, editors: *The lower extremity and spine in sports medicine,* St Louis, 1995, Mosby.

64. Ranawat CS et al: Long-term results of the total condylar knee arthroplasty, *Clin Orthop* 286:94, 1993.

65. Rand JA, Illstrup DM: Survivorship analysis of total knee arthroplasty. Cumulative rates of survival of 9200 total knee arthroplasties, *J Bone Joint Surg* 73A:397, 1991.

66. Ross M, Worrell TW: Thigh and calf girth following knee injury and surgery, *J Orthop Sports Phys Ther* 27(1):9, 1998.

67. Ross MD et al: *A comparison of quadriceps strength and girth between involved and uninvolved limbs in individuals with total knee arthroplasty,* research presentation, APTA Scientific Meeting, Orlando, June 1998.

68. Sahrmann SA: *Diagnosis and treatment of movement impairment syndromes,* course notes, San Francisco, June 1997.

69. Salter RB: The biological concept of continuous passive motion of synovial joints, *Clin Orthop* 242:12, 1989.

70. Savory CG: Total joint replacement patients should stick to low-impact sports, *Biomechanics* 5(3):71, 1998.

71. Shields RK et al: Reliability, validity, and responsiveness of functional tests in patients with total joint replacement, *Phys Ther* 75(3):169, 1995.

72. Smith LL: Acute inflammation: the underlying mechanism in delayed onset muscle soreness?, *Med Sci Sports Exerc* 23:542, 1991.

73. Spencer JD, Hayes KC, Alexander IJ: Knee effusion and quadriceps reflex inhibition in man, *Arch Phys Med Rehab* 65:171, 1984.

74. Stearn SH, Insall JN: Posterior stabilized prosthesis. Results after follow up of 9 to 12 years, *J Bone Joint Surg* 74A:980, 1992.

75. Tidius PM: Exercise and muscle soreness. In Torg JS, Welsh RP, Shephard RJ, editors: *Current therapy in sports medicine,* Toronto, 1990, Decker.

76. Tippett SR: Closed chain exercise, *Orthop Phys Ther Clin North Am* 1:253, 1992.

77. Toran MW: Pooling resources for sports medicine, *Adv Dir Rehab* 7(3):59, 1998.

78. Tropp H, Odenrick P: Postural control in single-limb stance, *J Orthop Res* 6:833, 1988.

79. Vince KG et al: Continuous passive motion after total knee arthoplarty, *J Arthroplasty* 2(4):281, 1987.

80. Walsh M et al: Physical impairments and functional limitations: a comparison of individuals one year after total knee arthroplasty with control subjects, *Phys Ther* 78(3):248, 1998.

81. http://www.aaos.org

82. Yashar AA et al: Continuous passive motion with accelerated flexion after total knee arthroplasty, *Clin Orthop* 345:38, 1997.

Chapter 17

Lateral Ligament Repair —————————

Richard Ferkel
Robert Donatelli
Will Hall

The ankle requires both static and dynamic stability. Mobility is crucial for normal ankle function in the midst of rapidly changing postures of the foot during sporting and everyday weight-bearing activities. Lateral ligament injuries of the ankle account for 13% to 56% of all injuries in sports requiring running or jumping such as soccer, basketball and volleyball.[8,10] The large majority of these injuries can be successfully treated conservatively with casting, bracing, nonsteroidal antiinflammatory medications, and physical therapy. Approximately 85% of all ankle sprains involve the lateral structures of the ankle.[7,18] The majority of ankle sprains heal without any residual functional instability.[7] Despite adequate trials of conservative measures, however, approximately 10% to 30% of all acute ligamentous injuries have recurrent symptoms of chronic pain, swelling, and instability with activities.[1,2,7,9,17] Functional instability of the ankle is reported to be as high as 20% after ankle sprains.[6] When conservative measures fail to produce satisfactory proprioceptive performance and mechanical stability, surgical repair or reconstruction of the injured lateral ligament structures should be considered.

Surgical Indications and Considerations

The etiology of the unstable ankle is usually a plantar flexion inversion injury that tears the anterior talofibular (ATF) ligament and possibly the calcaneofibular (CF) ligament and anterior inferior tibiofibular (AITF) ligament. The unstable ankle is generally caused by a traumatic event such as an ankle sprain. It also can be associated with ankle fractures but virtually never develops insidiously.

A lateral ankle reconstruction is an elective surgery used to treat chronic instability that results from a continuum of ankle injuries. Ankle injuries can result in permanent damage to the ligaments that support the lateral ankle. The surgical option is used when nonoperative treatments—including physical therapy, bracing, activity modification, and steroid injections—have failed. Postoperative physical therapy is a vital link in returning the patient to an active lifestyle.

Indications for reconstruction of the ankle's lateral ligaments include recurrent giving way with activities of daily living (ADLs) and sports that is refractory to conservative treatment, a positive physical examination, abnormal inversion, and/or positive anterior drawer stress x-rays (Fig. 17-1).

Patients of all ages and types are candidates for this type of surgery, but few patients older than 40 years undergo ankle reconstruction because of decreased activity levels and a decreased ability to adjust functions and lifestyle to avoid recurrent buckling episodes. Surgeons should take care when considering this procedure for patients with generalized ligamentous laxity and collagen disorders that may result in failure. In addition, advanced degenerative joint disease or arthrofibrosis may be relative contraindications to this surgery.

Surgical Procedures

More than 50 different surgical procedures for correction of lateral ankle instability have been described.* The majority of reconstructive procedures use part or all of the peroneal brevis tendon. Common procedures include the Watson-Jones, Evans, Chrisman-Snook, and Elmslie procedures and their modifications. Anatomic repair with direct suturing of the torn ligaments, imbrication, reinsertion to the bone, and in some instances augmentation with local tissue have increased in popularity recently.[6,12,15] Direct repair of the ATF and CF ligaments was described by Broström in 1966 and later modified by Gould in 1980.[3,12]

Direct repair of torn lateral ligaments has the advantage of being simple and reliable, avoiding the use of normal tendons. It restores the original anatomy, requires less exposure, and maintains full ankle motion.

Special consideration is given to Deborah Mandis Cozen, PT, and Richard B. Johnston III, MD, for their assistance in the preparation of this chapter.

*References 3, 5, 6, 9, 12, 15, 23.

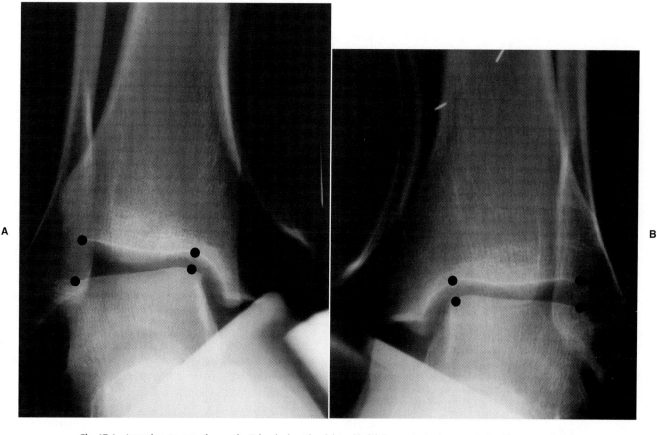

Fig. 17-1. Inversion stress testing on the Telos device. The right ankle **(A)** demonstrates increased talar tilt compared with the left ankle **(B)**.

Procedure

The patient is taken to the operating room and examined under anesthesia. If the surgeon has any questions about the degree of ankle instability, stress x-ray films (stressing the ankle in both inversion and anterior drawer) are taken. The thigh is then secured on a well-padded thigh holder in preparation for ankle arthroscopy, as described in Chapter 19. The lower extremity is prepared and draped in standard fashion. Arthroscopy is performed first; the authors of this chapter have found that 93% of patients have additional intraarticular ankle pathology associated with lateral ankle instability.[18] In addition, a similar report by Taga showed 95% of patients to have additional intraarticular pathology at the time of ankle reconstruction.[22]

The intraarticular pathology is identified and addressed through arthroscopic surgery. After the arthroscopy is completed, the nurse removes the thigh support and places the leg flat on the surgical table. The ankle is re-swabbed with a sterile antibacterial solution. An additional clean surgical drape is placed over the foot and ankle, and gloves are changed. New sterile instruments are used to perform the open portion of the procedure. Arthroscopic methods are available for surgical reconstruction of the lateral ankle liga-

ments, but at this time open stabilization as described by Broström gives a better, more reproducible result.

After arthroscopy the ankle is prepared and the tourniquet inflated. An incision is made over the lateral aspect of the ankle. This incision may be obliquely shaped in the skin folds or more vertical from the fibula toward the sinus tarsi, depending on the surgeon's preference and the clinical situation. Dissection is carried down through the subcutaneous tissues and the extensor retinaculum is carefully exposed because it is to be used for later reattachment. The surgeon must take care to avoid the intermediate dorsal cutaneous nerve, the lateral branch of the superficial peroneal nerve (which often lies near the end of the ATF ligament), and the sural nerve (which lies over the peroneal tendons). An oblique capsular incision is then made along the anterior border of the fibula from the AITF ligament to the CF ligament, leaving a small 3- or 4-mm cuff of tissue on the fibula for reattachment of the torn ligament complex (Fig. 17-2). The stretched ATF ligament is found as a thickening in the anterior capsule, and the CF ligament is found in the distal portion of the wound under the tip of the fibula, running deep to the peroneal tendons. The CF ligament often is attenuated or avulsed from the fibular tip.

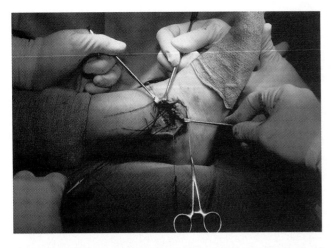

Fig. 17-2. An oblique capsular incision is made along the anterior border of the fibula from the AITF ligament to the CF ligament, leaving a small 3- to 4-mm cuff of tissue on the fibula for reattachment of the ligament complex.

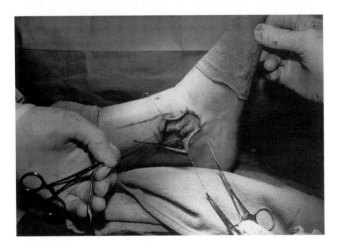

Fig. 17-3. The extensor retinaculum is pulled proximally over the repair and sutured to the fibular periosteum.

A "pants-over-vest" overlapping suture technique is used to imbricate or shorten the torn ligaments and provide a double layer of reinforcement to the repair. Suturing is done starting from the ligament portion attached to the talus, so that the knots are tied distal and inferior to the fibula. This helps prevent postoperative knot prominence and skin irritation with shoe wear. The sutures are tied with the ankle in neutral position, and a posterior drawer is applied to reduce the talus. The ankle is checked to make sure full range of motion (ROM) has been maintained during the repair. The extensor retinaculum is then pulled proximal over the repair and sutured to the fibular periosteum (Fig. 17-3). ROM is again checked, as is the stability of the ankle. The tourniquet is released, and bleeding tissues are coagulated. The subcutaneous tissue and skin are then closed in the standard fashion. The patient is placed in a short-leg well-padded cast that is split in the recovery room to allow for swelling.

Surgical Outcomes

A lateral ankle reconstruction is considered to be successful when the patient has full ROM and a pain-free ankle and can return to all ADLs and sports without restriction. Liu and Baker[19] studied the static restraints of various surgical procedures in 40 cadaveric ankles. They found no significant difference between the Watson-Jones and Chrisman-Snook procedures, but the modified Broström procedure produced the least anteroposterior (AP) displacement and talar tilt at all different forces tested.

Hennrikus[14] prospectively compared the Chrisman-Snook and modified Broström procedure in 40 patients. Although both produced 80% good to excellent results, the former procedure had a much greater proportion of complications and the latter procedure had a higher functional score. Hamilton performed the modified Broström procedure on 28 ankles; 54% of the patients were high-level ballet dancers.[13] At 64 months follow-up, he noted 27 out of 28 good to excellent results. Peters[20] reviewed the literature and found 460 ankles treated with anatomic modified Broström repairs had an average of between 87% and 95% good to excellent results.

Recently, Chams and Ferkel[4] reviewed the results of 21 patients who underwent the modified Broström procedure. The average patient age was 27.5 years and the average follow-up occurred at 57 months. They found 95% good to excellent results with an American Orthopaedic Foot and Ankle Society's (AOFAS) ankle/hindfoot score of 97.1.

Challenges

Despite having a stable ankle postoperatively, some patients still complain of pain, aching, swelling and crepitation.[22] Many of these complaints may be related to preexisting intraarticular pathology such as degenerative joint disease, loose bodies, chronic synovitis, and chronic scarring. Occasionally the ankle can be made too tight at the time of reconstruction; this severely limits the patient's ability to invert. This is the single most serious complication after ankle reconstruction. If a patient does not have full motion after surgery, especially full inversion and eversion, rehabilitation is significantly compromised and the patient tends to develop a painful valgus hindfoot.

Precautions and Contraindications

The physical therapist should increase the level of rehabilitation gradually for the patient after surgery. Too-vigorous exercise and the use of isokinetic machines can lead to increased pain, shear stress, and swelling that can last for weeks to months. If this occurs, the ultimate results can be compromised and the patient, physician, and physical therapist can all become quite frustrated. Every patient progresses at a different rate and the exercise program should be customized to the individual needs of each patient.

Rehabilitation Concerns

The therapist should contact the physician whenever pain appears to be out of proportion to expectations. In addition, any wound drainage, evidence of fever or infection, and increased laxity should alert the therapist to interact with the surgeon. If the patient has an acute episode of pain or feels a "pop" or significant change during rehabilitation or ADLs, the surgeon should be alerted immediately.

Therapy Guidelines for Rehabilitation

The first 6 weeks after surgery are important for the success of the surgery. Whether the reconstruction was done with primary ligamentous repair (as in the Broström procedure) or with tendon augmentation (as in the Chrisman-Snook procedure), the initial tissue healing stage is important.[14,17] The surgical reconstruction to correct the ligamentous instability is only as good as the stability gained from soft tissue healing. Soft tissue healing is considered the maximal protection stage.

Evaluation

The initial postoperative evaluation gives the therapist a baseline from which to proceed in returning the patient to desired function. Initial ROM measurements are taken both for active range of motion (AROM) and passive range of motion (PROM). PROM is measured within a pain-free range, especially that of inversion. The physical therapist has a responsibility to the surgeon and the patient to protect the lateral ligamentous reconstruction. Inversion ROM specifically stresses the reconstructed tissues and must be carefully engaged. Manual muscle testing to determine strength is part of the initial evaluation. However, inversion and eversion testing should be done with caution. The therapist should avoid having the patient perform a single-leg heel raise, which is usually advocated to determine normal gastrocnemius-soleus strength, because of decreased proprioception and the significant muscle deficits resulting from the effects of immobilization. The incision is assessed for mobility and hypersensitivity after complete healing has occurred. Operative damage to the sural nerve and the lateral branch of the superficial peroneal nerve has been reported as a cause of decreased sensation in the involved ankle.[6,16] Joint effusion and soft tissue edema can be factors in limited ROM, proprioception deficits, and the inability to strengthen the joint. Joint and soft tissue mobility also are assessed at the limits of ROM.

Phase I

TIME: Weeks 4-6 after surgery
GOALS: Decrease pain and swelling, restore joint and soft tissue mobility, increase strength in lower extremity and ankle, increase proprioception, normalize gait, maintain cardiovascular fitness, and provide patient education (Table 17-1)

During this maximal protection phase the patient is casted and allowed to progress from non–weight bearing to weight bearing. The patient remains non–weight bearing and the cast is removed at the first postoperative visit for wound inspection. A second cast is applied for an additional week and the stitches are removed. Weight bearing is initiated during the third week and the cast is removed at the sixth week. At this point the patient is placed in a controlled action motion (CAM) walker brace and compression stocking or in a small brace, depending on the individual patient. At 6 weeks the patient is started on ROM and strengthening exercises in physical therapy, as well as pool exercises.

Some authors have advocated a limited ROM of 10 degrees dorsiflexion and 10 degrees of plantar flexion, with partial weight bearing from 2 to 6 weeks after surgery.[21] Formal physical therapy is usually initiated at 6 weeks when the cast is removed. At this time the tissues should be adequately healed and ready to tolerate stresses within a pain-free ROM. Studies have shown that motion is beneficial to nourish cartilage, prevent soft tissue contractures, and restore joint mobility.[11]

After performing the initial evaluation, the physical therapist can implement appropriate treatment. Initially, the therapist performs PROM, especially inversion, within pain-free ranges. At 6 weeks after surgery the ligaments should have healed sufficiently to allow gentle active movement.[16] However, at this stage the soft tissue is unable to withstand significant forces into inversion.[7] The patient is able to perform AROM for plantar flexion and dorsiflexion using pain as a guide; submaximal multi-angle isometrics for all planes also are used at this stage of the rehabilitation. Soft tissue and joint mobilizations are started to reverse the effects of immobilization and surgical trauma. Effusion, pain, and soft tissue edema are treated with the appropriate modalities. Efforts to normalize full weight-bearing gait without assistive devices should include gait training

Table 17-1 Lateral Ligament Repair

Rehabilitation Phase	Criteria to Progress to this Phase	Anticipated Impairments and Functional Limitations	Intervention	Goal	Rationale
Phase I Postoperative 4-6 weeks	Postoperative Cleared by physician to begin rehabilitation	• Edema • Pain • Patient casted for 6 weeks • Limited weight bearing (non–weight bearing for 3 weeks then progressive weight bearing per physician) • Limited ROM • Limited strength	• Patients usually begin therapy at about 6 weeks • Modalities as needed • PROM—(stretches within pain-free ranges) Plantar flexion, dorsiflexion, and eversion; take care when stretching into inversion • Isometrics—Submaximal multi-angle exercises for all planes • AROM—Ankle—supine and seated plantar flexion and dorsiflexion • Progressive resistance exercises (PREs)—Hip—All ranges • Soft tissue mobilization • Joint mobilization as indicated • Gait training—Progress to full weight bearing using appropriate assistive device • Patient education	• Manage edema • Decrease pain • Increase ROM • Increase tolerance of muscle contraction	• Provide maximal protection in this phase: patient is casted for 6 weeks; communication with physician is imperative regarding weight-bearing status • Begin restoring joint and soft tissue mobility • Initiate muscle contraction and prepare for strengthening exercises • Improve hip strength to prepare for normal gait • Provide gait training to improve tolerance to accepting weight on involved leg • Avoid overstressing healing tissues; adapt program as symptoms dictate

drills. Proper foot mechanics throughout the stance phase of gait can be emphasized if pain is minimal or absent.

A home exercise program emphasizing increased frequency and decreased intensity of exercises should be initiated at this time. The therapist should clearly instruct the patient on precautions to protect healing tissues. The program may be altered as needed by the therapist.

Precautions. The therapist should take a few precautions during this phase. Careful monitoring of exercise progression and intensity of the workout session is crucial to avoid overstressing healing tissues. The therapist must caution the patient to avoid aggressive stretching or strengthening of lateral ankle tissues early in the rehabilitation program; progress should be cautious and slow. Exercises that cause increased symptoms in the lateral ankle complex must be modified or avoided.

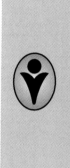

Q. Tricia is 32 years old. She tore her ATF ligament while playing soccer. She had an ATF ligament repair 8 weeks ago. Since then her physical therapy has consisted of massage, ultrasound, AROM and PROM exercises, cryotherapy, and a home exercise program. Her main complaint is pain during gait, while descending stairs, and during attempts to squat partially. Dorsiflexion is minimally limited and minimal swelling persists. What treatment is most likely to improve Tricia's dorsiflexion ROM?

Phase II

TIME: Weeks 6-8 after surgery
GOALS: Return gait within normal range, maintain normal ROM, increase strength, control pain and swelling, increase proprioception (Table 17-2)

Phase II is overlapped with phase I, as the patient's ROM begins to progress and therapeutic exercise options are expanded. At this stage rehabilitation is similar to that advocated in the literature for lateral ankle sprains.[7] Multiplane isometrics and AROM against gravity progress to exercises with appropriate grades of submaximal resistance using weights or rubber tubing. Peroneal strengthening is a major focus because repeated trauma resulting from the instability may lead to weakness of these muscles.[7] Activities to increase strength may occur on land or in a pool. On land, early proprioceptive activity is initiated with the use of a balance board; the patient progresses from sitting to stand-

ing, with bilateral and then unilateral support. One-leg standing also is initiated. Bilateral heel raises are started and progressed to unilateral as tolerated by the patient and according to the therapist's discretion. Proprioceptive neuromuscular facilitation (PNF) also is an excellent strengthening tool for the lower kinetic chain. In the pool, activities may include light jogging and jumping exercises in shallow water. Lunges and squats also are effective. The patient should continue with deep water running exercises for increased cardiovascular fitness. Gait training is an important aspect of the rehabilitation program and should be given priority. An aberrant pattern reinforces itself and leads to continued limitations in ROM and strength. Walking on a treadmill at a moderate speed with a low to moderate grade as tolerated aids in gait training.

A. A mobilization technique was performed at the talocrural joint. An AP movement was applied to the talus to increase dorsiflexion. This was followed by stretching and ROM exercises to reinforce dorsiflexion. Tricia's dorsiflexion PROM increased to 15 degrees. Pain with gait, stairs, and squatting was dramatically decreased after the first treatment.

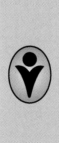

Q. Mary Kay is 19 years old. She plays basketball on the weekends. She tore her ATF ligament playing basketball when her ankle went into extreme inversion during a fall. She had an ATF ligament repair 10 weeks ago. Progress with exercises has decreased because of pain during many of the closed-chain exercises such as single-leg stance, double-heel lifts, mini-squats, and walking more than 8 minutes on the treadmill. What types of closed-chain exercises can Mary Kay do to progress with her strengthening?

Phase III

TIME: Weeks 8-10 after surgery
GOALS: Focus on training to allow return to work and sports, continue ankle mobilization and passive stretching, prevent pain and swelling (Table 17-3)

When ROM and gait are within normal limits, isokinetic strengthening for inversion and eversion can be initiated. At this time the patient should be able to tol-

Table 17-2 Lateral Ligament Repair

Rehabilitation Phase	Criteria to Progress to this Phase	Anticipated Impairments and Functional Limitations	Intervention	Goal	Rationale

Phase II
Postoperative
6-8 weeks
	No increase in pain
	No loss of ROM
	Improved tolerance to weight bearing
		• Mild edema
		• Mild pain
		• Limited strength
		• Limited ROM
		• Limited gait
			Continuation of Phase I interventions as indicated
			• Isometrics—
			  Multiplane submaximal inversion and eversion (pain-free)
			• AROM—
			  Ankle—all ranges against gravity
			  Standing bilateral heel raises
			  Squats and lunges
			• Treadmill
			• Stationary bicycle (using low resistance)
			• Elastic tubing (light resistance) exercises initiated late phase II; dorsiflexion, plantar flexion, inversion, and eversion
			• Balance board progressed from seated to standing with bilateral, then unilateral, support
			• Proprioceptive neuromuscular facilitation (PNF)
			• Pool therapy—
			  Deep water running and light jumping
				• Control edema and pain
				• Increase strength
				• Promote equal weight bearing with sit-stand
				• Minimize gait deviations on level surfaces
				• Increase tolerance to single-limb stance
				• Improve proprioception and stability of ankle
				• Increase tolerance to advanced activities
					• Continue modalities to control edema and pain
					• Improve strength and stability of ankle joint in numerous directions
					• Improve strength with mild resistance initially
					• Progress exercises incorporating functional activities
					• Maintain consistent cadence and work on endurance
					• Later in phase II ankle should be able to tolerate increased resistance with inversion and eversion motions
					• Proprioception exercises with varying degrees of weight bearing and manual resistance aids in return of proprioception
					• Buoyancy effect of water aids progression of more advanced activities

Table 17-3   Lateral Ligament Repair

Rehabilitation Phase	Criteria to Progress to this Phase	Anticipated Impairments and Functional Limitations	Intervention	Goal	Rationale
Phase III Postoperative 8-10 weeks	No loss of ROM No increase in pain Continued progress in therapy	• Limited gait on uneven surfaces • Limited ROM • Limited strength • Mild edema and pain associated with increased activity	Continue interventions as in phase I and II (joint and soft tissue mobilization performed as indicated) • Elastic tubing (mild to moderate resistance) Ankle—All ranges • Isotonics— Ankle—All ranges • Isokinetics— Performed at pain-free intensities	• Full AROM and PROM • 80% ankle strength • Self-management of edema and pain	• By the end of this phase the patient should have full ROM and hands-on care can be eliminated • Exercises should use a combination of varying resistance in different positions to acquire proprioceptive strength and stability • Exercises are progressed to include activity-specific drills emphasizing specificity of training principles

erate a submaximal strengthening program without exacerbation of symptoms. Resistive exercises for plantar flexion and dorsiflexion are initiated at 8 weeks. Inversion and eversion resistive exercises must be performed to the tolerance of the patient. All resistive exercises should be performed without pain. The ability to perform pain-free weight training and isokinetic

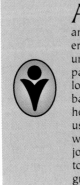

A. The therapist explained to Mary Kay that any activities that cause prolonged pain and swelling must be stopped. Any painful exercises should be eliminated or safely altered until she can perform them correctly without pain. Mary Kay was able to perform the following closed-chain exercises: forward lunges, backward lunges, lateral lunges, and single-heel raises performed on a leg press machine using 80 lb. She could also perform backward walking, minimal walking on a treadmill, and jogging or running in the pool. As strength and tolerance to exercise increased, Mary Kay progressed to more challenging exercises.

training is a good indication that soft tissue strength is progressing well. The therapist must monitor the progression of resistive exercises to ensure that symptoms are not exacerbated.

The patient may be ready for discharge after phase III or may progress to phase IV depending on the prior level of fitness or activity and goals.

Phase IV

TIME: Weeks 11-18 after surgery
GOAL: Return to sporting activities (Table 17-4)

The goal of rehabilitation is generally for the patient to return to sporting activity 11 to 18 weeks after surgery; an ankle brace is used initially on return to sporting activities.[6,14] Exercise should continue with the therapist monitoring patient progress. Exercises in this phase are more advanced, and chances of re-injury are greater. In this final phase of rehabilitation the patient should be able to perform all exercises safely and correctly, with proper form and technique and with little verbal cuing from the therapist.

After the AROM and PROM are within normal limits and strength has returned to normal, sport-specific and functional training can be implemented. Exercise

options include plyometrics, trampoline activities, box drills, figure-eight drills, carioca, slide board, and lateral shuffles (Figs. 17-4 through 17-7). Many of the initial ankle injuries resulted from sporting activities such as cutting activities and movements requiring quick reflexes and balance. These activities should be incorporated into the rehabilitation program.

Suggested Home Maintenance for the Postsurgical Patient

An exercise program has been outlined at the various phases. The home maintenance box on page 300 outlines rehabilitation suggestions the patient may follow. The physical therapist can use it in customizing a patient-specific program.

Troubleshooting

Limited dorsiflexion can be a problem with most patients because of limited talar tibia-fibula mobility as a result of joint restrictions and soft tissue tightness. If restrictions exist at the talocrural joint, long axis distraction thrust techniques are useful (see Fig. 18-5). In addition, mobilization of the talus, tibia, and fibula can be useful. Anterior and posterior glides to these bones help restore dorsiflexion (see Fig. 18-6).

The gastrocnemius and soleus muscle group can be the major limiting factor in dorsiflexion ROM. Low-load prolonged stretching techniques can be beneficial in increasing soft tissue extensibility. The load of the stretch is to the patient's tolerance for 20 to 30 minutes, one or two times per day.

Another method to prevent chronic ankle sprains is to use biomechanical foot orthotics. In theory, biomechanical foot orthotics are designed to enhance joint position, increasing the shock-absorbing capabilities of the lower limb and improving muscle function.

Summary

A successful outcome for lateral ligamentous reconstruction includes no recurrent instability, normal ROM and strength, and no pain with weight-bearing activities. A successful functional outcome is achieved if the patient experiences no instability on returning to daily activities or sporting activities. The first step toward a good outcome is adequate postoperative stabilization. However, the success of the surgical procedure depends on postoperative rehabilitation in which the patient, surgeon, and therapist work closely to achieve a functional ankle.

Table 17-4   Lateral Ligament Repair

Rehabilitation Phase	Criteria to Progress to this Phase	Anticipated Impairments and Functional Limitations	Intervention	Goal	Rationale
Phase IV Postoperative 11–18 weeks	Good progression through previous phases with the need to return to higher-level activities and sports Normal ROM Normal strength	• Limited strength and tolerance to higher-level activities	Continuation of exercises from phases I through III as indicated • Use ankle brace as appropriate • Plyometrics, trampoline activities, box drills, figure-8 drills, carioca, slide board, and lateral shuffle • Increase demand of pivoting and cutting exercises	• Prevent reinjury with return to sport • Discharge to gym program • Return to sport	• Patient's opportunity for re-injury is highest with the addition of advanced exercises; clinicians should ensure proper performance of drills (plyometrics, pivoting, cutting) • Functional training for sports • After patients can perform drills safely and adequately they are discharged with communication to coaches and trainer

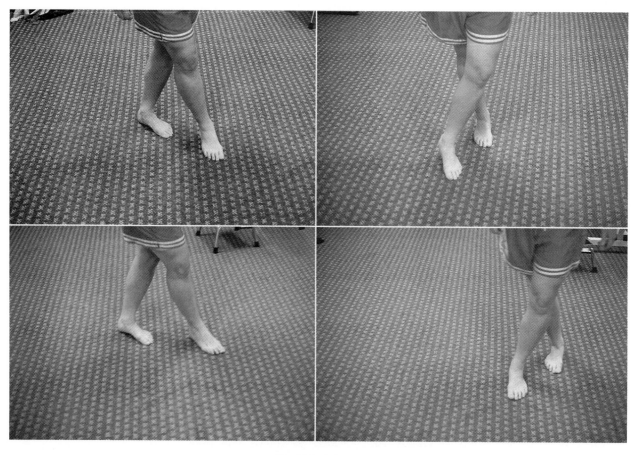

Fig. 17-4. Carioca.

Fig. 17-5. Trampoline stork standing.

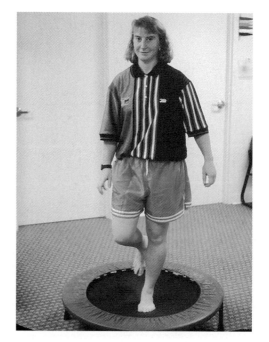

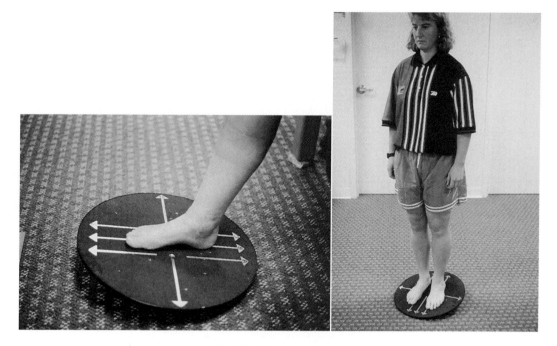

Fig. 17-6. Balance board exercise.

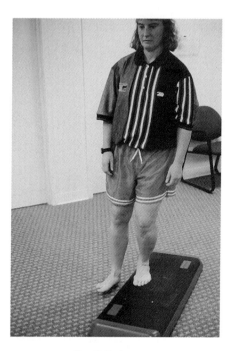

Fig. 17-7. Step-ups.

❧ Suggested Home Maintenance for the Postsurgical Patient

Weeks 6-8

GOALS FOR THE PERIOD: Improve gait, increase ROM to normal, gradually increase strength, control pain and swelling, and increase proprioception
1. AROM in plantar flexion, dorsiflexion, and eversion
2. Isometrics for plantar flexion, dorsiflexion, and eversion
3. Towel calf non–weight-bearing stretch for gastrocnemius-soleus muscle group
4. Towel-crunching exercise
5. Four-way hip non–weight-bearing exercise to initiate total lower extremity strength
6. Seated heel and toe raises

Weeks 8-10

GOALS FOR THE PERIOD: Maintain normal ROM, continue to increase strength and improve proprioception
1. Rubber tubing with appropriate resistance for dorsiflexion and plantar flexion
2. Submaximal isometric exercises of inversion and eversion (performed without pain)
3. Stationary bicycle
4. Heel raises (bilateral)
5. Step-ups, step-downs

Weeks 11-18

GOALS FOR THE PERIOD: Progress with strengthening, increase endurance, and return to previous level of function (sport activity)
1. Standing gastrocnemius-soleus stretch
2. Increased resistance of rubber tubing
3. Straight-ahead running if gait is normal
4. Heel raises, progressing to single-leg raises
5. Sports-specific training
6. Functional training
7. Return to sport as cleared by the therapist and physician with ankle bracing

---

REFERENCES

1. Bahr R, Fetal P: Biomechanics of ankle ligament reconstruction: an in vitro comparison of the Bronström repair, Watson-Jones reconstruction, and a new anatomic reconstruction technique, *Am J Sports Med* 25:424, 1997.
2. Balduini FC et al: Management and rehabilitation of ligamentous injuries to the ankle, *Sports Med* 4:364, 1987.
3. Broström L: Sprained ankles VI. Surgical treatment of "chronic" ligament ruptures, *Acta Chir Scand* 132:551, 1966.
4. Chams RN, Ferkel RD: Long term follow-up of the modified Broström procedure after arthroscopic evaluation, submitted for publication.
5. Chrisman OD, Snook GA: Reconstruction of lateral ligament tears of the ankle: an experimental study and clinical evaluation of seven patients treated by a new modification of the Elmslie procedure, *J Bone Joint Surg* 51A:904, 1969.
6. Colville MR, Grondel RJ: Anatomic reconstruction of the lateral ankle ligaments using a split peroneus brevis tendon graft, *Am J Sports Med* 23:210, 1995.
7. DeMaio M, Paine R, Drez D: Chronic lateral ankle instability-inversion sprains: part I & II, *Orthopedics* 15:87, 1992.
8. Ekstrand J, Trapp H: The incidence of ankle sprains in soccer, *Foot Ankle* 11:41, 1990.
9. Evans DL: Recurrent instability of the ankle: a method of surgical treatment, *Proc R Soc Med* 46:343, 1953.

10. Garrick JG: The frequency of injury, mechanism of injury and epidemiology of ankle sprains, *Am J Sports* 5(6):241, 1977.

11. Gebhard JS et al: Passive motion: the dose effects on joint stiffness, muscle mass, bone density, and regional swelling, *JBJS* 75A:163, 1993.

12. Gould N, Seligson D, Gassman J: Early and late repair of lateral ligament of the ankle, *Foot Ankle* 1:84, 1980.

13. Hamilton WB, Thompson FM, Snow SW: The modified Broström procedure for lateral ankle instability, *Foot Ankle* 13:1, 1993.

14. Hennrikus WL et al: Outcomes of the Chrisman-Snook and modified-Broström procedures for chronic lateral ankle instability. A prospective, randomized comparison, *Am J Sports Med* 24:400, 1996.

15. Karlsson J et al: Reconstruction of the lateral ligaments of the ankle for chronic lateral instability, *J Bone Joint Surg* 70A:581, 1988.

16. Karlsson J et al: Comparisons of two anatomic reconstructions for chronic lateral instability of the ankle joint, *Am J Sports Med* 25:48, 1997.

17. Keller M, Grossman J: Lateral ankle instability and the Broström-Gould procedure, *Foot and Ankle* 35:513, 1996.

18. Komenda G, Ferkel RD: Arthroscopic findings associated with the unstable ankle, *Foot Ankle Intern* 20(11):708, 1999.

19. Liu SH, Baker CL: Comparison of lateral ankle ligamentous reconstruction procedures, *Am J Sports Med* 22:313, 1994.

20. Peters WJ, Trevino SG, Renstrom PA: Chronic lateral ankle instability, *Foot Ankle* 12:182, 1991.

21. Sammarco GJ, Carrasquillo HA: Surgical revision after failed lateral ankle reconstruction, *Foot & Ankle International* 16:748, 1995.

22. Taga I et al: Articular cartilage lesions in ankles with lateral ligament injury. An arthroscopic study, *Am J Sports Med* 21:120, 1993.

23. Watson-Jones R: *Fractures and other bone and joint injuries,* Baltimore, 1940, Williams & Wilkins.

Chapter 18

Open Reduction and Internal Fixation of the Ankle

Richard Ferkel
Robert Donatelli
Will Hall

The treatment of ankle fractures dates back to antiquity. Evidence of healed ankle fractures has been noted in the remains of mummies from ancient Egypt.[8] Hippocrates recommended that closed fractures be reduced by traction of the foot, but few other advances in the understanding and treatment of ankle fractures were made until the middle of the eighteenth century.[10,12,15] Operative treatment of ankle fractures was popularized by Lambotte and Danis; the AO group began a systematic study of fracture treatment in 1958.[2,6,13,22] Since these original investigators, significant progress has been made in the treatment of ankle fractures.

An ankle fracture is a debilitating injury, especially if the fracture is unstable. The treatment of choice for an unstable ankle fracture is open reduction and internal fixation (ORIF). As technology and surgical techniques have advanced, so have the outcomes for ORIF.[18] Anand and Klenarman[3] report that in a sample of 80 patients older than 60 years, 88.5% were satisfied with their postoperative outcome.

Much of the current understanding of the mechanism of ankle fractures has developed from the work of Lauge-Hansen.[16] In his system the position of the foot (pronation or supination) at the time of the injury is described first and the direction of the deforming force is described second. Ankle fractures currently are classified most commonly by two systems: Lauge-Hansen and Danis.[22] The latter system is based on the level of the fracture of the fibula. Fractures also are classified by the number of bones that are affected—that is, a bimalleolar fracture involves injury to two areas of the ankle, whereas a trimalleolar fracture indicates that the medial, lateral, and posterior malleoli have all been fractured.

Surgical Indications and Considerations

Ankle fractures are treated conservatively if minimal displacement has occurred with little rotation and shortening of the fracture fragments. The ankle mortise must be secure with the medial clear space (the space between the medial malleolus and talus) measuring 3 mm or less. In addition, the lateral clear space (the space between the lateral fibula and the lateral dome of the talus) also must measure 3 mm or less. Moreover, the talus must be reduced beneath the tibial plafond and not subluxated forward or backward. If the fracture is felt to be stable, it can be treated in a cast, usually below the knee, extending to the tips of the toes with the foot in an appropriate position for the type of fracture deformity. In some instances, after swelling resolves, the fracture can displace; in this case ORIF should be performed. Generally ORIF should be performed on all patients, regardless of age, gender, activity level, or vocation, as long as they are healthy enough to undergo the procedure. However, exceptions do exist, including paraplegics and quadriplegics and patients who are nonambulatory and lack sensation to the lower extremities.

Preoperative variables that predict a successful outcome include an otherwise healthy patient who is well motivated to recover after surgery. Systemic diseases such as osteoporosis, diabetes, alcoholism, and tobacco abuse can all affect the ultimate outcome of surgery. These variables affect wound healing as well as the healing of the fracture itself.

Surgical Procedure

Surgical Options

The currently accepted method for fracture ORIF is the AO (Association for the Study of Internal Fixation [ASIF]) technique developed in Switzerland. This technique emphasizes the use of plates and screws and wires as needed to achieve rigid fixation. A careful preoperative assessment of not only the patient's health, but also the fracture and the patient's swelling and skin tension is important to a successful outcome. In some cases surgery may have to be delayed for as long as 14 days to allow swelling to resolve so the skin can be

Special consideration is given to Deborah Mandis Cozen, PT, and Richard B. Johnston III, MD, for their assistance in the preparation of this chapter.

closed at the end of surgery without a wound slough. Recently a foot and ankle pump device has been used to reduce swelling rapidly to permit earlier surgery and fewer complications.

Initially, patients may be too swollen to wear a cast. In this instance a bulky dressing with cast padding and bias-type compression wrap is applied with a posterior splint. The patient remains non–weight bearing with crutches and elevates the injured ankle above the heart to promote reduction of swelling.

Procedure

Four criteria must be fulfilled to achieve the best possible functional results in the treatment of ankle fractures:
1. Dislocations and fractures should be reduced as soon as possible.
2. All joint surfaces must be precisely reconstituted.
3. Reduction of the fracture must be maintained during the period of healing.
4. Motion of the joint should be instituted as early as possible.

The patient is taken to the operating room and either epidural or general anesthesia is provided. Prophylactic antibiotics are administered and the injured extremity is prepared and draped as described in Chapter 17. Recent research at the Southern California Orthopedic Institute (SCOI) indicates that a high percentage of patients have intraarticular pathology associated with ankle fractures.[17] Almost 75% of patients with displaced ankle fractures have an osteochondral lesion of the talus that is not evident on preoperative x-ray films and can only be seen on arthroscopy before ORIF. Based on these results and Lantz's research[14] (which found a 49% incidence of injuries to the talar dome articular cartilage in isolated malleolar fractures), the authors recommend arthroscopy before ORIF of all ankle fractures.

The arthroscopic evaluation is done as described in Chapter 17. All intraarticular pathology is documented and appropriately treated. The surgeon must examine carefully for osteochondral lesions of the talus, tears of the deltoid ligament, and dislocations of the posterior tibial tendon, which may impede fracture reduction. After the arthroscopic portion of the procedure is completed, the ankle is prepared and draped again, gloves are changed, and new sterile instruments are used.

Incisions are made over the lateral, medial, or posterior malleolus, depending on the nature of the fractures. When a fracture apparently involves only the medial malleolus, the surgeon should search for an injury to the syndesmosis with subsequent tearing of the interosseous membrane, which may result in a high fibular fracture. This type of fracture, which also is known as a Maisonneuve type of fracture, could even occur at the fibular head and may be missed if the surgeon is not diligent. In this instance the medial malleolar fracture is reduced anatomically, usually with two screws inserted proximally through a small incision from the tip of the medial malleolus. The deltoid ligament is split in line with its fibers, and the two screws are inserted parallel to each other under fluoroscopic control. If the syndesmosis and interosseous membrane have been torn and are unstable, a syndesmotic screw is inserted through the fibula and tibia, exiting the medial border of the tibia with the foot in maximal dorsiflexion. This screw is not placed with compression because compressing the syndesmosis restricts motion postoperatively. When both the medial and lateral malleoli have been fractured, the lateral malleolus is approached first (Fig. 18-1). The surgeon makes an incision over the fracture site and extends it proximally and distally. Dissection is carried down to the periosteum and the fracture site. The fracture is exposed and the periosteum is elevated with sharp dissection (Fig. 18-2). The surgeon uses a curette to remove the hematoma and applies reduction clamps to assist in reducing the fracture. Reduction of the fracture usually also requires traction and rotation of the foot and ankle. When anatomic reduction has been achieved, frequently one or two lag screws are used to provide interfragmentary compression across the fracture site. After this is accomplished, an appropriately sized plate is centered over the fracture site and stabilized with screws (Fig. 18-3). An incision is then made over the medial malleolus as previously described, the fracture site is exposed, the hematoma is removed, and the fracture is reduced. The surgeon inserts one or two screws. Postoperative x-ray films are taken to verify anatomic reduction of the fractures and appropriate positioning of the screws and plate (Fig. 18-4).

In ORIF of a trimalleolar fracture the lateral and medial malleoli are addressed as previously mentioned. Using the fluoroscope, the surgeon then reduces the posterior malleolar fracture by manipulating the fragment into place and making a small incision along the anterolateral aspect of the distal tibia. Two guide pins are inserted to reduce the fragment and one or two cannulated screws are inserted from anterior to posterior to hold the posterior malleolar fragment in place. Generally, posterior malleolar fracture fragments do not require internal fixation if they involve less than 30% of the articular surface.

Postoperative Considerations

After surgery the patient is placed in a well-padded short-leg cast; the cast is split in the recovery room to allow for swelling. The procedure can be done on an outpatient basis if the pain level is not too severe, but in some instances the patient may be required to stay 1 or 2 days in the hospital. After discharge the patient is non–weight bearing on crutches. The cast is changed

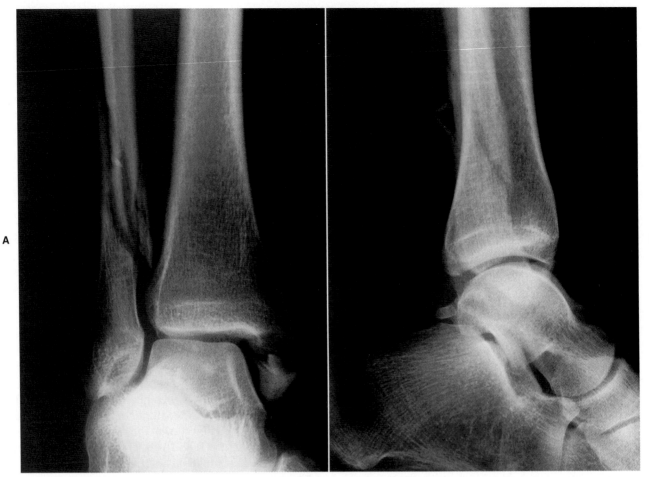

Fig. 18-1. Bimalleolar ankle fracture. Anteroposterior (**A**) and lateral (**B**) x-rays demonstrating fractures of the medial and lateral malleoli.

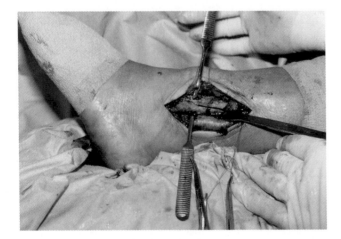

Fig. 18-2. The malleolus fracture of the left ankle is exposed and the periosteum is elevated with sharp dissection.

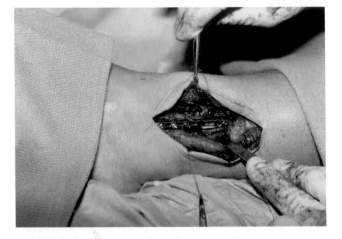

Fig. 18-3. Lag screws are used to provide interfragmentary compression across the fracture site. An appropriately sized plate is then centered over the fracture site and the fracture is stabilized with screws.

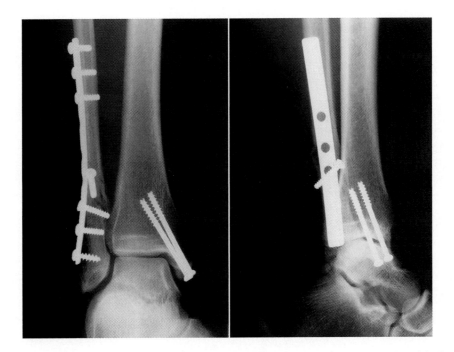

Fig. 18-4. Postoperative anteroposterior and lateral x-ray films are taken to verify anatomic reduction of the fractures with appropriate positioning of the screws and plate.

at 1 week after surgery, the wound is inspected, and all new dressings are applied. At 2 weeks after surgery the stitches are removed and a new short-leg cast is applied for 2 additional weeks. At 4 weeks after surgery, another short-leg cast is applied and the patient starts partial weight bearing, gradually increasing to full weight bearing without crutches. After the fracture has healed, the patient can wear a supportive brace and start pool and then land physical therapy. In patients with stable, reliable fixation, sometimes early motion can be initiated after the third or fourth postoperative week to facilitate early return of motion and strength.[9]

When a syndesmosis screw has been inserted, the patient must be non–weight bearing for 6 to 8 weeks; the screw is removed at 10 to 12 weeks postoperatively. The screw will break with weight bearing if it is left in place. Physical therapy is started 6 to 8 weeks after surgery. After the screw is removed, the patient can be full weight bearing and initiate physical therapy.

Surgical Outcomes

A successful outcome is defined as a fully healed fracture with the patient achieving near full or complete range of motion (ROM) with normal strength and function. Function is defined differently for each patient—an athlete's function is different from that of a sedentary, elderly patient. Several different grading systems, including subjective, objective, and functional data, are used to evaluate ankle fracture results. However, ankle fracture results are difficult to compare because of the multitude of fracture patterns and different circumstances of treatment. Results can be affected by many things, including severity and type of injury, associated intraarticular problems, preexisting arthritis, age and reliability of the patient, quality of the bone, and other site injuries.

Therapy Guidelines for Rehabilitation

The physical therapist normally evaluates the patient approximately 6 weeks after the surgery. In most cases the patient has been casted for those 6 weeks and has had partial weight bearing status between 2 and 4 weeks. Ahl et al[1] report that clinical outcomes may be improved in patients with trimalleolar fractures who have full weight bearing status in an ankle orthosis between 2 to 4 weeks after surgery. Some authors also suggest early active range of motion (AROM) for plantar flexion and dorsiflexion as soon as the surgical incision has healed.[1,11]

Evaluation

The initial evaluation establishes the baseline deficits from which further goals and treatment are formulated. AROM and passive range of motion (PROM) are assessed within the patient's tolerance. ROM is a primary limitation noted at the initial evaluation. Joint effusion and soft tissue edema are evaluated as well. The patient's ambulation is assessed to determine abnormal movement patterns secondary to an antalgic gait.

Table 18-1 Ankle ORIF

Rehabilitation Phase	Criteria to Progress to this Phase	Anticipated Impairments and Functional Limitations	Intervention	Goal	Rationale
Phase I Postoperative 6-8 weeks	• Cleared by physician to begin rehabilitation • Postoperative	• Limited weight bearing per physician • Pain • Edema • Limited ROM • Limited strength	• Encourage use of compression stocking • Cryotherapy • Electrical stimulation (with pads carefully placed) • Elevation • PROM—(pain-free)—Ankle—Plantar flexion, dorsiflexion, inversion, eversion • Isometrics (submaximal)—Ankle—Plantar flexion, dorsiflexion, inversion, eversion • AROM (pain-free)—Ankle—Plantar flexion, dorsiflexion, inversion, eversion • Proprioceptive neuromuscular facilitation (PNF) patterns • Weight-shifting exercises • Stationary bicycle • Balance board activities (seated) • Soft tissue mobilization • At 8 weeks initiate joint mobilization • Gait training as indicated by weight-bearing status • Home exercise program	• Manage edema • Decrease pain • Increase PROM • Increase strength • Decrease gait deviations, improve tolerance to weight bearing • Improve soft tissue mobility • Improve joint mobility	• Control edema and decrease pain using electrical stimulation, rest, ice, compression, and elevation • Improve ROM in pain-free ranges to avoid increase in edema or pain; movement nourishes the articular cartilage and improves tolerance to exercise • Weight-bearing status must be given by physician in order to progress gait; weight-shifting exercises and intermittent loading (bicycle) can be useful in progressing tolerance of the ankle and foot to compression • Soft tissue and joint mobilization is useful in restoring ROM and gating pain • Self-manage exercises

At this stage the patient may have acute pain and be in a fracture boot or other type of orthosis. The physical therapist inspects and evaluates scar mobility. Joint and soft tissue mobility is assessed with an emphasis on the way restrictions limit ROM and function. For example, posterior glide of the talus is often markedly restricted and has been correlated to restrictions in dorsiflexion and normal gait.

After evaluation and discussion, the physical therapist and patient formulate a treatment plan and goals. Belcher et al[5] reported impaired function as long as 24 months after an ORIF surgery for a trimalleolar fracture.

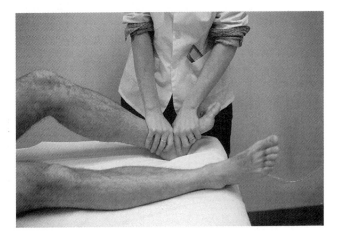

Fig. 18-5. Long-axis distraction of the talus.

Q. Sharon is 45 years old. She fell off a ladder while cleaning windows and sustained a bimalleolar fracture. She underwent an ORIF procedure on her ankle 8 weeks ago. She has full weight bearing status and walks with a boot. When she is on her feet for more than 30 minutes she has prolonged soreness. Yesterday she was intermittently on her feet throughout the morning and afternoon. She is a mother with small children and cannot always rest. Today she is in for a treatment. She has moderate swelling and complains of minimal to moderate pain with weight-bearing activities. What type of treatment should Sharon receive today?

Fig. 18-6. Posteroanterior glide of the talus.

Phase I

TIME: Weeks 6-8 after surgery
GOALS: Minimize pain and swelling, normalize ROM, initiate AROM and therapeutic exercises, normalize gait, increase joint and soft tissue mobility, maintain cardiovascular fitness, and provide patient education (Table 18-1)

Treatment goals initially are to decrease pain and swelling, increase ROM and strength, and normalize gait. AROM and PROM are initiated immediately for all planes of movement under the supervision of the physical therapist.

AROM can progress from movement with lessened gravity (e.g., in a pool) to movement using gravity as resistance. Soft tissue mobilization of restricted structures is particularly useful in decreasing pain and increasing ROM. Around 8 weeks joint mobilization of the ankle is implemented using distraction and glide maneuvers (Figs. 18-5 and 18-6).[7]

The rehabilitation program also includes gait training and lower extremity strengthening in shallow and deep water in addition to land therapy. Ankle AROM exercises also are initiated in the pool. The patient should avoid jumping and running exercises in shallow water at this time. However, if lack of ROM and gait are significant problems at the time of the patient's initial physical therapy evaluation, the therapist may decide to begin land therapy in combination with pool therapy to address specific problems and monitor the patient more closely.

A compressive stocking is useful to help control soft tissue edema and joint effusion, especially during initial weight-bearing activities. The patient is instructed in a home exercise program incorporating ice, elevation, compression, and light active exercises such as stationary bicycling or active ROM exercises to reduce soft edema and joint effusion. Pain and swelling are managed with appropriate modalities such as pulsed ultrasound or electrical stimulation. However, care must be taken to avoid placing these modalities over the metal implants.

Table 18-2 Ankle ORIF

Rehabilitation Phase	Criteria to Progress to this Phase	Anticipated Impairments and Functional Limitations	Intervention	Goal	Rationale

Phase II Postoperative 9–12 weeks	• No signs of infection
	• No loss of ROM
	• No significant increase in pain
		• Edema and pain present but under control
		• Limited ROM
		• Limited strength
		• Gait deviations
			• Continue interventions in phase I as indicated
			• Modalities as before
			• PROM (stretches)—Gastrocnemius-soleus
			    Tibialis anterior and posterior
			• AROM—Sitting heel raises (bilateral progressed to single leg and from sitting to standing)
			• Isotonics or elastic tubing exercises
			    Ankle—Plantar flexion, dorsiflexion, inversion, and eversion
			• Treadmill
			• Stationary bicycle
			• Stair-climbing machine
			• Closed-chain exercises (see Chapter 14)
			    Leg press machine
			    Heel raises
			    Step-ups and step-downs
			    Mini-squats
			    Partial lunges
			• Isokinetics (submaximal)—120°–180° per second
			• Balance exercises (balance board)
				• Self-manage edema
				• Decrease pain
				• Increase ROM
				• Increase strength
				• Decrease gait deviations
				• Improve functional strength of gait
				• Increase endurance
				• Increase proprioception and prevent re-injury
					• Progress home exercises and use modalities as indicated
					• Provide specific stretches for muscles
					• Improve tolerance to body weight as resistance for exercises
					• Use varying resistance to progress strength
					• Use gym equipment to progress functional strength and endurance; progress to cardiovascular levels when able
					• Use closed-chain and balance exercises to strengthen foot intrinsic and ankle muscles in a weight-bearing position

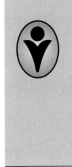

A. When pain or swelling limits the progress of rehabilitation, the intensity of rehabilitation needs to be altered. The therapist focused on controlling pain and decreasing swelling. Joint mobilization using glides and distraction maneuvers was performed on the talocrural joints. Gentle PROM was performed. No resisted or AROM exercises were done today because of pain and swelling. Massage was done to promote circulation and decrease swelling. Ice packs were used in conjunction with a compression device. Swelling and pain decreased after treatment. The patient was strongly encouraged to avoid aggravating her symptoms.

Phase II

TIME: Weeks 9-12 after surgery
GOALS: Minimize pain and swelling, normalize ROM, normalize gait, decrease soft tissue restrictions, increase strength of intrinsic and extrinsic foot and ankle muscles (Table 18-2)

The second phase is initiated after pain and swelling have subsided, usually 9 to 12 weeks after surgery. The second phase of treatment blends with the first as ROM and gait progress to normal. Progressive resistive exercises (PREs) are used to strengthen the anterior and posterior tibialis, peroneals, and gastrocnemius and soleus muscle groups. A home program using elastic tubing for resistance is helpful to augment supervised physical therapy in the office. Treatment options for strengthening exercises include the stationary bicycle, stair-climbing machine, step-ups, step-downs, calf raises, and isokinetic exercises. Specific muscle strengthening for the gastrocnemius and soleus muscles is important to examine because of the likelihood of muscle atrophy. A total lower extremity strengthening program is indicated as well as a program to maintain cardiovascular fitness. Joint and soft tissue mobilization is continued as indicated. Submaximal isokinetics can be implemented using high speeds such as 120 to 180 degrees per second. The higher velocities prevent excessive resistance that could exacerbate the patient's symptoms. Proprioceptive activities are increased as the patient begins to demonstrate increased balance; use of a balance board is helpful in developing proprioception. The patient progresses heel raises from sitting to standing to single-leg standing. Modalities such as compression wraps and ice packs are used as indicated for post-exercise pain and swelling. Electrical stimulation may be used if the pads are appropriately placed away from plates and pins. The intensity of the rehabilitation should be altered if pain or swelling limit the rehabilitation progression.

Q. Curt sustained a bimalleolar fracture. He had an ORIF surgery on his ankle 14 weeks ago. Curt has been progressing with therapy, but dorsiflexion ROM is still limited. How could the physical therapist attempt to gain increased dorsiflexion motion?

Phase III

TIME: Weeks 13-18
GOALS: Maintain normal limits of ROM, joint and soft tissue mobility, gait, and muscle strength; increase coordination for higher-level activities; improve balance and proprioception (Table 18-3)

The third phase of rehabilitation begins approximately 13 to 18 weeks from the time of surgery. The fracture is usually healed by this phase of rehabilitation.[11] The patient has progressed to normal ROM and demonstrates a normal gait and increased strength with manual muscle testing. Before progressing to a more aggressive program the patient should be cleared by the surgeon. Therapeutic exercises should progress to include strengthening exercises that are 60% to 70% of maximal effort. This submaximal effort is best determined by the patient's ability to lift a specific amount of weight 10 times. The ninth and tenth repetitions should be difficult for the patient. Isokinetic strengthening programs can be initiated. The use of various speeds during the workout session is referred to as *velocity spectrum*. The authors of this chapter have found velocity spectrum training useful in promoting strength and power of the extrinsic muscles of the foot and ankle.

Functional training should be initiated for the patient wishing to return to sporting activities or vigorous work. Treadmill walking on an incline or retrograde can be an excellent method of training for the endurance athlete. Pool activities can be used initially for running and jumping.

A. If ROM is limited because of joint restrictions, specific joint mobilizations for increasing dorsiflexion can be used (see Fig. 18-7). If muscle tightness or other soft tissue tightness is restricting dorsiflexion, a low-load, prolonged stretch for dorsiflexion over 2 to 30 minutes in combination with moist heat or ultrasound can be used. If both factors are limiting ROM, treatment is directed at both the joint and the soft tissues.

Phase IV

TIME: Week 19 and beyond

GOALS: Return to sporting activities or daily activities without restrictions (see Table 18-3)

Table 18-3   Ankle ORIF

Rehabilitation Phase	Criteria to Progress to this Phase	Anticipated Impairments and Functional Limitations	Intervention	Goal	Rationale
Phase III Postoperative 13-18 weeks	Continued progression with phase II activities No loss of ROM No increase in pain	• Limited strength • Limited gait • Limited with jumping and running	Continuation of phase I-II interventions as indicated • Treadmill using incline and retrograde • Isokinetic velocity spectrum • Agility drills—Lateral shuffles, carioca, and plyometrics • Pool therapy—Running and jumping in chest- to waist-deep water as indicated	• Full ROM • No gait deviations • Ankle muscle strength 80%-90% • Increase coordination, balance, and proprioception • Prepare for return to sport	• Progress exercises from phases I-II as indicated; discontinue reliance on modalities to control pain • Use uneven surface ambulation and agility drills to improve tolerance of the ankle and foot to the community environment, and return to sport • Progress isokinetics to train ankle to duration activities • Use water to aid in progression of tolerance to advanced activities while unweighted
Phase IV Postoperative 19+ weeks	Continued progress in phases I-III	• Limited with higher-level activities	Continuation of exercises from phases I-III as indicated • Work and sport simulated exercises • Functional capacity evaluation (FCE)	• Return to work and sport activities	• Use specificity of training principles to return to previous activities • Use FCE to determine work tolerances if activity is in question

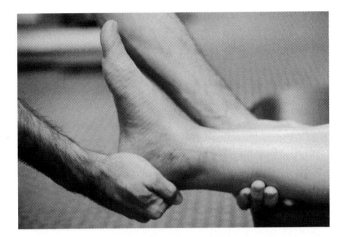

Fig. 18-7. Calcaneal distraction.

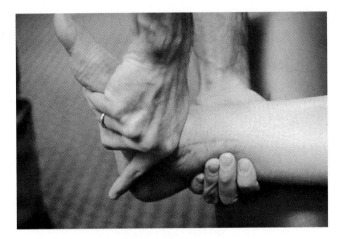

Fig. 18-8. Post-talus glides.

Phase IV is the last phase, starting at 19 weeks after surgery. This phase is used to condition the patient for a return to sports, work, or any activity requiring vigorous movement. Sport-specific activities are carefully implemented with the use of an ankle brace.

Plyometric exercises simulate many sporting activities because of the pre-stretch to the muscle before contraction. Some examples of plyometric exercises include depth jumping, trampoline, hopping, and jumping over obstacles. However, plyometric exercises are stressful to joints and soft tissue structures and should be initiated after normal muscle strength is obtained throughout the lower limb.

Precautions

A trimalleolar fracture is a serious injury. Secondary problems and complications can occur during postoperative rehabilitation. Occasionally low back or sacroiliac pain develops as a result of the antalgic gait with the cast or fracture boot. This is treated symptomatically with emphasis on the need to normalize gait as soon as possible or restrict ambulation activities.

Overuse injuries such as plantar fasciitis secondary to a preexisting over-pronation may be treated with modalities and foot orthosis. Because limited dorsiflexion is sometimes an issue, a low-load prolonged stretch for dorsiflexion over 2 to 30 minutes is effective. This can be done in conjunction with moist heat or ultrasound to the gastrocnemius and soleus muscle group. Specific joint mobilizations are shown in Figs. 18-7 and 18-8.

Suggested Home Maintenance for the Postsurgical Patient

An exercise program has been outlined at the various phases. The home maintenance box on page 312 outlines rehabilitation suggestions the patient may follow. The physical therapist can use it in customizing a patient-specific program.

Troubleshooting

Residual problems after surgical anatomic restoration of the ankle joint include chronic pain, loss of motion, recurrent swelling, and perceived instability. The cause of such poor outcomes is often unclear, but it may be related to missed occult intraarticular injury.[4,19,20,21] Other postoperative problems that can develop include malunion or nonunion, loosening or fracture of the internal fixation devices, infection, and wound problems. These complications are rare. Unless contraindicated, the physical therapist must work on mobilization of the scar or scars as well as general stretching and mobilization of the joint. Care should be taken to increase soft tissue and ankle flexibility gradually and not to stretch or stress the joint excessively to gain more rapid and improved ROM. Pool therapy should be used with some land therapy initially; as the patient progresses, land therapy increases and pool therapy is diminished. The physical therapist also must take care to avoid pushing the ankle too hard, resulting in increased swelling, pain, and subsequent loss of motion.

The physician should be notified immediately if the patient develops significantly increased pain, swelling, loss of motion, or wound healing problems. In addition, if signs of infection or loosening of the internal fixation develop, the physician should be notified immediately.

Summary

In the next century, continued advances in surgical techniques and rehabilitation will allow patients to return earlier to their work and sports activities. As additional physicians and physical therapists specialize in foot and ankle problems, more basic and clinical research will be carried out to "push the envelope" of progress to improve foot and ankle care.

❧ Suggested Home Maintenance for the Postsurgical Patient

Weeks 6-8

GOALS FOR THE PERIOD: Minimize pain and swelling, improve ROM, initiate AROM and therapeutic exercises, improve gait, and maintain cardiovascular fitness
1. AROM of the ankle (plantar flexion, dorsiflexion, inversion, and eversion)
2. Stretching exercises for the gastrocnemius-soleus muscle groups in a non–weight-bearing position (use of a towel or strap to stretch these muscles is recommended)
3. Seated heel and toe raises
4. Ice, elevation, and compression
5. Lower extremity conditioning using the stationary bicycle and/or pool

Weeks 9-12

GOALS FOR THE PERIOD: Normalize ROM and gait, increase strength of the intrinsic and extrinsic foot and ankle musculature, and improve cardiovascular condition
1. Standing heel raises
2. Resistive exercises using elastic bands or tubing for all ankle movements
3. Step-ups and step-downs
4. Single-leg standing progressed to standing on a pillow with eyes open and then with eyes closed (for balance and proprioception)
5. Walking program, including hills as appropriate
6. Lower extremity conditioning using a stationary bicycle, stair-climbing machine, treadmill, pool, leg press, and toe raises
7. Weight-bearing stretching exercises to the posterior calf muscles

Weeks 13-18

GOALS FOR THE PERIOD: Maintain normal ROM, gait, and strength; increase coordination for higher-level activities; improve balance and proprioception; and transition to sporting activities
1. Strengthening exercises with increasing resistance
2. Pool activities such as jumping, running, and cutting drills
3. Agility drills such as side shuffles, backward walking, and carioca
4. Lower extremity conditioning continued from phase II

Week 19 and Beyond

GOALS FOR THE PERIOD: Return to previous level of function (sport- and activity-specific exercises) without restrictions
1. Maximal strengthening of lower extremity muscles
2. Land-based functional activities such as running, jumping, and cutting
3. Sports simulated activities

REFERENCES

1. Ahl T et al: Early mobilization of operated on ankle fractures, *Acta Orthop Scand* 64:95, 1993.
2. Allgower M, Muller ME, Willenegger H: *Technique of internal fixation of fractures,* Berlin, 1965, Springer-Verlag.
3. Anand N, Klenarman L: Ankle fractures in the elderly: MVA versus ORIF, *Injury* 24:116, 1993.
4. Anderson IF et al: Osteochondral fractures of the dome of the talus, *J Bone Joint Surg* 71A:1143, 1989.
5. Belcher GL et al: Functional outcome analysis of operatively treated malleolar fractures, *J Orthop Trauma* 11:106, 1997.
6. Danis R: Le vrai but et les dangers de l'ostesynthese, *Lyon Chirurgie* 51:740, 1956.
7. Donatelli R: *Biomechanics of the foot and ankle,* Philadelphia, 1996, FA Davis.
8. Elliot S, Wood J: *The archeological survey of the Nubia report,* 1907-1908, vol 2, Cairo, 1910.
9. Godsiff SP et al: A comparative study of early motion and immediate plaster splintage after internal fixation of unstable fractures of the ankle, *Injury* 24:116, 1993.
10. Adams F: *The genuine works of Hippocrates,* London, 1849, C and J Adlard.
11. Hovis WD, Bucholz RW: Polyglycolide bioabsorbable screws in the treatment of ankle fractures, *Foot & Ankle Internat* 18(3):128, 1997.
12. Hughes SPF: A historical view of fractures involving the ankle joint, *Mayo Clin Proc* 50:611, 1975.
13. Lambotte A: *Chirurgie operatoire des fractures,* Paris, 1913, Masson & Cie.
14. Lantz BA et al: The effect of concomitant chondral injuries accompanying operatively reduced malleolar fractures, *J Orthop Trauma* 5:125, 1991.
15. Lauge N: Fractures of the ankle. Analytic historic survey as the basis of new experimental, roentgenologic and clinical investigations, *Arch Surg* 56:259, 1948.
16. Lauge-Hansen N: "Ligamentous" ankle fractures: diagnosis and treatment, *Acta Chir Scand* 97:544, 1949.
17. Loren GJ, Ferkel RD: Arthroscopic assessment of occult intraarticular injury in acute ankle fractures, accepted for publication in *Arthroscopy.*
18. Michaelson J, Curtis M, Magid D: Controversies in ankle fractures, *Foot & Ankle* 14:170, 1993.
19. Renström Per AFH: Persistently painful sprained ankle, *J Am Acad Orthop Surg* 2:270, 1994.
20. Stone JW: Osteochondral lesions of the talar dome, *J Am Acad Orthop Surg* 4:63, 1996.
21. Taga I et al: Articular cartilage lesions in ankles with lateral ligament injury. An arthroscopic study, *Am J Sports Med* 21:120, 1993.
22. Weber BG: *Die verletzungen des oberon Sprunggellenkes, Aktuelle Probleme in der Chirurgie,* Bern, 1966, Verlag Hans Huber.

Chapter 19

Ankle Arthroscopy

Richard Ferkel
Deborah Mandis Cozen

The first arthroscopic inspection of a cadaveric joint was performed by Takagi in Japan in 1918.[15] In 1939 he reported on the arthroscopic examination of an ankle joint in a human patient.[15] With the advent of fiberoptic light transmission, video cameras, instruments for small joints, and distraction devices, arthroscopy has become an important diagnostic and therapeutic modality for disorders of the ankle. Arthroscopic examination of the ankle joint allows direct visualization during stress testing of intraarticular structures and ligaments about the ankle joint. Various arthroscopic procedures have been developed with less attendant morbidity and mortality to patients.[1,3,4,5-7,13]

Surgical Indications and Considerations

Diagnostic indications for ankle arthroscopy include unexplained pain, swelling, stiffness, instability, hemarthrosis, locking, and abnormal snapping or popping. Operative indications for ankle arthroscopy include loose body removal, excision of anterior tibiotalar osteophytes, debridement of soft tissue impingement, and treatment of osteochondral lesions, synovectomy and lateral instability (Fig. 19-1). Other indications include arthrodesis for posttraumatic degenerative arthritis and treatment for ankle fractures and post-fracture defects.

Absolute contraindications for ankle arthroscopy include localized soft tissue or systemic infection and severe degenerative joint disease. With end-stage degenerative joint disease, successful distraction may not be possible, precluding visualization of the ankle joint. Relative contraindications include reflex sympathetic dystrophy, moderate degenerative joint disease with restricted range of motion (ROM), severe edema, and tenuous vascular supply.

Methods

Ankle arthroscopy is usually performed in one of three ways: in the supine position, with the knee bent 90 degrees over the end of the table, or in the decubitus position. The method of choice is determined by the surgeon and surgical circumstances. Different types and sizes of arthroscopic equipment can be used depending on surgeon preference and availability.

Surgical Procedure

The procedure described is that used most commonly by the author of this chapter; a more detailed description of ankle arthroscopy can be found in his textbook.[6] The patient is taken to the operating room and placed in the supine position. The hip is flexed to 45 degrees, and the leg is placed on to a well-padded thigh support. The thigh support is placed proximal to the popliteal fossa and distal to the tourniquet. The lower extremity is then prepared and draped so that good access is available posteriorly. A tourniquet is applied as needed.

A noninvasive distraction strap is placed over the foot and ankle. Distraction is used to separate the distal tibia from the talus so that at least 4 mm of joint space opening is obtained (Fig. 19-2). Without distraction the surgeon has difficulty positioning the arthroscopic instruments in the ankle without scuffing the articular cartilage; visualizing the central and posterior portions of the ankle also is difficult without adequate joint separation. The distraction device is carefully positioned so as not to injure the neurovascular structures, and approximately 30 lb of force is placed across the ankle for no more than 60 to 90 minutes.

Before applying the distraction strap, the surgeon should identify and outline the dorsalis pedis artery, the deep peroneal nerve, saphenous vein, tibialis anterior tendon, peroneus tertius tendon, and superficial peroneal nerve and its branches on the skin with a marker. Identification of the superficial peroneal nerve and its branches is facilitated by inverting and plantar flexing the foot and flexing the toes.

The surgeon uses three primary portals or access areas to insert the arthroscope and instrumentation (Fig. 19-3). These include the anteromedial, anterolateral, and posterolateral portals. Accessory portals can be used as needed, but are rarely required. Portals are made by nicking the skin only and then spreading with a clamp through the subcutaneous tissue and into the ankle joint. The surgeon must take great care to avoid injuring the neurovascular and tendinous structures.

The anteromedial portal is established first and a 2.7-mm, 30-degree oblique small joint videoscope is inserted. The surgeon establishes the anterolateral por-

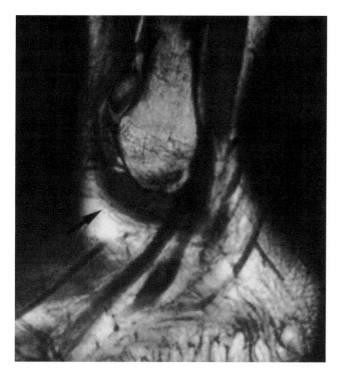

Fig. 19-1. Sagittal T-weighted magnetic resonance image showing low signal intensity consistent with anterolateral soft tissue impingement of the ankle.

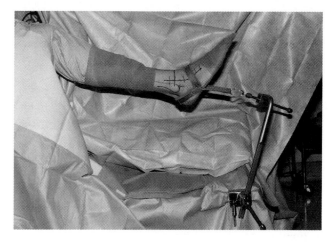

Fig. 19-2. Noninvasive distraction is used to increase the space between the distal tibia and the talus.

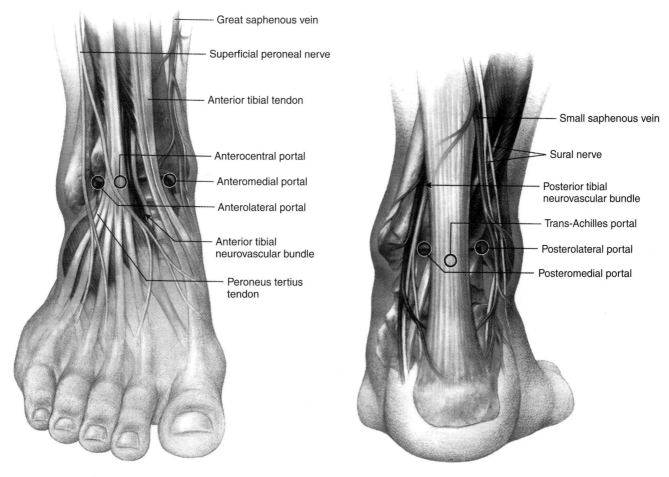

Great saphenous vein

Superficial peroneal nerve

Anterior tibial tendon

Anterocentral portal

Anteromedial portal

Anterolateral portal

Anterior tibial neurovascular bundle

Peroneus tertius tendon

Small saphenous vein

Sural nerve

Posterior tibial neurovascular bundle

Trans-Achilles portal

Posterolateral portal

Posteromedial portal

Fig. 19-3. Anteromedial, anterolateral, and posterolateral portals are commonly used for insertion of the arthroscopic instrumentation. (From Ferkel RD, Scranton P: Current concepts review: arthroscopy of the ankle and foot, *J Bone Joint Surg* 75A:1233, 1993.)

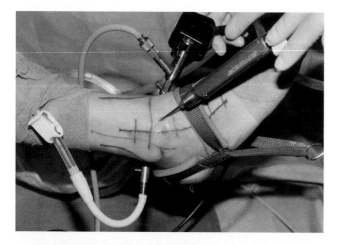

Fig. 19-4. Synovectomy performed with an intraarticular shaver.

tal under direct vision, using extreme care to avoid injuring the superficial peroneal nerve branches. The arthroscope is then positioned in the posterior portion of the ankle so the posterolateral portal can be made just lateral to the Achilles tendon, entering the ankle beneath the posterior ankle ligaments.

A 21-point arthroscopic examination of the ankle is performed to ensure a systematic evaluation.[6] After completing the arthroscopic evaluation, the surgeon identifies the pathology and treats it accordingly, using small joint instrumentation ranging in size from 1.9 to 3.5 mm. These instruments include baskets, knives, intraarticular shavers, and burrs. Scar tissue is removed using baskets and an intraarticular shaver. Synovectomy is performed with an intraarticular shaver (Fig. 19-4). Osteochondral lesions of the talus are carefully evaluated and, if they are found to be loose, excised with a ring curette and banana knife. The surgeon can use trans-talar drilling, abrasion arthroplasty, or microfracture techniques to promote fibrocartilage formation and new circulation in the avascular area. Acute ankle fractures can be evaluated arthroscopically; the surgeon can perform percutaneous screw insertion while monitoring fracture reduction arthroscopically.

After the procedure is performed, the wounds are closed with nonabsorbable suture and a compression dressing and posterior splint are applied. The patient remains non–weight bearing on crutches for 1 week. The splint and the stitches are then removed. If an osteochondral lesion has been treated with one of the previously mentioned methods, the patient may be required to be non–weight bearing for 4 to 6 weeks. During this time the patient is initially in a removable splint and is allowed to exercise the ankle actively to promote new fibrocartilage formation. Weight-bearing status and rehabilitation are determined by the type of arthroscopic procedure performed and individual patient goals.

Surgical Outcomes

Numerous papers have been published regarding the outcome of arthroscopic surgery of the ankle. Results vary depending on the type of procedure and the study that was undertaken.[2,8-11,14] Generally, a large percentage of patients should achieve a successful outcome depending on the nature of the pathology. Expectations after surgery include a full ROM, strength, and full function. Results are heavily influenced by the preoperative ROM, strength, and severity of the pathologic condition surgically addressed.

Therapy Guidelines for Rehabilitation

Several factors must be considered in planning a successful rehabilitation. Rehabilitation guidelines may vary greatly for the same injury or surgery depending on patient age, severity of injury, healing rate of tissue, and previous level of activity. The physician, physical therapist, and patient must work together as a team to develop an appropriate treatment plan to achieve the same goals. The phases in each of the following rehabilitation protocols may overlap by 1 to 3 weeks depending on the factors mentioned previously and therefore may need to be modified to meet the needs of each patient.

The physical therapist should consider six basic rehabilitation principles when planning an ankle rehabilitation protocol:

1. Never over-stress healing tissue.
2. Ankle rehabilitation involves more than just strengthening. Control of acute symptoms and sufficient increase in joint mobility need to be addressed before efficient ankle strengthening can be accomplished. Also, increased proprioception should be emphasized in all ankle rehabilitation programs.
3. The effects of immobilization must be minimized.
4. Neutral position of the subtalar joint during exercise is important for efficient strengthening of the intrinsic and extrinsic muscle groups of the ankle joint.
5. The ultimate goal of rehabilitation is not only to return the patient to the previous level of function safely, but also to prevent re-injury. Therefore patient education should be addressed from the moment rehabilitation begins until the time of discharge.
6. Avoid isolating treatment to only the joint involved. The entire lower kinetic chain should be assessed to identify dysfunctional links within the chain that may have contributed to the original injury.

The following rehabilitation program is designed for a patient who developed chronic sprain pain after an inversion basketball injury and underwent arthroscopic debridement for anterolateral soft tissue impingement of the ankle.

Table 19-1	Ankle Arthroscopy				
Rehabilitation Phase	Criteria to Progress to this Phase	Anticipated Impairments and Functional Limitations	Intervention	Goal	Rationale
Phase I Postoperative 1 week	Postoperative and cleared by physician to initiate therapy • There may be specific pre-cautions de-pending on the stability of fix-ation (com-municate with physician)	• Non–weight bearing	• Splint extremity to prevent re-injury	• Protect surgical site and promote adequate healing in preparation for physical therapy	• Patient is not yet ready for rehabili-tation exercises this soon after surgery; sufficient healing time is crucial

Phase I: Acute Phase

TIME: Week 1
GOALS: Provide adequate soft tissue and joint healing af-ter surgery in preparation for the appropriate rehabilita-tion protocol (Table 19-1)

Patient is placed in a splint and is non–weight bearing.

Phase II: Early Rehabilitation

TIME: Weeks 2-5
GOALS: Decrease inflammation and pain, restore normal gait, increase ankle joint ROM, restore soft tissue flexibility, increase strength and proprioception, maintain cardio-vascular fitness, increase patient knowledge and aware-ness (Table 19-2)

Rehabilitation program. The splint is removed and the patient is progressed to full weight bearing. Exer-cises are performed on land two to three times per week. Pool exercises are indicated only if the patient has difficulty with full weight bearing, has persistent problems with pain and swelling, or is unable to tol-erate land exercise two times per week.
DECREASE INFLAMMATION AND PAIN. The follow-ing modalities are useful in treating and decreasing pain and swelling:
- Ice and elevation
- Electrical stimulation
- Soft tissue massage
- Phonophoresis

- Grade I and II ankle and forefoot joint mobilizations
- Active ankle circles and pumps

Passive accessory movements are performed by the clinician to decrease pain and swelling and increase joint mobility within the anatomic limit of the joint's ROM. After ankle immobilization, sustained stretch techniques can be used as a beginning technique to stretch a tight joint capsule. Sustained stretch uses the gliding component of the joint motion to restore joint play and improve mobility. Gentle oscillatory distrac-tion can be used to reduce swelling and pain (grades I and II). After pain and swelling have been reduced, more specific capsular stretching can be initiated to improve limited joint ROM (grades III and IV).

The following accessory joint mobilizations are per-formed according to specific joint limitations and indi-vidual patient needs:
- Medial and lateral glides of the subtalar joint to in-crease ankle inversion and eversion
- Posterior glide of the talocrural joint to increase dorsiflexion (see Fig. 18-8)
- Anterior glide of the talocrural joint to increase plan-tar flexion
- Distraction of the subtalar joint (see Fig. 18-7)
- Distraction of the talocrural joint to increase joint play at the ankle mortise (see Fig. 18-5)
- Talar rock to increase general calcaneal movement medially and laterally
- Forefoot metatarsal anterior and posterior glides
RESTORE NORMAL GAIT. Full weight bearing empha-sizing heel-toe gait and sufficient push-off with gait train-ing drills helps the patient learn a normal gait pattern.

Table 19-2   Ankle Arthroscopy

Rehabilitation Phase	Criteria to Progress to this Phase	Anticipated Impairments and Functional Limitations	Intervention	Goal	Rationale
Phase II Postoperative 2–5 weeks	Splint removed Weight-bearing status progressed to full weight bearing as tolerated Physician's orders to begin physical therapy	• Pain • Swelling • Decreased ROM and flexibility • Decreased proprioception • Decreased weight-bearing ability	• Land therapy two times a week (or land therapy two times a week and pool therapy one time a week) • Pain control modalities • Joint mobilization and passive ROM (PROM) • Active ROM (AROM) • Gait training • Progressive resistive exercises (PREs) using Theraband or manual resistance • Intrinsic muscle strengthening (e.g., towel curls) • Biomechanical Ankle Platform System (BAPS) board and balancing exercises • Cardiovascular conditioning: Stationary bicycle Upper body ergometer Deep water pool running • Closed-chain exercises: Bilateral heel raises Partial squats Leg press machine Lunges After 4 weeks step-ups, step-downs, slide board, mini-trampoline, treadmill, and stair climber may be added • Home exercise program • Patient education	• Decrease pain and swelling • Increase ankle joint ROM • Increase strength and proprioception • Restore normal gait to full weight bearing • Increase soft tissue flexibility • Maintain cardiovascular fitness • Increase patient knowledge and awareness of injury and rehabilitation	• Modalities decrease pain and swelling • Joint mobilizations decrease pain and increase ankle ROM • AROM and PREs increase strength • BAPS board and balancing exercises increase proprioception and coordination • Stabilize metatarsophalangeal joints for effective propulsion • Improve cardiovascular fitness • Provide functional strengthening • Home exercise programs and education improve patient follow-through at home

INCREASE ANKLE JOINT ROM AND RESTORE SOFT TISSUE FLEXIBILITY. The following exercises can be used to help the patient increase ROM and improve flexibility:

- Passive range of motion (PROM) to ankle joint and forefoot
- Active range of motion (AROM) exercises in all directions
- Grade II to III ankle and forefoot joint mobilizations
- Hamstring and Achilles tendon stretching (non–weight bearing)

INCREASE STRENGTH. The following exercises are useful in helping the patient increase strength in the lower extremity and ankle intrinsic and extrinsic muscle groups:

- Manual resistance as tolerated (light to moderate) in all planes of motion
- Active resistive exercises using Theraband (starting with light-resistance red bands)
- Intrinsic muscle strengthening (e.g., towel curls)
- "Windshield wipers"
- Upper extremity and general hip and knee strengthening on isotonic gym equipment
- Toe push-ups

Intrinsic muscle strengthening (e.g., towel curls) entail closed-chain exercise to increase strength and endurance in the long and short toe flexors. The function of the intrinsic muscles is to stabilize the metatarsophalangeal (MTP) joints for effective propulsion, converting the toes into rigid beams to provide stability and terminal stance. The patient sits with both feet on the ground with hips and knees flexed to 90 degrees. The heels are directly under the knees, with the feet placed on a towel spread over a smooth surface. The patient flexes the toes repeatedly to curl the towel up and under the arches and then fully extends the toes. Flexion of the knees to 90 degrees emphasizes the long tow flexors; flexion of less than 90 degrees emphasizes the short toe flexors.

Windshield wipers are a closed-chain exercise to strengthen and increase endurance in the ankle extrinsic stabilizing muscles, the posterior tibialis and peroneus longus. The patient sits with the hips and knees flexed to 90 degrees. Both feet are flat on the ground, shoulder width apart. The patient places both fists between the knees to stabilize them, then pivots on the heels and moves the feet inward and outward, keeping the feet *completely* flat against the ground.

Upper and lower extremity strengthening and endurance training are done to maintain fitness in other areas of the body while the foot and ankle joint is healing. The physical therapist must address the entire lower kinetic chain (i.e., hip, knee, ankle joints) for successful rehabilitation to occur. Abnormalities and weaknesses in one link of the chain (e.g., the hip) directly affect the mechanism of the foot and ankle, leading to re-injury or insufficient strengthening. Before patients achieve full weight-bearing status, physical therapists can help them build and maintain strength in the hip and knee joints with traditional exercises that do not involve the ankle joint. After the patient has full weight-bearing status, closed kinetic chain exercise should be emphasized for lower extremity strengthening. These exercises provide decelerated training for the large lower extremity muscle groups, as well as enhanced neuromuscular training benefits of speed, balance, and coordination. Closed kinetic chain exercises are performed with the distal segment of the extremity fixed, allowing motion to occur at the proximal segments. In the beginning of phase II these exercises include partial squats, leg presses, lunges, elastic resistive bands, and heel raises. At the end of phase II (4 weeks), step-ups and step-downs, stair climbing, treadmill walking, slide boards, and mini-trampoline can be added to the program.

INCREASE PROPRIOCEPTION. The following exercises encourage increased proprioception:

- Biomechanical Ankle Platform System (BAPS) board—start with non–weight bearing in sitting (all planes) and progress to weight bearing as tolerated in standing
- Balance exercises, including single-limb stance (i.e., stork exercises)

MAINTAIN CARDIOVASCULAR FITNESS. The following exercises can be used by the patient to increase cardiovascular fitness:

- Stationary bicycle
- Upper body ergometer (UBE)
- Deep-water pool running

INCREASE PATIENT KNOWLEDGE AND AWARENESS. The physical therapist should provide the following to the patient to increase knowledge and awareness:

- Home exercise program
- Specific instructions concerning pathology of injury, precautions and limitations with activities, rate of progression, and specific goals

Phase III: Advanced Rehabilitation

TIME: Weeks 6-8
GOALS: Alleviate pain and swelling, improve ROM, strength, and proprioception (Table 19-3)

Rehabilitation program

ALLEVIATE PAIN AND SWELLING. The patient should continue with modalities only as needed for control of pain and swelling. Iontophoresis can be used for specific or localized pain.

RETURN ROM TO WITHIN NORMAL LIMITS. The physical therapist should continue with manual ankle joint mobilizations as needed until full ROM has been achieved. General lower extremity stretching should

Table 19-3   Ankle Arthroscopy

Rehabilitation Phase	Criteria to Progress to this Phase	Anticipated Impairments and Functional Limitations	Intervention	Goal	Rationale
Phase III Postoperative 6–8 weeks	• Patient progressing well with decreased pain and minimal swelling • Improved strength from $^{3+}/_5$ to $^4/_5$ and near normal ROM • Full weight bearing with very slight gait deviations	• Localized pain • Persistent swelling • Minimal limitations in ROM • Decreased strength and proprioception	• Iontophoresis • Ankle joint mobilization grades III and IV • Proprioceptive neuromuscular facilitation (PNF) • Resistance exercises • Closed-chain exercises, advancing as able • Mini-trampoline and advanced balancing exercises	• Alleviate pain and swelling • Decrease use of modalities except for ice after high-level exercises • Improve ROM to within normal limits • Improve strength and proprioception to within normal limits	• Iontophoresis decreases localized pain • Aggressive ankle mobilization decreases end range tightness in ankle and forefoot • Exercises provide strengthening in functional patterns • Strengthening of extrinsic muscles improves function • Advanced functional strengthening speeds the return to previous level of function • Advanced trampoline and balancing exercises develop functional proprioceptive skills

Table 19-4   Ankle Arthroscopy

Rehabilitation Phase	Criteria to Progress to this Phase	Anticipated Impairments and Functional Limitations	Intervention	Goal	Rationale
Phase IV Postoperative 9-12 weeks	No pain or swelling Normal strength ($^5/_5$) Good proprioception Full ankle ROM in all planes Normal gait without deviations	• Patient requires sport-specific training to increase functional strength, endurance, and proprioception for a safe return to sport	• Sport-specific drills and exercises emphasizing power, agility, and speed • Running • Plyometric • Duplication of sport activities	• Full return to sports without limitations • Excellent patient knowledge and performance of home exercises and clear understanding of the pathology of injury	• Advanced sport-specific training helps ensure a safe return to sport

be continued before and after exercise. The patient can add posterior tibialis, anterior tibialis, and peroneal stretching, if indicated.

IMPROVE STRENGTH. The following exercises are recommended to help the patient increase in strength:
- Ankle proprioceptive neuromuscular facilitation (PNF), using moderate to maximal resistance
- Increased Theraband resistance
- Increased resistance in windshield wipers and towel curls
- Concentric and eccentric gastrocnemius and soleus strengthening in weight bearing with resistance
- Step-ups and step-downs
- Retro stair-climbing machine (Retro rehabilitation is the performance of certain activities in reverse direction. This decreases knee joint loading while increasing quadriceps strength and power. Stability is decreased, and therefore proprioception is more difficult to control.)
- Treadmill walking
- Closed kinetic chain exercises with sports cord (begin with light resistance)
- Slide board
- Front and side lower extremity lunges, with weight if tolerated
- Continued upper extremity strengthening to maintain strength and endurance for return to sports

IMPROVE PROPRIOCEPTION. The following exercises promote improved proprioception:
- BAPS board, weight bearing and with weights
- Trampoline drills that incorporate balance exercises and weight shifting
- Stork exercises with dynamic movement of uninvolved side and applied external resistance

Phase IV: Specificity of Sport

TIME: Weeks 9-12
GOALS: Provide sport-specific training to return to basketball, prepare for discharge from physical therapy to a structured sport-specific home exercise program, have patient demonstrate good knowledge and technique with home exercise program and good awareness of physical limitations to avoid re-injury (Table 19-4)

The time of this final phase of rehabilitation varies greatly depending on the patient's progression through the earlier phases of rehabilitation. Additionally, before implementing this advanced phase of rehabilitation, the patient must be free of pain and swelling and have proprioception and ROM within normal limits.

Rehabilitation program. During this phase the patient works on advanced strengthening and proprioceptive training. Exercises are tailored to the specific sport. Exercises that are useful for a basketball player in phase IV follow:
- Running and side-stepping on a treadmill
- Cross-over stepping on a stair-climbing machine
- Squat jumping on a trampoline
- Lower extremity plyometric exercises
- Running and agility drills with a sport cord (forward, backward, side-to-side)
- Agility drills on basketball court (or a simulated court outside), including figure eights, cutting drills, and cariocas
- Advanced trampoline exercises with resistance (e.g., throwing plyoball, using body blade)
- Videotaping patient playing basketball and reviewing tape with patient to assess weaknesses

and biomechanical problems with form that may lead to re-injury or other related injuries in the future

Advanced mini-trampoline exercises in single-limb stance with added external resistance are used to incorporate sport-specific activities. The soft surface of the trampoline provides an element of instability, thus requiring more control in the weight-bearing lower extremity. The patient maintains balance using a single-limb stance while performing upper extremity skills such as throwing, batting, and dribbling. He or she can then progress to incorporate walking (swinging leg), specific dance moves, and kicking actions performed by the non–weight-bearing leg.

Before ending the formal rehabilitation program, the physical therapist should review proper training technique and the home exercise program with the patient in detail.

Suggested Home Maintenance for the Postsurgical Patient

A home maintenance program for ankle exercises has been outlined in Chapter 18. The reader is referred to page 312.

Troubleshooting

Patients after ankle arthroscopy may experience soreness or numbness and tingling over the portal sites. In addition, residual swelling and discoloration may occur. Patients are started on physical therapy 2 or 3 weeks after surgery. If rehabilitation is begun too soon, significant swelling and pain may develop with loss of motion and strength; these sequelae may be difficult to reverse. If formal physical therapy is delayed for at least 2 to 3 weeks, the author of this chapter has found these problems to be significantly diminished. The rest period allows for gentle ROM and strengthening, promotes soft tissue healing, and gives the residual swelling, edema, and soreness time to abate. Some patients may require additional special precautions depending on the type of procedure performed; the physical therapist should consult with the physician after reviewing the operative report for specific cautions and guidelines.

Conclusion

The therapist should notify the physician immediately if any wound opening, drainage, redness, or increased swelling and pain occurs. In addition, if physical therapy has been progressing well and suddenly the patient develops problems with rehabilitation, the therapist should notify the physician. If the patient does not attend physical therapy, is not cooperative, or tries to rush the program, this also should be discussed with the physician.

REFERENCES

1. Andrews JR, Previte WJ, Carson WG: Arthroscopy of the ankle: technique and normal anatomy, *Foot Ankle* 6:29, 1985.
2. Baker CL, Andrews JR, Ryan JB: Arthroscopic treatment of transchondral talar dome fractures, *Arthroscopy* 2:82, 1986.
3. Chen Y: Arthroscopy of the ankle joint. In Watanabe M, editor: *Arthroscopy of small joints,* New York, 1985, Igaku-Shoin.
4. Drez D, Jr, Guhl JF, Gollehon DL: Ankle arthroscopy: technique and indications, *Foot Ankle* 2:138, 1981.
5. Ferkel RD: Arthroscopy of the ankle and foot. In Mann RA, Coughlin M, editors: *Surgery of the foot and ankle,* ed 6, St Louis, 1993, Mosby.
6. Ferkel RD: *Arthroscopic surgery: the foot and ankle,* Philadelphia, 1996, Lippincott-Raven.
7. Ferkel RD, Fischer SP: Progress in ankle arthroscopy, *Clin Orthop* 240:210, 1989.
8. Ferkel RD et al: Arthroscopic treatment of anterolateral impingement of the ankle, *Am J Sports Med* 19:440, 1991.
9. Ferkel RD, Sgaglione NA: Arthroscopic treatment of osteochondral lesions of the talus: long term results, *Orthop Trans* 14:172, 1990.
10. Johnson LL: *Diagnostic and surgical arthroscopy,* ed 2, St Louis, 1981, Mosby. Operatively reduced malleolar fractures, *J Orthop Trauma* 5:125, 1991.
11. Liu SH et al: Arthroscopic treatment of anterolateral ankle impingement, *Arthroscopy* 10:215, 1994.
12. O'Connor RL: *Arthroscopy,* Kalamazoo, MI, 1977, Upjohn.
13. Parisien JS, Shereff MJ: The role of arthroscopy in the diagnosis and treatment of disorders of the ankle, *Foot Ankle* 2:144, 1981.
14. Parisien JS, Vangsness T: Operative arthroscopy of the ankle: three years experience, *Clin Orthop* 199:46, 1985.
15. Takagi K: The arthroscope, *J Jpn Orthop Assoc* 14:359, 1939.

Chapter 20

Achilles Tendon Repair and Rehabilitation

Bert Mandelbaum
Jane Gruber
James Zachazewski

Achilles tendon injuries, whether acute or chronic, occur in many individuals. The severity of these injuries varies from mild, overuse-related inflammatory responses to acute, traumatic tendon rupture. This chapter describes current trends in surgical intervention, outlines rehabilitative guidelines and techniques, and details the rationales associated with treating Achilles tendon ruptures.

Surgical Indications and Considerations

Anatomy

The Achilles tendon complex is composed of contributions from the gastrocnemius, soleus, and plantaris (collectively known as the *triceps surae*) and inserts directly into the central third of the posterior calcaneal surface. During dorsiflexion, the tendon articulates with the superior third of the calcaneus. This articulation is cushioned by the retrocalcaneal bursa, which lies between the tendon and the superior third of the calcaneus.

The Achilles tendon does not possess a true synovial sheath. The peritendinous structures of the Achilles are composed of a triple-layered tissue.[85] The superficial layer of tissue is the most durable and is analogous to the deep fascia. This layer comprises the posterior boundary of the superficial posterior compartment. The middle layer, the mesotendon, provides the major blood supply for the central portion of the Achilles tendon. The deepest layer of tissue is quite delicate and thin; however, it can always be isolated from the most superficial layer of the tendon, the epitenon.

The Achilles tendon is supplied with blood and nutrients by three different sources.[85] The most abundant supply is at the proximal and distal portions of the tendon, and the poorest in the central portion of the tendon. As originally demonstrated by Lagerrgren and Lindholm[57] and corroborated by others,[2,10] a gradual decrease occurs in the number of blood vessels in the central part of the tendon 2 to 6 cm proximal to the calcaneal insertion (Fig. 20-1).

Nutrient branches emanate directly from the muscle to nourish the distal gastrocnemius aponeurosis and proximal portion of the tendon.[83] The insertion of the Achilles tendon is supplied by anastomotic branches between the periosteal vessels and the tendon vessels. As already noted, the major blood supply comes from the mesotendon. Vessels enter the tendon itself via a network of fine connections with the deepest peritendinous layer. These vessels come off the deepest layer radially and enter the tendon perpendicular to its long axis. They then course proximally and distally. Because of the external forces that may be encountered by the posterior aspect of the tendon as a result of friction supplied by the skin, most of these fine vessels are found along the anterior aspect of the tendon, where they are afforded more protection (Fig. 20-2).

Pathogenesis

Based on clinical and histologic findings, Achilles tendon pathology may be classified into three different categories: paratendinitis, paratendinitis with tendinosis, and pure tendinosis.[61,80]

Paratendinitis involves inflammation only in the paratenon, regardless of whether it is lined by synovium. The paratenon thickens, and adhesions may form between the paratenon and the tendon.[56] This condition is most commonly referred to as *Achilles tendinitis*.

Paratendinitis with tendinosis involves not only inflammation of the paratenon, but also a degenerative change within the substance of the tendon. Paddu et al[80] and Kvist and Kvist[56] have noted thickening, softening, and yellowing of the tendon, as well as cleavage planes and vascular budding, at surgery for this condition. As in tendinitis, pain also is commonly noted because of the inflammatory process.

Pure tendinosis is usually asymptomatic, showing itself only with acute ruptures of the Achilles tendon.[58] Histopathologic changes such as hypoxic and mucoid degeneration, lipomatous infiltration, and calcifying tendinopathy have been noted at the time of surgical

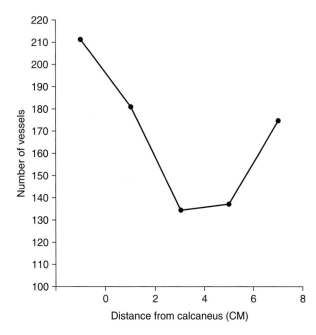

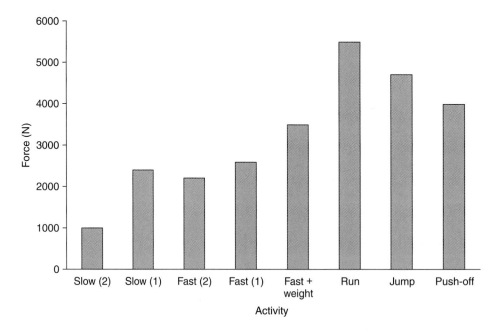

Fig. 20-1. The number of intratendinous vessels of the Achilles tendon varies depending on the distance from the calcaneus. (From Carr AJ, Norris SH: The blood supply of the calcaneal tendon, *Br J Bone Joint Surg* 71B:100, 1989.)

Fig. 20-2. Diagram of the blood vessels of the Achilles paratenon, showing supply for the osseous junction *(A)*, the mesotendon *(B)*, and the musculotendinous junction *(C)*. (From Carr AJ, Norris SH: The blood supply of the calcaneal tendon, *Br J Bone Joint Surg* 71B:100, 1989.)

Fig. 20-3. Increasing Achilles tendon forces during toe-raising exercises over the edge of a step and three sports-related activities. *Slow (2),* Weight on both feet, slow speed; *Slow (1),* weight on one foot, slow speed; *Fast (2),* weight on both feet, fast speed; *Fast (1),* weight on one foot, fast speed; *Fast + weight,* extra weight added to body; *Run,* spring running; *Jump,* landing from 50 cm; *Push-off,* change in direction from backward to forward running. The slow and fast movements represent progressive steps in the clinical exercise program to treat Achilles tendinitis. (From Curwin SL: Tendon injuries: pathophysiology and treatment. In Zachazewski JE, Magee DG, Quillen WS, editors: *Athletic injuries and rehabilitation,* Philadelphia, 1996, WB Saunders.)

repair of acute ruptures.[50,80] These degenerative and histopathologic changes have been commonly noted in the tendons of persons older than 35 years who have suffered spontaneous rupture.[50]

The precise etiology of Achilles tendon ruptures has been debated since the first report of the injury in 1575 by Ambrose Pare. Pare was the preeminent anatomist of his time and made a number of important anatomic and surgical advancements.[70,85] Theories that implicate the degenerative changes that take place in the Achilles with the increased mechanical loads associated with various activities are the most common explanations of the pathogenesis of these ruptures.[69,70] A combination of hypovascularity and repetitive microtrauma results in degenerative changes and inflammation, putting the tendon at risk for rupture. Healing and regeneration are hindered or halted because of poor blood supply to the tendon and recurrent microtrauma. The combination of these factors may account for the fact that most ruptures occur 2 to 6 cm proximal to the tendon's insertion into the calcaneus. Associated intrinsic factors of age (which further compromise vascularity to this area)[40,91] and endocrine function and nutrition[21] and extrinsic factors of compression and friction on the posterior aspect of the tendon (from the skin and inappropriately compressive footwear) further hinder vascularity, healing, and regeneration.

Normally, tendons are able to tolerate high forces associated with daily activities and athletics. However, if degenerative changes take place, the mechanical load usually tolerated may exceed the tendon's physiologic capacity. Mechanically, a tendon may be damaged or ruptured by a sudden application of force. This often involves a forceful lengthening or eccentric muscle contraction. Sudden maximal muscle activation results in a larger than normal force that is applied rapidly to the tendon, causing the rupture. The high load forces that cause such rupture are usually associated with vigorous activities such as sports. The forces to which the Achilles tendon is exposed during activities such as running and jumping have been calculated to be between 4000 and 5500 N;[19,37] they are summarized in Fig. 20-3.[21] Arner and Lindholm[3] describe three activities that can rupture a tendon:

1. Pushing off with weight bearing on the forefoot while extending the knee (running, sprinting, jumping)
2. Sudden dorsiflexion with full weight bearing as might occur with a slip, fall, or sudden deceleration
3. Violent dorsiflexion when jumping from a height and landing on a plantar-flexed foot

The theoretical explanation for tendon injuries suggests a continuum of events, including hypovascularity and repetitive microtrauma, that results in localized tendon degeneration and weakness and ultimately rupture with the application of an otherwise normal load that now exceeds the tendon's physiologic capacity. The possible progression of tendon injury is best summarized by Curwin (Fig. 20-4).[21]

Epidemiology

Reports regarding the incidence, etiology, and conservative, surgical, and postoperative management of Achilles tendon ruptures have increased during the past 50 to 60 years. The number of cases reported may be attributed not only to the observation and diligence of the health care community in publishing their research and thus improving patient care, but also to the fact that the general population has increased its level of participation in recreational activity.

Although spontaneous tendon ruptures are rare, the Achilles tendon appears to be the one that is most frequently ruptured. Kannus and Jozsa[50] report that 44.6% (397 out of 891) of tendon ruptures treated surgically between 1968 and 1989 involved the Achilles tendon, whereas the biceps brachii accounted for 33.9%. Achilles tendon ruptures are usually traumatic and occur between the ages of 30 and 40 years,[4,14,48] which is younger than for other tendon ruptures (Fig. 20-5).

Most ruptures are suffered by recreational athletes rather than highly competitive, very active athletes. Of the 105 patients with Achilles ruptures described by Nistor,[79] only 9 participated in competitive sports. Of the remaining patients, 35 exercised twice a week, 41 once a week, 20 took walks and occasionally exercised, and two were physically inactive. Of the 111 patients who ruptured their Achilles tendon while participating in a sports activity in Cetti et al's report,[14] 92 (83%) averaged only 3.6 hours of athletic activity per week. Of the 292 Achilles tendon ruptures documented by Jozsa et al,[48] 59% occurred during recreational athletic activity—141 of these (83.2%) in men and 29 (16.8%) in women. No patients in Jozsa et al's study participated in competitive athletics. In their study, more than 625 of the Achilles tendon ruptures occurred in professional or white-collar workers who tended to have generally sedentary lifestyles except when involved in sports. A review of numerous studies demonstrates that athletic activities that require sudden acceleration or deceleration are most likely to cause a rupture (Table 20-1). Ruptures not attributed to athletic activity are usually caused by falls or stumbles that also produce sudden acceleration and deceleration movements. Overall, Achilles tendon ruptures have been demonstrated to be more common in men than in women. Ratios of 2:1,[9] 4:1,[17] 1.6:1,[43] 8.7:1,[79] 10:1,[4] and 12:1[80] have been reported.

Diagnosis of Acute Achilles Tendon Rupture

In most situations the history is diagnostic. Patients describe hearing a "pop" as though someone had shot

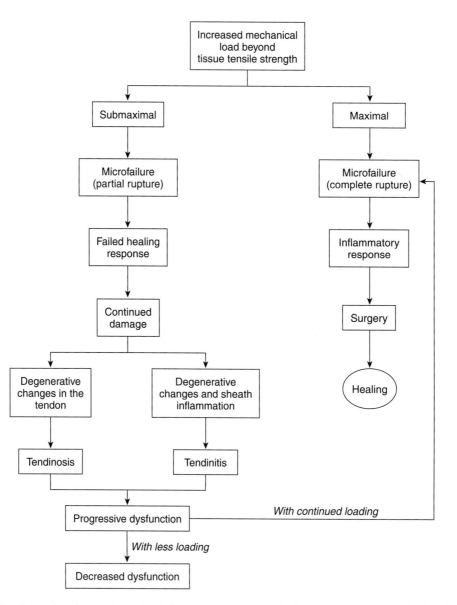

Fig. 20-4. Progression of tendon injury. The inflammatory response may be limited and barely noticed by the athlete, even as degenerative changes continue. As the remaining collagen fibers are overloaded and more are damaged, the inflammatory response recurs, possibly weeks or months after the initial injury. After the tendon is in the inflammatory stage, it can be treated as an acute injury and should heal normally. In rare cases the tendon may rupture because applied forces exceed the tensile strength of the now-weakened tendon. (Adapted from Curwin SL: Tendon injuries: pathophysiology and treatment. In Zachazewski JE, Magee DG, Quillen WS, editors: *Athletic injuries and rehabilitation*, Philadelphia, 1996, WB Saunders.)

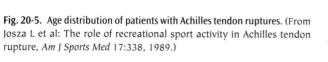

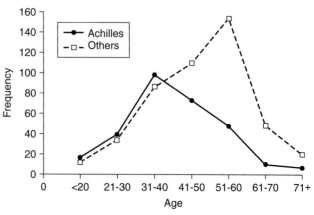

Fig. 20-5. Age distribution of patients with Achilles tendon ruptures. (From Josza L et al: The role of recreational sport activity in Achilles tendon rupture, *Am J Sports Med* 17:338, 1989.)

Table 20-1 Distribution of Achilles Tendon Ruptures According to Sport

Sport	Frings[30] 1969 Germany	Nillius et al[78] 1976 Sweden	Inglis[44] 1981 USA	Cetti and Christenson[13] 1983 Denmark	Holz[41] 1983 Germany	Schedl[84] 1983 Austria	Zolinger[97] 1983 Switzerland	Kellam et al[52] 1985 Canada	Jozsa et al[49] 1987 Hungary	Cetti et al[13] 1983 Denmark	Soldatis et al[88] 1997 USA	Karjalainen et al[51] 1997 Finland
Soccer	102	35	18	7	168	13	300	33	58	10	3	2
Handball	32	9	4	19	57				10	7		1
Volleyball			4		6	14		5	3	3	4	2
Basketball			29		6				23		10	1
Badminton	4	38		20						58		7
Tennis	5	15			23	4			12	3	3	3
Table tennis	4		20						2			
Other ball games	9	5	20						5			
Gymnastics	43	19		5	47	7	230		12	10		
Running	46	6			42	5	110		14			
Jumping	31		5		18			17	14			1
Climbing				1								
Rock climbing									3			
Weight lifting									6			
Trampoline				1								
Bicycling			1		39				3			
Skiing	6		12		73	19	570	4	4			1
Dancing			10						7	1		
Jogging			9									
Racquetball											2	
Aerobics												1
Baseball											4	
Others	30	7			6	6	30			19	4	1
Total	317	134	131	53	479	68	1240	59	173	111	30	20

Adapted from Jozsa L et al: The role of recreational sport activity in Achilles tendon rupture. A clinical, pathoanatomical, and sociological study of 292 cases, *Am J Sports Med* 17(3):338, 1989.

them in the back of the ankle. The rupture commonly occurs in the "watershed area," between 2 and 6 cm proximal to the calcaneus.[57] Avulsion fractures of the calcaneus are relatively uncommon.[2] The physical examination is characterized by palpation of the defect and documentation by Thompson's test,[93] which indicates discontinuity and loss of plantar flexion when the calf is squeezed. Radiographic evaluation rules out the presence of a bony injury. Magnetic resonance imaging (MRI) can be helpful in demonstrating the presence, location, and severity of tears of the Achilles tendon. MRI also is helpful in assessing the status of an Achilles tendon repair.[73] Ultrasonography (US) has been used to define Achilles tendon discontinuity[39] in countries where MRI is not routinely used.

After an accurate diagnosis is made, definitive treatment can be implemented by establishing the objectives for management. If any questions remain regarding the diagnosis or severity of the tear, MRI and US can be used to enhance diagnostic accuracy. The physical therapist should define the patient's functional and athletic goals, personal needs, and temporal priorities before making therapeutic judgments.

Nonoperative Versus Operative Management

Treatment for Achilles tendon ruptures was nonoperative until the twentieth century. It included immobilization with strapping, wrapping, and braces for varying periods of time.[95] In 1929 Quenu and Stoianovitch[82] stated that a rupture of the Achilles tendon should be operated on without delay. Christensen[17] in 1953 and Arner et al[2] in 1958 compared patients treated surgically and those managed nonoperatively; the surgical group had better results. As the field of sports medicine progressed with new surgical techniques, including rigid internal fixation combined with rehabilitation, the optimal treatment for Achilles tendon rupture became controversial. Some studies supported nonoperative management of Achilles ruptures,[59,79] as shown in the following editorial statement made in 1973: *"In view of the excellent results obtainable by conservative treatment, it is doubtful whether surgical repair in closed rupture of the Achilles tendon can be justified."*[22] However, other studies,[43,46] including a recent report by Cetti,[14] demonstrated superior results with surgery.

Recently an emphasis has been placed on postoperative management of Achilles tendon repair. These postoperative treatment programs avoid cast immobilization and are well tolerated, safe, and effective with well-motivated athletes and patients who especially desire the highest functional outcome.*

In summary, early nonoperative options were well accepted and tolerated. But in the past 20 years, pa-

tient expectations and functional goals have increased, so that surgical options have gained acceptance and preference. Indications for nonoperative treatment include concomitant illness in the patient, a sedentary lifestyle, or lower functional and athletic goals. In contrast, the patient selected for operative repair should be an individual who is extremely interested in optimal functional restoration.

Acute Care of the Achilles Tendon Rupture

In the past century the literature has proposed numerous approaches to the management of acute Achilles tendon ruptures. The most important design principles of the option selected should include the following:

1. The option and procedure are safe and effective.
2. The method allows the patient to accomplish realistic goals.
3. The surgeon can execute the method successfully.
4. The risks of the method are acceptable to the patient and surgeon.

The categorical options for the surgical treatment of acute Achilles tendon rupture include repair, repair with augmentation, and reconstruction.

Surgical Procedure

Repair

The rationale for any repair method is to restore continuity of the ruptured tendon end, facilitate healing, and restore muscle function. The technical difficulty is taking relative "mop ends" and opposing them in a stable fashion. Bunnell and Kessler[8,53] were the first to popularize the end-to-end suture technique for ruptured tendons. Ma and Griffith described a percutaneous repair in 1977;[67] however, a higher re-rupture rate also occurred in their series. Beskin introduced the three-bundle suture,[4] and Cetti demonstrated the suture weave in 1988,[12] which was further modified by Mortensen and Saether in 1991 as a six-strand-suture technique.[74] Nada described the use of external fixation for Achilles tendon ruptures in 1985.[77] Each of these techniques has advantages and disadvantages, hence the wide spectrum of options. The surgeon's selection of a method should be based on technical training, an accurate pathoanatomic diagnosis, and the patient's goals and desires.

Repair with Augmentation

Historically, augmentation procedures evolved to supplement the repair construct of "mop ends" plus suture. Most augmentation procedures involved the local use of gastrocnemius fascia flaps or the plantaris tendon if available. Christensen[17] described the use of the gastrocnemius aponeurosis flap to augment Achilles

---

*References 12, 15, 18, 64, 70, 72.

tendon repair in 1981. Silfverskiold described a central rotation gastrocnemius flap, and Lindholm devised a method of two turn-down flaps.[65,87] Lynn in 1966 used the plantaris tendon, fanning it out to use the membrane to reinforce the repair.[66] Kirschembaum and Kellman modified the technique in 1980 by placing the fascial flaps centrally rather than separating them. Chen and Wertheimer in 1992 demonstrated the use of Mitek distally at the calcaneus to repair the gastrocnemius turn-down flap with semi-rigid fixation.[16] Overall, these methods can facilitate the continuity and strength of the repair construct when doubt persists concerning the repair's integrity. In practice these techniques are applied only in limited situations, but they should still be in the surgeon's armamentarium.

Reconstruction

Acute ruptures are usually managed with the repair techniques already described with or without augmentation. Usually these are appropriate to promote continuity and healing of acute ruptures. Neglected, chronic ruptures, however, require reconstruction with endogenous or exogenous materials. Endogenous materials include fascia lata,[7] peroneus brevis transfer,[92] flexor digitorum longus,[71] and flexor hallucis longus.[94] Exogenous materials include carbon fiber,[47] Marlex mesh,[42] Dacron vascular grafts,[64] PLA implant, and a polypropylene braid.[36] Once again, the surgeon must be familiar with these procedures and understand their advantages and disadvantages before applying them in appropriate scenarios.

New Concepts of Achilles Tendon Repair

Prolonged cast immobilization has been used with both operative and nonoperative treatment of Achilles tendon ruptures. Although cast immobilization may promote healing, it also promotes one or more of the following manifestations of "cast disease":[76]

- Muscle atrophy
- Joint stiffness
- Cartilage atrophy
- Degenerative arthritis
- Adhesion formation
- Deep venous thrombosis

Immobilization after tendon surgery was termed the single factor most responsible for postsurgical complications as long ago as 1954.[3,17,67] Various clinical studies in the literature document residual isokinetic strength deficits between 10% and 16% after cast immobilization of Achilles tendon injuries, regardless of whether they were managed operatively or nonoperatively.[6,44,63,79,86]

The A-O Group of Switzerland found that stable and rigid internal fixation of bone fractures allows early range of motion (ROM) and maximal rehabilitation,

thus minimizing atrophy and the manifestations of cast disease. This principle indicates that early mobilization of tendon ruptures should be promoted as long as stable fixation is ensured. In support of this concept, it has been demonstrated that early motion limits atrophy,[5] promotes fiber polymerization to collagen,[81] and increases the organization of collagen at the repair site, leading to increased strength.[24-26,33] Krackow et al initially described a suture technique that allows "rigid" internal fixation without tendon necrosis.[55] This technique, coupled with complete repair of the peritenon, should result in progressive and successful healing of the Achilles tendon rupture without postoperative cast immobilization.

Mandelbaum et al[70] recently reported on the successful use of the Krackow modified suture technique in a series of 29 athletes with acute Achilles tendon rupture. Postoperatively the patients were not rigidly immobilized and were started on early ROM and conditioning programs. No patients in this series experienced re-rupture, persistent pain, frank infection, or skin necrosis as a complication. By 6 weeks postoperatively, 90% of patients had full ROM. By 6 months, 92% had returned to sports participation, and strength deficits were less than 3% on isokinetic testing. "Rigid" internal fixation of Achilles tendon tears allowed a more functional rehabilitation process in this series, including early motion and weight bearing. This method of management proved to be safe and highly effective at returning the athlete and patient to activities of daily life and sport with the highest level of function.[69,70,90]

Surgical Technique

Ideally the surgical technique is performed in an outpatient setting about 1 week after rupture. This delay allows consolidation of the tendon ends, making repair technically easier. Surgery is performed with the patient in the prone position under general, regional, or local anesthesia. In selected cases, both feet are prepared in the field to allow accurate side-to-side comparison of tendon length. An anteromedial incision is made just medial to the gastrocnemius. A direct incision is made through the peritenon, which is split and tagged. Each end of the tear is sewn with a #2 nonabsorbable suture using the Krackow suture technique (Fig. 20-6). The sutures are tied with the ankle in a neutral position to achieve appropriate tension. If any doubt exists regarding the amount of tension, the contralateral side may be used for comparison. The suture knots are passed to the anterior aspect of the tendon and secured. The peritenon is then closed anatomically with 4-0 absorbable suture. The ankle is taken through a ROM to evaluate the stability of the repair construct. The wound is closed with dermal mattress sutures with the knots based on the medial side to protect the tendon, and a posterior splint is applied. On the second day after surgery, the splint is

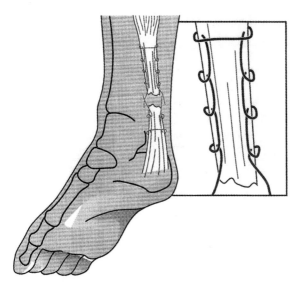

Fig. 20-6. Krackow suture technique. (Courtesy Santa Monica Orthopaedic and Sports Medicine Group, Santa Monica, CA.)

removed and the ankle is taken gently through active range of motion (AROM). Gentle ROM exercises are begun. The sutures are removed by about day 14, and a progressive weight-bearing program is initiated using a walker boot.

A phasic therapy program successfully allows ROM and progressive exercises with accelerated weight bearing. The ongoing rehabilitation of Achilles tendon injuries must be specific and continue in a cyclic progression. *Overuse can occur at any time, so attention to the signs of overuse during the retraining phase is essential.* Early in the rehabilitation program patients are encouraged to increase their weight bearing as progressive ROM exercises continue. Cross-training with bicycle and stair-climbing machine starts as soon as possible; however, an overly aggressive stair-climbing progression should not be used. By the third month, the patient begins jogging; by the sixth month a systematic progression returns the patient to full participation in athletics. Performance parameters include single-leg toe raises at 3 months and full isokinetic strength measurement by 6 months. The objective is full return to safe and effective performance.[70]

Potential Complications

The major complication with nonoperative treatment is a higher re-rupture rate and an incomplete return of function and performance. Complications associated with the surgical technique include infection, anesthetic problems, re-rupture, deep vein thrombosis, and an incomplete return of function. Infection can be a disastrous complication because soft tissue coverage is a major problem and can only be resolved with vascularized flaps and a reconstructive tendon procedure.[62]

Therapy Guidelines for Rehabilitation

Consideration Toward the Healing Tendon

The use of early motion during postoperative rehabilitation requires the physical therapist to have a working knowledge of the process of tissue healing. With this knowledge, the therapist can apply appropriate amounts of stress at the correct times, progressing the rehabilitation program at an optimal pace and ensuring a good clinical outcome. Extensive summaries by Leadbetter[61] and Curwin[19,21] fully describe tendon physiology and healing.

Fig. 20-7 summarizes the stages of the healing process and the implications they have for traditional postoperative management of Achilles tendon repairs and motion in the early postoperative period. Tendon healing occurs in four consecutive, related phases, with somewhat overlapping time frames.

Stages of Healing

Inflammatory response. Minutes after injury, laceration, or the initiation of surgical repair, a coagulation response occurs, triggering the formation of a fibrin clot. This clot contains fibronectin, which is essential to reparative cell activity. Fibronectin eventually creates a scaffold for cell migration and supports fibroblastic activity. Soon after this clot forms, polymorphonuclear leukocytes and macrophages invade the area to clear cellular and tissue debris. The resulting arachidonic acid cascade is the primary chemical event during this stage. This stage is usually complete in less than 6 days unless infection and wound disturbance occur.

Repair and proliferation. The repair and proliferation stage may begin as early as 48 hours after injury and may last for 6 to 8 weeks. Tissue macrophages are the key factors early in this stage. The macrophage is mobile and capable of releasing various growth factors, chemotactants, and proteolytic enzymes when necessary or appropriate for the activation of fibroblasts and tendon repair.[61] Fibroblastic proliferation continues and produces increasing amounts of collagen. Type III collagen, which has poor crosslink definition, small fibril size, and poor strength, is initially deposited rapidly. As the repair process continues, collagen deposition shifts to type I collagen, which has greater crosslink definition, fibril size, and strength. The deposition of type I collagen accelerates and continues throughout this stage and well into the remodeling and maturation stage.

Changes in the postoperative internal structure of 21 surgically repaired Achilles tendons have been documented by Karjalainen et al[51] during the healing process using MRI. After surgery, patients were casted in equi-

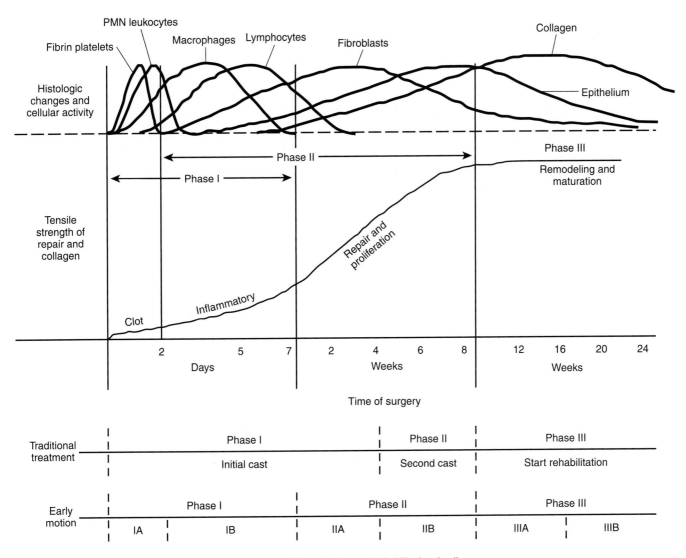

Fig. 20-7. Phases of tissue healing and rehabilitation timelines.

nus position for 3 weeks without weight bearing and for another 3 weeks in a short walking cast in neutral position, with weight bearing as tolerated. After cast removal, patients began AROM and walking exercises. MRI was repeated at 3 weeks, 6 weeks, 3 months, and 6 months after repair to document changes (Fig. 20-8). During this stage the postoperative cross-sectional area of repaired Achilles tendon increased dramatically, measuring 2.9 and 3.4 times the size of the uninjured contralateral tendon at 3 and 6 weeks, respectively. Diffuse, high-intensity heterogeneous signal was present at the repair site for all 21 tendons at 3 weeks and in 13 of 21 tendons at 6 weeks. In the other eight tendons, early formation of high-intensity intratendinous signal was present in the center of the tendon at the level of repair.

Remodeling and maturation. Remodeling and maturation of collagen fibrils and crosslinks characterize the third healing stage. Overall a trend toward decreased

cellularity and synthetic activity, increased organization of the extracellular matrix, and a more normal biochemical profile is evident.[60] Functional linear alignment of the collagen fibrils is usually present by 2 months.[61] Although maturation appears to be complete a number of months after the injury, biochemical differences in collagen type and arrangement, water content, deoxyribonucleic acid (DNA) content, and glycosaminoglycan content persist indefinitely. The material properties of these scars never become identical to those of intact tendon.[1] Biomechanical properties can be reduced by as much as 30% despite the completion of all stages of healing and maturation.[1,19,32,34]

Karjalainen et al[51] found that the cross-sectional area of the tendon continues to increase. The area is 6.1 times the size of the unaffected tendon at 3 months and 5.6 times the size at 6 months. A variably sized, high-intensity signal demonstrating a central intratendinous lesion was detected in 19 of 21 repaired ten-

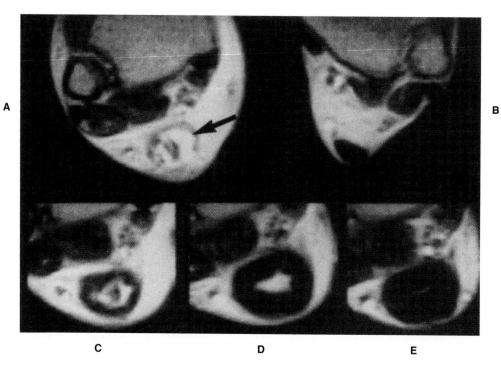

Fig. 20-8. T_2 weighted MRI (TR, 2000 msec; TE, 80 msec) of the normal reunion process of ruptured and surgically repaired Achilles tendon. **A,** The affected tendon shows a high-intensity signal *(arrow)* with a peripheral thin of low-intensity signal area and also low-intensity elements centrally. **B,** The unaffected side. **C,** At 6 weeks the intratendinous lesion and the margin of the Achilles tendon are better visualized. **D,** At 3 months the periphery of the healing tendon has returned to its normal low-intensity signal level. The intratendinous lesion inside the tendon is rather small. The cross-sectional area is seven times as large as the unaffected side (**B**). **E,** At 6 months the scar is barely visible and the edema around the tendon has decreased compared with previous images. (From Karjalainen PT et al: Magnetic resonance imaging during healing of surgically repaired Achilles tendon ruptures, *Am J Sports Med* 25(2):164, 1997.)

dons at 3 months. The development of an intratendinous lesion appears to be a normal part of the healing process after surgical repair and casting.

Postoperative Management: Traditional Immobilization and Remobilization Versus Early Motion

Since surgical repair of Achilles tendon ruptures began almost 50 years ago,[95] the most common method of postoperative management has traditionally been to immobilize the repair in a plaster cast or other type of restrictive device until healing is considered complete, and then begin ROM and strengthening exercises.* This method continues to be used today.[14,29,35,88] Based on an understanding of connective tissue physiology and the success achieved with other types of surgical repairs, such as anterior cruciate ligament (ACL) reconstruction, several authors have begun using early postoperative motion to minimize the deleterious effects of immobilization on joints (e.g., stiffness and loss of muscle strength, endurance, and flexibility)[5,34,68,96] and facilitate an earlier return to preoperative functional levels.†

Q. Kerry had an Achilles tendon repair 7 weeks ago. She is partial weight bearing and uses a fixed protective splint. At 9 weeks she will initiate non–weight bearing stretching exercises for all ankle motions. During phases I and II (weeks 1 through 8) of the healing process, fibroblastic proliferation continues, producing a rapid increase in the amount of collagen. Even though collagen amounts are increased, the repaired tissue is weak and requires protection (e.g., restricted weight bearing and nonaggressive ROM stretches). Why do the healing tissues remain weak despite the increase in collagen fibers?

---

*References 14, 29, 35, 43, 52, 88.
†References 11, 28, 64, 69, 70, 89.

Guidelines for Traditional Immobilization and Remobilization

Phases I and II

TIME: Weeks 1-8
GOALS: Minimize deconditioning, control edema and pain, encourage independent gait (non–weight bearing until cleared by the physician to progressive weight bearing, usually at 4 weeks) with assistive device as appropriate

During traditional postoperative rehabilitation of surgically repaired Achilles tendon ruptures, a cast is in place throughout phases I and II of the healing process (Table 20-2). The physical therapist can do little to influence healing and affect the outcome of the surgical repair. Casting, usually for 6 to 9 weeks, incorporates varying degrees of plantar flexion to protect the repair from stress. Casts that were initially applied with the foot in plantar flexion are usually changed to neutral (0 degrees dorsiflexion) for the final 3 to 4 weeks of immobilization. During this period a conditioning program is designed to maintain the patient's general strength and cardiovascular conditioning. After the cast is removed, the physical therapist can further protect the tendon from full stress by using a heel lift of varying heights for as long as 8 weeks, if needed. Crutches with progressive weight bearing also may be used to control mechanical stress.

 **A.** Type 3 collagen is deposited; it has poor crosslink definition, small fibril size, and poor strength. As the repair process continues the collagen deposition shifts to type 1 collagen, which has better crosslink definition, fibril size, and strength.

Phase III

TIME: Weeks 9-16
GOALS: Normalize gait, increase ROM and strength, improve scar mobility

With the traditional approach, the rehabilitation program does not truly begin until phase III. The scar and tissue have begun to mature and therefore ROM, joint mobilization, stretching, strengthening, gait training, and return to function may progress as tolerated (see Table 20-3). The sequence of treatment depends more on resolving the patient's physical impairments and functional limitations than on the timeline of healing. Impairments are resolved to reestablish function, develop skills, and return the patient to full activity and sports participation.

The initial goal is to restore ROM. Restoration of mobility must occur before the patient can begin to work on strength. Active exercises in the sagittal (dorsiflexion and plantar flexion) and transverse (inversion and eversion) planes are initiated and progressed with the knee flexed and extended. The therapist should use joint mobilization techniques to assist in gaining joint ROM and stretching exercises to gain muscle flexibility and improve joint ROM (see Figs. 18-5 through 18-8). *Any symptoms of pain and swelling that occur must be controlled during this phase through the use of appropriate modalities and adjustments in the intensity of the treatment plan and home program.* Soft tissue mobilization can be used to reduce scar adhesion. These adjuncts for restoring ROM, muscle and tendon flexibility, and strength are continued throughout the program as appropriate (Table 20-3).

Phase IV

TIME: Weeks 17-20
GOALS: Demonstrate normal gait on level surfaces, initiate running program, have full ROM, increase strength, improve balance and coordination

The therapist can initiate strengthening as ROM progresses. Initially, isometric techniques are used for all motions. Strength training then progresses to the use of elastic tubing and manual resistive techniques, such as proprioceptive neuromuscular facilitation (PNF). Isokinetic exercise and body weight resistance can be added if symptoms do not arise from the other techniques. The patient should begin double-heel raises before single-heel raises to reduce tensile stress and the potential for symptoms such as pain and swelling. The heel raises should initially be performed on a level, flat surface, after which the patient can progress to doing them over the edge of a stair to use the full ROM available. Proprioceptive and balance activities (see Figs. 14-3 and 17-4 through 17-7) should be initiated concurrently with strengthening. The physical therapist can begin a running progression, sport-specific skill development, and functional activities after the patient has a normal gait and full ROM and can rapidly perform heel raises. Isokinetic measurement of strength, power, and endurance at 4 to 6 months may *assist* in the determination of return to sport activity, but it is not the determining factor.

The success of Achilles tendon repair using traditional immobilization and rehabilitation has been favorably measured, primarily by re-rupture rates, strength, calf circumference, tendon width, and return to previous activity levels. Re-rupture rates have been reported at an average of less than 2%.[95] Strength measurements include the ability to perform single-toe raises, manual muscle tests, and isokinetic strength measurements. Authors using peak torque measurements of isokinetic plantar flexion strength have reported that the gastrocnemius-soleus strength of the

Table 20-2 Achilles Tendon Repair (Traditional Rehabilitation)

Rehabilitation Phase	Criteria to Progress to this Phase	Anticipated Impairments and Functional Limitations	Intervention	Goal	Rationale
Phase I Postoperative 1–4 weeks	Postoperative	• Edema • Pain • Non–weight bearing • Cardiovascular and muscular deconditioning	• Cast in equinus • Provide elevation and ice • Instruct and monitor non–weight-bearing crutch gait on all surfaces • Design and implement cardiovascular and muscular conditioning program	• Control edema and pain • Protect repair • Minimize deconditioning	• Immobilization in equinus minimizes stress on surgical repair during healing process • Elevation and ice assist in minimizing pain and swelling • Non–weight-bearing status protects repair • Maintenance of cardiovascular and muscular conditioning is crucial to general health and return to preoperative level of function when out of cast
Phase II Postoperative 5–8 weeks	• Stable edema and pain • Well healed incision present at cast change	• Abolished or diminishing postoperative pain and swelling • Atrophy of lower leg and foot muscles • Progressive weight-bearing status allowed • Cardiovascular and muscular deconditioning	• Recasted in neutral dorsiflexion • Elevation and ice as needed • Instruct in progressive weight bearing to full weight bearing using appropriate assistive devices • Modify cardiovascular and muscular conditioning program as appropriate	• Control symptoms of edema and pain if they occur • Continue to protect repair • Encourage full weight bearing during gait cycle • Minimize deconditioning	• Decreased rate of atrophy occurs when muscles are immobilized in a lengthened position[34] • Progressive weight bearing to full weight bearing allows loading and proprioceptive input • Conditioning program should be progressed as the patient's condition allows

Table 20-3   Achilles Tendon Repair (Traditional Rehabilitation)

Rehabilitation Phase	Criteria to Progress to this Phase	Anticipated Impairments and Functional Limitations	Intervention	Goal	Rationale
Phase III Postoperative 9-16 weeks	• Out of cast • No increase in pain • No increased loss of ROM • Incision healed	• Altered gait cycle (pre-swing phase of gait) • Limited joint ROM and muscle flexibility • Atrophy and limited strength • Soft tissue edema and joint swelling • Tendon hypertrophy • Scar tissue adhesion • Limited cardiovascular fitness	• Ice, elevation, and nonsteroidal antiinflamma-tory drugs (NSAIDs) • US and/or whirlpool • Passive range of motion (PROM) (stretches)—Gastrocnemius-soleus, peroneals, tibialis anterior, tibialis posterior • Exercises, pool therapy and joint mobilization as listed under the early motion program • AROM and isometrics in all directions, progressing to resisted exercises using tubing or manual resistance (proprioceptive neuromus-cular facilitation [PNF]) • Gait training—Heel lift if required; return to progressive weight bearing with appropriate assistive devices (crutches or cane) to obtain normal gait cycle if necessary to avoid secondary overuse/tendinitis syndrome; progress as indicated based on symptoms and gait cycle	• Control edema and pain if they occur • Initiate normalization of gait cycle • Obtain full ROM • Improve strength of all foot and ankle musculature • Reduce scar tissue adhesion • Promote cardiovascular and muscular conditioning	• Modalities have been demonstrated to improve the ease of tissue deformation when used in conjunction with mobilization and stretching • Restore normal ROM • Initiate strength through ROM to improve overall function • Increase strength and endurance • Gait deficits in the pre-swing phase may result from limited dorsiflexion and decreased plantar flexion strength—heel lifts assist in reducing stress on musculotendinous structures in the foot and ankle during the early gait cycle out of cast; heel lift can be decreased or eliminated as indicated • Overuse symptoms should be addressed as appropriate to minimize their severity and longevity

Continued

Table 20-3　Achilles Tendon Repair (Traditional Rehabilitation)—cont'd

Rehabilitation Phase	Criteria to Progress to this Phase	Anticipated Impairments and Functional Limitations	Intervention	Goal	Rationale
Phase IV Postoperative 17-20 weeks	• No symptoms from ROM, flexibility, and strengthening exercises initiated during weeks 9-16 • Able to sustain isometric single-leg toe raise and lower body weight eccentrically under control • AROM dorsiflexion 5° • PROM dorsiflexion 10° • Symmetric plantar flexion, inversion, and eversion • No assistive devices required for ambulation	• Mild or minimal alteration in gait cycle without assistive devices • Restricted joint ROM and muscle flexibility • Unable to do repeated single-leg heel raise • Limited strength • Limited proprioception • Soft tissue edema • Tendon hypertrophy • Minimal scar tissue adhesion • Cardiovascular and muscular deconditioning	• Continue interventions from phase III as indicated • Continue joint mobilization techniques as appropriate • Continue stretching exercises; initiate body weight stretching over edge of step • Continue strength program for foot and ankle musculature as listed in early motion program • Modify cardiovascular and muscular conditioning program as needed • Isokinetics and body weight resistance exercises such as heel raises (if no increase in symptoms occurs with previous exercises) • Balance and proprioceptive activities (e.g., BAPS board, single-leg balance activities) • Near the end of the phase (see criteria on p. 333), begin running progression and sport-specific skill development	• Normal gait cycle on level surfaces; initiate running program when normal gait cycle is evident • Full symmetric ankle joint ROM and muscle flexibility • Continue to improve foot and ankle strength; repeated single-leg heel raise • Symmetric single-limb balance • Reduce scar tissue adhesion • Promote cardiovascular and muscular conditioning	• Progress intensity of rehabilitation program as indicated • Restore arthrokinematics • Promote patient self-management of stretching program • Prepare for discharge • Promote symmetric strength of foot and ankle via single-limb balance, isokinetic testing, and progressive plyometric program initiated in water and progressed to land • Continue and progress based on each patient's response to intervention • Provide a good cardiovascular maintenance program based on patient's needs • Increase strength and improve function • Improve balance and coordination on uneven surfaces • Transition into high-level occupational activities or sports

repaired Achilles tendon ranges from 83% to 101% of the uninvolved extremity.[95] Outcome measures in studies that have been reported in the literature are difficult to use in comparing various studies.[95] These studies used different operational definitions, set forth different methodologies, and collected data at different times, making meaningful comparison difficult.

Guidelines for Early Motion

As early as 1984, in an effort to reduce the effects of immobilization, various authors began to present methods of repair that would allow early motion and rehabilitation.[28,64,70,75] All these techniques described some type of augmentation to strengthen the repair (synthetic materials such as mesh,[28] graft[64] or wire[75] or specialized suturing).[70] Newly developed orthoses have been used to protect the repair postoperatively.[11,75,89] Despite the fact that some type of augmentation is used, rehabilitation programs that emphasize early motion must consider the strength and integrity of the repaired Achilles tendon as it changes during the various stages of healing.

Phase Ia

> TIME: Days 1-2
> GOALS: Prevent infection, control edema and pain, increase AROM, prevent complications, promote independent gait using assistive device as appropriate

Phase Ib

> TIME: Days 3-7
> GOALS: Demonstrate AROM dorsiflexion to 5 degrees and plantar flexion 50% of uninvolved side, control edema and pain

When using an early motion program for postoperative rehabilitation, the therapist must keep in mind the phases of tissue healing and the degree to which tissues can tolerate tensile stress. During phase Ia and Ib (Table 20-4) of the early motion program, the primary concerns are evaluating wound status, decreasing swelling, and initiating ROM exercises. However, ROM should not be pushed aggressively. The patient should work through PROM within the limits of pain and swelling intermittently throughout the day. The physical therapist may prescribe ice, compression, and elevation to decrease swelling.

Phase IIa

> TIME: Weeks 2-4
> GOALS: Increase AROM and PROM, strength, and weight-bearing tolerance (on day 14) to partial weight bearing

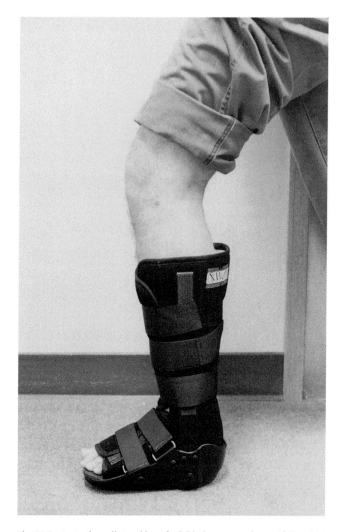

Fig. 20-9. Protective splint and boot for initiating progressive and full weight bearing. A fixed hinge should be used.

During phase IIa (Table 20-5) of the early motion program, emphasis is placed on gaining active dorsiflexion past neutral, following a full weight-bearing program in a protective splint or boot with a fixed hinge (Fig. 20-9), and initiating a gentle strength training program of all the muscle groups in a range that minimizes tensile stress on the repair.

During phases I and IIa US can be used to assist in the healing response. In some instances US has been shown to increase collagen synthesis and tensile strength in experimentally repaired rabbit Achilles tendon.[23,27,31,45] Enwemeka[23,27] has reported favorable results that enhanced the healing response using 1 MHz at dosages of 0.5 W/cm^2 and 1 W/cm^2 for 5 minutes during nine consecutive treatments. Jackson et al[45] noted changes in collagen synthesis and breaking strength as early as 5 days after injury when giving continuous US at 1.5 W/cm^2 for 4 minutes over 8 consecutive days and then every other day for up to 21

Table 20-4 Achilles Tendon Repair (Early Motion)

Rehabilitation Phase	Criteria to Progress to this Phase	Anticipated Impairments and Functional Limitations	Intervention	Goal	Rationale

Phase Ia Postoperative 1-2 days	Postoperative	• Pain
		• Soft tissue and joint edema
		• Altered weight bearing, non–weight bearing with crutches
			• Instruct in surgical site protection
			• Provide ice, compression, and elevation
			• Teach toe curls and pumps
			• AROM (out of splint)—
			  Ankle
			    Dorsiflexion
			    Plantar flexion within pain limits two times a day
			• Patient Education
			  Instruction and monitoring of non–weight-bearing crutch gait
				• Monitor wound status for drainage
				• Prevent wound infection
				• Control pain and swelling
				• Increase AROM
				• Prevent complications
					• Surgical site inspection and cleanliness is crucial when patient is out of splint for ROM
					• Ice, compression, and elevation with a Cryocuff over sterile wound dressing minimizes swelling
					• Toe curls and AROM dorsiflexion and plantar flexion provide muscle pump to minimize edema

Phase Ib Postoperative 3-7 days	No signs of infection	• Pain • Soft tissue and joint edema • Altered weight bearing, non–weight bearing with crutches until day 14	• Monitor wound for infection • Provide ice, compression, and elevation • AROM—Increase frequency to three times a day for dorsiflexion and plantar flexion • US • Instruction and monitoring of non–weight-bearing crutch gait	• Minimize joint stiffness • Facilitate healing • Reduce soft tissue and joint swelling • Active dorsiflexion to −5° • 50% active plantar flexion ROM compared with opposite side	• As in phase Ia • US has been demonstrated to assist in fibroblastic proliferation and facilitate collagen development along lines of stress.[23,27,31]

Table 20-5   Achilles Tendon Repair (Early Motion)

Rehabilitation Phase	Criteria to Progress to this Phase	Anticipated Impairments and Functional Limitations	Intervention	Goal	Rationale
Phase IIa Postoperative 2-4 weeks	Absence of wound drainage and infection Stable edema and pain levels Diminishing postoperative pain No increase in pain with touchdown weight bearing using crutches *A well-healed incision should be present by week 3 to progress to the more active interventions (pool therapy) outlined in this phase*	• Diminishing postoperative pain • Diminishing soft tissue and joint swelling • Scar adhesion • Touchdown and progressive weight-bearing status • Restricted ROM • Decreased strength • Altered cardiovascular endurance and conditioning	Continue interventions as noted in phase I • Joint mobilization progress techniques for distraction–anteroposterior and medial–lateral glides • Progressive soft tissue mobilization and scar massage • Progressive weight-bearing exercises and gait training in walking splint • Start touchdown weight bearing on day 8; progress from partial to full weight bearing as pain and symptoms allow, beginning on day 14 • Isometrics— Out of splint Ankle in neutral—inversion and eversion Start plantar flexion isometrics in late phase IIa	• Minimize joint stiffness • Facilitate healing • Decrease edema • Minimize scar adhesion • Increase weight-bearing tolerance to full weight bearing, beginning on day 14 • Initiate isometric strength program • Improve general muscular strength and endurance	• US is most effective in first 3 weeks and less effective thereafter; it is discontinued by late phase IIa • Repair is strong enough and symptoms are stable enough to initiate full weight bearing in protective brace; reduce weight-bearing status as necessary based on symptom fluctuation and patient activity pattern • Isometrics to facilitate strengthening and diminish edema and atrophy are performed in neutral position to reduce stress on repair • Pool exercises facilitate ROM and strength in non–weight-bearing environment

Continued

Table 20-5 Achilles Tendon Repair (Early Motion)—cont'd

Rehabilitation Phase	Criteria to Progress to this Phase	Anticipated Impairments and Functional Limitations	Intervention	Goal	Rationale
Phase IIa Postoperative 2-4 weeks—cont'd			• Pool therapy—Walk or run under full buoyancy conditions *Non–weight bearing only!* • AROM—Out of splint Ankle— Early phase IIa, all directions, knee flexed and extended Late phase IIa *Gentle* dorsiflexion stretching with towel or strap, knee flexed and extended towel curls with toes • Gait training wearing protective splint, with weight bearing to tolerance • Elastic tubing or band exercises—Inversion, eversion and plantar flexion and dorsiflexion Progress as tolerated if pain and symptoms allow • Isotonics—Weight training program for all unaffected muscle groups • Cardiovascular exercise using stationary bicycle to tolerance in walking splint	• Early phase IIa: Active dorsiflexion to 0° with knee extended, 5° with knee flexed • Late phase IIa: Active dorsiflexion to 0°-5° with knee extended, 5°-10° with knee flexed • Minimize cardiovascular deconditioning	• Sufficient strength present at repair site based on healing and surgical technique to allow AROM to 0° dorsiflexion and all other motions to symptom tolerance with knee flexed and extended • Towel curls facilitate muscle pump action to diminish edema and atrophy • By 4 weeks, sufficient strength to allow start of plantar flexion isometrics and isotonics within symptom limits, using light resistance; performed in non–weight bearing • Maintenance of general muscular strength and cardiovascular endurance necessary to resume full activities of daily living and recreational activities when feasible; walking splint protects repair during activity

days. Freider et al[31] reported similar results in partially ruptured, nonsurgically repaired Achilles tendons of Marland rats that received continuous US at 1.5 W/cm^2 three times a week for either a 2- or a 3-week period. Although the results of studies using animal models may not be directly applicable to the human response, the therapeutic use of US in the inflammatory and proliferative stages could prove beneficial. Using US during these stages is a common clinical intervention.

Phase IIb

TIME: Weeks 5-8
GOALS: Demonstrate normal gait on level surfaces, encourage full ROM (symmetric), increase strength and proprioception

During phase IIb (Table 20-6) the patient should strive to obtain full symmetric ROM, achieve a normal gait cycle on level surfaces and in controlled environments without the protective boot, progress the strength program, and initiate proprioceptive training.

Phase IIIa

TIME: Weeks 9-16
GOALS: Demonstrate normal gait for all activities, have full weight bearing, increase strength and endurance, initiate walking or jogging program, isokinetics, and pool therapy plyometrics as appropriate (toward end of phase)

Phase IIIb

TIME: Weeks 17-20
GOALS: Return to preoperative level of activity or sport

During phase IIIa (Table 20-7) emphasis is on increasing the velocity of activity, increasing the patient's strength to perform a repeated single-leg heel raise, and improving the endurance of the gastrocnemius-soleus group to tolerate a functional progression. During phase IIIb (Table 20-8) a full functional progression is initiated to return the patient to the desired level of function.

All authors using the early motion program, regardless of the type of augmentation used during surgery, have reported excellent results. Success was measured by the same methods as for traditional rehabilitation. Limitation of ROM for dorsiflexion and plantar flexion are rare; patients are able to walk heel-toe and do single-leg raises at the time of follow-up examination. In addition, isokinetic peak torque levels are within 5% of the uninvolved side.[11,70] Reruptures are rare and are usually attributed to lack of retraining before a return to sports.[75] However, these outcomes are also difficult to compare for the same reasons as cited for traditional rehabilitation programs.

The superiority of early motion for Achilles tendon repairs compared with traditional postoperative casting cannot yet be fully determined. Although studies reported to date state that the results are excellent, the different rehabilitation philosophies cannot be compared critically because of differences in operational definitions, criteria monitored, postoperative time when the data are collected, and surgical technique. Although the ultimate level of function achieved appears to be the same regardless of the rehabilitative program, the authors of this chapter believe that using early motion after Achilles tendon repair enables the patient to obtain a more independent and active quality of life sooner than that seen with traditional postoperative casting. However, patient compliance and ongoing oversight of the rehabilitation program are crucial factors that must always be considered.

Suggested Home Maintenance for the Postsurgical Patient

Adherence to a home exercise program is crucial for a successful return to full activities of daily living and recreational function after Achilles tendon repair. The suggestions provided in this chapter do not constitute a fixed protocol. The home program for any patient must be individually determined based on the patient's postoperative condition, anticipated follow-through, and individual needs. Frequency, sets, and repetitions are determined similarly based on the therapist's professional opinion of what is needed in a particular situation (see home maintenance box on pp. 345-347).

Table 20-6   Achilles Tendon Repair (Early Motion)

Rehabilitation Phase	Criteria to Progress to this Phase	Anticipated Impairments and Functional Limitations	Intervention	Goal	Rationale

Phase IIb Postoperative 5-8 weeks	No loss of ROM
	No increase in symptoms
	Full weight bearing in walking splint
	Incision healed
	Mild edema
	Pain controlled
	AROM
	Dorsiflexion to neutral or better
	Plantar flexion, inversion, eversion symmetric
		• Minimal postoperative pain
		• Limited ROM
		• Limited strength
		• Tendon hypertrophy and continued soft tissue swelling
		• Altered gait cycle out of walking splint
		• Unable to do a single-leg heel raise
		• Altered proprioception and joint reaction time
			• Continue interventions as listed in phases I-II
			• PROM—Initiate weight-bearing dorsiflexion stretch with knee extended and flexed
			• AROM (out of splint)
			• Gait training out of walking splint to tolerance
			• Strength training—
			  Initiate double-leg heel raises
			• Isokinetics—
			  Submaximal velocity spectrum
			  Plantar flexion and dorsiflexion, emphasizing endurance
			• Weight training program for all unaffected muscle groups
			• Stationary bicycle to tolerance without walking splint
			• Pool therapy for ROM (walking or running under totally buoyant conditions); heel raises in waist- to chest-deep water
				• Full symmetric ROM in all motions
				• Normal gait cycle on level surfaces and controlled environments out of walking splint
				• Initiate isokinetic and isotonic strength training program for gastrocnemius-soleus complex
				• Improve cardiovascular conditioning
				• Improve muscular strength and endurance
				• Improve proprioception and joint reaction time
					• Continue mobilizations to increase soft tissue strength and mobility and restore joint ROM sufficient to initiate gait training out of splint; gait should be practiced in controlled environment out of splint for safety as appropriate; discontinue use of splint at physician's and therapist's discretion
					• Weight-bearing dorsiflexion required for normal activities of daily living; repair should be sufficiently strong; discontinue if symptoms occur
					• Gastrocnemius-soleus and repair initially conditioned with isometrics; repair is now strong enough to tolerate increased strength training on a progressive weight and force basis

Table 20-7   Achilles Tendon Repair (Early Motion)

Rehabilitation Phase	Criteria to Progress to this Phase	Anticipated Impairments and Functional Limitations	Intervention	Goal	Rationale

Phase IIIa Postoperative 9–16 weeks	• No longer requires walking splint for activity of daily living gait; may require use of splint for extended ambulatory periods in early parts of phase
	• Pain-free gait during activities of daily living walking out of splint
	• Minimal difference in dorsiflexion ROM versus uninvolved side
	• Full plantar flexion, inversion, and eversion
		• Gait deviations in pre-swing phase of gait resulting from limited plantar flexion, strength, and endurance, not insufficient dorsiflexion
		• Unable to perform single-leg heel raise
		• Unable to jump and run
		• Mild pain and muscle and tendon fatigue at end of day if walking for a significant period
		• Limited tolerance to tendon-loading activities (concentric and eccentric)
			• Continue interventions from phases I–II as indicated, especially weight-bearing dorsiflexion stretch
			• AROM—
			  Single-leg heel raises
			  Add resistance up to 1.5 times body weight as symptoms dictate
			• Gait training—
			  Treadmill walking on level surfaces and slight incline
			  Uneven surface walking
			  Stair climbing
			  Progress to jogging toward end of phase if symptom free
			  No sprinting, cutting, or jumping activities
			• Jogging on mini-trampoline
			• Isokinetics—
			  Submaximal effort velocity spectrum plantar flexion and dorsiflexion
			• Pool therapy (waist-deep)—
			  Plyometrics: hopping, bounding, and jumping in waist-deep water
			• Cardiovascular exercises
				• Discontinue use of walking splint
				• Repeated single-leg heel raise from level surface
				• Normal gait cycle for all activities of daily living
				• Full symmetric weight-bearing dorsiflexion
				• Initiate fast walking or jogging program
				• Decrease complaints of mild pain or muscle and tendon fatigue at end of day with walking activities
				• Increase plantar flexion strength and endurance
				• Improve plantar flexion strength and endurance at maximal velocities
				• Prepare for land-based agility drills
				• Improve cardiovascular fitness level
					• Plantar flexion weakness will compromise gait; emphasis is placed on improving functional plantar flexion strength and endurance (single-leg heel raise); higher gait velocities will be affected until late in this phase or into phase IIIb
					• Incline treadmill use will develop strength and endurance of gastrocnemius–soleus muscles
					• Uneven surface and stair training improves proprioception and community ambulation
					• Jogging and running must be initiated only if patient is symptom free, has a normal gait, and is able to perform multiple single-leg heel raises at moderate to high velocities to avoid overloading tendon and initiating an inflammatory cycle
					• Use of mini-trampoline will facilitate achievement of dorsiflexion at varying velocities, simulate higher-level function, and develop higher-velocity eccentric load tolerance
					• Continued development of strength and endurance required throughout this phase to achieve full activities of daily living and recreational function
					• Plyometric activities in the pool facilitate functional use without full weight-bearing stress
					• Use gait training activities and stair machine to provide aerobic training

Table 20-8   Achilles Tendon Repair (Early Motion)

Rehabilitation Phase	Criteria to Progress to this Phase	Anticipated Impairments and Functional Limitations	Intervention	Goal	Rationale
Phase IIb Postoperative 17–20 weeks	Normal gait on all surfaces and inclines Able to fast walk or jog without gait deficits Able to do repeated single-leg heel raises with moderate to high velocities Asymptomatic with all activities of daily living, treadmill walking, and jogging	• Unable to hop or jump on single leg without perform-ance deficit or compensatory movement • Difficulty with sprinting or cutting during higher-level recreational activities	• Review of past rehabilitation program to address areas that may not have been appropriately addressed • Development of individualized strength, flexibility, ROM, and functional progression program to alleviate impairments and functional limitations	• Resolve all impairments and functional limitations that limit full return to preoperative level of function	• Most patients and athletes have only minor performance deficits by this time; deficits (which may continue to exist) require individualized attention based on their presentation and the way they affect the athlete or patient in question; these areas may not have been appropriately addressed earlier or the patient/athlete might have tried to progress too fast; any impairments or functional limitations are usually resolved within this phase and time period

Suggested Home Maintenance for the Postsurgical Patient—Traditional Rehabilitation Program

Weeks 1-4

GOALS FOR THE PERIOD: Manage edema, improve function
1. For edema: Use ice and elevation; perform toe curls and pumps
2. For function: Use non–weight-bearing crutch gait

Weeks 5-8

GOALS FOR THE PERIOD: Manage edema, improve function
1. For edema: Use ice, compression, and elevation as needed; perform toe curls and pumps as needed
2. For function: Progress to full weight bearing to tolerance with appropriate assistive devices if needed

Weeks 9-16

GOALS FOR THE PERIOD: Improve ROM, continue strength training, and achieve functional improvement
1. For ROM:
    a. Initiate non–weight-bearing stretching exercises for all ankle motions (dorsiflexion, plantar flexion, inversion, and eversion)
    b. Initiate weight-bearing dorsiflexion stretch with knee flexed and extended
2. For strength training:
    a. Initiate isometric and elastic band strengthening exercises for all muscle groups
    b. Progress to double-leg heel raises as tolerated
3. For function:
    a. Begin ambulation out of cast to symptom tolerance
    b. Use heel lift and cane or crutches as appropriate to limit symptoms

Weeks 17-20

GOALS FOR THE PERIOD: Improve ROM, continue strength training, and achieve functional improvement
1. For ROM: Continue all stretching exercises
2. For strength training:
    a. Initiate single-leg heel raises
    b. Progress to additional weight heel raises with up to 1.5 times body weight provided no symptoms of pain, swelling, or inflammation develop
3. For function:
    a. Initiate walking on all types of surfaces and inclines and declines
    b. Progress to fast walking and jogging toward the end of this phase if no symptoms have occurred and patient is able to do single-leg toe raises repeatedly
    c. *NO sprinting, cutting, or jumping allowed*

Week 20 and Beyond

GOALS FOR THE PERIOD: Continue strength training, achieve functional improvement
1. For strength training:
    a. Do single-leg heel raises over the edge of a step
    b. Do weight lifting to tolerance
2. For function:
    a. Initiate jogging when able
    b. Initiate hopping, skipping, and jumping activities
    c. Return to all recreational and sports activities

❦ Suggested Home Maintenance for the Postsurgical Patient—
Early Motion Program

Week 1

GOALS FOR THE WEEK: Manage edema, improve ROM, and begin work on function
1. For edema: Use ice, compression, and elevation; perform toe curls and pumps
2. For ROM: Perform AROM three times daily; perform plantar flexion and dorsiflexion out of the splint within pain limits with the knee flexed and extended
3. For function: Use non–weight-bearing crutch gait

Weeks 2-4

GOALS FOR THE PERIOD: Manage edema, improve ROM, continue strength training, work on function
1. For edema: Use ice, compression, and elevation as needed; perform toe curls and pumps as needed
2. For ROM in early phase IIa (days 7-21): Perform AROM three times daily in all directions out of the splint (plantar flexion, dorsiflexion, inversion, and eversion) with the knee flexed and extended
3. For ROM in late phase IIa (days 21-28): Perform *gentle* dorsiflexion stretching with a towel or strap with the knee flexed and extended three times daily
4. For strength training in early phase IIa (days 7-21): Perform isometric inversion and eversion in neutral dorsiflexion
5. For strength training in late phase IIa (days 21-28): Perform isometric plantar flexion and dorsiflexion; progress to light elastic band exercises if free of pain and swelling
6. For function (*NOTE: Use a walking boot at all times*): Start touchdown weight bearing on day 8; perform progressive weight bearing at day 14 if no increase in pain and symptoms is noted

Weeks 5-8

GOALS FOR THE PERIOD: Improve ROM, continue strength training, and improve function
1. For ROM:
    a. Continue phase IIa activities as appropriate
    b. Initiate weight-bearing dorsiflexion stretch with knee flexed and extended
2. For strength training:
    a. Continue phase IIa activities as appropriate
    b. Initiate double-leg heel raises
3. For function:
    a. Begin ambulation out of the walking splint to symptom tolerance
    b. Use heel lift and cane as appropriate to limit symptoms

Weeks 9-16

GOALS FOR THE PERIOD: Improve ROM, continue strength training, and improve function
1. For ROM: Continue phase IIb activities as appropriate to gain full ROM
2. For strength training:
    a. Initiate single-leg heel raises
    b. Progress to additional weight heel raises with up to 1.5 times body weight if no symptoms of pain, swelling, or inflammation occur
3. For function:
    a. Initiate walking on all types of surfaces and inclines and declines
    b. Progress to jogging toward end of phase if no symptoms have occurred
    c. *NO sprinting, cutting, or jumping allowed*

❧ Suggested Home Maintenance for the Postsurgical Patient— Early Motion Program—cont'd

Weeks 17-20

GOALS FOR THE PERIOD: Continue strength training and achieve functional improvement
1. For strength training:
   a. Do single-leg heel raises over the edge of a step
   b. Perform weight lifting to tolerance
2. For function:
   a. Initiate hopping, skipping, and jumping activities
   b. Return to all recreational and sports activities

REFERENCES

1. Amadio PC: Tendon and ligament. In Cohen IK, Diegelmann RF, Lindblad WJ, editors: *Wound healing: biochemical and clinical aspects,* Philadelphia, 1992, WB Saunders.

2. Arner O, Lindholm A, Orell SR: Histologic changes in subcutaneous rupture of the Achilles tendon, *Acta Chir Scand* 116:484, 1958/1959.

3. Arner O, Lindholm A: Avulsion fracture of the os calcaneus, *Acta Chir Scand* 117:258, 1959.

4. Beskin JL et al: Surgical repair of Achilles tendon ruptures, *Am J Sports Med* 15:1, 1987.

5. Booth FW: Physiologic and biochemical effects of immobilization on muscle, *Clin Orth* 219:15, 1987.

6. Bradley JP, Tibone JE: Percutaneous and open surgical repairs of Achilles tendon ruptures, *Am J Sports Med* 18:188, 1990.

7. Bugg EI, Jr, Boyd BM: Repair of neglected rupture or laceration of the Achilles tendon, *Clin Orth* 56:73, 1968.

8. Bunnell S: Primary repair of severe tendons, *Am J Surg* 47:502, 1940.

9. Carden DG et al: Rupture of the calcaneal tendon. The early and late management, *J Bone Joint Surg* 69B:416, 1987.

10. Carr AJ, Norris SH: The blood supply of the calcaneal tendon, *J Bone Joint Surg* 71B(1):100, 1989.

11. Carter TR, Fowler PJ, Blokker C: Functional postoperative treatment of Achilles tendon repair, *Am J Sports Med* 20:459, 1992.

12. Cetti R: Ruptured Achilles tendon. Preliminary results of a new treatment, *Br J Sports Med* 22:6, 1988.

13. Cetti R, Christensen SE: Surgical treatment under local anesthesia of Achilles rupture, *Clin Orthop* 173:204, 1983.

14. Cetti R et al: Operative versus nonoperative treatment of Achilles tendon rupture. A prospective randomized study and review of the literature, *Am J Sports Med* 21(6):791, 1993.

15. Cetti R, Henriksen LO, Jacobsen KS: A new treatment of ruptured Achilles tendons, *Clin Orthop* 308:155, 1994.

16. Chen DS, Wertheimer SJ: A new method of repair for rupture of the Achilles tendon, *J Foot Surg* 31:440, 1992.

17. Christensen IB: Rupture of the Achilles tendon: analysis of 57 cases, *Acta Chir Scand* 106:50, 1953.

18. Crolla RMPH et al: Acute rupture of the tendo calcaneus, *Acta Orthop Belgica* 53:492, 1987.

19. Curwin S, Stanish W: *Tendinitis: its etiology and treatment,* Lexington, MA, 1984, Collamore Press.

20. Curwin SL: *Force and length changes of the gastrocnemius and soleus muscle-tendon units during a therapeutic exercise program and three selected activities,* master's thesis, Halifax, Nova Scotia, Canada, 1984, Dalhousie University.

21. Curwin S: Tendon injuries: pathology and treatment. In Zachazewski JE, Magee DJ, Quillen WS, editors: *Athletic injuries and rehabilitation,* Philadelphia, 1996, WB Saunders.

22. Achilles tendon rupture (editorial), *Lancet* 1:189, 1973.

23. Enwemeka CS, Rodriguez O, Mendosa S: The biomechanical effects of low intensity ultrasound on healing tendons, *Ultrasound Med Biol* 16:801, 1990.

24. Enwemeka CS, Spielholz NI, Nelson AJ: The effect of early functional activities on experimentally tenotomized Achilles tendon in rats, *Am J Phys Med Rehabil* 67:264, 1988.

25. Enwemeka CS: Connective tissue plasticity: ultrastructural, biomechanical, and morphometric effects of physical factors on intact and regenerating tendons, *J Ortho Sports Phys Ther* 14(5):198, 1991.

26. Enwemeka CS: Inflammation, cellularity, and fibrillogenesis in regenerating tendon: implications for tendon rehabilitation, *Phys Ther* 69:816, 1989.

27. Enwemeka CS: The effect of therapeutic ultrasound on tendon healing. A biomechanical study, *Am J Phys Med Rehab* 67:264, 1988.

28. Fernandez-Fairen M, Gimeno C: Augmented repair of Achilles tendon ruptures, *Am J Sports Med* 25(2):177, 1997.

29. Fitzgibbons RE, Hefferon J, Hill J: Percutaneous Achilles tendon repair, *Am J Sports Med* 21(5):724, 1993.

30. Frings H: Uber 317 falle von operrierten subkutanen Achillesrupturen be sportiern und sportlerinnen, *Arch Orthop Unfall-Chir* 67:64, 1969.

31. Freider S et al: A pilot study: the therapeutic effect of ultrasound following partial rupture of Achilles tendons in male rats, *J Ortho Sports Phys Ther* 10(2):39, 1988.

32. Gamble JG: *The musculoskeletal system: pathological basics,* New York, 1988, Raven Press.

33. Gelberman RH et al: Flexor tendon repair in vitro: a comparative histologic study of the rabbit, chicken, dog, and monkey, *J Orthop Res* 2:39, 1984.

34. Gelberman RH et al: Effects of early intermittent passive mobilization on healing canine flexor tendons, *J Hand Surg* 7(2):170, 1982.

35. Gerdes MH et al: A flap augmentation technique for Achilles tendon repair, postoperative strength and functional outcome, *Clin Orthop* 280:241, 1992.

36. Giannini S et al: Surgical repair of Achilles tendon ruptures using polypropylene braid augmentation, *Foot & Ankle* 15:372, 1994.

37. Gregor RV, Komi PV, Jarvinen M: Achilles tendon forces during cycling, *Int J Sports Med* 8(suppl):9, 1987.

38. Haggmark T et al: Calf muscle atrophy and muscle function after non-operative vs. operative treatment of Achilles tendon ruptures, *Orthopaedics* 9(2):160, 1986.

39. Harcke H, Grisson LE, Finkelstein MS: Evaluation of the musculoskeletal system with sonography, *AJR* 150:1253, 1988.

40. Hastad K, Larsson HG, Lindholm A: Clearance of radiosodium after local deposit in the Achilles tendon, *Acta Chir Scand* 116:251, 1958/1959.

41. Holz U: Die Achilles shenen ruptur–klinische und ultrastrukturturelle aspekte. In Chapchal G, editor: *Sportverletzungen und Sportschagen,* Stuttgart, 1983, Georg Tieme.

42. Hosey G et al: Comparison of the mechanical and histologic properties of Achilles tendons in New Zealand white rabbits secondarily repaired with Marlex mesh, *J Foot Surg* 30:214, 1991.

43. Inglis AE et al: Ruptures of the tendo Achilles, *J Bone Joint Surg* 58A:990, 1976.

44. Inglis AE, Sculco TP: Surgical repair of ruptures of the tendo Achilles, *Clin Orthop* 156:160, 1981.

45. Jackson BA, Schwane JA, Starcher BC: Effect of ultrasound on the repair of Achilles tendon injuries in rats, *Med Sci Sports Exerc* 23(2):171, 1991.

46. Jacobs D et al: Comparison of conservative and operative treatment of Achilles tendon rupture, *Am J Sports Med* 6:107, 1978.

47. Jenkins DHR et al: Induction of tendon and ligament formation by carbon implants, *J Bone Joint Surg* 59B:53, 1977.

48. Jozsa L et al: The role of recreational sport activity in Achilles tendon rupture. A clinical, pathoanatomical, and sociological study of 292 cases, *Am J Sports Med* 17(3):338, 1989.

49. Jozsa L et al: Pathological alterations of human tendons, *Morphol Igazsagugy: Orr Sz* 27(2):106, 1987.

50. Kannus P, Jozsa L: Histopathological changes preceding spontaneous rupture of a Achilles tendon, *J Bone Joint Surg* 73A(10):1507, 1991.

51. Karjalainen PT et al: Magnetic resonance imaging during healing of surgically repaired Achilles tendon ruptures, *Am J Sports Med* 25(2):164, 1997.

52. Kellam JF, Hunter GA, McElwain JP: Review of the operative treatment of Achilles tendon rupture, *Clin Orthop* 201:80, 1985.

53. Kessler I: The grasping technique for tendon repair, *Hand* 5:253, 1973.

54. Kirschembaum SE, Kellman C: Modification of the Lindholm procedure for plastic repair of ruptured Achilles tendon: a case report, *J Foot Surg* 19:4, 1980.

55. Krackow KA, Thomas SC, Jones LC: A new stitch for ligament-tendon fixation. Brief note, *J Bone Joint Surg* 68A:764, 1986.

56. Kvist H, Kvist M: The operative treatment of chronic calcaneal paratendonitis, *J Bone Joint Surg* 62B(3):353, 1980.

57. Lagerrgren C, Lindholm A: Vascular distribution in the Achilles tendon: an arteriographic and microangiographic study, *Acta Chir Scand* 116:491, 1958/1959.

58. Landvater SJ, Renstrom PA: Complete Achilles tendon ruptures, *Clin Sports Med* 11(4):741, 1992.

59. Laseter JT, Russell JA: Anabolic steroid-induced tendon pathology: a review of the literature, *Med Sci Sports Exerc* 23:1, 1991.

60. Laurant TC: Structure, function and turnover of the extracellular matrix, *Adv Microcir* 13:15, 1987.

61. Leadbetter WB: Cell matrix response in tendon injury, *Clin Sports Med* 11(3):533, 1992.

62. Leppilahti J et al: Free tissue coverage of wound complications following Achilles tendon rupture surgery, *Clin Orthop* 328:171, 1996.

63. Leppilahti J et al: Isokinetic evaluation of calf muscle performance after Achilles rupture repair, *Int J Sports Med* 17:619, 1996.

64. Levy M et al: A method of repair for Achilles tendon ruptures without cast immobilization, *Clin Orthop* 187:199, 1983.

65. Lindholm A: A new method of operation in subcutaneous rupture of the Achilles tendon, *Acta Chir Scand* 117:261, 1959.

66. Lynn TA: Repair of the torn Achilles tendon, using the plantaris tendon as a reinforcing membrane, *J Bone Joint Surg* 48A:268, 1966.

67. Ma GW, Griffith TG: Percutaneous repair of acute closed ruptured Achilles tendon; a new technique, *Clin Orthop* 128:247, 1977.

68. Malone TR, Garrett WE, Zachazewski JE: Muscle: deformation, injury, repair. In Zachazewski JE, Magee DJ, Quillen WS, editors: *Athletic injuries and rehabilitation,* Philadelphia, 1996, WB Saunders.

69. Mandelbaum BR, Hayes WM, Knapp TP: Management of Achilles tendon ruptures, *Foot and Ankle* 2(3):1, 1997.

70. Mandelbaum BR, Myerson MS, Forster R: Achilles tendon ruptures, a new method of repair, early range of motion, and functional rehabilitation, *Am J Sports Med* 23(4):392, 1995.

71. Mann RA et al: Chronic rupture of the Achilles tendon: a new technique of repair, *J Bone Joint Surg* 73A:214, 1991.

72. Marti RK, Weber BG: Achillessehnenruptur-functionalle Nachbehandlung, *Helv Chir Acta* 4:293, 1974.

73. Mink JH, Deutsch AL, Kerr R: Tendon injuries of the lower extremity: magnetic resonance assessment, *Top Magn Reson Imaging* 3:23, 1991.

74. Mortensen NHM, Saether J: Achilles tendon repair: a new method of Achilles tendon repair tested on cadaverous materials, *J Trauma* 31:381, 1991.

75. Motta P, Errichiello C, Pontini I: Achilles tendon rupture. A new technique for easy surgical repair and immediate movement of the ankle and foot, *Am J Sports Med* 25(2):172, 1997.

76. Muller ME et al: General considerations. In Muller ME et al, editors: *Manual of internal fixation: techniques recommended by the AO-Group*, Berlin, 1979, Springer-Verlag.

77. Nada A: Rupture of the calcaneal tendon, *J Bone Joint Surg* 67B(3):449, 1985.

78. Nillius SA, Nilsson BE, Westin WE: The incidence of Achilles tendon rupture, *Acta Orthop Unfall Chir* 67:1, 1976.

79. Nistor L: Surgical and non-surgical treatment of Achilles tendon rupture, *J Bone Joint Surg* 63A(3):395, 1981.

80. Paddu G, Ippolito E, Postacchini F: A classification of Achilles tendon disease, *Am J Sports Med* 4(4):145, 1976.

81. Pepels WRJ, Plasmans CMT, Sloof TJH: The course of healing of tendons and ligaments (abstract), *Acta Orthop Scand* 54:952, 1983.

82. Quenu J, Stoianovitch I: Les ruptures du tendon d'Achilles, *Rev Chir Paris* 67:647, 1929.

83. Schatzker J, Branemark PI: Intravital observation of the microvascular anatomy and microcirculation of tendon, *Acta Ortho Scand Suppl* 126:3, 1969.

84. Schedl R, Fasol P, Spangler H: Die Achillessehnen-ruptur als sportverletzung. In Chapchal G, editor: *Sportverletzungen und Sportschagen*, Stuttgart, 1983, Georg Tieme.

85. Schuberth JM: Achilles tendon trauma. In Scurran BL, editor: *Foot and ankle trauma*, ed 2, New York, 1996, Churchill Livingstone.

86. Shields CL et al: The Cybex II evaluation of surgically repaired Achilles tendon ruptures, *Am J Sports Med* 6:369, 1978.

87. Silfverskiold N: Uber die subkutane totale Achillessehnenruptur und deren Behandlung, *Acta Chir Scand* 84:393, 1941.

88. Soldatis JJ, Goodfellows DB, Wilber JH: End to end operative repair of Achilles tendon rupture, *Am J Sports Med* 25(1):90, 1997.

89. Solveborn S-A, Moberg A: Immediate free ankle motion after surgical repair of acute Achilles tendon ruptures, *Am J Sports Med* 22(5):607, 1994.

90. Soma CA, Mandelbaum BR: Repair of acute Achilles tendon ruptures, *Orth Clin NA* 26(2):239, 1995.

91. Strocchi R et al: Human Achilles tendon: morphological and morphometric variations as a function of age, *Foot Ankle* 12:100, 1991.

92. Teuffeur AP: Traumatic rupture of the Achilles tendon. Reconstruction by transplant and graft using the lateral peroneus brevis, *Orth Clin North Am* 5:89, 1974.

93. Thompson TC, Doherty JH: Spontaneous rupture of tendon of Achilles: a new clinical diagnostic test, *J Trauma* 2:126, 1962.

94. Wapner KL, Hecht PJ, Mills RH, Jr: Reconstruction of neglected Achilles tendon injury, *Orthop Clin North Am* 26:249, 1995.

95. Wills CA et al: Achilles tendon rupture. A review of the literature comparing surgical versus non-surgical treatment, *Clin Orthop* 207:156, 1986.

96. Zachazewski JE: Muscle flexibility. In Scully R, Barnes ML, editors: *Physical therapy*, Philadelphia, 1989, JB Lippincott.

97. Zolinger H, Rodriquez M, Genoni M: Zur atiopathogenese-und diagnostik der Achillesehnenrupturen im sport. In Chapchal G, editor: *Sportverletzungen und Sportschagen*, Stuttgart, 1983, Georg Tieme.

Transitioning the Throwing Athlete Back to the Field

Luga Podesta

Injuries to athletes happen every day. Some can be easily treated, while others require surgery and/or lengthy rehabilitation. An arm injury to a baseball player is potentially career ending and therefore needs very special attention. Every baseball player knows the demands put on an arm in training and competition, so we also realize the need for very intense and specialized rehabilitation. During my playing career I had three serious shoulder injuries. Much time and energy was spent on the strengthening of my shoulder, but the critical time of rehabilitation was the transition from physical therapy into a throwing program. An aggressive full-body conditioning program, including plyometrics, was essential in assisting my shoulder to function correctly when throwing a baseball. This program paved the way for a smooth transition onto the field and a successful return to competition.

Mike Scioscia
Anaheim Angels

A great deal of literature exists detailing the surgical technique and postoperative rehabilitation of the injured shoulder. However, little has been written on the difficult task of transitioning the throwing athlete from the rehabilitation setting back to throwing sports after surgery. This appendix outlines a program to return the throwing athlete back to his or her sport after surgery.

Numerous surgical procedures can be performed on a throwing athlete's shoulder for a variety of pathologic conditions (e.g., glenohumeral instability, labral tears, rotor cuff tears, impingement syndrome, acromioclavicular joint injury). Because one short appendix cannot describe each surgical procedure and the postoperative rehabilitation course recommended for it, the program described in this appendix is based on the assumption that the athlete has already been cleared to begin an advanced throwing and conditioning program.

Assessment

Regardless of the surgical procedure performed, the physical therapist must assess the athlete's overall physical condition before beginning a more aggressive conditioning and throwing program. Knowledge of the athlete's flexibility, strength, and endurance is essential for the development of a program specific for his or her needs. The athlete's throwing mechanics must be carefully evaluated throughout rehabilitation and the transition back to throwing sports.

Strengthening and Conditioning

In the past a great deal of emphasis was placed on developing mobility in the postoperative shoulder and developing strength in the shoulder-supporting musculature, including the rotator cuff and scapular stabilizers. Very little attention was given to the remainder of the musculature that plays a significant role in permitting the athlete to throw effectively and without injury.

Dynamic stability of the throwing shoulder requires fine, coordinated action of the glenohumeral and scapulothoracic stabilizers to facilitate synchronous function of the glenohumeral joint. After surgery, proper neuromuscular control must be reestablished to prevent asynchronous muscle firing patterns, which can result in dysfunction.[3,6]

Neuromuscular control is defined as a purposeful act initiated at the cortical level.[23] Payton et al[23] stated that motor control is an involuntary associated movement organized subcortically that results in a well-learned skill operating without conscious guidance. The fine coordinated activity necessary for propelling a ball rapidly and accurately requires subcortical control of the muscles responsible for throwing.

Kinesthesia is the ability to discriminate joint position, relative weight of body parts, and joint movement, including speed, direction, and amplitude.[21] Proprioception is the ability to discriminate joint position. The ability to throw requires that joint proprioceptors (muscle and joint afferents present in ligament and synovial tissues) function normally. Joint proprioceptors within the glenohumeral joint are responsible for signaling a stretch reflex when the glenohumeral capsule is taut to prevent translation at extremes of motion.[9] Many throwers recovering from surgery, especially those who have undergone procedures for instability, complain of stiffness and tightness in their shoulders. Neuromuscular controls may have been arrested by trauma and surgery, resulting in a new subcortical sense of joint tightness during throwing that was not present before the shoulder stabilization procedure.

The upper extremity and shoulder represent the last link in the kinetic chain during the overhead throwing motion, which begins distally as ground reactive forces are transferred caudally. Biomechanical analysis shows that tremendous forces are generated and extreme motion occurs in the shoulder with overhand throwing. Angular velocities in excess of 7000 degrees/second have been recorded during the transition from external rotation to internal rotation when throwing.[22,24] Shearing forces on the anterior shoulder are estimated at 400 N.[22] Approximately 500 N of distraction force occurs during the deceleration phase of the throwing motion.[22] These forces are short in duration, develop quickly, occur at extremely high intensity, and must be performed repeatedly. The direction and magnitude of the forces generated when throwing a ball cause anteroposterior translational and distraction vectors that stress the glenohumeral constraints.

However, these forces are not entirely generated in the shoulder. The shoulder-supporting musculature is not capable of generating the forces and motions measured at the shoulder during throwing. Throwing a ball effectively requires the athlete to generate, summate, transfer, and regulate these forces from the legs through the throwing hand. To generate the forces measured with throwing, the shoulder relies on its position at the end of the kinetic chain. It has been reported that 51% to 55% of the kinetic energy created is generated in the lower extremities.[5,28] Use of ground reaction forces sequentially linked with the activity of the large lower extremity and trunk muscles generate a significant proportion of the forces measured. Biomechanical data show that the shoulder itself contributes relatively little of the overall total energy necessary to the throwing motion. However, it provides a relatively high contribution to the total forces (21%), indicating that the shoulder, because of its position at the end of the kinetic chain, must effectively transfer and concentrate the developed energy. Conditioning of the shoulder and upper extremity musculature is important in returning throwing athletes back to their sports. Moreover, the trunk and lower extremity musculature must be adequately conditioned to

Box A-1   Basic Conditioning Principles

Develop muscle synergy
Train for performance, not work capacity
Train for muscle balance
Train movements, not muscles
Develop structural (core) strength before extremity strength
Use body weight resistance before external resistance
Build strength before strength endurance
Develop synergists before prime movers
Promote joint integrity before mobility
Teach fundamental movement skill before specific sport skill

provide the foundation to generate the forces required for effective and safe throwing.

When designing a program to return a throwing athlete back to sports, the physical therapist should consider two primary objectives: enhancing current performance levels and preventing injury. Gambetta[17] has outlined ten key principles that are basic to the development of a conditioning program for the throwing athlete (Box A-1). The many components of the program must work together to produce optimal performance. The quality of the effort and the overall intensity should be emphasized first. The clinician should monitor each exercise and eventually scrutinize the throwing technique to ensure optimal training effect and minimize the potential for injury.

The development of muscle balance is essential for coordinated, efficient movement to occur, especially around the shoulder where muscle imbalance can easily develop. Muscles (e.g., rotator cuff) cannot simply be trained solely and in isolation, as in the early phases of most postoperative programs. After base strength has been developed in the postoperative shoulder, functional activities and more sport-specific exercises must be added to mimic the activities the athlete will be performing.

The development of core strength in the abdominals, trunk, and spinal-stabilizing muscles cannot be overemphasized. Without adequate core strength, the throwing athlete becomes vulnerable to improper postural alignment, which can lead to compensatory movements that place even greater stress on the shoulder, further predisposing the athlete to injury. After adequate strength has been achieved in the shoulder-supporting musculature, abdominals, spinal stabilizers, and lower extremities, endurance training can be added.

Only after sufficient strength and endurance are developed and normal, synchronous muscle firing patterns are reestablished can a more functional and sport-specific activity such as throwing be added. The ulti-

Table A-1   Jobe's Shoulder Exercises

Exercise*	Weight (in pounds)	Sets/Repetitions
Shoulder flexion	3-5	3-4/10-15
Shoulder elevation	3-5	3-4/10-15
Shoulder abduction	3-5	3-4/10-15
Military press	3-5	3-4/10-15
Horizontal abduction	3-5	3-4/10-15
Shoulder extension	3-5	3-4/10-15
External rotation I (side-lying)	1-5	3-4/10-15
External rotation II (prone)	1-5	3-4/10-15
Internal rotation	1-5	3-4/10-15
Horizontal adduction	3-5	3-4/10-15
Rowing	3-5	3-4/10-15

Modified from Jobe FW et al: *Shoulder and arm exercises for the athlete who throws,* Inglewood, CA, 1996, Champion Press.
*All exercises should be performed three times a week.

Table A-2   Isotonic Core Strengthening Exercises

Exercise*†	Sets/Repetitions
Chest	
Bench press (close grip)	2-3/8-10
Legs	
Squats	2-3/8-10
Leg press	2-3/8-10
Knee extensions	2-3/8-10
Leg curls	2-3/8-10
Lunges	2-3/8-10
Calf press	2-3/8-10
Toe raises	2-3/8-10
Back	
Latissimus pull-downs	2-3/8-10
Shoulder shrugs	2-3/8-10
Seated rows	2-3/8-10
Bent-over rows	2-3/8-10
Abdominals	
Crunches (to be performed in sequence)	
Feet flat	3/15, rest 30 seconds
Weight on chest	3/15, rest 60 seconds
Knees bent	1/25, rest 60 seconds
Knees up with weight	1/25

*Wide-grip bench press, behind-neck pull-down, deep squats, and behind-neck military press should *not* be performed.
†All exercises should be performed two to three times a week.

mate success of the training program depends on its overall design in introducing a variety of training stimuli to maximize total conditioning. An ideal conditioning program should contain a preparation period, an adaptation period, and an application period.[17] The preparation period should consist of general work, including strength and endurance training. Specialized work incorporating joint dynamics of the sport occurs during the adaptation period. Finally, the application period incorporates the specific joint actions and movements required to perform the sport.

Isotonic Exercises

A progressive weight and functional training program should start with body weight exercise. This allows the athlete to develop the proper exercise techniques and regain the synchronous muscle firing patterns required to perform the overhand sport. This method of training also is adaptable to the more advanced plyometric exercises that follow after base strength has been gained.

Weight training is one of the most popular methods of training and can be performed with either free weights or machines. Free weight training with dumbbells is preferable because it allows for unilateral training while permitting a full range of motion (ROM) of the extremity. Machines are better used in training the lower extremities. The use of rubber tubing or bands is another popular method of early strength training for the overhand-throwing athlete. These exercises can be performed as a warm-up for more strenuous weight resistance exercises or as a cool-down exercise; they can accommodate all muscle actions. Rubber tubing or band exercises also allow for unilateral training of the extremity through a full ROM. They can be performed during the rehabilitation period and should continue when the thrower returns to play. Isotonic strengthening can be tailored to each athlete's needs and can be used to maintain strength in all muscle groups. Jobe's upper extremity exercise program is the most popular group of isotonic exercises performed. They can be initiated early in the rehabilitation period and continue throughout the athlete's career. However, they *must* be performed correctly to maximize their benefit (Table A-1).

Core strength should first be developed using isotonic training. Only after base strength is developed should the intensity of the exercise program be increased (Table A-2).

Plyometric Exercises

Plyometric training was first introduced in the late 1960s by Soviet jump coach Yuri Verkhoshanski.[29] American track coach Fred Wilt first introduced plyometrics in the United States in 1975.[32] The majority of the literature concerning plyometric exercise discusses its use in the lower extremities. Adapting these principles to the conditioning of throwing athletes is logical, considering the maximal explosive concentric contractions and rapid decelerative eccentric contractions that occur with each throwing cycle. Controversy exists regarding the optimal use of plyometric exercise in the training program, although agreement surrounding the benefits of this form of exercise is well documented.[7,8,19,25]

Plyometric exercise can be broken down into three phases: the eccentric (or setting) phase, the amortization phase, and the concentric response phase. The setting phase of the exercise is the preloading period; it lasts until the stretch stimulus is initiated. The amortization phase of the exercise is the time that occurs between the eccentric contraction and the initiation of the concentric contraction. During the concentric phase the effect of the exercise (a facilitated contraction) is produced and preparation for the second repetition occurs.

Physiologic muscle performance is believed to be enhanced by plyometric exercise in several ways. The faster a muscle is loaded eccentrically, the greater the resultant concentric force produced. Eccentric loading of a muscle places stress on the elastic components, increasing the tension of the resultant force produced.

Neuromuscular coordination is improved through explosive plyometric training. Plyometric exercise may improve neural efficiency, thereby increasing neuromuscular performance.

Finally, the inhibitory effect of the Golgi tendon organs, which serve as a protective mechanism limiting the amount of force produced within muscle, can be desensitized by plyometric exercise, thereby raising the level of inhibition. This desensitization and the resultant raise in the inhibition level ultimately allows increased force production with greater applied loads.

Through neural adaptation the throwing athlete can coordinate the activity of muscle groups and produce greater net force output (in the absence of morphologic change within the muscles themselves). The faster the athlete is able to switch from eccentric or yielding work to concentric overcoming work, the more powerful the resultant response. Effective plyometric training requires that the amortization phase of the exercise be quick, limiting the amount of energy wasted as heat. The rate of stretch rather than the length of stretch provides a greater stimulus for an enhanced training effect. With slower stretch cycles the stretch reflex is not activated.

Before implementing a plyometric training program, the patient must have an adequate level of base strength to maximize the training effect and prevent injury. Remedial shoulder exercises focusing on the rotator cuff and shoulder-supporting musculature are continued to develop and maintain joint stability and muscle strength in the arm decelerators. These exercises also should be used to warm up before the plyometric drill and cool down after it has been concluded.

Plyometric exercise is contraindicated in the immediate postoperative period, in the presence of acute inflammation or pain, and in athletes with gross shoulder and/or elbow instability. Plyometric training also is contraindicated in athletes who do not have an adequate degree of base strength and those who are not participating in a strength training program. This form of exercise is intended to be an advanced form of strength training. Post-exercise muscle soreness and delayed-onset muscle soreness are common adverse reactions that the clinician should be aware of before beginning an athlete on this type of exercise. Tremendous amounts of stress occur during plyometric exercises. Therefore they should not be performed for an extended period. A plyometric program should be used during the first and second preparation phases of training.

The plyometric training program for the upper extremity can be divided into four groups of exercise as described by Wilk[31] (Table A-3):
1. Warm-up exercises
2. Throwing movements
3. Trunk extension and flexion exercises
4. Medicine ball wall exercises

Warm-up exercises are performed to provide the shoulder, arms, trunk, and lower extremities an adequate physiologic warm-up before beginning more intense plyometric exercise. The facilitation of muscular performance through an active warm-up has been ascribed to increased blood flow, oxygen use, nervous system transmission, muscle and core temperature, and speed of contraction.[1,2,11,15,20] The athlete should perform two to three sets of 10 repetitions for each warm-up exercise before proceeding to the next group of exercises.

Throwing-movement plyometric exercises attempt to isolate and train the muscles required to throw effectively. Movement patterns similar to those found with overhead throwing are performed. These exercises provide an advanced strengthening technique at a higher exercise level than that of more traditional isotonic dumbbell exercises. The exercises in this group are performed for two to four sets of six to eight repetitions two to three times weekly. Adequate rest times should occur between each session for optimal muscle recovery.

Plyometric exercises for trunk strengthening include medicine ball exercises for the abdominals and trunk extensor musculature. The athlete performs two to four sets of eight to ten repetitions two to three times weekly.

The final group of exercises, the plyoball wall exercises, require the use of 2- and 4-pound medicine balls

Table A-3   Plyometric Exercises

Exercise*	Equipment	Sets/Repetitions
Warm-Ups		
Medicine ball rotation	9-pound ball	2-3/10
Medicine ball side bends	9-pound ball	2-3/10
Medicine ball wood chops	9-pound ball	2-3/10
Tubing		
Internal and external rotation and 90-degree shoulder abduction	Medium tubing	2-3/10
Diagonal patterns (D2)	Medium tubing	2-3/10
Biceps	Medium tubing	2-3/10
Push-ups		2-3/10
Throwing Movements		
Medicine ball soccer throw†	4-pound ball	2-4/6-8
Medicine ball chest pass†	4-pound ball	2-4/6-8
Medicine ball step and pass†	4-pound ball	2-4/6-8
Medicine ball side throw†	4-pound ball	2-4/6-8
Tubing plyometrics		
Internal and external rotation		6-8 repetitions
Diagonals		6-8 repetitions
Biceps		6-8 repetitions
Push-ups	6-8 inch box	10 repetitions
Trunk Extension and Flexion Movements		
Medicine ball sit-ups	4-pound ball	2-3/10
Medicine ball back extension	4-pound ball	2-3/10
Medicine Ball Exercises (Standing and Kneeling)		
Soccer throw	4-pound ball	2-4/6-8
Chest pass	4-pound ball	2-4/6-8
Side-to-side throw	4-pound ball	2-4/6-8
Backward side-to-side throws	4-pound ball	2-4/6-8
Forward two hands through legs	4-pound ball	2-4/6-8
One-handed baseball throw	2-pound ball	2-4/6-8

Modified from Wilk KE, Voight ML: Plyometrics for the shoulder complex. In Andrews JR, Wilk KE, editors: *The athlete's shoulder,* New York, 1994, Churchill Livingstone.
*All exercises should be performed two to three times a week.
†Throw with partner or pitch-back device

or plyoballs and a wall or pitch-back device to allow the athlete to perform this group of exercises without a partner. This group of drills starts with two-handed throws with a heavier 4-pound ball and concludes with one-handed plyometric throws using the lighter 2-pound ball. All the exercises in this phase of the program should be performed in the standing and kneeling positions to increase demands on the trunk, upper extremity, and shoulder girdle and eliminate the use of the lower extremities. The same number of repetitions and sets should be performed two to three times weekly (Fig. A-1).

Plyometric training of the lower extremities is essential in developing the throwing athlete's explosive strength needed for speed, lateral mobility, and acceleration. Lower extremity plyometric training also helps develop the coordination and agility necessary to compete effectively. High demands are placed on the musculature supporting the hips, knees, and ankle joints during plyometric jump exercises. The physical therapist *must* monitor exercise loads performed and allow adequate recovery time between sets. Proper technique in performing these exercises is vital to prevent injury. A variety of jump exercises can be used to train the

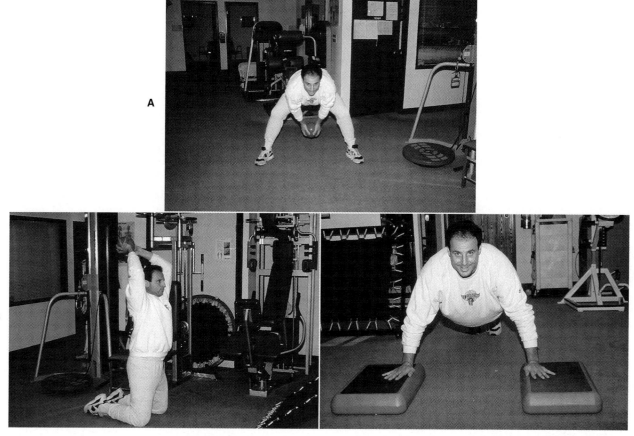

Fig. A-1. **A,** Medicine ball wood chop warm-up exercises. **B,** Medicine ball soccer throw exercises from the knees. **C,** Plyometric push-up. (Photos by Dr. Luga Podesta, Oxnard, CA.)

Table A-4	Lower Extremity Plyometric Exercises		
Exercise*		**Equipment**	**Sets/Repetitions**
Rapid box jumps (alternating height)		Boxes of varying heights	2-3/8-10
Box jumps		12- to 24-inch boxes	3-4 sets
Depth jump and sprint†		24-inch box	5-8 repetitions
Depth jump and base steal†		24-inch box	5-8 repetitions

*All exercises should be performed two to three times per week.
†Jump from a 24-inch box followed by an immediate 10-yard sprint

lower extremities when preparing the throwing athlete to return to athletic competition (Table A-4).

Rapid box jumps are performed to develop explosive power in the calf and quadriceps musculature. An explosive but controlled jump up onto the box then down off the box is performed; box height can be increased as the exercise is mastered. The athlete should immediately jump back on the box, spending as little time as possible on the ground.

Alternating-height box jumps train the quadriceps, hamstrings, gluteals, and calf muscles and help de-velop explosive power. Box jumps are performed using three to five plyometric boxes of varying heights (from 12 to 24 inches) placed in a straight line two feet apart from one another. Starting at the smallest box, the athlete performs controlled jumps from the box to the ground to the next tallest box, spending as little time on the ground as possible; the athlete should rest for 15 to 20 seconds between sets.

The depth jump and sprint and the depth jump with base steal focus on teaching muscles to react force-fully from a negative contraction to an explosive pos-

---

Box A-2   Aerobic Conditioning Exercises

Running
Bicycling
Versa-Climber
Stair-climbing machine
Elliptical runner
Cross-country ski machine
Rowing machine
Swimming

---

itive contraction. The athlete immediately explodes into a 10-yard sprint or 10-yard base steal after jumping off a 24-inch box.

Aerobic Conditioning

Although the initial postoperative emphasis is on rehabilitation of the shoulder, the transition from formal therapy to return to play requires the throwing athlete to regain the pre-injury aerobic condition. Therefore the aerobic conditioning component of the training program must not be neglected. Aerobic fitness can be developed using a variety of exercises (Box A-2).

For any method of aerobic activity to be effective, the exercise should be performed continuously for 20 to 40 minutes four to five times weekly. Because this type of conditioning is long and repetitive, the athlete should enjoy the activity being performed.

Throwing

The overhead throwing motion is not unique to throwing a baseball. Similar muscular activity is required to throw a softball, football, or javelin. However, the majority of research performed on overhead throwing has been conducted on the overhead pitch.

The clinician must appreciate the highly dynamic nature of the throwing motion to be effective in preparing and progressing the rehabilitating athlete through a safe throwing program. A thorough understanding of normal and abnormal throwing mechanics and the biomechanical forces placed on the throwing arm are essential for the therapist wishing to implement a throwing program in the rehabilitation setting.

Pitching a baseball is the most violent and dynamic of all overhead throwing activities, producing angular velocities in excess of 7000 degrees/second across the shoulder. Maximal stability of the glenohumeral joint occurs at 90 degrees of shoulder elevation.[26] Because muscle weakness can result in abnormal compression and shear forces, muscle balance is necessary to maintain stability of the humeral head in the glenoid fossa. A favorable balance between compression and shear

forces occurs at 90 degrees of shoulder elevation, placing the shoulder in the optimal position for joint stability.[3,23,26,27] All throwers therefore should maintain 90 degrees of glenohumeral elevation relative to the horizontal surface regardless of technique or pitching style.

Dynamic control of the glenohumeral joint during throwing depends on the rotator cuff and biceps muscle strength.[3,6] An abnormal throwing pattern can result from glenohumeral instability and inadequate control of the rotator cuff and biceps tendon. Neuromuscular conditioning and control of the glenohumeral joint allows for safer throwing by facilitating the dynamic coordination of the rotator cuff and scapulothoracic stabilizers.

The throwing or pitching motion can be divided into six phases (Fig. A-2):

1. Wind-up
2. Early cocking
3. Late cocking
4. Acceleration
5. Deceleration
6. Follow-through

Wind-up is the preparatory phase of the throwing motion. Relatively little muscle activity occurs during this phase. From a standing position the athlete initiates the throw by shifting the weight onto the supporting back leg. The weight shift from the stride leg to the supporting leg sets the rhythm for the delivery. Wind-up ends when the ball leaves the gloved nondominant hand (Fig. A-3, *A*).

During early cocking the shoulder abducts to approximately 104 degrees and externally rotates to 46 degrees.[11] The scapular muscles are active in positioning the glenoid for optimal contact with the humeral head as the arm is abducted. The supraspinatus and deltoid muscles work synergistically to elevate the humerus. The deltoids position the arm in space, and the supraspinatus stabilizes the humeral head within the glenoid[10] (Figs. A-3, *B* through *H*, and A-4).

The stride forward is initiated during the early cocking phase of throwing. The athlete should keep the trunk and back closed as long as possible to retain the energy stored, which later results in velocity.

As the stride leg moves toward the target, the ball breaks from the glove and the throwing arm swings upward in rhythm with the body. The positioning of the breaking hands followed by the downward then upward rotation of the throwing arm ensures optimal positioning of the arm (Fig. A-5). Establishing this synchronous muscle firing pattern is one of the most crucial aspects of the throw. If the throwing arm and striding leg are synchronized properly, the arm and hand will be in the early cocked position when the stride foot contacts the ground (see Figs. A-3, *H*, and A-4, *D*).

The direction of the stride should either be directly toward the target or slightly closed (to the right side of

Text continued on p. 363

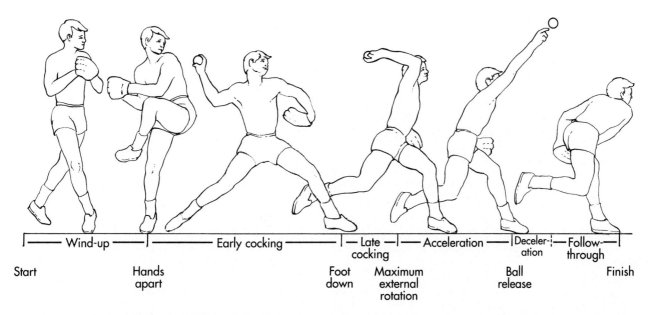

Fig. A-2. Phases of the baseball pitch. (From Jobe FW: *Operative techniques in upper extremity sports injury,* St Louis, 1996, Mosby.)

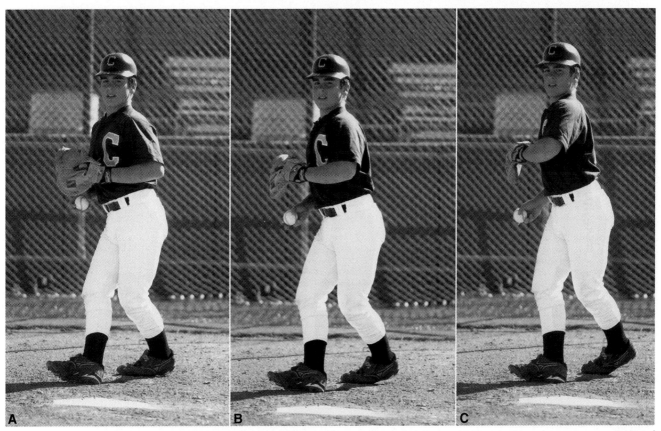

Continued

Fig. A-3. Front view of the throwing motion. **A** through **E,** The "crow-hop" step begins the throwing motion. The pelvis and chest are rotated 90 degrees from the target. The hands separate as weight is shifted to the back leg. **F** through **J,** During the cocking phase of throwing the throwing arm is elevated and externally rotated. The front foot is planted in a slightly closed position as the pelvis begins to rotate. **K** through **L,** During the acceleration phase the elbow is above the height of the shoulder and weight is shifted to the front foot as the pelvis rotates. **M** through **O,** The deceleration and follow-through phases. (Photos by Marsha Gorman, Camarillo, California.)

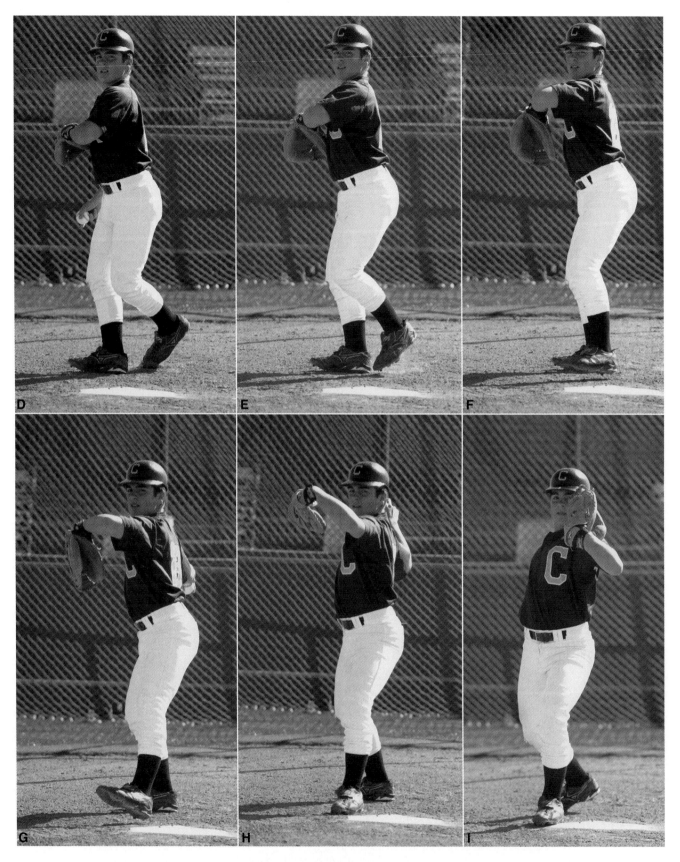

Fig. A-3, cont'd For legend see p. 357.

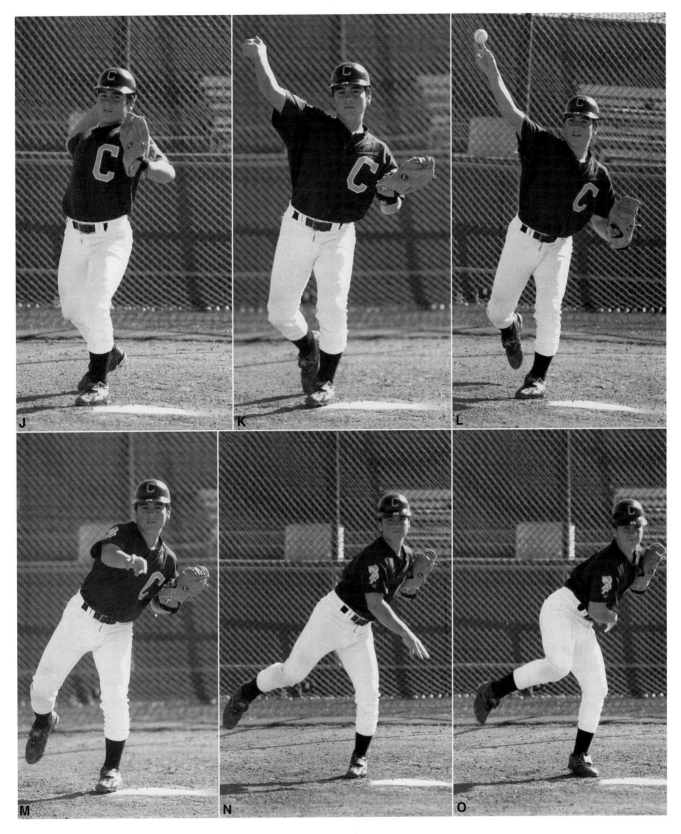

Fig. A-3, cont'd For legend see p. 357.

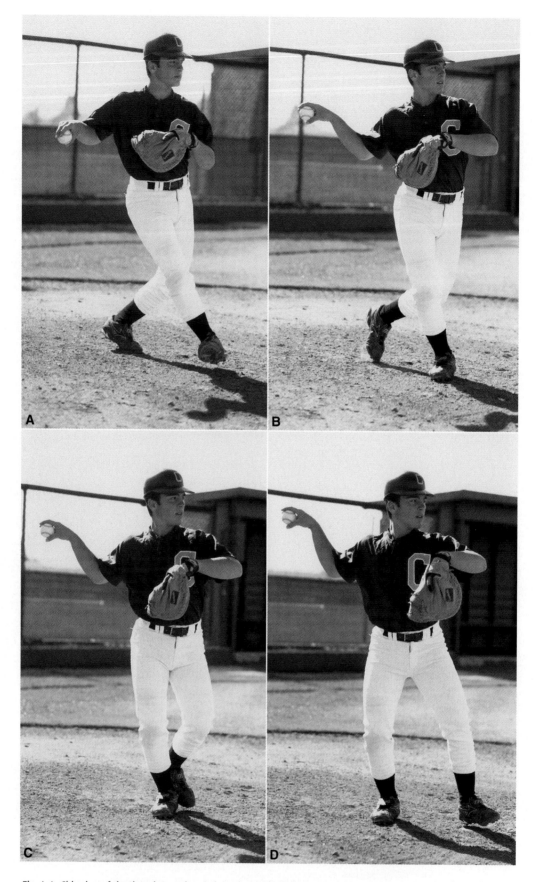

Fig. A-4. Side view of the throwing motion. **A** through **G**, The wind-up and cocking phases of throwing. **H** through **J**, The acceleration phases. **K** through **L**, The deceleration and follow-through phases. (Photos by Marsha Gorman, Camarillo, California.)

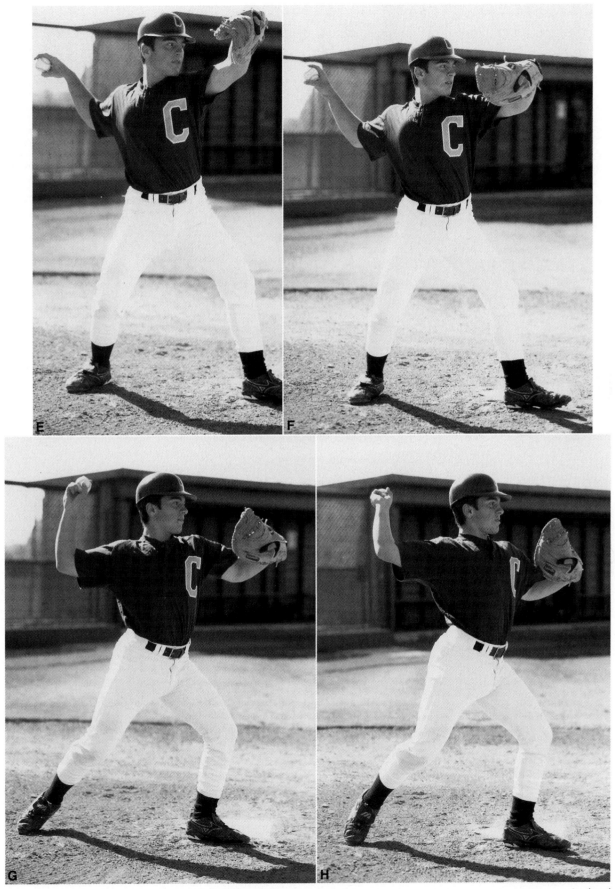

Continued

Fig. A-4, cont'd For legend see opposite page.

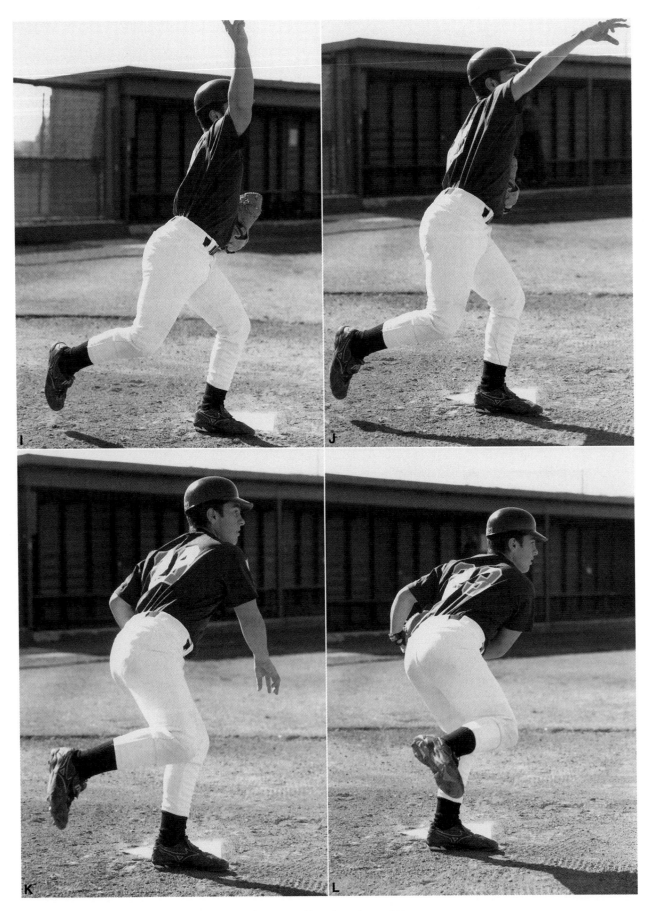

Fig. A-4, cont'd For legend see p. 360.

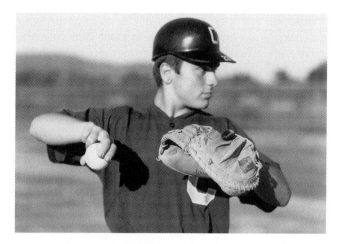

Fig. A-5. The proper technique for gripping the ball and releasing it from the glove. The ball is gripped loosely across four seams in the fingertips of the index and middle fingers. The thumb is placed under the ball, with the index and middle fingers held together. The hands separate with a supinating motion of the forearms forcing the thumbs of both the glove and ball hand downward. (Photo by Marsha Gorman, Camarillo, California.)

a right-handed thrower) (see Figs. A-3, *H*, and A-4, *E*). When the stride is too closed, the hips are unable to rotate and the thrower is forced to throw across the body, losing kinetic energy from the lower extremities. When the stride is too open (i.e., the stride foot lands too far to the left of a right-handed thrower), the hips rotate too early, forcing the trunk to face the batter too early and dissipating stored kinetic energy. This also places tremendous stress on the anterior shoulder. After the stride leg contacts the ground, the stride is completed and cocking of the throwing arm is initiated.

During the late cocking phase of throwing the humerus maintains its level of abduction while moving into the scapular plane. The arm externally rotates from 46 degrees to 170 degrees.[11] In this position the humeral head is positioned to place an anterior-directed force, potentially stretching the anterior ligamentous restraints.

The trunk moves laterally toward the target, and pelvic rotation is initiated. As the trunk undergoes rotation and extension, the elbow is flexed and the shoulder externally rotates. When the trunk faces the target, the shoulder should have achieved maximal external rotation. At the end of this phase, only the arm is cocked as the legs, pelvis, and trunk have already accelerated (see Figs. A-3, *I* and *J*, and A-4, *F* and *G*).

During the acceleration phase the humerus internally rotates approximately 100 degrees in 0.005 seconds. Tremendous torque and joint compressive forces and high angular velocities across the glenohumeral joint are present at this time.[11,16,22]

The acceleration phase begins when the humerus begins to internally rotate. Just before the beginning of internal rotation, the elbow should begin to extend (see Figs. A-3, *K*, and A-4, *H* and *I*). When ball release occurs, the trunk is flexed, the elbow reaches almost full extension, and the shoulder undergoes internal rotation (see Figs. A-3, *L*, and A-4, *J*). At ball release the trunk should be tilted forward with the lead knee extending. Acceleration ends with ball release.

The deceleration phase of the throwing motion is the first third of the time from ball release to the completion of arm motion (see Figs. A-3, *M* and *N*, and A-4, *K*). During deceleration excess kinetic energy that was not transferred to the ball is dissipated. High calculated forces and torque also occur during this phase.[4,13]

Follow-through occurs during the final two thirds of the throwing motion, during which time the arm continues to decelerate and eventually stops (see Figs. A-3, *O*, and A-4, *L*). After ball release, the throwing arm continues to extend at the elbow and internally rotates at the shoulder. Internal angular velocities drop from their maximal level at ball release to zero. A proper follow-through is crucial in minimizing injury to the shoulder during this violent stage of throwing. Follow-through is completed when the throwing shoulder is over the opposite knee. This is achieved by allowing the supporting leg to rotate forward, finishing the rotation of the trunk across the body.

Interval Throwing Program

The purpose of the interval throwing program is to return motion, strength, and confidence gradually to the throwing arm after injury or surgery. The interval throwing program allows the throwing patient the opportunity to reestablish timing, movement patterns, coordination, and synchronicity of muscle firing before returning to competition.[30] This is accomplished by slowly increasing the throwing distances and eventually the velocity of the throws. The program should be individualized to each athlete. No set timetable is prescribed for the completion of the program; each patient's time spent completing the program may vary. The throwing program is designed to minimize the chance of injury by emphasizing proper pre-throwing warm-up, stretching, and cool-down. It should be performed in the presence of a coach, trainer, or therapist knowledgeable in throwing mechanics. Careful supervision cannot be over-stressed. The participants must resist the temptation to increase the intensity of the throwing program and understand that this may increase the incidence of re-injury, which would greatly retard the rehabilitation process.

Before initiating the interval throwing program the athletic patient must exhibit the following criteria:
1. Full and painless ROM
2. No pain or tenderness
3. Satisfactory muscle strength and conditioning
4. Normal or clinically stable examination

Box A-3   Throwing Evaluation Checklist

Foot position—"Crow hop," back foot 90 degrees to the target

Body position—Non-dominant hip and shoulder to the target

Hand break—Ball release from glove, thumbs down

Ball hand and glove position—Ball facing away from the target, glove side elbow points to target flexed 90 degrees, glove down

Arm position—Elbow above shoulder level

Front foot plant—Step toward the target, "toes to target," slightly closed

Trunk rotation—Hips rotate before shoulders

Balance—Stand tall, weight back

Finish—Stride foot posts, back leg and hip rotate through

Specific attention throughout the interval throwing program to the maintenance of proper throwing mechanics is crucial (Box A-3). Participants in the rehabilitation program may find videotaping throwing sessions extremely helpful in assisting with the analysis of the athlete's throwing mechanics.

Proper warm up before beginning to throw cannot be overemphasized. A common mistake is for the thrower to begin throwing to warm up. Instead, the thrower should increase the blood flow to muscles and joints before throwing. This can be accomplished by running or jogging long enough to break a sweat. The athletic patient must warm up to throw, not throw to warm up.

A "crow-hop" throwing technique uses a hop, skip, and throw to accentuate lower extremity and trunk involvement in the throw. The use of the crow-hop method simulates the throwing motion and empha-

---

Box A-4   Progressive Interval Throwing Program

Warm-up
Run to break sweat
Stretching

45-Foot Phase (Half the Distance to First Base from Home Plate)

Step 1: a. Warm-up throwing—25 feet
         b. 45 feet (25 throws)
         c. Rest 10-15 minutes
         d. Warm-up throwing
         e. 45 feet (25 throws)

Step 2: a. Warm-up throwing
         b. 45 feet (25 throws)
         c. Rest 10 minutes
         d. Warm-up throwing
         e. 45 feet (25 throws)
         f. Rest 10 minutes
         g. Warm-up throwing
         h. 45 feet (25 throws)

60-Foot Phase (Distance from Home Plate to Pitching Mound)

Step 3: a. Warm-up throwing
         b. 60 feet (25 throws)
         c. Rest 10-15 minutes
         d. Warm-up throwing
         e. 60 feet (25 throws)

Step 4: a. Warm-up throwing
         b. 60 feet (25 throws)
         c. Rest 10 minutes

Step 4: cont'd d. Warm-up throwing
                e. 60 feet (25 throws)
                f. Rest 10 minutes
                g. Warm-up throwing
                h. 60 feet (25 throws)

90-Foot Phase (Distance from Home Plate to First Base)

Step 5: a. Warm-up throwing
         b. 90 feet (25 throws)
         c. Rest 10-15 minutes
         d. Warm-up throwing
         e. 90 feet (25 throws)

Step 6: a. Warm-up throwing
         b. 90 feet (25 throws)
         c. Rest 10 minutes
         d. Warm-up throwing
         e. 90 feet (25 throws)
         f. Rest 10 minutes
         g. Warm-up throwing
         h. 90 feet (25 throws)

120-Foot Phase (Distance from Home Plate to Second Base)

Step 7: a. Warm-up throwing
         b. 120 feet (25 throws)
         c. Rest 10-15 minutes
         d. Warm-up throwing
         e. 120 feet (25 throws)

Modified from Wilk KE, Arrigo CA: Interval sport programs for the shoulder. In Andrews JR, Wilk KE, editors: *The athlete's shoulder,* New York, 1994, Churchill Livingstone.

sizes proper throwing mechanics (see Figs. A-3, *A* through *F*, and A-4, *A* through *D*). Throwing flat-footed encourages improper throwing mechanics and places increased stress on the throwing shoulder.

The throwing athlete progresses through each step of the program, throwing every other day, or three times weekly. The thrower progresses to the next step after the prescribed number of throws can be completed without pain or residual pain. If pain or difficulty throwing occurs, the athlete should regress to the previous level or attempt the same level during the next session. The ultimate goal is for the athlete to throw 75 repetitions at 180 feet without pain for positional players and 150 feet for pitchers. Box A-4 illustrates a progressive interval throwing program.[30]

Pattern throwing (Fig. A-6) also can be implemented to develop arm strength:[17]

1. Proper warm up before throwing (i.e., jogging, running, bicycling)

2. Throwing from a kneeling position, facing the direction of the throw with the arm already in the abducted position for a distance of 20 feet, easy effort, for 10 repetitions, with emphasis on proper grip

3. Kneeling on one knee facing the target with the arm in the abducted position (right-handed thrower on the right knee, left-handed thrower on the left knee) from a distance of 30 feet, easy effort, 10 repetitions with emphasis on hitting the target and maintaining proper follow-through

4. Standing with the feet in a straddle position facing the target with the shoulders turned and the ball in the glove at a distance of 40 feet, medium effort, with emphasis on follow-through

5. Standing in a regular throwing position at a distance of 40 feet, throwing medium effort for 10 repetitions with emphasis on staying closed and pointing the front shoulder to the target

---

Box A-4   Progressive Interval Throwing Program—cont'd

120-Foot Phase (Distance from Home Plate to Second Base)—cont'd

Step 8: a. Warm-up throwing
         b. 120 feet (25 throws)
         c. Rest 10 minutes
         d. Warm-up throwing
         e. 120 feet (25 throws)
         f. Rest 10 minutes
         g. Warm-up throwing
         h. 120 feet (25 throws)

150-Foot Phase (Distance from Home Plate to Grass Behind Second Base)

Step 9: a. Warm-up throwing
         b. 150 feet (25 throws)
         c. Rest 10-15 minutes
         d. Warm-up throws
         e. 150 feet (25 throws)

Step 10: a. Warm-up throwing
         b. 150 feet (25 throws)
         c. Rest 10 minutes
         d. Warm-up throwing
         e. 150 feet (25 throws)
         f. Rest 10 minutes
         g. Warm-up throwing
         h. 150 feet

180-Foot Phase (Distance from Home Plate to the Outfield)

Step 11: a. Warm-up throwing
         b. 180 feet (25 throws)
         c. Rest 10-15 minutes
         d. Warm-up throwing
         e. 180 feet (25 throws)

Step 12: a. Warm-up throwing
         b. 180 feet (25 throws)
         c. Rest 10 minutes
         d. Warm-up throwing
         e. 180 feet (25 throws)
         f. Rest 10 minutes
         g. Warm-up throwing
         h. 180 feet (25 throws)

Step 13: a. Warm-up throwing
         b. 180 feet (25 throws)
         c. Rest 10 minutes
         d. Warm-up throwing
         e. 180 feet (25 throws)
         f. Rest 10 minutes
         g. Warm-up throwing
         h. 180 feet (25 throws)

Step 14: Return to position or begin throwing from the mound (see Box 3-1)

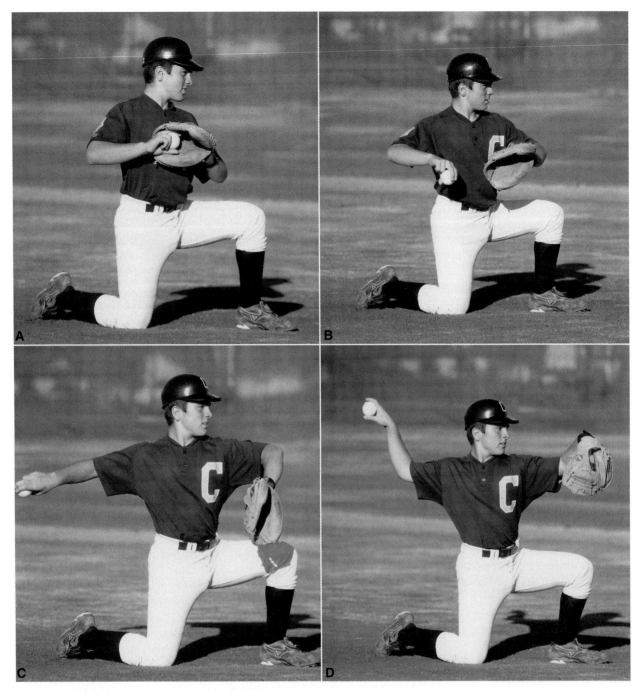

Fig. A-6. Pattern throwing from the kneeling position. Emphasis is placed on proper positioning of the hand, elbow, shoulder, and trunk throughout the entire throwing motion. (Photos by Marsha Gorman, Camarillo, California.)

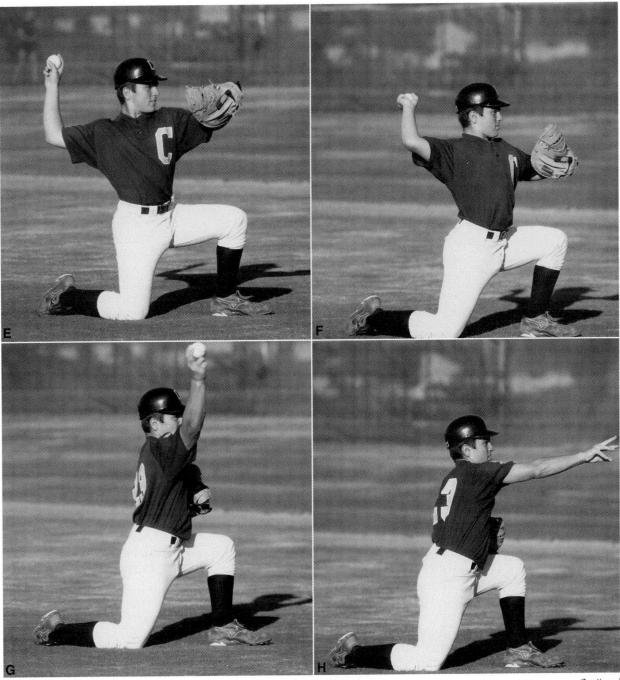

Continued

Fig. A-6, cont'd For legend see opposite page.

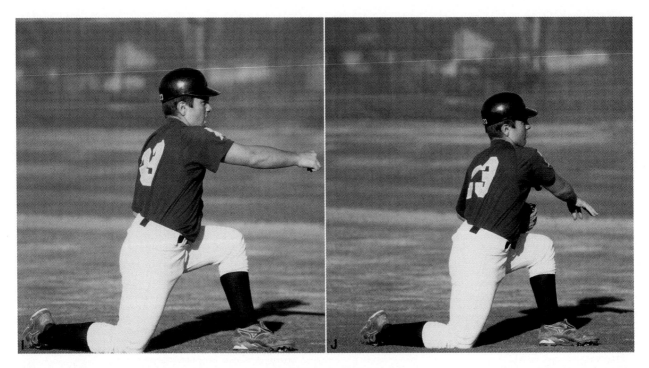

Fig. A-6, cont'd For legend see p. 366.

Summary

Rehabilitation goals for the shoulder after surgery emphasize pain management, reestablishing ROM, and developing strength in the shoulder-supporting musculature. To return the throwing athlete to sports after surgery requires further intense strengthening and conditioning to regain pre-injury form and performance. Progressive strengthening followed by aerobic conditioning helps prepare the thrower recovering from surgery for an eventual return to throwing. After throwing has been introduced into the rehabilitation regimen, careful attention to throwing technique is imperative to prevent re-injury. An interval throwing program is followed to establish a time frame for a safe, gradual, and progressive return to throwing.

The program described in this appendix should only serve as a guide for the progressive return of the thrower to throwing; it is not a specific postoperative protocol applicable to all patient athletes. Each patient's program requires individualization and should progress at its own rate.

REFERENCES

1. Adams T: An investigation of selected plyometric training exercises on muscle leg strength and power, *Track Field Q Rev* 84:36, 1984.

2. Astrand P, Rodahl K: *Textbook of work physiology,* New York, 1970, McGraw-Hill.

3. Atwater AE: Biomechanics of overarm throwing movements and of throwing injuries, *Exerc Sport Sci Rev* 7:43, 1979.

4. Browne AO et al: Glenohumeral elevation studied in three dimensions, *J Bone Joint Surg* 72B:843, 1990.

5. Broer MR: *Efficiency of human movement,* Philadelphia, 1969, WB Saunders.

6. Cain PR, Mutschler TA, Fu FH: Anterior instability of the glenohumeral joint: a dynamic model, *Am J Sports Med* 15:144, 1987.

7. Cavagna G, Disman B, Margari R: Positive work done by a previously stretched muscle, *J Appl Physiol* 24:21, 1968.

8. Chu D: Plyometric exercise, *Nat Strength Cond Assoc J* 6:56, 1984.

9. Dickoff-Hoffman SA: Neuromuscular control exercises for shoulder instability. In Andrews JR, Wilk KE, editors: *The athlete's shoulder,* New York, 1994, Churchill Livingstone.

10. DiGiovine N et al: An electromyographic analysis of the upper extremity in pitching, *J Shoulder Elbow Surg* 1(1):15, 1992.

11. Feltner M, Dapena J: Dynamics of the shoulder and elbow joints of the throwing arm during a baseball pitch, *Int J Sports Biomech* 2:235, 1986.

12. DeVries HA: *Physiology of exercise for physical education and athletics,* Dubuque, IA, 1974, WC Brown.

13. Ferrari D: Capsular ligaments of the shoulder anatomical and functional study to the anterior superior capsule, *Am J Sports Med* 18(1):20, 1990.

14. Fleisig GS, Dillman CJ, Andrews JR: *A biomechanical description of the shoulder joint during pitching,* symposium on clinical biomechanics of the shoulder, ACSM Annual Meeting, Dallas, May 1992.

15. Franks BD: Physical warm up. In Morgan WP, editor: *Ergogenic aids and muscular performance,* Orlando, FL, 1972, Academic Press.

16. Gainor BJ et al: The throw: biomechanics and acute injury, *Am J Sports Med* 8:114, 1980.

17. Gambetta V: Conditioning of the shoulder complex. In Andrews JR, Wilk KE, editors: *The athlete's shoulder,* New York, 1994, Churchill Livingstone.

18. Jobe FW et al: *Shoulder and arm exercises for the athlete who throws,* Inglewood, CA, 1996, Champion Press.

19. Lundin PE: A review of plyometrics, *Nat Strength Cond Assoc J* 7:65, 1985.

20. McArdle WD, Katch FL, Katch VL: *Exercise physiology; energy, nutrition, and human performance,* Philadelphia, 1981, Lea & Febiger.

21. Newton R: Joint receptor contributions to reflexive and kinesthetic responses, *Phys Ther* 62:22, 1982.

22. Pappas AM, Zawaki RM, Sullivan TJ: Biomechanics of baseball pitching, a preliminary report, *Am J Sports Med* 13:216, 1985.

23. Payton OD, Hirt S, Newton RA: *Scientific bases for neurophysiologic approaches to therapeutic exercise,* Philadelphia, 1972, FA Davis.

24. Perry J: Anatomy & biomechanics of the shoulder in throwing, swimming, gymnastics, and tennis, *Clin Sports Med* 2:247, 1973.

25. Scoles G: Depth jumping-does it really work? *Athletic J* 58:48, 1978.

26. Siewert MW et al: Isokinetic torque changes based on lever arm placement, *Phys Ther* 65:715, 1985.

27. Smith RL, Brunolli J: Shoulder kinesthesia after anterior glenohumeral dislocation, *Phys Ther* 69:106, 1989.

28. Toyoshima S et al: The contribution of the body parts to throwers performance. In Nelson R, Morehouse C, editors: *Biomechanics IV,* Baltimore, 1974, University Press.

29. Verkhoshanski Y: Perspectives in the improvement of speed-strength preparation of jumpers, *Yessis Rev Soviet Phys Educ Sports* 4:28, 1969.

30. Wilk KE, Arrigo CA: Interval sport programs for the shoulder. In Andrews JR, Wilk KE, editors: *The athlete's shoulder,* New York, 1994, Churchill Livingstone.

31. Wilk KE, Voight ML: Plyometrics for the shoulder complex. In Andrews JR, Wilk KE, editors: *The athlete's shoulder,* New York, 1994, Churchill Livingstone.

32. Wilt F: Plyometrics what it is and how it works, *Athletic J* 55:76, 1995.

Index

A

A/AROM; *see* Assisted, active range-of-motion exercise

Abdominal bracing
  in lumbar microdiscectomy, 131, 135, 138, 139
  in lumbar spine fusion, 157, 163, 164-165, 166

Abduction, hip, after ORIF, 202, 204

Abduction external rotation in rotator cuff repair, 56

Abduction pillow in total hip replacement, 180

Accessory lateral collateral ligament in elbow joint, 84

Accessory movements in ankle arthroscopy, passive, 317

Achilles paratenon blood vessels, 323, 324

Achilles tendinitis, 323

Achilles tendon, 323-349
  anatomy of, 323
  forces in, 324, 325
  pathogenesis of, 323-325
  progression of injury to, 326
  rupture of, 323; *see also* Achilles tendon repair
    acute care of, 328
    age and, 325, 326
    diagnosis of, 325-328
    epidemiology of, 325, 326
    etiology of, 325
    internal fixation in, 329
    nonoperative versus operative management of, 328
    repair and rehabilitation of, 323-349; *see also* Achilles tendon repair
    repeat, 329, 333, 341
    sports-related, 327

Achilles tendon repair, 323-349
  home maintenance in, 341, 345, 346
  incomplete return of function after, 330
  indications and considerations in, 323-328
  internal fixation in, 329
  normal reunion process in, 331, 332
  procedure for, 328-330
    endogenous and exogenous materials for, 329
    new concepts of, 329
    potential complications in, 330
    reconstruction, 329
    repair with augmentation, 328-329
    technique for, 329-330
  rehabilitation in, 330-332
    early motion, 332, 337, 346-347
    healing stages in, 330-332, 336
    phase I, 333, 334
    phase Ia, 337, 338
    phase Ib, 337
    phase II, 333, 334
    phase IIa, 337, 339-340
    phase IIb, 341, 342
    phase III, 333, 335
    phase IIIa, 341, 343
    phase IIIb, 341, 344
    phase IV, 333, 336
    postoperative management in, 332
    traditional immobilization in, 332, 333-341

ACL repair and reconstruction; *see* Anterior cruciate ligament repair and reconstruction

Acromioclavicular joint
  disease of; *see* Impingement syndrome
  mobilization of, 55
  osteoarthritis of, 65
  pain in, 55

Acromionizer, 14

Acromioplasty, 11-28
  indications for, 11-12
  open, 12

Acromioplasty—cont'd
  rehabilitation after, 15-23
    guidelines for, 14-24, 25-26
    phase I, 15-18
    phase II, 18-22
    phase III, 23
  in rotator cuff repair, 49
  subacromial decompression in, 12-14
  troubleshooting in, 24

Active range-of-motion exercise; *see also* Assisted, active range-of-motion exercise; Range of motion; Range-of-motion exercise
  in Achilles tendon repair rehabilitation, 330, 331, 338-343
  in ACL repair and reconstruction, 210, 213, 214
  in anterior capsular reconstruction, 31, 32, 33, 35
  in anterior capsulolabral reconstruction, 31
  in arthroscopy
    of ankle, 318, 319
    in lateral retinaculum release, 230
  assisted; *see* Assisted, active range-of-motion exercise
  in carpal tunnel syndrome surgery, 106, 107, 108, 110
  in extensor brevis release and lateral epicondylectomy, 73, 74, 75
  in lateral ligament repair, 291, 292, 293, 294
  in lumbar microdiscectomy, 138
  in meniscal repair, 245
  in open reduction and internal fixation
    of ankle, 305, 306, 307
    of hip, 197
    of patella, 261, 262-264
  in rotator cuff repair, 52, 56
  in total hip replacement, 180, 182
  in total knee replacement, 274, 275, 276, 278
  in UCL reconstruction, 88, 90

Active wrist flexion exercise, 111-114

Activity drills
  in lumbar microdiscectomy, 143
  in lumbar spine fusion, 166

Adduction
  across midline after femoral neck fracture repair, 190
  hip, after ORIF, 202, 204

Adductor isometric contractions after meniscal repair, 248

Adductor squeezes after hip ORIF, 196, 197, 198

Adhesions
  in immobilized connective tissue, 5
  muscle splay and, 8-9
  at porthole sites after meniscal repair, 249

Aerobic exercise; *see also* Cardiovascular exercise
  in carpal tunnel syndrome surgery, 116
  in lumbar microdiscectomy, 136

Agility drills
  in ankle arthroscopy, 321
  in ankle ORIF, 310
  in lumbar spine fusion, 165
  in meniscal repair, 252, 253

AITF; *see* Anterior inferior talofibular ligament

All-inside meniscal repair, 244

Analgesia, patient-controlled, in subacromial decompression, 13

Anconeus, 84

Anesthetic problems in Achilles tendon repair, 330

Ankle
  dorsiflexion of; *see* Dorsiflexion of ankle
  eversion of
    in Achilles tendon repair, 333, 339, 340

Ankle—cont'd
  eversion of—cont'd
    lateral ligament repair and, 292, 294, 295, 296
    in meniscal repair, 249
  fractures of
    Maisonneuve, 303
    open reduction and internal fixation for, 302, 303; *see also* Ankle, open reduction and internal fixation of
    trimalleolar, 303
  interosseous membrane tearing in, 303
  inversion of
    in Achilles tendon repair, 333, 339, 340
    lateral ligament repair and, 290, 294, 295, 296
    in meniscal repair, 249
  open reduction and internal fixation of, 302-313
    home maintenance after, 311, 312
    indications and considerations for, 302
    movement with and without gravity after, 307
    outcomes of, 305
    pain after, 309
    postoperative considerations in, 303-305
    precautions after, 311
    procedure for, 302-305
    rehabilitation after, 305-311
    troubleshooting after, 311
  plantar flexion of; *see* Plantar flexion of ankle
  syndesmosis injury to, 303
  unstable
    after total knee replacement, 284
    lateral ligament repair for, 288

Ankle arthroscopy, 314-322
  contraindications to, 314
  indications for, 314
  in ORIF, 303
  outcomes of, 316
  procedure for, 314-316
  rehabilitation after, 316-322
    phase I, 317
    phase II, 317-319
    phase III, 319-321
    protocol and principles in, 316
  troubleshooting in, 322

Ankle brace, lateral ligament repair and, 297

Ankle exercise; *see also* Ankle pumps
  in ankle arthroscopy, 317
  in meniscal repair, 249
  in total hip replacement, 181

Ankle ORIF, initial evaluation in, 305

Ankle proprioceptive neuromuscular facilitation after hip surgery, 196

Ankle pumps; *see also* Ankle exercise
  in Achilles tendon repair, 338
  in ACL repair and reconstruction, 210, 211, 213
  in arthroscopic lateral retinaculum release, 230
  in hip ORIF, 196
  in total hip replacement, 178, 179, 180, 181

Annular ligament in elbow joint, 84

Annulotomy in lumbar microdiscectomy, 126

Anterior capsular reconstruction, 29-45
  home maintenance after, 44
  indications and considerations for, 29-30
  procedure for, 30-31
  rehabilitation after, 31-38
    phase I, 33
    phase II, 33-36
    phase III, 36-38
  troubleshooting after, 44-45

Anterior capsulolabral reconstruction, 30-31
  Bankart lesion in, 30, 31
  capsule laxity in, 31

Anterior capsulolabral reconstruction—cont'd
  capsulotomy in, 30
  glenoid labrum absence in, 31
  splinting in, 31
Anterior cruciate ligament repair and reconstruction, 206-226
  age group of ruptures in, 206
  edema in, 211
  endoscopic BPB reconstruction in, 208-209
  extraarticular, 206
  graft fixation in, 207
  graft maturation in, 207-208
  graft selection in, 207
  home maintenance in, 221-222
  indications and considerations in, 206-208
  initial postoperative examination in, 211-212
  intraarticular, 206-207
  pain management in, 211
  postoperative guidelines and rationales in, 212-221
    number of treatments and, 213
    phase I, 213-217
    phase II, 217-218
    phase III, 219
    phase IV, 219-221
  preoperative management in, 209-211
  procedure for, 208-209
  rehabilitation in, 209-212
  treatment options in, 206-207
  troubleshooting after, 221, 223
Anterior inferior talofibular ligament, 288; *see also* Lateral ligament repair
Anterior lumbar interbody fusion, 153
Anterior talofibular ligament, 288; *see also* Lateral ligament repair
Anterolisthesis, lumbar spine fusion and, 151
Antiembolic exercises in meniscal repair, 245
Antiinflammatory medications in patella tilt, 227
Anti-thrombotic stockings; *see* Thromboembolic disease hose
Anti-vibration gloves in carpal tunnel syndrome, 116
Anxiety, lumbar spine fusion and, 162-163
Apprehension sign in shoulder instability, 29
Aquatic therapy
  in Achilles tendon repair, 335, 340, 342, 343
  in ACL repair and reconstruction, 222
  in ankle arthroscopy, 319
  in ankle ORIF, 310
  in lateral ligament repair, 294
  in meniscal repair, 246, 249
  in total hip replacement, 184, 185
  in total knee replacement, 280, 281
AROM exercise; *see* Active range-of-motion exercise
Arthritis
  in lumbar disc herniation, 123
  in total knee replacement, 268
Arthrodesis, lumbar; *see* Lumbar spine fusion
Arthrofibrosis
  in ACL repair and reconstruction, 221
  in meniscal repair, 249
Arthrography in rotator cuff repair, 48
Arthroplasty, resurfacing, in total hip replacement, 172
Arthroscope in subacromial decompression, 13
Arthroscopy
  in ACL repair and reconstruction, 206
  ankle; *see* Ankle arthroscopy
  glenohumeral, in rotator cuff repair, 49
  in lateral ligament repair, 289
  in lateral retinaculum release, 227-242; *see also* Lateral retinaculum release, arthroscopic
  in UCL reconstruction, 86
Articular cartilage degeneration after patella ORIF, 262
Assisted, active range-of-motion exercise
  in ACL repair and reconstruction, 210
  in anterior capsular reconstruction, 31, 32
  in rotator cuff repair, 51, 53, 56
  in total knee replacement, 274, 275, 276

ATF; *see* Anterior talofibular ligament
Atrophy in carpal tunnel syndrome, 102
Autografts
  quadruple-strand semitendinosus, 207
  sterilization of, 207
Axillary crutches in hip ORIF, 198
Axillary roll in anterior capsular reconstruction, 33
Axis of motion, shoulder, 66

B

Balance and proprioception exercises; *see also* Balance board
  in Achilles tendon repair, 333
  in ACL repair and reconstruction, 218
  in ankle arthroscopy, 318, 319
  in hip ORIF, 200
  in lumbar microdiscectomy, 145
  in meniscal repair, 250
  in total knee replacement, 280, 281
Balance board; *see also* Balance and proprioception exercises
  in ankle ORIF, 306, 308
  in lateral ligament repair, 294, 299
  in lumbar microdiscectomy, 140
  in meniscal repair, 250, 251
Baltimore Therapeutic Equipment, 77
Bankart lesion, 30, 31
BAPS; *see* Biomechanical Ankle Platform System
BAPs; *see* Balance and proprioception exercises
Basket-weave in connective tissue, 5
Bed mobility training
  in hip ORIF, 196, 197
  in lumbar spine fusion, 156, 158, 159
  in total hip replacement, 180, 182
  in total knee replacement, 274
Bending, lumbar microdiscectomy and, 133
Biceps brachii, 84
Biceps curls in carpal tunnel syndrome, 115
Bicycle, stationary; *see* Stationary bicycle
Bicycle riding after hip ORIF, 202, 205; *see also* Stationary bicycle
Biofeedback
  in arthroscopic lateral retinaculum release, 232
  in lumbar microdiscectomy, 134
Biomechanical Ankle Platform System, 318, 319, 321
Biomechanical foot orthotics, 296
Biomechanics, soft tissue healing and, 2-5
Bipolar hip replacement in femoral neck fractures, 189
Body blade in ankle arthroscopy, 321
Body mechanics training
  in lumbar microdiscectomy, 130, 133
  in lumbar spine fusion, 156, 157, 159-162
Body weight resistance in Achilles tendon repair, 333
Bone plugs, 208
Bone punch, 272, 273
Bone-morphogenic protein, 154
Bone-patella tendon-bone complex graft, 207, 208-209
Bony clearing in connective tissue, 9
Boot with fixed hinge, 337, 341; *see also* Splint
Box drills
  in ACL repair, 217, 218
  in lateral ligament repair, 296, 297
BPB graft; *see* Bone-patella tendon-bone complex graft
Braces
  in Achilles tendon rupture, 328
  in ACL repair and reconstruction, 213
  in arthroscopic lateral retinaculum release, 235
  hinged
    after patella ORIF, 262
    elbow, in collateral ligament reconstruction, 88, 89
    locked, in ACL repair, 213
  in lateral ligament repair, 291, 297
  in lumbar microdiscectomy, 130
Brachialis, 84

Brachioradialis, 84
Bridging in lumbar spine fusion, 140, 164, 166
Broström procedure, 290
Bursectomy in subacromial decompression, 13-14
Bursoscopy, subacromial, 49

C

Cages in lumbar spine fusion, 154
Calcaneofibular ligament, 288; *see also* Lateral ligament repair
Calcar replacement prosthesis, 190
Calcification in lateral epicondylitis, 71-72
Calf pumping after arthroscopic lateral retinaculum release, 231
Calf raises after ankle ORIF, 309
Calf stretching after hip ORIF, 200, 201
Callus in lumbar spine fusion, 155
CAM brace; *see* Controlled action motion walker brace
Cane
  after hip ORIF, 202
  after total hip replacement, 185
Cannulated screws
  in ACL repair and reconstruction, 207, 209
  in ankle ORIF, 303
  in bone-patella tendon-bone complex graft, 209
  in femoral neck fractures, 198
  in patella ORIF, 259
Capsule laxity in anterior capsulolabral reconstruction, 31
Capsulotomy in anterior capsulolabral reconstruction, 30
Cardiovascular exercise; *see also* Aerobic exercise
  in Achilles tendon repair, 334, 336, 340
  in ACL repair and reconstruction, 213
  in ankle arthroscopy, 319
  in hip ORIF, 202, 204
  in lumbar microdiscectomy, 136, 142, 143, 146
  in lumbar spine fusion, 155, 163, 166
  in meniscal repair, 251
  in rotator cuff repair, 53
  training heart rate in, 136
Caregiver training in total hip replacement, 182
Carioca
  in ankle ORIF, 310
  in lateral ligament repair, 296, 297, 298, 299
Carpal ligament division, 101, 102
Carpal tunnel syndrome, 101-118
  home maintenance in, 117-118
  patient history in, 104
  rehabilitation after surgery for, 104-117
    phase I, 105-111
    phase II, 111-116
  postoperative evaluation in, 104-105
  surgical indications in, 101-103
  surgical procedure for, 103-104
Carrying objects in lumbar spine fusion, 162
Cartilage degeneration after patella ORIF, 262
Cast
  in Achilles tendon repair, 329, 334
  in equinus, 334
  lateral ligament repair and, 291
  short-leg, in ankle ORIF, 303
Cast disease in Achilles tendon repair, 329
Catchers, rehabilitation program for, 40
Cellular proliferation in graft maturation, 207, 208
Cemented implant in total hip replacement, 172, 173
Central rotation gastrocnemius flap, 329
Cephalosporins, 268
Cerebral palsy, 176
Cervical spine evaluation in rotator cuff repair, 63-64
CF ligament; *see* Calcaneofibular ligament
Chair exercises in lumbar spine fusion, 158, 159
Chrisman-Snook procedure, 290
Circuit-training in lumbar spine fusion, 165
Clavicle excision, 14

Closed-chain exercises
  in ACL repair and reconstruction, 212-213
  in ankle arthroscopy, 319, 320, 321
  in arthroscopic lateral retinaculum release, 232, 234, 235, 237
  in meniscal repair, 248, 249, 250, 251
  in open reduction and internal fixation
    of ankle, 308
    of hip, 204
    of patella, 262, 265
  in rotator cuff repair, 57, 58
  in total hip replacement, 184
  in total knee replacement, 276, 278, 279
  in vastus medialis oblique and vastus lateralis surgery, 276
Coban, 109
Cobb periosteal elevator, 125
Co-contraction muscle contraction in meniscal repair, 245, 246, 248
Cold packs; see Cryotherapy
Collagen
  in connective tissue fibers, 2
  in extracellular matrix, 2
  in graft maturation, 207, 208
  in healing process, 330, 331, 332
  in remobilization, 5-6
Compartment syndrome, transverse muscle bending in, 9
Compression, Achilles tendon and, 325, 337, 338
Compression dressing
  in ankle arthroscopy, 316
  in extensor brevis release and lateral epicondylectomy, 73, 74
  in lumbar microdiscectomy, 136, 137
  in UCL reconstruction, 88
Compression glove in carpal tunnel syndrome, 109
Compression plate in subtrochanteric femoral neck fractures, 193
Compression screws, 190, 192, 193
Compression thromboembolic disease hose; see Thromboembolic disease hose
Computed tomography
  in lumbar disc herniation, 123
  and lumbar spine fusion, 151
Connective tissue
  classification of, 3
  creep in, 8
  ground substance in, 2
  histology and biomechanics of, 2-5
    extracellular matrix in, 2-3
  immobilization effects on, 5
  mobilization techniques in, 8-10
    bony clearing in, 9
    cross-friction in, 10
    muscle splay in, 8-9
    transverse muscle bending in, 9
  normal biomechanics in, 4-5
  remobilization effects on, 5-5
  scar and, 6-7
  short and long principles in, 8
  three-dimensionality of, 7
  trauma effects on, 6-7
  types of, 3-4
Continuous passive motion machine
  in ACL repair and reconstruction, 212
  in extensor brevis release and lateral epicondylectomy, 79
  in total knee replacement, 274, 275
Contractile tissue loading after acromioplasty, 24
Controlled action motion walker brace, 291
Cooper's ligament, 84
Corner wall stretch in rotator cuff repair, 58, 59
Corset in lumbar microdiscectomy, 130
Corticosteroids in lumbar disc herniation, 122
Cortisone injections
  in lateral epicondylitis, 71
  in rotator cuff tears, 48
Cough after total hip replacement, 180
Coumadin; see Warfarin
CPM machine; see Continuous passive motion machine

Creep, connective tissue and, 8
Crepitus
  arthroscopic lateral retinaculum release for, 227
  patellofemoral, preoperative, 211
Cross-country ski machine
  in ACL repair and reconstruction, 219
  in meniscal repair, 250, 251
  in total hip replacement, 184, 185
Crossed straight leg raise test in lumbar disc herniation, 122
Cross-friction in connective tissue, 10
Cruciate ligaments, anterior, repair of; see Anterior cruciate ligament repair and reconstruction
Crutches
  in Achilles tendon repair, 333, 334, 338
  in ACL repair and reconstruction, 214
  in arthroscopic lateral retinaculum release, 229
  in meniscal repair, 245
  in open reduction and internal fixation
    of hip, 198
    of patella, 260
  in total hip replacement, 178, 181
Cryocuff in ACL repair and reconstruction, 211
Cryotherapy
  in Achilles tendon repair, 334, 335, 337, 338
  in ACL repair and reconstruction, 210, 211, 213
  in acromioplasty, 16, 18
  in ankle arthroscopy, 317
  in ankle ORIF, 306, 307
  in anterior capsular reconstruction, 33
  in arthroscopic lateral retinaculum release, 230, 231, 235
  in carpal tunnel syndrome, 106, 107, 108, 109
  in extensor brevis release and lateral epicondylectomy, 73, 74
  in lumbar microdiscectomy, 129, 130, 136, 142, 146
  in lumbar spine fusion, 157, 162
  in meniscal repair, 245, 246, 247
  in rotator cuff repair, 48, 51, 52
  in UCL reconstruction, 88, 89, 97
CTS; see Carpal tunnel syndrome
Cubital tunnel, 85
Cutaneous nerve intermediate dorsal, 289
Cycling; see Stationary bicycle
Cyst formation, synovial, 123

D
de Quervain's syndrome, 115
Deep massage in arthroscopic lateral retinaculum release, 233
Deep venous thrombosis
  in Achilles tendon repair, 330
  in total knee replacement, 274, 275, 282
Degeneration
  in lumbar spine, 151, 152
  in rotator cuff, 46
Degenerative fibroneuromas, arthroscopic lateral retinaculum release for, 227
DeLorme strength progression protocol in meniscal repair, 249
Dense irregular connective tissue, 3
Dense regular connective tissue, 3
Dexterity evaluation of finger in carpal tunnel syndrome, 104
Diamon and Hughston internal fixation of unstable trochanteric fracture, 191
Dips in lumbar spine fusion, 164
Disc, intervertebral
  degenerative cascade in, 152
  extruded, 123
  herniation of, lumbar microdiscectomy in, 122
  subligamentous, 123
Discectomy in lumbar disc herniation, 123
Discharge planning
  in lumbar microdiscectomy, 146
  in total hip replacement, 183
Dislocation
  of patella, surgery for, 229
  in total hip replacement, 179

Displaced femoral neck fractures, 189-190
  minimally, 188-189
Distraction
  subtalar, 317
  talocrural, 317
Distraction device in ankle arthroscopy, 314, 315
Distraction-type fixation in lumbar spine fusion, 152
Dorsiflexion of ankle
  in Achilles tendon repair, 333, 337, 338, 340, 341, 342, 343
  in lateral ligament repair, 291, 292, 295, 296
    limited, 296
  in meniscal repair, 249
  in open reduction and internal fixation, 309, 311
  sudden or violent, Achilles tendon rupture and, 325
Double upright brace in ACL repair and reconstruction, 213
Double-limb squats in arthroscopic lateral retinaculum release, 235
Driving
  lumbar microdiscectomy and, 129, 132
  total hip replacement and, 185
Dural adhesions in lumbar microdiscectomy, 133
Dural nerve root stretches
  in lumbar microdiscectomy, 130, 133-134, 139
  in total knee replacement, 282, 283
DVT; see Deep venous thrombosis
Dying bug
  in lumbar microdiscectomy, 138, 139
  in lumbar spine fusion, 139, 164, 166
Dynamic compression hip screw in femoral neck fractures, 190, 192, 193
Dynamometer in carpal tunnel syndrome, 105

E
Eccentric elbow extension, 92
Eccentric elbow flexion, 92
Eccentric shoulder flexion, 55
ECRB; see Extensor carpi radialis brevis
ECU; see Extended care unit
Edema; see also Effusion
  in Achilles tendon repair, 337
  in ankle arthroscopy, 319
  in arthroscopic lateral retinaculum release, 231
  in carpal tunnel syndrome, 102, 104
  in extensor brevis release and lateral epicondylectomy, 73, 75, 79
  in hip ORIF, 205
  in knee, ACL repair and reconstruction and, 211, 212, 221; see also Knee, effusion of
  in meniscal repair, 249
  in total hip replacement, 185
Effusion; see also Edema
  arthroscopic lateral retinaculum release for, 227
  knee; see Knee, effusion of
Elastic band exercise in Achilles tendon repair, 340; see also Elastic tubing exercise
Elastic compression wrap in extensor brevis release and lateral epicondylectomy, 73, 74
Elastic cords in meniscal repair, 251
Elastic tubing exercise; see also Exercise tubing
  in Achilles tendon repair, 333, 340
  in ACL repair and reconstruction, 219
  in arthroscopic lateral retinaculum release, 235
  in lateral ligament repair, 294, 295
  in meniscal repair, 246, 249, 250
  in open reduction and internal fixation
    of ankle, 308, 309
    of hip, 199
    of patella, 264
Elasticity of connective tissue, 4
Elastin
  in connective tissue fibers, 2
  in extracellular matrix, 2

Elbow brace, hinged, in UCL reconstruction, 88, 89
Elbow extension
  in anterior capsular reconstruction, 33
  in carpal tunnel syndrome, 115
  in extensor brevis release and lateral epicondylectomy, 75
  in UCL reconstruction, 90
Elbow flexion
  in anterior capsular reconstruction, 33
  in extensor brevis release and lateral epicondylectomy, 75
  in UCL reconstruction, 90
Elbow flexion contracture in UCL reconstruction, 89
Elbow instability, 86
Elbow lying in lumbar microdiscectomy, 139
Elbow range-of-motion exercise in carpal tunnel syndrome, 106
Elbow valgus stress, 82-100
Electrical stimulation; see also Neuromuscular stimulation
  in ACL repair and reconstruction, 211, 213
  in ankle arthroscopy, 317
  in arthroscopic lateral retinaculum release, 230, 233
  in carpal tunnel syndrome, 108, 109
  in extensor brevis release and lateral epicondylectomy, 73, 74
  in lumbar microdiscectomy, 130, 136
  in meniscal repair, 245, 246
  in open reduction and internal fixation
    of ankle, 306, 307, 309
    of hip, 198
    of patella, 261, 262
  in rotator cuff repair, 51
  in total knee replacement, 275
  in UCL reconstruction, 97
Electrocautery in lumbar microdiscectomy, 125
Electromyography
  after total knee replacement, 283
  in lumbar microdiscectomy, 134, 138, 139
Electrosurgical lateral release electrode, 229
Electrotherapeutic modalities in lumbar disc herniation, 122
Elevation
  in Achilles tendon repair, 334, 335, 337, 338
  in ACL repair and reconstruction, 210, 211
  in ankle ORIF, 306, 307
  in arthroscopic lateral retinaculum release, 231
  in meniscal repair, 245
ELPS; see Excessive lateral pressure syndrome
Embolus
  exercises to prevent, in meniscal repair, 245
  pulmonary, after total knee replacement, 281, 282
Endocrine function, Achilles tendon and, 325
Endoprosthetic hip replacement in femoral neck fractures, 189
Endoscopic BPB reconstruction in ACL repair and reconstruction, 208-209
Endoscopic discectomy in lumbar disc herniation, 123
Endurance in shoulder, troubleshooting for, 44
Endurance training
  after acromioplasty, 23
  in meniscal repair, 251
Entrapment neuropathy, carpal tunnel syndrome as, 101
Envelope of function after acromioplasty, 24
Epicondylectomy, lateral, and extensor brevis release, 71-81
Epicondylitis in carpal tunnel syndrome, 115
Ergonomic keyboards, 115
Ergonomics
  in carpal tunnel syndrome, 115
  lumbar microdiscectomy and, 132
Evaluation
  in ACL repair and reconstruction, 211, 212
  in ankle ORIF, 305-307
  in carpal tunnel syndrome, 104-105
  functional capacity; see Functional capacity evaluation

Evaluation—cont'd
  of gait
    in ACL repair and reconstruction, 209-210, 217
    in meniscectomy and meniscal repair, 245
    in total knee replacement, 281, 283
  home safety in total hip replacement, 184
  in impingement syndrome, 12
  in lateral ligament repair rehabilitation in, 291
  in lumbar microdiscectomy, 146
  in lumbar spine fusion, 159
  in meniscal repair, 244-245, 245-247
    of flexibility, 245-247, 248, 250
    in meniscectomy and meniscal repair, 245, 247
  in patella ORIF, 259
  of range of motion after total knee replacement, 281
  of rotator cuff, 46-48, 48
  of scar in carpal tunnel syndrome, 105
  in subacromial decompression, 14
Eversion of ankle
  in Achilles tendon repair, 333, 339, 340
  in lateral ligament repair, 292, 294, 295, 296
  in meniscal repair, 249
Excessive lateral pressure syndrome in arthroscopic lateral retinaculum release, 227
Exercise
  in acromioplasty, troubleshooting for, 24
  in lumbar microdiscectomy, 133-136
  strengthening; see Strengthening exercise
  stretching; see Stretching exercise
Exercise tubing; see also Elastic tubing exercise
  in meniscal repair, 251
  in rotator cuff repair, 55, 56
Extended care unit, total knee replacement and, 276
Extensor brevis release and lateral epicondylectomy, 71-81
  home maintenance in, 79, 80
  indications for, 71-72
  outcome for, 72
  patient education in, 73
  procedure for, 72
  rehabilitation in, 73-78
    phase I, 73, 74
    phase II, 75-77
    phase III, 77, 78
  symptom recurrence after, 79
  troubleshooting in, 79
Extensor carpi radialis brevis, 84
  in lateral epicondylitis, 71-72
  repair of, 72
Extensor carpi radialis longus, 84
Extensor carpi ulnaris, 84
Extensor digiti minimi, 84
Extensor digitorum, 84
Extensor muscles, 84
Extensor-supinator muscles, 84
External rotation after acromioplasty, 18, 21, 25
  isometrics and, 25
External rotator exercises, resisted, 55
Extracellular matrix, 2-3

F
Facet arthritis, 123
Facet hypertrophy, 123
Facet joints, degenerative cascade in, 152
Fascia, bending, splaying, or movement of, 9
Fascia lata in Achilles tendon rupture repair, 329
Fasciitis, plantar, 310
Fear, lumbar spine fusion and, 162
Femoral condyles, guide to chamfer, 270, 271
Femoral neck fractures, 188-190
  nonunion of, 189
Femoral nerve in total hip replacement, 176
Femoral osteotomy in total knee replacement, 270, 271
Femoral tunnel in endoscopic bone–patella tendon–bone complex graft, 209
Femur
  anatomic and mechanical axes of, 268, 269
  osteotomy of in total knee replacement, 270, 271

Fibrofatty infiltrate in immobilized connective tissue, 5
Fibroneuromas, degenerative, 227
Fibroplastic phase of scar formation, 7
Fibula mobilization, lateral ligament repair and, 296
Figure-eight drills
  in ACL repair and reconstruction, 217, 218
  in lateral ligament repair, 296, 297
Finger dexterity evaluation, 104
Fixation of grafts with interference screw, 207
Flexibility after meniscal repair, 245-247, 248, 250
Flexion contracture in UCL reconstruction, 96
Flexion deformity in total knee replacement, 270
Flexion-relaxation phenomenon in lumbar microdiscectomy, 127
Flexor carpi, 84
Flexor carpi ulnaris, 84
Flexor digitorum superficialis, 84
Flexor hallucis longus, 329
Flexor muscles in elbow joint, 84
Flexor-pronator muscles in elbow joint, 84
Floor, rising from, after lumbar spine fusion, 158, 159, 163
Foot
  excessive pronation of, in arthroscopic lateral retinaculum release, 239
  mechanics of, in meniscal repair, 245
Foot cradle in total hip replacement, 180, 181
Foot drop after total knee replacement, 283
Foot orthotics, lateral ligament repair and, 296
Football drills in lumbar microdiscectomy, 144
Foraminal stenosis in lumbar disc herniation, 123
Forearm pronation
  in anterior capsular reconstruction, 33
  in carpal tunnel syndrome, 115
  in extensor brevis release and lateral epicondylectomy, 75
  in UCL reconstruction, 90
Forearm rotation in carpal tunnel syndrome, 106, 115
Forearm strengthening in carpal tunnel syndrome, 115
Forearm supination
  in anterior capsular reconstruction, 33
  in carpal tunnel syndrome, 113, 115
  in extensor brevis release and lateral epicondylectomy, 75
  in UCL reconstruction, 90
Forward step down in meniscal repair, 250
Forward step up in meniscal repair, 250
"4 quad" program in meniscal repair, 246, 249
Four-point cane after total hip replacement, 185
Four-wall elastic tubing exercise in arthroscopic lateral retinaculum release, 235
Fracture
  femoral neck, 188-190
  malleolus, medial and lateral, 304
  patellar, after ACL repair and reconstruction, 221
  trimalleolar, 303
Fracture boot in ankle ORIF, 307
Friction, Achilles tendon and, 325
Front-wheeled walker after hip ORIF, 196
Frostbite in cryotherapy, 211
Full-thickness tears in rotator cuff, 48-51
Functional capacity evaluation
  in ankle ORIF, 310
  in carpal tunnel syndrome, 116
  in lumbar microdiscectomy, 143
  in lumbar spine fusion, 166
Functional double-limb squats, 235
Functional status of patient in carpal tunnel syndrome, 105
Functional training
  in Achilles tendon repair, 341
  in acromioplasty, 23
  in ankle ORIF, 309
  in arthroscopic lateral retinaculum release, 235
  in lateral ligament repair, 296
  in lumbar microdiscectomy, 145

Fusion types in lumbar spine fusion, 152-154
    instrumentation vs noninstrumentation, 152-153
    posterior, 153-154

G

Gait; see also Gait training
    in Achilles tendon repair, 341
    in ACL repair and reconstruction, 209-210, 217
    in hip ORIF, 202
    in meniscectomy and meniscal repair, 245
    in total knee replacement, 281, 283
    Trendelenburg, after femoral neck fracture fixation, 190
Gait training
    in Achilles tendon repair, 335, 343
    in ACL repair and reconstruction, 210, 214, 217, 219
    in ankle arthroscopy, 317-319
    in lateral ligament repair, 292, 293
    in lumbar spine fusion, 156
    in meniscal repair, 246
    in open reduction and internal fixation
        of ankle, 306, 307
        of hip, 199, 202, 203
        of patella, 261, 262-264
    in total hip replacement, 180, 182, 184
    in total knee replacement, 274, 276
Gastrocnemius fascia flaps, 328
Gastrocnemius flaps, 328-329
Gastrocnemius-soleus stretches
    in ankle ORIF, 308
    in lumbar microdiscectomy, 135
    in meniscal repair, 246, 247-248
Genu recurvatum in total knee replacement, 270
Girth
    knee
        in ACL repair and reconstruction, 211, 212
        in meniscal repair, 245, 247
        mid-patellar, in ACL repair and reconstruction, 211, 212
Glenohumeral arthroscopy, 49
Glenohumeral instability
    in acromioplasty, 22
    in subacromial impingement syndrome, 11
Glenohumeral joint in subacromial decompression, 13
Glenohumeral ligament laxity in shoulder instability, 29
Glenoid labrum absence in anterior capsulolabral reconstruction, 31
Glides
    metatarsal, in ankle arthroscopy, 317
    patellar, 228
        in ACL repair and reconstruction, 214
    patellofemoral, 217
    subtalar, in ankle arthroscopy, 317
    talar, posterior, in ankle ORIF, 307
    talocrural, in ankle arthroscopy, 317
Gluteal nerve, superior, 176
Gluteal sets
    in hip ORIF, 196, 197
    in total hip replacement, 178, 179, 180, 181
    in total knee replacement, 274, 276
Gluteal stretches in lumbar microdiscectomy, 135
Gluteus maximus weakness after total hip replacement, 185
Gluteus medius inhibition or facilitation after total knee replacement, 284
Gluteus minimus weakness after total hip replacement, 185
Golfers
    lumbar microdiscectomy in, 145
    rehabilitation program for, 43
Gracilis
    grafts of semitendinosus, 207
    stretches of, in lumbar microdiscectomy, 142
Grafts
    bone–patella tendon–bone complex, 207
    BPB; see Grafts, bone–patella tendon–bone complex

Grafts—cont'd
    central third patellar tendon, 206-208
    fixation of, 207
    hamstring tendon, 206-208
    maturation of, 207-208
    quadruple-strand semitendinosus, 207
    selection of, 207
    semitendinosus gracilis, 207
    single-strand semitendinosus, 207
Granulation phase of scar formation, 6
Gravity in exercises after ankle ORIF, 307
Grip isometric exercise, 114
Grip strength
    in acromioplasty, 16
    in carpal tunnel syndrome, 101, 105
    in UCL reconstruction, 88, 97
Ground substance
    connective tissue, 2
    in extracellular matrix, 2
    in remobilization, 5-6
Guide pins in ankle ORIF, 303

H

Hamstring co-contraction
    in ACL repair and reconstruction, 210, 211
    in meniscal repair, 248
Hamstring exercise; see also Hamstring sets
    in ACL repair and reconstruction, 210, 211, 213, 214
    in lumbar microdiscectomy, 141
    in meniscal repair, 248, 250, 251
Hamstring isometrics in meniscal repair, 248
Hamstring sets; see also Hamstring exercise
    in ACL repair and reconstruction, 213, 214
    in arthroscopic lateral retinaculum release, 230
    in meniscal repair, 245, 246
    in open reduction and internal fixation
        of hip, 196
        of patella, 261, 262
    in total knee replacement, 274, 276
Hamstring stretches
    in arthroscopic lateral retinaculum release, 230
    in hip ORIF, 200, 201
    in lumbar microdiscectomy, 135
    in lumbar spine fusion, 163
    in meniscal repair, 246, 247, 248
Hamstring tendon grafts, 206-208
Hand exerciser, 33
Hand exercises in anterior capsular reconstruction, 33
Hand weakness in UCL reconstruction, 97
Hands-and-knees push-ups, modified, 36
Hands-behind-back exercise in rotator cuff repair, 58, 60
Harrington hook/rod construct, 152
Hawkins-Kennedy sign, 12
Healing stages, 330-332
    inflammatory response in, 330
    remodeling and maturation in, 331-332
    repair and proliferation in, 330-331
Heat therapy
    in arthroscopic lateral retinaculum release, 232, 233
    in carpal tunnel syndrome, 109
    in meniscal repair, 246
    in rotator cuff, 48
Heel cord stretches in hip ORIF, 200
Heel hangs in ACL repair and reconstruction, 213, 214, 215
Heel lifts
    in Achilles tendon repair, 333
    in lumbar spine fusion, 164, 166
Heel raises
    in Achilles tendon repair, 333, 341, 343
    in ACL repair and reconstruction, 214
    in lateral ligament repair, 293, 294
Heel slides
    in ACL repair and reconstruction, 210, 213, 214
    in hip ORIF, 197
    in meniscal repair, 245, 246, 247
    in total hip replacement, 181, 182

Heel ulcers in hip ORIF, 196
Hemarthrosis
    in ACL repair and reconstruction, 211, 222
    in arthroscopic lateral retinaculum release, 229-231
Hematoma in carpal tunnel syndrome, 102
Heparin in total knee replacement, 274
High-impact sports after total hip replacement, 185
High-voltage galvanic stimulation; see also Electrical stimulation
    in carpal tunnel syndrome, 109
    in extensor brevis release and lateral epicondylectomy, 73, 74
    in UCL reconstruction, 97
Hinge
    boot with fixed, 337, 341
    on brace after patella ORIF, 262
    in elbow brace, 88, 89
    hip, in lumbar spine fusion, 159, 160, 161
Hip abduction
    in ACL repair and reconstruction, 210
    in ORIF, 196, 197, 202, 204
    in total hip replacement, 179, 181, 182
Hip adduction
    in ACL repair and reconstruction, 210, 217
    in meniscal repair, 246
    in ORIF, 202, 204
Hip contractions in meniscal repair, 248
Hip extension
    in ACL repair and reconstruction, 217
    in total hip replacement, 179
Hip external rotator stretches in lumbar microdiscectomy, 135
Hip flexion
    in ACL repair and reconstruction, 210, 217
    in femoral neck fracture repair, 190
    in lumbar spine fusion, 163
    in ORIF, 196
    in total hip replacement, 178, 179
Hip hinge in lumbar spine fusion, 159, 160, 161
Hip lateral rotation after total knee replacement, 284
Hip mobility restriction in lumbar spine fusion, 163
Hip muscle strength testing in lumbar microdiscectomy, 132
Hip open reduction and internal fixation, 188-205
    indications for, 188
    procedures for, 188-195
        in displaced femoral neck fractures, 188-190
        in intertrochanteric fractures, 190-193
        in nondisplaced or minimally displaced femoral neck fractures, 188-189
        in subtrochanteric fractures, 193-195
Hip open reduction and internal fixation, rehabilitation in
    home phase of, 198-202
    hospital phase of, 196-198
    outpatient phase of, 202-205
Hip open reduction and internal(fixation, rehabilitation in, 196-205
Hip precautions after femoral neck fracture repair, 190
Hip proprioceptive neuromuscular facilitation in meniscal repair, 249
Hip replacement, total, 172-187; see also Total hip replacement
Hip rotator stretches
    in lumbar spine fusion, 163
    in ORIF, 202
Histology, soft tissue healing and, 2-5
History, carpal tunnel syndrome and, 104
Homans' sign after total knee replacement, 282
Home maintenance
    in Achilles tendon repair, 341, 345, 346
    in ACL repair and reconstruction, 221-222
    in acromioplasty, 24, 25-26
    in ankle ORIF, 311, 312
    in anterior capsular reconstruction, 44
    in arthroscopic lateral retinaculum release, 239, 240

Home maintenance—cont'd
   in carpal tunnel syndrome, 117-118
   in extensor brevis release and lateral
      epicondylectomy, 79, 80
   in lateral retinaculum release, arthroscopic,
      239, 240
   in lumbar microdiscectomy, 146-148
   in lumbar spine fusion, 168-169
   in meniscectomy and meniscal repair, 254-
      255
   in open reduction and internal fixation
      of ankle, 311, 312
      of hip, 198-202
      of patella, 264, 265
   in rotator cuff repair, 63, 67-68
   in total knee replacement, 282, 285
   in UCL reconstruction and ulnar nerve
      transposition, 96, 98-99
Home safety evaluation in total hip replacement, 184
Home therapy phase in total hip replacement,
   183-185
Homebound status, Medicare reimbursement
   and, 198
Hopping exercises in ACL repair and reconstruction, 221
Horizontal abduction
   in acromioplasty, 21, 26
   in rotator cuff repair, 56
Horizontal adduction in anterior capsular
   reconstruction, 36
Horizontal push-ups plus in anterior capsular
   reconstruction, 37
Hot pack in carpal tunnel syndrome, 108
Humeroulnar joint in elbow valgus stress, 82
HVGS; see High-voltage galvanic stimulation
Hyperactive muscles in total knee replacement,
   283-284
Hyporeflexia in lumbar disc herniation, 122
Hypovascularity of Achilles tendon, 325

I
Ice therapy; see Cryotherapy
Iliopsoas stretching in meniscal repair, 251
Iliotibial band, 227, 228, 230
Immobilization
   in Achilles tendon rupture, 329
   in acromioplasty, 18
   in patella ORIF, 262
   in soft tissue healing, 5
Impingement
   in carpal tunnel syndrome, 115
   of rotator cuff, 46, 47
   in shoulder instability, 29
   test for, 12
Impingement syndrome, subacromial, 11-28
   prevention of, carpal tunnel syndrome and,
      115
   surgical indications in, 11-12
      rehabilitation guidelines in, 14-24, 25-26
      subacromial decompression in, 12-14
      troubleshooting after, 24
Implant allergy after total hip replacement, 185
Incentive spirometer
   in hip ORIF, 196
   in total hip replacement, 180
Inclined sled in ACL repair and reconstruction,
   216, 217
Inclined squat machines in meniscal repair, 249
Infection
   in Achilles tendon repair, 330
   in ACL repair and reconstruction, 222
Infielders, rehabilitation program for, 40
Inflammation
   in acromioplasty, 18
   in ankle arthroscopy, 317
   in carpal tunnel surgery, 105-111
      healing and, 330
      scar formation in, 6
   in lumbar spine fusion, 162
Injury risk and pliability of tissue, 6
Instability test in impingement syndrome, 12
Insurance, homebound status and, 198
Interbody cages in lumbar spine fusion, 154

Interbody lumbar fusion, 153-154
Interference screw; see Cannulated screws
Interferential stimulation
   in carpal tunnel syndrome, 109
   in lumbar microdiscectomy, 136, 142
   in UCL reconstruction, 97
Intermediate dorsal cutaneous nerve, 289
Intermedullary nail fixation in subtrochanteric
   femoral neck fractures, 193-195
Intermittent claudication after total hip replacement, 185
Internal fixation and open reduction; see Open
   reduction and internal fixation
Internal rotation exercise
   in acromioplasty, 25
   in femoral neck fracture repair, 190
   resisted, in rotator cuff repair, 55
Interosseous membrane tearing, ankle ORIF
   and, 303
Intertrochanteric fractures, ORIF of, 190-193
Interval sport program in UCL reconstruction,
   91
Interval throwing program in UCL reconstruction, 91, 94, 95, 96
Intervertebral disc, degenerative cascade in,
   152
Intramedullary femoral guide in total knee
   replacement, 270
Intramedullary nail fixation in intertrochanteric
   femoral neck fractures, 190, 192
Inversion of ankle
   in Achilles tendon repair, 333, 339, 340
   in lateral ligament repair, 290, 294, 295, 296
   in meniscal repair, 249
Inward rotation after acromioplasty, 25
Iontophoresis
   in ankle arthroscopy, 319
   in carpal tunnel syndrome, 108
Ischemia in rotator cuff, 46
Isokinetic peak torque levels in Achilles tendon
   repair, 341
Isokinetic velocity spectrum in ankle ORIF, 310
Isokinetics
   in Achilles tendon repair, 333, 341, 343
   in ACL repair and reconstruction, 217, 218,
      219, 220
   in ankle ORIF, 308, 309, 310
   in anterior capsular reconstruction, 37, 38
   in arthroscopic lateral retinaculum release,
      234
   in lateral ligament repair, 293, 295
   in meniscal repair, 250, 251, 252
   in patella tilt, 227
   in rotator cuff repair, 57-60, 58
Isometrics
   in Achilles tendon repair, 339
   in ACL repair and reconstruction, 210, 213,
      214
   in acromioplasty, 16, 25
   in ankle ORIF, 306
   in arthroscopic lateral retinaculum release,
      230, 233
   in carpal tunnel syndrome, 108, 110-111, 114
   in extensor brevis release and lateral
      epicondylectomy, 76
   in lateral ligament repair, 291, 292, 293, 294
   in lumbar microdiscectomy, 138
   in lumbar spine fusion, 157, 166
   in meniscal repair, 245, 246, 248
   in patella ORIF, 261, 262
   in rotator cuff repair, 51, 52
   shoulder, in anterior capsular reconstruction,
      31, 32, 33
   in total hip replacement, 179, 180
   in total knee replacement, 274, 276
   in UCL reconstruction, 88
Isotonics
   in Achilles tendon repair, 340
   in acromioplasty, 18
   in ankle ORIF, 308
   in carpal tunnel syndrome, 113
   in extensor brevis release and lateral
      epicondylectomy, 78
   in lateral ligament repair, 250

Isotonics—cont'd
   in lumbar microdiscectomy, 143
   in meniscal repair, 250
   in rotator cuff repair, 56
   in UCL reconstruction, 90, 91
ITB; see Iliotibial band

J
Jewett nail, 192
Jogging in Achilles tendon repair, 330, 343
Joint congruity after patella ORIF, 257
Joint effusion
   in ACL repair and reconstruction, 211
   in meniscal repair, 249
   in total knee replacement, 283
Joint forces at tibiofemoral interface after total
   knee replacement, 281
Joint line pain in meniscal repair, 249
Joint mobilization
   in Achilles tendon repair, 333, 335, 336, 339
   in ACL repair and reconstruction, 210, 214,
      217, 218
   in ankle arthroscopy, 317, 318, 319, 320
   in lateral ligament repair, 291, 292, 293
   in lumbar microdiscectomy, 131
   in lumbar spine fusion, 157
   in open reduction and internal fixation
      of ankle, 306, 307, 309, 311
      of patella, 261, 262, 264
   in rotator cuff repair, 52, 58, 60
   in total knee replacement, 283, 284
Joint pain, arthroscopic lateral retinaculum
   release for, 227
Jumping exercise
   in ACL repair and reconstruction, 221
   in lumbar microdiscectomy, 144, 145

K
k wires; see Kirschner wires
Kerrison rongeurs, 125
Kinesthesia after acromioplasty, 23
Kinesthetic-proprioceptive coordination in lumbar microdiscectomy, 133
Kirschner wires, 257-259
Knee; see also Patella
   circumference measurement of; see Knee girth
   crepitus of, arthroscopic lateral retinaculum
      release for, 227
   effusion of
      in ACL repair, 211, 212, 222
      in arthroscopic lateral retinaculum release,
         227
      in meniscal repair, 249
   extensor mechanism of, after patella ORIF,
      259
   flexibility of, in meniscal repair, 245-247, 248,
      250
   instability of
      ACL repair and reconstruction for, 206
      in meniscal repair, 249
   lateral ligament repair of, 288-301; see also
      Lateral ligament repair
   locking of
      arthroscopic lateral retinaculum release for,
         227
      in meniscal repair, 249
   manipulation of, under anesthesia, after total
      knee replacement, 281
   meniscal repair of, 243-256; see also
      Meniscectomy and meniscal repair
   pain in
      in ACL repair and reconstruction, 211
      in meniscal repair, 249, 251, 253
      total knee replacement for, 268, 284
   stiffness of, after total knee replacement, 284
Knee extension
   in ACL repair and reconstruction, 210, 211,
      213, 214, 215
   in arthroscopic lateral retinaculum release, 234
   in total hip replacement, 182
   in total knee replacement, 274, 276, 278
Knee flexion
   in ACL repair and reconstruction, 210, 211, 212
   in arthroscopic lateral retinaculum release,
      234

Knee flexion—cont'd
    in meniscal repair, 250, 251
    in total hip replacement, 178
Knee girth
    in ACL repair and reconstruction, 211, 212
    in meniscal repair, 245, 247
Knee-to-chest exercises after hip ORIF, 202
Krackow suture technique, 329, 330
KT-1000, 208, 212, 219

L

Lachman's test, 206
Lag screws in ankle ORIF, 303
Lateral collateral ligament, 84
Lateral epicondylitis; see Extensor brevis release
        and lateral epicondylectomy
Lateral ligament repair, 288-301
    direct, for tears, 288
    home management in, 296, 300
    indications and considerations for, 288
    outcomes of, 290-291
    procedures for, 288-290
    rehabilitation in, 291-296
        evaluation in, 291
        phase I, 291-293
        phase II, 293, 294
        phase III, 293-296
        phase IV, 296, 297, 298, 299
        precautions in, 293
    troubleshooting after, 296
Lateral malleolus fractures, 304
Lateral patellotibial ligament release, 229
Lateral pulls in lumbar spine fusion, 164
Lateral retinaculum release, arthroscopic, 227-
        242
    home maintenance in, 239, 240
    indications for, 229
    patellofemoral taping in, 227-229
    procedure in, 229-231
    rehabilitation in, 231-239
        acute phase, 231-232
        advanced phase, 235-239
        subacute phase, 233-235
    troubleshooting in, 239-240
Lateral shuffles, lateral ligament repair and,
        296, 297
Lateral soft tissue structures, unloading of, 231
Lateral step-ups in meniscal repair, 250, 251
Lateral ulnar collateral ligament, 84
Leg bridging in lumbar microdiscectomy, 139,
        140
Leg length discrepancy after total hip replace-
        ment, 185
Leg presses
    in ACL repair and reconstruction, 214, 217
    in hip ORIF, 204, 205
    in meniscal repair, 249
    in patella ORIF, 264, 265
Leg raise
    in lumbar disc herniation, 122
    in total hip replacement, 179
Lido equipment, 77
Lifting
    from hip hinge, in lumbar spine fusion, 161
    in lumbar microdiscectomy, 133
Ligament balancing in total knee replacement,
        270
Ligaments in elbow joint, 83-84
Ligamentum flavum
    in lumbar disc herniation, 123
    in lumbar microdiscectomy, 126
Locked hinged brace in ACL repair, 213
Locking of knee
    arthroscopic lateral retinaculum release, 227
    in meniscal repair, 249
Log roll technique in lumbar spine fusion, 156
Loose irregular connective tissue, 4
Low back pain in lumbar disc herniation, 122
Lower extremity strengthening in ankle ORIF,
        307
Lower extremity stretch
    in lumbar spine fusion, 163
    in total hip replacement, 179
Low-molecular-weight heparin, 274

Lumbar arthrodesis; see Lumbar spine fusion
Lumbar disc herniation
    extruded, 123
    in lumbar microdiscectomy, 122
    subligamentous, 123
Lumbar flexion stretches in lumbar spine
        fusion, 163
Lumbar lordosis in lumbar microdiscectomy,
        130
Lumbar microdiscectomy, 122-150
    home maintenance in, 146-148
    indications for, 122
    lumbar evaluation in, 146
    procedure for, 123-127
    rehabilitation in, 127-146
        phase I, 129-137
        phase II, 137-146
Lumbar multifidi, 127, 134, 139
Lumbar pain syndrome in lumbar microdiscec-
        tomy, 127
Lumbar spine fusion, 151-170
    fusion types in, 152-154
        instrumentation vs noninstrumentation,
            152-153
        posterior, 153-154
    home maintenance in, 168-169
    indications for, 151-152
    procedure for, 154
    rehabilitation in, 154-168
        phase I, 155
        phase II, 155-165
        phase III, 165
        phases IV and V, 165-168
Lunges
    in ankle arthroscopy, 321
    in arthroscopic lateral retinaculum release,
        234, 235, 236
    in hip ORIF, 200
    in lateral ligament repair, 294
    in patella ORIF, 264, 265
Lying postures in lumbar spine fusion, 159

M

Macroadhesions in remobilization, 5-6
Magill Pain Questionnaire, 79
Magnetic resonance imaging
    in Achilles tendon rupture, 328, 332
    in lumbar disc herniation, 123
    in lumbar spine fusion, 151
    in rotator cuff, 48
Maisonneuve fracture, 303
Malleolus, fractures of, 303, 304, 309, 311
Manipulation under anesthesia after total knee
        replacement, 281
Manual labor after total hip replacement, 185
Manual muscle testing
    in hip ORIF, 202
    in lateral ligament repair, 291
Manual resistance
    in Achilles tendon repair, 333
    in ankle arthroscopy, 319
Manual therapy in lumbar disc herniation, 122
Massage
    in arthroscopic lateral retinaculum release,
        233
    in carpal tunnel syndrome, 108, 109
    in persistent joint effusion after total knee
        replacement, 283
    retrograde
        in carpal tunnel syndrome, 108, 109, 112
        in extensor brevis release and lateral
            epicondylectomy, 76
    scar
        in Achilles tendon repair, 339
        in carpal tunnel syndrome, 109, 111, 112
    soft tissue
        in ankle arthroscopy, 317
        in extensor brevis release and lateral
            epicondylectomy, 76
        in lumbar microdiscectomy, 138
        in lumbar spine fusion, 157
Maturation stage of healing, 7, 331-332
    in carpal tunnel surgery, 116-117
McConnell patellofemoral taping, 227, 231, 235,
        239; see also Patellofemoral taping

McCulloch frame retractor, 123, 124
Mechanical axis of femur, 268, 269
Mechanics of sport after anterior capsular
        reconstruction, 45; see also Sport-specific
        training
Medial malleolar fractures, 304
Median nerve, 84-85
    in carpal tunnel syndrome, 101, 108, 109
Medicare reimbursement, homebound status
        and, 198
Meniscal repair, 243-256; see also
        Meniscectomy and meniscal repair
    all-inside, 244
    inside-out, 243
    open, 243
    outside-in, 244
Meniscectomy and meniscal repair, 243-256
    evaluation for, 245
    home maintenance in, 254-255
    indications and considerations for, 243
    procedure for, 243-244
    rehabilitation in, 244-254
        advanced phase of, 252, 253
        initial phase of, 245-249
        intermediate phase of, 250, 251
        preoperative care and, 244-245
    visual examination for, 245
Microcurettes in lumbar microdiscectomy, 125
Microdiscectomy, lumbar, 122-150; see also
        Lumbar microdiscectomy
Microtrauma of Achilles tendon, 325
Midas-Rex AM-8 dissector, 124, 125, 126
Mid-patellar girth measurements, 211, 212
Military press in rotator cuff repair, 56
Minimally displaced femoral neck fractures,
        ORIF of, 188-189
Mini-squats
    in hip ORIF, 204
    in meniscal repair, 250, 251
    in patella ORIF, 264
Mini-trampoline
    in Achilles tendon repair, 343
    in ankle arthroscopy, 320, 321
Minivibrator in carpal tunnel syndrome, 109
MMT; see Manual Muscle Test
Mobility training
    in hip ORIF, 196, 197
    in total hip replacement, 180
Mobility work, goals in, after surgery, 7-8
Mobilization
    joint; see Joint mobilization
    soft tissue; see Soft tissue mobilization
    soft tissue healing and
        principles of, 7-8
        techniques in, 8-10
    spinal, in lumbar microdiscectomy, 136
    of talus, tibia, and fibula in lateral ligament
        repair, 296
Moist heat
    in arthroscopic lateral retinaculum release,
        232, 233
    in carpal tunnel syndrome, 109, 111
Motion
    limitation of, in ACL repair and
        reconstruction, 222
    range of; see Range of motion
Motor impairment in UCL reconstruction, 89
Movement testing in lumbar microdiscectomy,
        142
Movement without and with gravity in ankle
        ORIF, 307
MRI; see Magnetic resonance imaging
Multifidi, lumbar
    in lumbar microdiscectomy, 127, 134
    in lumbar spine fusion, 155
Multiplane isometrics in lateral ligament repair,
        293, 294
Muscle
    elbow joint and, 84
    hyperactive, after total knee replacement, 283
    inhibition of, after total knee replacement,
        283
    spinal, degenerative cascade in, 152
Muscle bending, transverse, 9

Muscle co-contraction in meniscal repair, 245, 246, 248
Muscle flexibility exercise, 245-247, 248, 250
Muscle imbalance
    in anterolateral total hip replacement, 176
    in total knee replacement, 283-284
Muscle splay in connective tissue, 8-9
Muscle strengthening
    in Achilles tendon repair, 334, 336
    in ankle arthroscopy, 319
    in arthroscopic lateral retinaculum release, 229
Muscle testing
    in carpal tunnel syndrome, 105
    in impingement syndrome, 12
Muscle weakness
    in carpal tunnel syndrome, 102
    in total hip replacement, 185
    in total knee replacement, 283
Musculocutaneous nerve, 84-85
Myotome weakness in lumbar disc herniation, 122

N
Nada-Chair, 132
Nail fixation in femoral neck fractures
    intertrochanteric, 190, 192
    subtrochanteric, 193-195
Necrosis in graft maturation, 207-208
Needle marker in Southern California Orthopedic Institute arthroscopic lateral release, 229
Neer impingement sign, 12
Nerve gliding
    in carpal tunnel syndrome, 109, 111
    in lumbar spine fusion, 162
Nerve mobilization
    in lumbar microdiscectomy, 138
    in lumbar spine fusion, 157
    in total knee replacement, 282, 283
Nerve palsy in ACL repair and reconstruction cryotherapy, 211
Nerve root impingement in lumbar disc herniation, 123
Nerve structures of elbow joint, 84-85
Nerve velocity test after total knee replacement, 283
Neural fibrosis in lumbar microdiscectomy, 133
Neural foramen, spinal, degenerative cascade in, 152
Neural tension
    in lumbar microdiscectomy, 132, 142
    in lumbar spine fusion, 159
    in rotator cuff repair, 64
Neuromuscular stimulation; see also Electrical stimulation
    in arthroscopic lateral retinaculum release, 230, 232, 233
    in total knee replacement, 275
Neuropathy in UCL reconstruction, 97
Neuropraxia, peroneal nerve, after total knee replacement, 270, 282, 283
Neutral spine concept in lumbar microdiscectomy, 134
Nirschl procedure, 72
NMES; see Neuromuscular stimulation
Noncemented implant in total hip replacement, 172
    modular, 173
Nondisplaced femoral neck fractures, ORIF of, 188-189
Nonsteroidal antiinflammatory drugs
    in Achilles tendon repair, 335
    in carpal tunnel syndrome, 101
    in rotator cuff tears, 48
Nonunion of femoral neck fractures, 189
Non-weight-bearing
    in Achilles tendon repair, 334, 338
    in ankle ORIF, 305
    in femoral neck fracture, 190
NSAIDs; see Nonsteroidal antiinflammatory drugs
Nutrition in Achilles tendon repair, 325
NWB; see Non-weight-bearing

O
One-leg standing
    in ankle arthroscopy, 319, 321
    in lateral ligament repair, 293, 298
Open meniscal repair, 243
Open reduction and internal fixation
    of ankle, 302-313; see also Ankle, open reduction and internal fixation of
    of hip, 188-205; see also Hip open reduction and internal fixation
    of patella, 257-267; see also Patella, open reduction and internal fixation of
Open-chain exercises
    in ACL repair and reconstruction, 212-213
    in meniscal repair, 248
Open-chain knee flexion in total knee replacement, 276, 278
Operating microscope in lumbar microdiscectomy, 123, 124
ORIF; see Open reduction and internal fixation
Orthotics in lateral ligament repair, 296
Osseous preparation in total knee replacement, 270-273
Osteoarthritis
    acromioclavicular, 65
    total knee replacement for, 268
Osteochondral lesion
    in ankle arthroscopy, 316
    in ankle ORIF, 303
Osteonecrosis of femoral neck fractures, 189
Oswestry Modified Low Back Pain Questionnaire, 132
Oswestry Pain Disability Scale, 127, 128
Outfielders, rehabilitation program for, 40
Outpatient clinic after total hip replacement, 185
Outside-in meniscal repair, 244
Outward rotation after acromioplasty, 25
Overuse injuries of ankle after ORIF, 311

P
Pain
    in ACL repair and reconstruction, 211, 221
    in acromioplasty, 18
    in ankle arthroscopy, 317, 319
    in ankle ORIF, 309
    in anterior capsular reconstruction, 38
        troubleshooting for, 44
    in arthroscopic lateral retinaculum release, 227, 231
    in carpal tunnel syndrome, 102, 114
    in extensor brevis release and lateral epicondylectomy, 79
    in hip ORIF, 205
    in impingement syndrome, 12
    in lateral epicondylitis, 71
    low back; see Low back pain
    in lumbar microdiscectomy, 127, 129
    in lumbar spine fusion, 162
    in meniscal repair, 249, 251, 253
    in patella ORIF, 261, 262, 263
    in rotator cuff surgery, 46-47, 48
    in total hip replacement, 185
    in total knee replacement, 268, 284
    in UCL reconstruction, 97
Palmaris longus, 84
    absence of, 86
Paper crunches in carpal tunnel syndrome, 110, 111, 114
Paratendinitis of Achilles tendon, 323
Paratenon, Achilles, blood vessels of, 323, 324
Paresthesia
    in carpal tunnel syndrome, 101
    in UCL reconstruction, 88
Partial lunges in meniscal repair, 250, 251
Partial patellectomy in fractures, 259-260
Partial sit-ups in lumbar microdiscectomy, 139
Partial squats
    in lumbar microdiscectomy, 136
    in meniscal repair, 249
Partial weight bearing
    in meniscal repair, 249
    in total hip replacement, 181

Passive accessory movements
    in ACL repair and reconstruction, 211
    in ankle arthroscopy, 317
Passive range-of-motion exercise
    in Achilles tendon repair, 335, 337, 342
    in ACL repair and reconstruction, 210, 213, 214
    in arthroscopy
        of ankle, 318
        in lateral retinaculum release, 230
    in carpal tunnel syndrome, 112
    in extensor brevis release and lateral epicondylectomy, 74, 76
    in lateral ligament repair, 291, 292
    in lumbar microdiscectomy, 130, 138
    in lumbar spine fusion, 157
    in meniscal repair, 246
    in open reduction and internal fixation
        of ankle, 305, 306, 308
        of hip, 199
        of patella, 260, 261, 262
    in rotator cuff repair, 51, 52, 58
    in total knee replacement, 274
Passive stretches in ACL repair and reconstruction, 213; see also Passive range-of-motion exercise
Pass-through sign in shoulder instability, 29
Patella; see also Knee
    entrapment of, in ACL repair and reconstruction, 222
    eversion of, in total knee replacement, 269
    fracture of
        in ACL repair and reconstruction, 221
        displaced or nondisplaced, 257
        tension band wiring in, 257-260
    instability of, in total knee replacement, 281
    open reduction and internal fixation of, 257-267
        home maintenance after, 264, 265
        indications and considerations for, 257
        joint mobilization in, 261, 262, 264
        postoperative complications after, 257
        procedures for, 257-260
        rehabilitation after, 260-264
        troubleshooting after, 266
    surgery on
        for dislocation, 229
        failure of previous, 229
        for subluxation, 229
Patella glides
    in ACL repair and reconstruction, 214
    in arthroscopic lateral retinaculum release, 228
Patella mobilization in arthroscopic lateral retinaculum release, 230, 231, 234, 235
Patella rotation taping, 228; see also Patellofemoral taping
Patella taping; see Patellofemoral taping
Patella template in total knee replacement, 272, 273
Patella tendinitis in meniscal repair, 249
Patella tilt, 228-229
    treatment of, 227
Patella tracking in total knee replacement, 273
Patellar tendon
    in endoscopic bone–patella tendon–bone complex graft, 208
    grafts of, 206-208
Patellectomy
    in irreducible comminution of fracture fragments, 257
    partial, in patellar fractures, 259-260
Patellofemoral crepitus, 211
Patellofemoral glide, 217, 228
Patellofemoral joint
    in ACL repair and reconstruction, 212
    in meniscal repair, 247
    palpation assessment of, 212
    in patella ORIF
        long-term strengthening and, 264
        taping and, 262, 263, 264, 265
    in total knee replacement, 281
Patellofemoral mobility in ACL repair and reconstruction, 211

Patellofemoral pain
in ACL repair and reconstruction, 221
in arthroscopic lateral retinaculum release, 227
Patellofemoral taping
in arthroscopic lateral retinaculum release, 227-229, 230, 231, 232, 234, 235
glide component in, 228
tilt component in, 228-229
weaning program for, 239-240
in meniscal repair, 249
Patellofemoral tilt component, 228-229
Patellotibial ligament, lateral, release of, 229
Patient education
in ankle arthroscopy, 319
in carpal tunnel syndrome, 113
in extensor brevis release and lateral epicondylectomy, 73, 78
in lumbar spine fusion, 155, 162-163
Patient-controlled analgesia in subacromial decompression, 13
Pedicle screw constructs in lumbar spine fusion, 152-153
Pelvic rock in lumbar microdiscectomy, 131, 135
Pelvic tilt in hip ORIF, 196, 202
Pendulum exercise
in acromioplasty, 25
in rotator cuff repair, 51, 52
Percutaneous discectomy in lumbar disc herniation, 123
Performance parameters in Achilles tendon repair, 330
Peripheral neural facilitation patterns; *see* Proprioceptive neuromuscular facilitation
Peroneal nerve
in lateral ligament repair, 289
neuropraxia of, after total knee replacement, 270, 282, 283
Peroneal strengthening, lateral ligament repair and, 293
Peroneus brevis transfer in Achilles tendon rupture repair, 329
Persistent joint effusion in total knee replacement, 283
PF joint; *see* Patellofemoral joint
Phonophoresis
in ankle arthroscopy, 317
in carpal tunnel syndrome, 108, 109
in meniscal repair, 249
Physical therapy
after patella ORIF, 260-264
in total knee replacement, 273-280
Pick-up walker in hip ORIF, 196
Pillar pain in carpal tunnel syndrome, 114
Pinch measurement in carpal tunnel syndrome, 105
Pinch meter in carpal tunnel syndrome, 105
Pinch weakness in carpal tunnel syndrome, 101
Pitchers, rehabilitation throwing program for, 38-39
Pituitary forceps, 125
Plantar fasciitis, 310
Plantar flexion of ankle
in Achilles tendon repair, 328, 333, 338, 339, 340, 341, 342, 343
in lateral ligament repair, 288, 291, 292, 294, 295, 296
in meniscal repair, 249
Plantaris tendon, 328, 329
Platform walker in hip ORIF, 196
Pliability of tissue, risk of injury and, 6
Plyoball in ankle arthroscopy, 321
Plyometrics
in Achilles tendon repair, 343
in ACL repair and reconstruction, 221
in ankle arthroscopy, 321
in ankle ORIF, 310, 311
in lateral ligament repair, 296, 297
in lumbar microdiscectomy, 144
in rotator cuff repair, 58, 60
in UCL reconstruction, 91, 93
Pneumatic intermittent compression, 73, 74
PNF; *see* Proprioceptive neuromuscular facilitation

Pool exercise; *see* Aquatic therapy
Pool therapy; *see* Aquatic therapy
Portals for ankle arthroscopy, 314-316
Posterior capsule stretch in rotator cuff repair, 58, 59
Posterior lumbar interbody fusion, 153
Posterior shoulder pain, troubleshooting in, 44
Posteroanterior standing films before total knee replacement, 268
Posterolateral lumbar fusion, 153
Postural alignment in arthroscopic lateral retinaculum release, 239
Posture
lumbar microdiscectomy and, 132
rotator cuff repair and, 64
Pregnancy, carpal tunnel syndrome and, 101
PREs; *see* Progressive resistance exercises
Press fit implant in total hip replacement, 172
Pressure biofeedback in lumbar microdiscectomy, 134
Pressure sores in hip ORIF, 196
Prevention of impingement syndrome, 24
Progressive resistance exercises
in ACL repair and reconstruction, 214, 217, 218, 220
in acromioplasty, 18, 19, 25
in ankle arthroscopy, 318, 319
in ankle ORIF, 309
in anterior capsular reconstruction, 37
in carpal tunnel syndrome, 108, 114
in extensor brevis release and lateral epicondylectomy, 78
in lateral ligament repair, 292, 296
in lumbar microdiscectomy, 131
in lumbar spine fusion, 166
in meniscal repair, 246
in rotator cuff repair, 56, 57, 58, 60
Progressive steps up and down in total knee replacement, 276, 279
Progressive weight bearing in Achilles tendon repair, 334, 339
Proliferation phase of healing
in Achilles tendon, 330-331
in carpal tunnel surgery, 111-116
PROM exercise; *see* Passive range-of-motion exercise
Pronation of foot, excessive, in arthroscopic lateral retinaculum release, 239
Pronator teres, 84
Prone heel hangs in ACL repair and reconstruction, 213, 214, 215
Prone knee flexion in total knee replacement, 278
Prone lying, three-quarter, in lumbar spine fusion, 159
Proprioception exercise; *see also* Proprioceptive neuromuscular facilitation
in Achilles tendon repair, 333, 341
in acromioplasty, 23
in ankle arthroscopy, 319, 321
in ankle ORIF, 309
in lateral ligament repair, 293
in lumbar microdiscectomy, 145
Proprioceptive neuromuscular facilitation; *see also* Proprioception exercise
in Achilles tendon repair, 333
in ACL repair and reconstruction, 217
in ankle arthroscopy, 320, 321
in lateral ligament repair, 293, 294
in open reduction and internal fixation
of ankle, 306
of hip, 196
in rotator cuff repair, 51-54, 53, 55
in UCL reconstruction, 91, 93
Prosthesis in femoral neck fractures, 190
Provocative discography, 151-152
Pull-downs in lumbar spine fusion, 166
Pulling an object in lumbar spine fusion rehabilitation, 161
Pulmonary embolus in total knee replacement, 281, 282
Pulmonary hygiene exercise in total hip replacement, 179

Pumps
ankle; *see* Ankle pumps
calf; *see* Ankle pumps
calf, in arthroscopic lateral retinaculum release, 231
Pushing an object in lumbar spine fusion, 161
Pushing off, Achilles tendon rupture and, 325
Push-ups in lumbar spine fusion rehabilitation, 164, 166
Putty exercise in carpal tunnel syndrome, 113

Q

Quadriceps co-contraction
in ACL repair and reconstruction, 210, 211
in meniscal repair, 248
Quadriceps exercises
in arthroscopic lateral retinaculum release, 233, 240
in meniscal repair, 249
Quadriceps inhibition in arthroscopic lateral retinaculum release, 239
Quadriceps sets
in ACL repair and reconstruction, 211, 213, 214
in arthroscopic lateral retinaculum release, 229, 230, 233
in hip ORIF, 196, 197, 198
in meniscal repair, 245, 246, 248
in patella ORIF, 261, 262
in total hip replacement, 178, 179, 180, 181
in total knee replacement, 274, 276
Quadriceps stretches
in hip ORIF, 200-202
in lumbar microdiscectomy, 141
in lumbar spine fusion, 163
in meniscal repair, 251
Quadriceps weakness after total knee replacement, 283-284
Quadruped with arm and leg raise in lumbar spine fusion, 164, 166
Quadruple-strand semitendinosus grafts, 207

R

Radial collateral ligament, 84
Radial nerve, 84
Radicular syndrome, acute unilateral, 122
Radioulnar joint, 82-83
Range of motion, evaluation of
in ACL repair and reconstruction, 211
in anterior capsular reconstruction, 44
in carpal tunnel syndrome, 105
in extensor brevis release and lateral epicondylectomy, 79
in impingement syndrome, 12
in lumbar spine fusion, 159
in meniscal repair, 244-245, 245-247
in patella ORIF, 259
in rotation cuff repair and reconstruction, 66
in rotator cuff, 48
in total knee replacement, 281
Range-of-motion exercise; *see also* Active range-of-motion exercise; Passive range-of-motion exercise
in acromioplasty, 16, 17, 18
in anterior capsular reconstruction, 37
in arthroscopic lateral retinaculum release, 229
in meniscal repair, 245
in patella ORIF, 260-265
in rotator cuff repair, 55, 64
in total knee replacement, 274-276, 280-281
Reconditioning exercise in lumbar spine fusion, 163
Reflex quadriceps inhibition in arthroscopic lateral retinaculum release, 239
Reflex sympathetic dystrophy in ACL repair and reconstruction, 221, 222
Regional block, scalene, in subacromial decompression, 13
Rehabilitation throwing program for pitchers, 38-39; *see also* specific surgical procedure
Reinjury in ACL repair and reconstruction, 222
Relocation sign in shoulder instability, 29
Relocation test in shoulder instability, 29
Remobilization in soft tissue healing, 5-6

Remodeling stage of healing, 331-332
  in carpal tunnel surgery, 116-117
Repair phase in Achilles tendon healing, 330-331
Repetitive motion injury in carpal tunnel syndrome, 101
Resistance exercises, progressive; see Progressive resistance exercises
Resistant weight training in patella tilt, 227
Resisted external rotation, 25
Resisted internal rotation, 25
Resisted scaption, 25
Resisted scapular protraction, 25
Resisted scapular retraction, 25
Resistive gripping exercise, 114
Resistive leg press, 235
Resistive pinching exercise in carpal tunnel syndrome, 114
Resurfacing arthroplasty and total hip replacement, 172, 173
Reticulin
  in connective tissue fibers, 2
  in extracellular matrix, 2
Retinacula
  lateral, arthroscopic release of, 227-242; see also Lateral retinaculum release, arthroscopic
  in patella ORIF, 259
Retinacula strain, arthroscopic lateral retinaculum release for, 227
Retro stair-climbing machine in ankle arthroscopy, 321
Retrograde massage
  in carpal tunnel syndrome, 108, 109, 112
  in extensor brevis release and lateral epicondylectomy, 76
Revascularization in graft maturation, 207, 208
Reverse rows in rotator cuff repair, 56
Rice gripping in carpal tunnel syndrome, 110, 114
Richards compression screw-plate device, 194
Roland-Morris Functional Disability Questionnaire, 132
Rosenberg's view for x-ray before total knee replacement, 268
Rotational trunk stability in lumbar microdiscectomy, 145
Rotator cuff exercises
  in rotator cuff repair and rehabilitation, 48; see also Rotator cuff tears, repair and rehabilitation in
  in UCL reconstruction, 90, 97
Rotator cuff tears, 46, 48-51
  arthroscopic technique in, 50-51
  clinical evaluation of, 46-48
  degeneration in, 46
  deterioration process in, 47
  diagnostic signs in, 48
  full-thickness tears in, 48-51
  home maintenance in, 63, 67-68
  impingement in, 46, 47
  ischemia in, 46
  massive tendon defects in, 50
  open surgical technique in, 49-50
  pain in, 46-47
  procedure in, 48-51
    indications for, 46-48
  repair and rehabilitation in, 46-70, 51-63
    phase I, 51
    phase II, 51-54
    phase III, 55-57
    phase IV, 57-60
    phase V, 60
    phase VI, 60-63
    troubleshooting in, 63-66
  treatment options in, 48
Rotator cuff tendon
  tendonitis of, in UCL reconstruction, 97
  transosseous repair of, 43-44
Rowing
  in lumbar microdiscectomy, 146
  in lumbar spine fusion, 164, 166
  in rotator cuff repair, 55
Rubor
  in hip ORIF, 205
  in total hip replacement, 185

Rugby drills in lumbar microdiscectomy, 144
Running program
  in Achilles tendon repair, 333
  in ACL repair and reconstruction, 219, 220
  in ankle arthroscopy, 321
  in meniscal repair, 251
Russell-Taylor interlocking nail technique, 194

S
SAD; see Subacromial decompression
Safe transfer techniques; see Transfer techniques
SAQs exercises; see Short arc quadriceps exercises
Scalene block
  in acromioplasty, 18
  in subacromial decompression, 13
Scaption
  in acromioplasty, 18, 21-22, 26
  in rotator cuff repair, 53, 54, 56
Scapula exercises in rotator cuff repair, 55, 56, 57
Scapular depression in lumbar spine fusion, 164, 166
Scapular protraction in acromioplasty, 25
Scapular retraction in acromioplasty, 16, 17, 25
Scapular slide test in acromioplasty, 22
Scapular stabilizers in acromioplasty, 22
Scapular winging in rotator cuff repair, 65
Scapulothoracic concerns
  in acromioplasty, 24
  in rotator cuff repair, 65-66
Scar conformer in carpal tunnel syndrome, 108, 109-110, 112, 116
Scar deformation, 8
Scar desensitization in carpal tunnel syndrome, 108, 109, 111, 112
Scar management
  in Achilles tendon repair, 333
  in carpal tunnel syndrome, 105, 108-112, 116
  connective tissue and, 6-7
  in extensor brevis release and lateral epicondylectomy, 75, 79
Scar massage
  in Achilles tendon repair, 339
  in carpal tunnel syndrome, 109, 111, 112
Scar mobility
  in ankle ORIF, 307, 311
  in lumbar spine fusion, 163
Scar remodeling in extensor brevis release and lateral epicondylectomy, 75-77
Scar tissue removal in ankle arthroscopy, 316
Sciatic nerve
  in total hip replacement, 174
  in total knee replacement, 282
SCOI technique of arthroscopic lateral release; see Southern California Orthopedic Institute technique
Screws
  cannulated
    in ankle ORIF, 303
    in femoral neck fractures, 198
    in patella ORIF, 259
  compression, 190, 192, 193
  interference, fixation of grafts with, 207
  lag, in ankle ORIF, 303
  sliding compression, in femoral neck fractures, 190, 192
  syndesmotic, 303, 305
  tag, 303
  with washer and barbed staple, 207
Seated knee flexion in ACL repair and reconstruction, 210
Seated push-ups on rotator cuff repair, 58, 62
Segmental mobility of thoracic spine, 163-164
Semitendinosus grafts, 207
Semmes-Weinstein Pressure Esthesiometer Kit, 105
Sensibility testing in carpal tunnel syndrome, 105
Sensory loss in lumbar disc herniation, 122
Serratus anterior strengthening, 57
Sexual activity after total hip replacement, 185
Shoes after total hip replacement, 185

Short and long principles in connective tissue, 8
Short arc quadriceps exercises in meniscal repair, 249
Short-leg cast in ankle ORIF, 303
Shoulder abduction
  isometric, in anterior capsular reconstruction, 34
  in rotator cuff repair, 56
  in UCL reconstruction, 88
Shoulder exercises
  in anterior capsular reconstruction, 33, 34, 35, 36
  in rotator cuff repair, 53, 54, 56
  in UCL reconstruction, 88
Shoulder extension
  in anterior capsular reconstruction, 33, 34, 36
  in UCL reconstruction, 88
Shoulder external rotation
  in anterior capsular reconstruction, 36
  isometric, in anterior capsular reconstruction, 34
  in rotator cuff repair, 53, 54
Shoulder flexion
  after acromioplasty, 18
  in anterior capsular reconstruction, 34
  in rotator cuff repair, 53, 54, 56
  in UCL reconstruction, 88
Shoulder girdle depressions, 58, 63
Shoulder horizontal abduction, 33, 35
Shoulder horizontal adduction, 33, 35
Shoulder impingement syndrome, 115
Shoulder instability; see Anterior capsular reconstruction
Shoulder internal rotation
  in anterior capsular reconstruction, 34
  in UCL reconstruction, 88
Shoulder pain, troubleshooting in, 44
Shoulder range-of-motion exercise, 106
Shoulder serratus anterior exercise, 36
Showering in lumbar microdiscectomy, 129
Side-lying, supported, in lumbar spine fusion, 159
Signs, Trendelenburg, 205
Silicon gel sheet in extensor brevis release and lateral epicondylectomy, 75, 76
Single-leg heel raise in Achilles tendon repair, 341, 343
Single-leg hop in ACL repair and reconstruction, 221
Single-leg toe raise in lateral ligament repair, 291
Single-limb squats in arthroscopic lateral retinaculum release, 235
Single-point cane in total hip replacement, 185
Single-strand semitendinosus grafts, 207
Sit-stand in patella ORIF, 264
Sitting in lumbar microdiscectomy, 132
Sitting up
  in hip ORIF, 196
  in total hip replacement, 181
Sit-to-stand exercises
  in arthroscopic lateral retinaculum release, 235
  in total knee replacement, 276, 279
Sit-ups
  diagonal, in lumbar spine fusion, 164
  in lumbar microdiscectomy, 138
  partial
    in lumbar microdiscectomy, 139, 140
    in lumbar spine fusion, 164, 166
Skilled nursing facility, 276
Skill-specific training in arthroscopic lateral retinaculum release, 238
Skin flaps in total knee replacement, 269
Skin temperature in ACL repair and reconstruction, 212
SLAP; see Superior labral anteroposterior lesion
Sled, inclined, in ACL repair and reconstruction, 216, 217
Sleeping posture in lumbar microdiscectomy, 132
Slide board
  in ankle arthroscopy, 321
  in lateral ligament repair, 296, 297

Sliding compression screw in femoral neck fractures
  intertrochanteric, 190, 192
  subtrochanteric, 193
Sling in acromioplasty, 18
Slump testing in lumbar microdiscectomy, 132
SNF; see Skilled nursing facility
Soft tissue healing after surgery, 2-10
  histology and biomechanics in, 2-5
  immobilization, remobilization, and trauma in, 5-7
  mobilization principles in, 7-8
  mobilization techniques in, i-10
  surgery defined in, 2
Soft tissue massage
  in ankle arthroscopy, 317
  in extensor brevis release and lateral epicondylectomy, 76
  in lumbar microdiscectomy, 138
  in lumbar spine fusion, 157
Soft tissue mobilization; see also Tissue mobilization
  in Achilles tendon repair, 339
  in ankle ORIF, 306, 307
  in arthroscopic lateral retinaculum release, 232, 233
  in lateral ligament repair, 291, 292
  in lumbar microdiscectomy, 140-142, 145
  principles of, 7-8
  in rotator cuff repair, 53, 54
Southern California Orthopedic Institute technique
  of ankle ORIF, 303
  of arthroscopic lateral release, 229
Spasticity in anterolateral total hip replacement, 176
Spider killers, 213, 215
Spine; see also specific spinal region
  mobilization of, 136, 142, 145
  stabilization of, 134
Spirometer, incentive
  in hip ORIF, 196
  in total hip replacement, 180
Splint
  in Achilles tendon repair, 337
  in ankle arthroscopy, 316, 317
  in anterior capsular reconstruction, 33
  in anterior capsulolabral reconstruction, 31
  in carpal tunnel syndrome, 108, 109
  in extensor brevis release and lateral epicondylectomy, 73, 79
  in UCL reconstruction, 88, 89, 97
Spondylolisthesis, 151
Spondylolysis, 151
Sports, high-impact, after total hip replacement, 185
Sport-specific training
  in Achilles tendon repair, 333
  in ankle arthroscopy, 321
  in ankle ORIF, 310, 311
  in anterior capsular reconstruction, 37, 38, 45
  in extensor brevis release and lateral epicondylectomy, 77, 78
  in lateral ligament repair, 296
  in lumbar microdiscectomy, 143, 145
  in rotator cuff repair, 60
Sprinting drills in meniscal repair, 252, 253
Squat jumping in ankle arthroscopy, 321
Squat machines, inclined, in meniscal repair, 249
Squats
  in lateral ligament repair, 294
  in lumbar microdiscectomy, 136, 140, 141
  in lumbar spine fusion, 141, 163, 164
Stabilization exercise
  in lumbar microdiscectomy, 145
  in lumbar spine fusion, 155, 163
Stabilization taping in arthroscopic lateral retinaculum release, 227, 231
Stair hopple in functional evaluation for ACL repair, 221
Stairs and stair-climbing machine
  in Achilles tendon repair, 330, 343
  in ankle arthroscopy, 321

Stairs and stair-climbing machine—cont'd
  in ankle ORIF, 308, 309
  in arthroscopic lateral retinaculum release, 235
  in hip ORIF, 199, 202, 204
  in lumbar spine fusion, 157, 164, 166
  in meniscal repair, 250, 251
  in total hip replacement, 183, 185
Standing and walking in lumbar microdiscectomy, 132-133
Standing balance exercises in hip ORIF, 204
Standing elastic tubing exercise in arthroscopic lateral retinaculum release, 235
Standing hamstring curls in ACL repair and reconstruction, 213, 214
Staples, removal of
  in hip ORIF, 200
  in total hip replacement, 183
Stationary bicycle
  in Achilles tendon repair, 330, 342
  in ACL repair and reconstruction, 214, 217, 219
  in ankle arthroscopy, 319
  in arthroscopic lateral retinaculum release, 235
  in lateral ligament repair, 294
  in lumbar microdiscectomy, 136
  in meniscal repair, 246, 249, 250, 251
  in open reduction and internal fixation
    of ankle, 306, 307, 308, 309
    of hip, 203
    of patella, 263
  in total hip replacement, 185
Step-down exercises
  in ACL repair and reconstruction, 216, 217
  in ankle arthroscopy, 321
  in ankle ORIF, 309
  in arthroscopic lateral retinaculum release, 235, 237, 239
  in meniscal repair, 250
  in patella ORIF, 264
  in total knee replacement, 276, 279
Step-over-step stair climbing; see Stairs and stair-climbing machine
Step-to gait exercise in total hip replacement, 183
Step-up exercises
  in ACL repair and reconstruction, 214, 216, 217
  in ankle arthroscopy, 321
  in ankle ORIF, 309
  in hip ORIF, 202
  in lateral ligament repair, 299
  in meniscal repair, 250
  in total knee replacement, 276, 279
Sterilization of autografts, 207
Sternoclavicular degeneration, 65
Steroids
  in carpal tunnel syndrome, 101-102
  in lumbar disc herniation, 122
Stiffness
  in extensor brevis release and lateral epicondylectomy, 79
  in impingement syndrome, 12
  in UCL reconstruction, 96
Stork standing
  in ankle arthroscopy, 319, 321
  in lateral ligament repair, 293, 298
Straight leg raise
  in arthroscopic lateral retinaculum release, 229
  in lumbar disc herniation, 122
  in meniscal repair, 249
  in total hip replacement, 179
Strength in shoulder after anterior capsular reconstruction, 44
Strength testing
  in Achilles tendon repair, 333-337
  in lumbar microdiscectomy, 132
  in lumbar spine fusion, 159
  in meniscal repair, 244-245
Strengthening exercise
  in Achilles tendon repair, 333
  in ankle arthroscopy, 320
  in ankle ORIF, 307, 309
  in arthroscopic lateral retinaculum release, 233

Strengthening exercise—cont'd
  in extensor brevis release and lateral epicondylectomy, 77
  progression of, 21
Stress
  in lumbar spine fusion, 155
  and viscoelasticity of connective tissue, 4-5
Stretch cords in rotator cuff repair, 48
Stretching exercise
  in Achilles tendon repair, 335, 336
  in ACL repair and reconstruction, 210, 213
  in ankle ORIF, 308
  in anterior capsular reconstruction, 44
  in arthroscopic lateral retinaculum release, 234, 235
  in lumbar microdiscectomy, 140
  in patella ORIF, 265
  in UCL reconstruction, 91, 96
Stroke, anterolateral total hip replacement and, 176
Subacromial bursoscopy, 49
Subacromial decompression in impingement syndrome, 12-14
Subacromial impingement syndrome, 11-28
  surgery for, 11-12
    rehabilitation after, 14-24, 25-26
    subacromial decompression in, 12-14
    troubleshooting after, 24
Subacromial space, 14
Subluxation of patella, 229
Subtrochanteric fractures, 193-195
Superior labral anteroposterior lesion, 29
Superman in lumbar spine fusion, 164, 166
Supinator of elbow joint, 84
Supine flexion in acromioplasty, 25
Supine heel slides in ACL repair and reconstruction, 213
Supine knee extension in ACL repair and reconstruction, 214
Supine leg press in ACL repair and reconstruction, 214
Supine lying, supported, in lumbar spine fusion, 159
Supine passive knee extension in ACL repair and reconstruction, 213
Supine sit-stand in lumbar spine fusion, 156, 158, 159
Supine wall slides in ACL repair and reconstruction, 213, 214
Supraspinatus exercises in anterior capsular reconstruction, 33, 35
Sural nerve, 289
Surgery
  defined, 2
  soft tissue healing in, 2-10
Surgical retractor in lumbar microdiscectomy, 123, 124
Suture technique, Krackow, 329, 330
Swelling; see Edema
Swimming
  in hip ORIF, 202, 205
  in lumbar microdiscectomy, 136
Swiss ball
  in lumbar microdiscectomy, 138, 140
  in rotator cuff repair, 58, 63
Syndesmosis, injury to, 303
Syndesmotic screw, 303, 304
Synovectomy in ankle arthroscopy, 316
Synovial cyst formation in lumbar disc herniation, 123
Synovial resector, 13
Synovitis in ACL repair and reconstruction, 222

T

"T kicks" in meniscal repair, 250, 251, 253
T_2 weighted magnetic resonance imaging in Achilles tendon rupture, 328, 331, 332
Tag screw, 303
Tai Chi, 202, 205
Talar rock in ankle arthroscopy, 317
Talus
  mobilization of, lateral ligament repair and, 296
  posterior glide of, ankle ORIF and, 307

Taping, patellofemoral; *see* Patellofemoral taping
Tear
  of interosseous membrane in ankle, 303
  in rotator cuff; *see* Rotator cuff tears
TED hose; *see* Thromboembolic disease hose
Tendinitis
  Achilles, 323
  patellar, in meniscal repair, 249
  rotator cuff, 97
Tendinosis of Achilles tendon
  paratendinitis with, 323
  pure, 323-325
Tendon defects in rotator cuff repair, 50
Tendon gliding exercise in carpal tunnel syndrome, 106-107, 109, 111
Tendon graft in UCL reconstruction, 87
Tendon-bone healing in ACL repair and reconstruction, 208
Tendonitis; *see* Tendinitis
Tennis elbow; *see* Extensor brevis release and lateral epicondylectomy
Tennis players, rehabilitation program for, 41-43
TENS; *see* Transcutaneous electrical nerve stimulation
Tension band wiring in patellar fractures, 257-260
  complications of, 260
Terminal knee extensions
  in total hip replacement, 182
  in total knee replacement, 274, 276, 278
Thenar muscle atrophy, 101
Theraband
  in ankle arthroscopy, 319, 321
  in hip ORIF, 196
  in UCL reconstruction, 97
Thigh pain
  in hip ORIF, 205
  in total hip replacement, 185
Thoracic extension in rotator cuff repair, 62
Thoracic spine mobility
  in lumbar spine fusion, 163-164
  in rotator cuff repair, 64
Three-point stance in lumbar microdiscectomy, 144
Thromboembolic disease hose
  in ankle ORIF, 306, 307
  in hip ORIF, 196, 205
  in lateral ligament repair, 291
  in total hip replacement, 179
  in total knee replacement, 268, 273, 282
Thrombosis, deep venous
  in Achilles tendon repair, 330
  total knee replacement and, 274, 275, 282
Thrower's Ten program in UCL reconstruction, 97
Throwing program
  in rotator cuff repair, 60
  in UCL reconstruction, 91, 97
Tibia, mobilization of, in lateral ligament repair, 296
Tibia-femoral glides in ACL repair and reconstruction, 214
Tibial stem punch, 272, 273
Tibial template, 272, 273
Tibial tubercle, pain over, 221
Tibial tunnel in endoscopic bone–patella tendon–bone complex graft, 209
Tibiofemoral interface, joint forces at, 281
Tilt, patella, 228-229
  treatment of, 227
Tilt compression syndrome, arthroscopic lateral retinaculum release in, 227
Tinel's testing, 105
Tiny steps in lumbar spine fusion, 157, 163
Tiptoes, bilateral, in hip ORIF, 200
Tissue, misapprehending quality of, 44
Tissue mobilization; *see also* Soft tissue mobilization
  in ACL repair and reconstruction, 210
  in arthroscopic lateral retinaculum release, 232
  in lumbar spine fusion, 163
Tissue protection in acromioplasty, 18
TKEs; *see* Terminal knee extensions
TKR; *see* Total knee replacement
Toe curls in Achilles tendon repair, 338

Toe push-ups in ankle arthroscopy, 319
Toe raises in meniscal repair, 249, 250, 251
Toe touch weight bearing in total hip replacement, 181
Torn lateral ligaments, direct repair of, 288
Torque in immobilized connective tissue, 5
Total hip replacement
  in femoral neck fractures, 189
  indications for, 172
  procedures for, 172-178
  rehabilitation in, 178-185
    phase I, 178-179
    phase IIa, 179-181
    phase IIb, 181-183
    phase III, 183-185
  teaching of precautions in, 178, 181
  troubleshooting in, 185-186
Total knee replacement, 268-287
  home maintenance after, 282, 285
  indications and considerations for, 268
  medical complications after, 282-284
  outcomes of, 284
  procedure for, 268-273
    exposure in, 269
    ligament balancing in, 270
    osseous preparation in, 270-273
    preoperative evaluation before, 268
    technique in, 268-273
  rehabilitation guidelines after, 273-282
    extended care unit, 276
    inpatient, 275-276
    outpatient, 276-282
    skilled nursing facility, 276
  troubleshooting after, 282-284
Touch down weight bearing after femoral neck fracture repair, 190
Towel curls
  in Achilles tendon repair, 340
  in ankle arthroscopy, 319, 321
Towel squeeze in ACL repair and reconstruction, 214
Track running in meniscal repair, 252, 253
Traction in lumbar disc herniation, 122
Training heart rate in cardiovascular conditioning, 136
Trampoline
  in ACL repair and reconstruction, 219, 220
  in ankle arthroscopy, 321
  in lateral ligament repair, 296, 297, 298
  in meniscal repair, 250, 251
Transcutaneous electrical nerve stimulation
  in ACL repair and reconstruction, 211
  in carpal tunnel syndrome, 109
  in extensor brevis release and lateral epicondylectomy, 79
  in lumbar microdiscectomy, 136
  in lumbar spine fusion, 162
  in UCL reconstruction, 97
Transfer techniques
  in hip ORIF, 196, 197
  in lumbar microdiscectomy, 133
  in total hip replacement, 178, 180, 182
  in total knee replacement, 274
Transtrochanteric approach in total hip replacement, 172
Transverse carpal ligament division in carpal tunnel syndrome, 102
Transverse muscle bending in connective tissue, 9
Transversus abdominis, 134, 135
Trauma
  in carpal tunnel syndrome, 101
  in shoulder instability, 29
  in soft tissue healing, 6-7
Treadmill
  in Achilles tendon repair, 343
  in ankle arthroscopy, 321
  in ankle ORIF, 308, 309
  in hip ORIF, 203, 205
  in lateral ligament repair, 293, 294
  in lumbar microdiscectomy, 145
  in meniscal repair, 250, 251
  in total hip replacement, 184
Trendelenburg gait, 190

Trendelenburg sign
  in hip ORIF, 205
  in total hip replacement, 185
Triceps brachii, 84
Triceps dips in lumbar spine fusion, 166
Trimalleolar fracture, 303, 311
Triple jump in ACL repair and reconstruction, 221
Trochanteric osteotomy, 176
Trochlear groove, 227
Trunk and leg strengthening exercise in rotator cuff repair, 58
Trunk flexion in lumbar microdiscectomy, 130
Trunk rotation in hip ORIF, 202
Trunk stabilization exercise in hip ORIF, 203
T-sign in elbow instability, 86
Tumors in carpal tunnel syndrome, 101
Turn-down plantaris tendon flap, 329
Two-point discrimination testing in carpal tunnel syndrome, 105
Typing, recommendations for, in carpal tunnel syndrome, 115

U

UCL; *see* Ulnar collateral ligament
Ulnar collateral ligament, 82; *see also* Ulnar collateral ligament reconstruction and ulnar nerve transposition
  tensile strength of, 86
Ulnar collateral ligament reconstruction and ulnar nerve transposition, 82-100
  home maintenance in, 96, 98-99
  indications for, 82-86
  procedure for, 86-87, 88
  rehabilitation in, 89-96
    phase I, 89-90
    phase II, 91
    phase III, 91
    phase IV, 91-96
  troubleshooting in, 96-97
Ulnar nerve, 85
  neuropathy of, 97
  transposition of, 87
Ultrasonography
  in Achilles tendon repair, 337-341
  in Achilles tendon rupture, 328
  in ankle ORIF, 307
  in arthroscopic lateral retinaculum release, 232, 233
  in carpal tunnel syndrome, 108
  in meniscal repair, 249
ULTT; *see* Upper limb tension tests
Uneven surface walking in Achilles tendon repair, 343
Unloading devices in lumbar microdiscectomy, 145
Unstable ankle lateral ligament repair for, 288
Upper body ergometer
  in ankle arthroscopy, 319
  in anterior capsular reconstruction, 33
  in hip ORIF, 203, 204
  in lumbar spine fusion, 164, 166
  in rotator cuff repair, 55, 58
Upper extremity exercise
  in hip ORIF, 196
  in total hip replacement, 182
Upper extremity stretches in carpal tunnel syndrome, 114
Upper limb tension tests, 64-65
US; *see* Ultrasonography

V

Valgus deformity in total knee replacement, 270, 283
Valgus stress and medial elbow instability, 85
Varus deformity in total knee replacement, 270
Vasopneumatic compression, 230, 231
Vastus lateralis, 276
Vastus medialis oblique
  in arthroscopic lateral retinaculum release, 233, 240
  in total knee replacement, 276
Velocity spectrum training in ankle ORIF, 309, 310; *see also* Isokinetics

Vertical jump in ACL repair and reconstruction, 221
Vibrator in carpal tunnel syndrome, 109, 112
Viscoelasticity of connective tissue, 4
Viscosity of connective tissue, 4
VL; see Vastus lateralis
VMO; see Vastus medialis oblique
Volumeter in carpal tunnel syndrome, 104

W

Waddell signs, 129-132
Walker
    in hip ORIF, 196
    in total hip replacement, 178, 181
Walker boot in Achilles tendon repair, 330
Walking
    in Achilles tendon repair, 331, 343
    in ACL repair and reconstruction, 218
    in ankle ORIF, 309
    in hip ORIF, 196, 202, 205
    in lateral ligament repair, 293
    in lumbar microdiscectomy, 129, 131, 132-133, 136
    in lumbar spine fusion, 157, 163, 164, 166
    in meniscal repair, 251
Walk-run program in lumbar microdiscectomy, 146
Wall push-ups in anterior capsular reconstruction, 36
Wall push-ups plus
    in anterior capsular reconstruction, 37
    in rotator cuff repair, 58

Wall slides
    in ACL repair and reconstruction, 210, 213, 214
    in arthroscopic lateral retinaculum release, 235, 237
    in hip ORIF, 200, 201
    in meniscal repair, 246, 247
    in patella ORIF, 262, 264
Wall squats
    in hip ORIF, 204
    in meniscal repair, 250, 251
Wand exercises
    in anterior capsular reconstruction, 32, 33
    in rotator cuff repair, 56
Warfarin, 274
Warm-up in acromioplasty, 18
Watson-Jones procedure for lateral ligament repair, 290
Weakness
    in carpal tunnel syndrome, 102
    in impingement syndrome, 12
Weight bearing
    in Achilles tendon repair, 334, 337, 339, 342
    in intermedullary reconstruction nailing, 190, 195
    in patella ORIF, 260
    in total hip replacement, 178, 181
Weight shifting in open reduction and internal fixation
    of ankle, 306
    of hip, 198
    of patella, 261
Weight training
    in lumbar spine fusion, 165
    in patella tilt, 227

Weight well in carpal tunnel syndrome, 114
Weights, lunges with, 234, 235
Wilson frame in lumbar microdiscectomy, 126
Windshield wipers in ankle arthroscopy, 319, 321
Work, return to
    in lumbar microdiscectomy, 129
    in lumbar spine fusion, 165
Work activity simulation
    in ankle ORIF, 310
    in carpal tunnel syndrome, 113, 116-117
    in extensor brevis release and lateral epicondylectomy, 77, 78
Work splints in carpal tunnel syndrome, 116
Work-hardening activities in lumbar microdiscectomy, 145
Workstation ergonomics
    in carpal tunnel syndrome, 115
    in lumbar microdiscectomy, 132
Wound care in lumbar microdiscectomy, 136
Wound infection after total knee replacement, 282
Wrist exercises
    in anterior capsular reconstruction, 33
    in carpal tunnel syndrome, 113, 114
    in extensor brevis release and lateral epicondylectomy, 75
    in UCL reconstruction, 88
Wrist splint in carpal tunnel syndrome, 102, 108, 109
Wrist tumors in carpal tunnel syndrome, 101

X

X-ray before total knee replacement, 268